'If life is a journey of learning, then flower essences are simple aids to help us effortlessly on the journey of learning about ourselves. This encyclopedia is an excellent and thorough text on the whole subject of using flower essences, the why, the how, the what and the when. Packed with useful tips and original insights (such as the concept of long, slow, shock), every practitioner, user and explorer of essence work will find help in abundance.'

— Dr Andrew Tresidder, Somerset GP and Educator, Life President of the British Flower and Vibrational Essence Association

'This updated and revised edition of Clare G. Harvey's *The Practitioner's Encyclopedia of Flower Remedies* has to be one of the most thoroughly and painstakingly researched books on flower remedies published. Covering all the essential information on what flower remedies are, their benefits, history and development, Harvey gives clear instructions on how best to use individual remedies and combinations for a wide range of conditions. The comprehensive section covering all the many different flower remedies currently available is a valuable resource for both complementary therapists and interested individuals. An important book.'

— Gill Farrer-Halls, Aromatherapist, Principal Teacher and Examiner with the International Federation of Aromatherapists, Author of The Spirit in Aromatherapy, The Aromatherapy Bible *and several other books*

'Clare G. Harvey has written the definitive text for practitioners and students of flower essences. A beautifully illustrated journey through the theory and application of flower remedies. Quite simply the most comprehensive and well-written book on the subject.'

— Steve Flood, All About Natural Medicine

'Flower essences came into my life more than forty years ago, and are for me an essential provider of emotional, mental and physical balance. Clare G. Harvey has put a lifetime of study and personal experience into this wonderful book, which has arrived at a time when it is so needed. It's a rare combination of perfect research tool and a thing of beauty which will inspire any who wish to explore subtle healing. We now have the map; the journey is up to us.'

— Martin Shaw, Actor and Lifetime President of the British Flower and Vibrational Essences Association

The Practitioner's Encyclopedia of
FLOWER REMEDIES

of related interest

Culpeper's Medicine
A Practice of Western Holistic Medicine New Edition
Graeme Tobyn
ISBN 978 1 84819 121 1
eISBN 978 0 85701 126 8

Fragrance and Wellbeing
Plant Aromatics and Their Influence on the Psyche
Jennifer Peace Rhind
ISBN 978 1 84819 090 0
eISBN 978 0 85701 073 5

The Spirit in Aromatherapy
Working with Intuition
Gill Farrer-Halls
ISBN 978 1 84819 209 6
eISBN 978 0 85701 159 6

Ayurvedic Medicine
The Principles of Traditional Practice
Sebastian Pole
ISBN 978 1 84819 113 6
eISBN 978 0 85701 091 9

Ayurvedic Healing
Contemporary Maharishi Ayurveda Medicine and Science
2nd edition
Hari Sharma, MD and Christopher Clark, MD
ISBN 978 1 84819 069 6
eISBN 978 0 85701 063 6

The Compassionate Practitioner
How to create a successful and rewarding practice
Jane Wood
ISBN 978 1 84819 222 5
eISBN 978 0 85701 170 1

Principles of Bach Flower Remedies
What it is, how it works, and what it can do for you
Stefan Ball
Part of the Discovering Holistic Health series
ISBN 978 1 84819 142 6
eISBN 978 0 85701 120 6

The Practitioner's Encyclopedia of

FLOWER REMEDIES

THE DEFINITIVE GUIDE TO ALL FLOWER ESSENCES, THEIR MAKING AND USES

CLARE G. HARVEY

Preface by Dr George Lewith
Foreword by Richard Gerber, MD

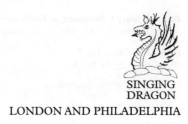

SINGING DRAGON

LONDON AND PHILADELPHIA

Figure 8.1 on page 110 and excerpts in Chapter 9 and Section A are reproduced with kind permission of Andreas Korte. The excerpt on page 108 "Women's Problems" is reproduced with kind permission of Ian White. The excerpt on pages 108-9 "Cancer Study using Petite Fleur Range" is reproduced with kind permission of Dr Judy Griffin. The "Flower Essence Society (FES)" section on page 338 is adapted with kind permission from writings by Patricia Kaminski. Images in the colour plate are reproduced with kind permission of the artists/photographers, as detailed in the individual image captions; all other images in the plate are the author's own.

This edition published in 2015
by Singing Dragon
an imprint of Jessica Kingsley Publishers
73 Collier Street
London N1 9BE, UK
and
400 Market Street, Suite 400
Philadelphia, PA 19106, USA

www.singingdragon.com

This is the expanded, revised and updated edition of *The New Encyclopedia of Flower Remedies* published in 2007 by Watkins Publishing, which was first published as *Encyclopaedia of Flower Remedies* in 1996 by Thorsons. The second edition was published in the UK in 2007 by Watkins Publishing, Sixth Floor, Castle House, 75–76 Wells Street, London W1T 3QH, Clare G. Harvey (Author) and Eliana Harvey (Editor), 2007.

The Author wishes to thank Amanda Cochrane for her invaluable work and contribution to *The Encyclopaedia of Flower Remedies* originally published by Thorsons (an imprint of HarperCollins) in 1996, substantial passages of which have been included in the second and third edition

Copyright © Clare G. Harvey 2015
Preface copyright © George Lewith 2015
Foreword copyright © Richard Gerber 2015

Front cover image source: Shutterstock®.

Library of Congress Cataloging in Publication Data
Harvey, Clare G.
  [Encyclopaedia of flower remedies]
  The practitioner's encyclopedia of flower remedies : the definitive guide to all flower essences, their
making and uses / Clare G. Harvey. -- 3rd edition.
    pages cm
  Revision of: Encyclopaedia of flower remedies.
  Includes bibliographical references and index.
  ISBN 978-1-84819-173-0 (alk. paper)
  1. Flowers--Therapeutic use--Encyclopedias. 2. Essences and essential oils--Therapeutic use--
Encyclopedias. 3. Homeopathy--Materia medica and therapeutics--Encyclopedias. I. Title.
  RX615.F55H35 2015
  635.903--dc23
                         2014031616

British Library Cataloguing in Publication Data
A CIP catalogue record for this book is available from the British Library

ISBN 978 1 84819 173 0
eISBN 978 0 85701 126 8

Printed and bound in Great Britain

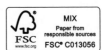

To my grandmother, who taught me the wonders of the remedies when I was young and continues to whisper in my ear to encourage me to explore further!

To the late J. Krishnamurti and Dr David Bohm for their friendship and influence in my life.

To all the flower girls and boys that have shared the journey with me when being taught by the flowers and all those who have been captured by the passion that working with flower essences brings.

DISCLAIMER

While the Author and the Publisher have taken every care to ensure the accuracy of information included in this book, it is offered with no guarantees. If there are any errors or omissions we will, if informed, make corrections to any future editions. Neither the Publisher nor Author accept any responsibility for any ill effects resulting from the use or misuse of the information contained in this book.

CONTENTS

LIST OF PLATES

FOREWORD

We are living during a unique period in human history. Over the past 50 years, science has discovered many ways of looking at the world and, in the process, has redefined the very nature of what it means to be human. Revolutionary discoveries in medical science have given us an understanding of the way in which the body works and how intricately linked the body and mind truly are. But a new breed of spiritual scientists has begun to explore the links between the body, the mind and the spiritual nature of human beings. Vibrational medicine is the evolving field of healing research that focuses on these links. Although the principles behind vibrational medicine are quite ancient, the development of modern technologies which can visualize and quantify the energetic nature of the links between body, mind and our spiritual anatomy are very new.

The concept that human beings are multidimensional energy systems is an idea that stems, in part, from the Einsteinian realization that matter and energy are dual expressions of the same universal substrate that makes up all things. Quantum physicists have begun to awaken to the concept that the subatomic particles that make up the entire universe, including people, are actually patterns of frozen energy and light. Many other scientists have begun to see the world in a similar light, having been led there by science instead of pure spirituality and intuition. We are literally beings of light and energy assembled in a way that is fundamentally hidden from our limited physical senses. The vibrational medicine perspective ascribes to this light/energy link by viewing humans as multidimensional beings consisting of far more than a physical brain and body. The new field of vibrational medicine is actually a fusion of science and spirituality which has defined the energy networks linking the physical body and its energetic substrates to the more rarefied world of spirit. Vibrational medicine views the world from the perspective of vibration and energy with an eye towards how this understanding of our energetic natures can lead to many new and wonderful forms of diagnosis and healing.

Our physical bodies are controlled by many biochemical cellular systems which are, in turn, finely tuned by subtle energy systems including the acupuncture meridian system and the chakra system. While our physical body is nurtured by physical nutrients and oxygen, it is also fed by subtle environmental energies such as Qi and *prana* which we absorb through the meridian and chakra networks. These subtle energetic forms of nutrition, understood by the ancients of China and India, are just as important as food and water to sustaining life. The subtle energy networks also connect the physical body to another type of energy system – the etheric body – which is a holographic energy template that invisibly guides human growth and development. Scientific evidence for the existence of subtle energy systems is growing. Modern technology has begun to validate ancient wisdom in a marriage of science and spirituality, the like of which has not been seen on this planet for thousands of years.

It is only through a fuller appreciation of a multidimensional model of human functioning that subtle energy therapies, such as flower essences, can be truly understood. Modern medicine has become rigid and locked into a mechanistic model of the body, and the model does not explain how subtle life energies can affect cellular machinery. It is only when one takes into account the larger picture of human beings from a newly evolving multidimensional perspective that flower essences as a healing modality begin to make sense. Flower essences do not work like drugs in which molecular patterns often bind to specialized receptors throughout the cells of the body. Instead they work by influencing the subtle energy structures that feed life energy into the body/mind. Flower essences modify energy flow through the acupuncture meridians, the chakras and the subtle bodies with the end result of affecting the very energetic patterns that influence consciousness.

The essences of flowers have been used in healing for hundreds (and possibly thousands) of years. Dr Edward Bach was one of the first modern pioneers of healing with flower essences. Bach was a medical practitioner as well as a psychic who experienced disturbing emotional patterns within himself when he was near a particular flower. Bach came to learn that taking an essence of the nearby flower would neutralize his psychically induced emotional disturbance. He discovered that the same flower essence would heal similar emotional patterns in others. Bach was among the first vibrational healers of the 20th century to realize how healing the emotions would contribute to the healing of any physical illness, regardless of the cause. It is in this regard, the energetic healing and repatterning

of emotional energies, that flower essences have a wide spectrum of applications.

Since Dr Bach's pioneering work in the first half of the 20th century, flower essence usage has undergone a veritable explosion of interest. Working groups that study the effects of local flower essences have sprung up all over the world, from England and North America to the outback of Australia. The merging of healing traditions has also begun to occur as practitioners have learned to apply principles of acupuncture to healing with flower essences by applying them to specific acupoints on the body. The wide variety of flower essence applications in healing has become an entire subspecialty within vibrational medicine.

It is because of this renaissance of interest in flower essences that *The Practitioner's Encyclopedia of Flower Remedies* is of great importance. Clare G. Harvey has performed an invaluable service by compiling the knowledge and wisdom of healing with flowers from around the world. It has been said that the answers to curing all of humanity's ills lie within nature. This book is an important step towards revealing the incredible healing wisdom within nature that we have only begun to discover. After all, modern medicine does not have all the answers to healing the afflictions of our techno-industrialized society. Perhaps the real answers to curing modern ailments exist within an exploration of our ancient past in order to synthesize a healing science of the 21st century.

I encourage you to read this book and experiment with the healing and transforming life energy of flower essences. The study and usage of flower essences and flower remedies will allow us to rediscover new ways of healing and remember our true inner spiritual nature as evolving beings of light. Those who take this journey will be richly rewarded for their efforts.

Richard Gerber, MD
Author of *Vibrational Medicine:
New Choices for Healing Ourselves*

PREFACE

ACKNOWLEDGEMENTS

I am delighted to be asked to provide an up-dated preface to the third edition of Clare G. Harvey's *Encyclopedia of Flower Remedies*. She has diligently updated this comprehensive text and it provides an up-to-date, thorough, exceptionally well-researched resource for those practitioners who are interested in flower essences.

In spite of their long history, flower essences began to be used by homeopaths in the West in the 1920s. This was largely due to the excellent effective range of flower remedies initially developed by Edward Bach in the early part of this century. His painstaking research, based on a combination of intuition and detailed case observation, has resulted in a now-rapidly expanding body of knowledge which will allow the practitioner to treat both physical and mental problems through the unique approaches offered by flower essences. These remedies provide a whole new dimension for medicine – in particular homeopathic medicine. They allow for the treatment of both mental and physical problems in a safe and well-judged manner.

The Encyclopedia represents a compilation of various flower remedies available throughout the world, their indications and the clinical experiences that have been used to define their use and support their prescription.

It is my hope that over the coming years more people will use these powerful treatments and more detailed evaluation will become available. At present our knowledge is largely empirical, based exclusively on the clinical observation of individual patients. I believe that it is possible to translate this body of knowledge into approaches that will allow its evaluation in more exacting scientific terms. From my own clinical experience I believe the flower essences offer a powerful approach to the treatment of illness, particularly mental symptoms. If this could be further established in a more scientific context then we may begin to see a real revolution in medical care.

Dr George Lewith, MA,
DM, FRCP, MRCGP
The Centre for Complementary
& Integrated Medicine, 2014

ACKNOWLEDGEMENTS

A big thank-you to all those in the world of flower essences for their generosity of spirit and support throughout this venture.

To dear Andreas who was happy to collaborate with me and add his invaluable insight and unique contribution to create an even more in-depth and inspirational book for all who love and are passionate about the healing power of flowers!

I would particularly like to thank the following for their continued support: Andreas Korte (Amazon, African, Cactus, Mushrooms, Gems, etc.); Julian Barnard (Healing Herbs, Bach); Shabd-Sangeet Khalsa (Dancing Light); Fred Rubenfeld (Pegasus); Tanmaya (Himalayan Enhancers); Philippe Deroide (Deva); Steve Johnson (Alaskan); Patricia Kaminski and Richard Katz (Flower Essence Society); Franchelle Ofsoské-Wyber (First Light Flower Essences of New Zealand); Susie Morvan (Channel Island Flower Essences); New Hope Farm (Bermuda, Desert Flower Essences); Vasudeva and Kadambii Barnao (Living Essences of Australia); Judy Griffin (Petite Fleur); Sabina Pettitt (Pacific); Drs Rupa and Atul Shah (Himalayan Aditi); Simon Lilly and Sue Griffin (Green Man); Cynthia Athina Kemp Scherer (Desert Alchemy); Arthur Bailey (Bailey); Lila Devi (Spirit in Nature/Masters); Mimi Buttacavoli (Amazonian Shamanic Sacred Tree Essences); Marion Leigh (Findhorn); Ellie Webb (Harebell); Paul Strode (Wild Flower Essences); Vivien Williamson and Jane Stevenson (Sun, Animal Essences); the late Laurence Harry (Aurora Borealis photo); Peter Aziz (Habundia Essences); Bram and Miep Zaalbergís (Bloesem Essences); Star Riparetti and Roger Valencia (Peruvian Essences); Eric Pelham (Butterfly Essences); Colette Prideaux-Brune (Soundwave Essences); Eliana Harvey (our joint venture with Jaguar Is Calling Essences); Cathie Welchman (Hawaiian Essences); Angie Jackson and Adam Rubinstein (Mediterranean Essences), Sheila Hicks Balgobin (Spirit of Makasuti Essences); Molly Sheehan for the Green Hope Farm section; and Ingrid Porter for her German/English translation.

Thanks also to Dr Masaru Emoto (Messages from Water); Harry Oldfield and Erik Pelham for their invaluable input; to Gregory Valmis and Marion Bielby for their insight and input on Bach; to Zhixing Wang (Qigong Master); Burgs (Meditation Teacher); Peter Tadd (Clairvoyant Adviser); Vladimir Raipolov (Russian Herbalist) for their words of wisdom; Maura McClean for her invaluable insights (Spiritual Advisor); Corrine Cyster for her wonderful illustration of the Orchid Flower Deva (Psychic Artist), Lisa Clark and all at JKP Singing Dragon and Susan Mears, my friend and agent, for their faith and encouragement.

Special thanks to Dr Richard Gerber and Dr George Lewith for giving their valuable time to write the Foreword and the Preface.

I would also like to honour the Aboriginal Elders for keeping their flower essence tradition alive and for being the grandfathers and custodians of the art!

Finally, to Dr Edward Bach, for being the father of the flower remedies, our inspiration, and for rekindling awareness of the healing powers of flowers.

INTRODUCTION

I am delighted to present the third revised and greatly expanded edition of my encyclopedia, this time titled *The Practitioner's Encyclopedia of Flower Remedies*. It is not only targeted for the first time towards the budding practitioner but also reflects the exciting growth, development and usage of flower remedies over the last 20 years and the rapid growth spurt that the field has experienced within the last five years, clearly indicating their need and relevance in our lives today. This is something that Dr Bach predicted, when he said to my grandmother that although his essences were complete within themselves, with all the stresses to come, in the future there will be the need for more essences sourced from all over the world to cope with today's needs.

I have chosen a broad range of essence lines, almost all of which I have used in my practice, as well as some exciting new lines and I am sure as the journey with essences is ever evolving there will be more to be birthed in the future. In this third edition there are some lines that are now not included simply because either they are no longer being made or the quality and integrity has no longer been maintained.

I have also collaborated with and include a whole section of the invaluable and insightful research and work of my dear friend Andreas Korte and his wonderful essences; see Chapter 9 and Section A of the Encyclopedia.

In this edition I have revealed more of my journey with the flowers and the lines of vibrational essences that I have been inspired (or rather instructed) to bring into being, including essences for women (see Flowers of the Orient page 190, Sound Wave Essences page 454, and Jaguar Calling Essences page 439).

I cannot imagine a life without flowers and the magic and joy that they bring. Have you ever felt happier and uplifted by surrounding yourself with fresh flowers, and have been especially attracted to certain kinds of blooms, or found solace strolling among fields or gardens filled with flowering plants? If so, you have already experienced the therapeutic power of flowers.

Since the dawn of time we have instinctively known that flowers can lift our spirits and make us feel well again. Flowers and their remedies feature in the traditional healing practices of many cultures around the world. They play an important role in restoring or evoking a sense of harmony in mind, body and spirit. This concept of wholeness is a recurring theme in many ancient philosophies, and we are now rediscovering its relevance to us. We are at last emerging from a time when good health is interpreted as the absence of disease. True wellbeing is something that lies beyond this limited concept, encompassing contentment and security, peace of mind and an abundance of vitality that is essential if our lives are to be enjoyable and fulfilling.

Many ancient and native cultures believe that everything in nature is infused with a vital energy, the spark of life. Wise men living several thousands of years ago proposed that when mind, body and spirit are perfectly integrated, this life force abounds, bringing with it a real sense of health and happiness. The way to attain such inner harmony, they claimed, is to respect nature and her ways.

Symbolizing love and friendship, flowers have always been a source of pleasure and happiness – of healing in its quintessential form. From the sensuous rose to the humble daisy, the delicate blooms adorning gardens, fields, hedgerows, mountainsides, woodlands and jungles throughout the world possess special qualities that can ease emotional distress, boost self-confidence, lift energy levels, increase resilience to all kinds of illness and even enrich our relationships. Most importantly, they offer the perfect antidote to stress in its many different guises.

Our existence is becoming increasingly artificial. Cocooned in towns and cities, it is easy to feel isolated from the natural environment. We no longer rely on the flowering of different plants to tell us what time of year it is as our distant ancestors once did. In severing the bond with nature, we risk losing our sense of wholeness. When this happens we become increasingly vulnerable to stress. Stress is recognized as a major source of unhappiness and ill health. Too many people feel completely at its mercy, powerless either to avoid or conquer its disruptive effects. Orthodox medicine offers little in the way to relieve stress-induced turbulence. Drugs such as tranquillizers may ease the discomfort by dulling our perceptions and reactions, but they do not really help us to stay afloat in this sea of turmoil. This is where flower remedies come to our rescue.

Flower essences are not like other medicines. They do not contain active chemicals or possess pharmaceutical properties. They are best described as a sort of liquid energy, a vibrational medicine that brings about benefits by influencing each person's own life force. Taking these remedies can be likened to surrounding yourself with exquisite flowers which never fade or die.

The state of the world has altered dramatically in the last 50 years and many new sources of stress have arrived on the scene.

Horrific events such as wars, famines, tragic accidents, violent incidents and natural disasters may not be new, but thanks to television, radio and newspapers we are now bombarded with their details on a regular basis. We may try not to think about them, but still they often shake us to the core.

Overpopulation in many areas creates competition for vital resources and work, leading to widespread greed and insecurity. Meanwhile the breakdown of close-knit communities leaves many people feeling lonely and isolated.

Stress tends to be infectious: if you work in an office full of anxious, frazzled people, it will be difficult to keep calm. Add the pressures of feeling hemmed in due to overcrowding, the constant noise of traffic and the almost stifling levels of pollution in some cities and it is hardly surprising that stress has become the 20th-century ailment. It not only plays havoc with our nervous systems, but also weakens our immunity, leaving us easy prey to the new so-called 'super bugs' that keep appearing on the scene. Flower remedies are needed now more than ever.

Responding to this cry for help, certain people have set out to research and rediscover the therapeutic properties of indigenous flowers growing in countries all over the world. The new flower essences are made from an extraordinarily diverse variety of flora, ranging from the modest hedgerow and alpine flowers to romantic Roses, exotic Orchids and the blossoms of fruits such as the Banana and Avocado. Some flowers, especially those from the Australian Bush and Himalayan mountains, have a long tradition of being used in natural healing. The beneficial properties of others are only just being discovered. While some flower essences free us from negative moods and emotions, others go further, helping us to recognize and let go of behaviour patterns that generate negative feelings.

When we feel confused about a situation or relationship in our lives, flower essences help us to see things from an entirely different perspective – just as escaping to a place of stunning natural beauty leaves you feeling that your problems and worries are less daunting than you had imagined. Some essences act at the physical level, strengthening and rebalancing various areas of the body such as the immune system. Others offer protection against new sources of environmental stress. Many aspire to more spiritual realms, helping us to find our true direction and purpose in life.

Although I have been a professional flower remedy consultant for more than 20 years, I actually grew up with this form of healing. As a child I would watch my grandmother working with the Bach Flower Remedies and I have always been amazed by the profound ways in which people respond to this gentle form of treatment. I have witnessed the emergence of the newer flower essences and steadily added them to my own repertoire of remedies. Using specially chosen combinations of essences from around the world, I have helped people who were suffering from all kinds of illnesses back to health. Typical conditions I have treated include infertility, premenstrual tension, hay fever, arthritis and nervous exhaustion. I firmly believe that what sets flower essences apart from other forms of remedies and therapies is their ability to address physical, mental, emotional and spiritual aspects of ourselves simultaneously, bringing about complete healing.

The beauty of flower remedies is that they are relatively inexpensive, easy to use and totally free from any unpleasant side-effects. Furthermore, you can prescribe them for yourself and now that there are ready-made combinations addressing common problems they are very accessible. We all have different needs, and the flowers that may benefit one person will differ from those that can help another. You may notice that you are instinctively attracted or drawn to certain flowers such as roses, just as you may choose to use certain herbs when cooking. These are very often the flowers that you probably need.

As you begin to use the flower essences you will embark on a journey of self-discovery.

You will become aware of your strengths and weaknesses as well as any stress patterns you have acquired over the years. These are reactions and responses to situations and people that, if left unchecked, consistently undermine your health and happiness.

The remedies will give you the strength and support you need to cope with change in your life, as well as with the more far-reaching upheavals occurring on this Earth. There is no doubt that anything that calls for a shift in our lives and thinking will generate stress and the more we resist the challenges and transitions we have to face, the more painful the experience of change tends to be. Flower essences can help us to go with the flow, to be more flexible and enable us to respond appropriately to the increasing demands made upon us.

In these testing times, let flower essences help you regain control of your life and destiny, to find the vitality you need to pursue your dreams and goals, and, above all, to rediscover the true joy of living.

HOW TO USE THIS BOOK

This book is for anyone who wishes to explore the benefits of using flower remedies, but especially for practitioners from all healing modalities, both complementary and orthodox.

Part I tells you what flower remedies are and how they work. You will discover how to choose remedies that can help you and others, as well as help practitioners choose remedies for their clients in Part II, along with a chapter of case histories in which I have used remedies successfully to combat a variety of conditions, and further advice for flower essence practitioners.

Part III is made up of an encyclopedia of 11 families of flower essences from around the world, giving a brief description of the properties and benefits of more than 2000 remedies, combinations, mists and creams. It also includes recipes you can make up for your own use (such as my Stress Buster and Infection Fighter combinations).

The Appendices at the end of the book contain an Ailment Chart for easy reference, covering a range of typical physical, emotional/psychological and spiritual problems with suggested remedies that can help to relieve them, as well as useful contacts and further reading.

Note: Abbreviations for all essence ranges used in brackets throughout this book can be found on pages 123–4.

PART I

THE POWER OF FLOWERS

CHAPTER ONE

THE HISTORY OF HEALING FLOWERS

The idea that flowers possess healing powers may seem new and revolutionary. It is, however, a very ancient concept, the origins of which can be traced back into the mists of time. For at least 40,000 years the Aborigines of Australia have been using flowers as part of their natural healing system. In other parts of the world where folk medicine is still alive, the tradition of utilizing flowering plants and their essences to restore wellbeing to body, mind and spirit has continued down the centuries to the present day.

Many of us instinctively turn to flowers to lift our spirits and make us feel better. It is second nature to bring bouquets to those who are sick or ailing. Without floral decorations, festive occasions or religious ceremonies would seem soulless and incomplete.

The task before us is to uncover and rediscover knowledge about the natural world that has existed for aeons.

TALES OF A GOLDEN AGE
Lemuria and Atlantis

Legend has it that flower essences were first used for healing some 500,000 years ago in a mythical place called Lemuria or Mu. Located in an area now covered by the Pacific Ocean, Lemuria was reputedly a veritable 'garden of Eden'. The land was lush and, thanks to a near-perfect climate, all kinds of exquisite flowering plants flourished.

It is said that the inhabitants of this civilization were gentle, sensitive souls who truly appreciated the beauty of their environment and were content to live close to the Earth. They were also aware of the natural empathy that exists between human and plant life. To them, every plant was special and had its own personality, and some believe these people were ethereal beings who could sense the energy or vibration of all living things. It has been suggested that, to them, all living things including plants appeared as luminous or shimmering objects.

These people realized that the highest concentration of life force in a plant is found in its flowers. Just by being close to a delicate bloom they became aware of its particular healing qualities. The Lemurians were not, however, troubled by physical disease – indeed it is said they lived for around 2000 years. Instead they used flower essences to evolve spiritually, to attain enlightenment.

According to the myth, Lemuria gave way to Atlantis. Those who believe or suspect there was a civilization known as Atlantis think it probably existed between 12,000 and 150,000 years ago. Unlike the Lemurians, the Atlanteans were reputedly not content to live in harmony with nature. They wanted to dominate and manage it to their advantage. As their society became increasingly technologically advanced, stress seeped into their lives bringing with it all kinds of new physical, emotional and mental diseases.

At this time, so the legend goes, flower essences were first used as a complete system of medicine.

Ancient Egypt, Crete and India

The ancient Egyptians certainly harnessed the healing powers of flowers; they did, after all, perfect the art of aromatherapy. Within magnificent temples high priests built laboratories where they distilled flowers to obtain aromatic essential oils. These were then blended to create medicinal formulations for treating a wide variety of illnesses. It should be stressed that essential oils are not the same as flower essences, although the Egyptians recognized the therapeutic benefits of both, for they also collected the dew from flowers and exposed it to sunlight to increase its potency.

The Lotus flower, which grew in abundance along the banks of the Nile, was sacred to the Egyptians. In their mythology it was the first living thing to appear on Earth. When its petals unfurled, the supreme god representing intellectual rulership was revealed to them. Its flower essence was used in rituals, as were those of other indigenous plants such as bamboo and papyrus. It has been suggested that the Egyptians imparted thoughts to certain plants, knowing they would reach and help us today.

The Minoans of Crete were another highly cultured people who recognized the healing potential of flowers. They are said to have held rituals devoted to the quest for spiritual understanding during which they would place a splendid flowering plant such as a wild rose in the centre of the ceremonial chamber, and place flowers or sprigs of plants floating in bowls of water around the room. Participants would sip the water or eat the petals to cleanse themselves of any disturbing thoughts or feelings during the ceremony.

At about this time, many miles away in the remote Himalayan mountains, flowers were playing their part in Ayurveda ('science of life'), an ancient system of natural medicine dating back at least 5000 years. We know of it because the Ayurvedic principles have been handed down from generation to generation and are still alive today. Flowers with spiritual significance such as the Lotus continue to be used in Ayurvedic healing ceremonies. The petals were traditionally sprinkled into bowls of water, which were then drunk and used to anoint various parts of the body.

FLOWERS AND FOLK MEDICINE

If we look at the folk medicines practised by native peoples around the world, most make use of the flowers and plants growing in each region.

The Australian Aborigines

The Aborigines have always turned to their exotic flora for help in healing mind, body and spirit. They collect the dew that settles on petals at dawn, believing it to enhance emotional wellbeing and help them enter into the 'dreamtime'. In some instances they may also eat the flowers themselves.

The Aboriginal story of how flowers were born and came by their healing powers was handed down from generation to generation and is told here by Ken Colbung of the Bibulmun people:

> The Aborigines living in the southwest of Western Australia are known as the Bibulmun people. Their legends were given to them by the *Demmagoomba* – the spirits of the old people who lived here previously. According to the *Demmagoomba*, the creator (also known as the *Gujub*, God, Supreme Being or senior spirit) sent the Rainbow Snake, *Waugal*, down to Earth as a life-giving element. It landed at a place in the southwest of Bibulmun country known as Broiungarup.
>
> Rainbow colours of the Rainbow Snake gave the flowers their colour at the time of creation. At Broiungarup you will always see beautiful rainbows. Some of the smallest and rarest flowers are only found in this one area.
>
> The *Broiunga* is a clan. It is where you get your spirituality and your mortal being. You

can be clan to birds, to a tree or to flowers. Your *Broiunga* is a special being for which you are responsible. If your *Broiunga* is a flower, then you must maintain this flower. It also has a responsibility to you. It gives you a beautiful feeling of colour, of its essence, which is the link to the Rainbow Snake.

The flowers of the Earth have different link-ups for different people's needs. There are a lot of occasions when the body needs to be associated with the different types of flowers. The essences are important for our own spirit, or *Djugubra*. So we have what is known as *Kaba nij nyoong* (*Kaba* is the flower essences, *nij* is the 'I', and *nyoong* is the understanding of the person). We must be aware that when we first see a flower it will bring us happiness; when we have the essence from that flower it will bring us health and with health and happiness we have wealth – the wealth of the spirit *Djugubra*.

The flower sauna is a unique feature of traditional Aboriginal healing and is arguably one of the earliest forms of flower essence therapy, dating back around 10,000 years. The ceremony, still performed the same way today, is conducted by the Maban, a man or woman who is healer and Keeper of the Law. The sauna is prepared by lining a shallow pit with hot coals which are then covered with a layer of earth. Steam is created by sprinkling water over the hot earth. Clay blended with crushed flowers (specially chosen for the occasion) is then smeared onto the body of the person being healed – this helps the flower essence penetrate the skin.

The Maban takes charge of the patient, who enters the pit and is then covered with an animal skin to seal in the warmth. The patient remains there until sunrise the next day when he or she emerges, renewed with the spirit of the flowers.

Another ritual sees people sent to sit among a clump of flowers so that their souls may be purified and they become 'spiritually reborn'.

Native Americans

In ancient times, the native peoples of North America were blessed with the ability to draw energy from flowers and plants. When they lost this gift they turned to imbibing the therapeutic properties of flowers in the form of teas and extractions. Some spiritual medicine people can still utilize this energy, but always request the flower's permission first. The Native Americans match the energy of the flower to the particular part of the body that is out of balance and needs healing. Indeed, in their version of the creation story, when humans came into being much of their physical body was derived from the plants, rocks and waters of Mother Earth, while their spirit or soul came from the heavens or sky. To them this explains why certain plants have a special affinity for certain areas of the body. This idea is echoed in the legends relating to Lemurian times and in the creation myths of other indigenous peoples.

Russian medicine men

Across the Atlantic in Russia, medicine men or shamans also practise a natural form of healing handed down to them by their forefathers. All knowledge is passed on by word of mouth; nothing is committed to print. The medicine people living in the richest floral area of the Caucasus Mountains are called the Koldum. Nearly half the flowers growing here are unique to this area. These indigenous flowers are taken in the form of essences and tinctures. So famous are these remedies that people have been known to travel for miles to this region, even the infamous Genghis Khan, who made his pilgrimage from Mongolia. He reputedly prescribed them to his men to give them strength for battle.

The mystical Paracelsus

Healing with flowers was introduced into Europe during the 15th century by the renowned physician and mystic Philippus

Aureolus Theophrastus Bombast von Hohenheim, better known as Paracelsus.

While still in his early twenties Paracelsus left his home in Austria to embark on a ten-year adventure which took him to Russia, England and North Africa, where he encountered different kinds of folk medicines.

It is said that Paracelsus, aware of planetary energies and the healing power of flowers, gathered dew on glass plates exposed under various astrological configurations, believing that water when captured, concentrates and holds within it the plant as well as planetary energies. There is some question as to him prescribing the early morning dew from flowers to treat emotional disturbance in others but he would certainly have been exposed to the practice on his travels and exploration of indigenous peoples' use of plants and healing methods. Paracelsus was also responsible for reviving the old 'Doctrine of Signatures', a system of equating certain features of a flower or plant – its shape, colour, scent, taste or natural habitat – to its healing properties. For example, Eyebright, a blue flower with a yellow centre, looks like an eye and is said to help treat eye problems. Similarly the Skullcap flower, resembling the shape of a human skull, may be used to treat headaches and insomnia, while the bark of Willow, a tree that grows in wet places, eases rheumatism and other conditions that worsen in damp weather. We now know that Willow bark contains an anti-inflammatory substance called salicin which eases the pain of rheumatism as well as headaches. Its synthetic form is taken by millions each day as aspirin.

Paracelsus also believed that plants tend to grow where they are needed most; dock leaves, which can be used to treat nettle rash, always grow near nettles, while plants for easing fevers can often be found close to swamps.

THE LANGUAGE OF FLOWERS

With the birth of modern medicine, belief in the healing power of flowers appeared to die out. But this was not so; it simply became channelled into the popular notion that certain qualities or virtues are associated with flowers. From the earliest times the Rose has been a symbol of love. Cleopatra placed such faith in its romantic charm that she reputedly carpeted her bedroom with millions of fresh rose petals to help her seduction of Marc Anthony. Today, the Rose is still a symbol of love and romance, which is why lovers give each other red roses on St Valentine's Day.

Centuries before the slogan 'Say it with flowers', people intuitively knew the special meanings of different blooms. In ancient Egypt the Iris was seen as an emblem of power. It adorned the brow of the Sphinx of Giza and the sceptres of kings. To the Egyptians flowers also represented certain thoughts and feelings; just as we might send telegrams or cards to wish someone good health during an illness or to show our affection or love, they would send an appropriate flower.

Flowers had their own language and meaning to the ancient Greeks and Romans too, and it should come as no surprise that the Rose is associated with Aphrodite/Venus, the goddess of love. But the Rose is by no means the only flower linked to love. Others include the Iris, which is named after the goddess of the rainbow who guided the souls of women to their final resting place. Carnations also express pure love and constancy, while the Tulip denotes a declaration of love.

Many of the classical gods, goddesses and nymphs such as Hyacinthus, Narcissus and Iris are remembered today because they gave their name to flowers. Narcissus owes its name to the young man who, it was prophesied, would have a long and happy life unless he caught sight of his reflection and fell in love with his own beauty. To his cost he did indeed become enraptured by himself. Thus in most books about the language of flowers the Narcissus represents egotism. In the Middle East, however, it is traditionally linked with love, the beginning of new relationships and the enhancement of existing ones.

Flower symbolism occurs throughout the world. In India flowers are associated with various deities and ceremonies, *pujas*, prayers and certain festive occasions. A sprig of the magical Mimosa is often suspended above the bed to ward off ill fortune. Its yellow flowers give a sweet aroma which is also said to evoke psychic dreams. To the Chinese, Jasmine represents feminine sweetness, while in India it is considered sacred. The flower of sensuousness and physical attraction, the Jasmine is believed to enhance self-esteem and is always used in traditional bridal wreaths.

Flowers often have religious significance. The Lotus flower is recognized as a symbol of spirituality all over the world. It is not only sacred to the Ancient Egyptians, but throughout Asia, and the Far East especially, it is associated with Buddhism and the state of enlightenment. The figure of Buddha is often depicted sitting on a Lotus flower.

Good fortune, protection and strength have also traditionally been associated with flowers. For this reason they have often been adopted by kings and leaders. The Sunflower became the symbol of Atahualpa, King God of the Incas, for it was believed to hold great magical properties. Like the sun itself it has a strong life force, encouraging action and strengthening willpower.

The English Plantagenets derived their name from *Planta genista* (Latin for Broom) after Geoffrey Count of Anjou wore it as an emblem on his helmet when he went into battle in 1140. The sweet scent of its fresh flowers is said to purify thoughts and feelings. Inhaling the aroma also instils a sense of peace and tranquillity. And the people of Shakespeare's day were well acquainted with the ancient meanings associated with plants and flowers, as demonstrated by Ophelia in *Hamlet* as she cries, 'There's rosemary, that's for remembrance'.

However, it was not until more than 200 years later that the language of flowers really took shape. In 1817 the first real flower dictionary, *Le Langage des Fleurs* by Madame Charlotte de la Tour, was published in Paris. It proved so popular and sparked such great interest that other versions followed. With the help of these flower dictionaries,

shy Victorians found ways to express what they would not say in words. They sent each other bouquets in which every blossom, leaf and stem was fraught with significance. The language of flowers flourished, and was even given the special name 'florigraphy'.

At the beginning of that century, 'flower fairies' epitomizing the personality or character of various blossoms and buds also became fashionable. These tiny ethereal beings with gossamer wings reputedly lived among the flowers at the bottom of the garden. They captured the imagination of writers such as J.M. Barrie, who conjured up Peter Pan's rather wayward guardian angel, Tinkerbell. Sherlock Holmes' creator, Arthur Conan Doyle, was also fascinated by these nature spirits – as his book *The Coming of the Fairies* reveals. Legend has it that these nature spirits, or devas, first made their appearance in Lemurian times. Each fairy was entrusted with a different flower, and together they were said to be responsible for teaching us how to live in harmony with nature.

Folklore tells us that if we wish to see the fairy kingdom we should make a concoction of Rose water, Marigold water and wild Thyme. Leave this lotion in the sunlight for three days, apply it to the eyes and the windows of the fairy world will magically open!

FLOWERS AND SIGNS OF THE ZODIAC

When astrology became fashionable, flowers, like gem stones, were also attributed to the signs of the zodiac, as follows:

Aries: Geranium, Honeysuckle

Taurus: Rose, Violet

Gemini: Forsythia, Morning Glory

Cancer: Acanthus, Jasmine

Leo: Marigold, Sunflower

Virgo: Anemone, Melissa

Libra: Columbine, Orchid

Scorpio: Gentian, Hyacinth

Sagittarius: Pinks, Dandelion

Capricorn: Pansy, Tulip

Aquarius: Orchid, Primrose

Pisces: Clematis, Hydrangea

REDISCOVERING THE HEALING POWER OF FLOWERS

In the 1930s, healing with flowers was rediscovered by a remarkable man called Dr Edward Bach. Thanks to his pioneering work, flower essences have come to the rescue of millions of people throughout the world.

Bach was born near Birmingham, England in 1886. Even at an early age he was fascinated by nature and loved going for walks in the countryside. He pursued a career in medicine specializing in pathology and bacteriology. In 1920 he established a successful practice in Harley Street, London.

During the next few years he became increasingly disenchanted with the orthodox medical approach, which he felt focused on relieving the symptoms of disease rather than its true cause. At the same time he felt increasingly drawn towards the homeopathic principle of treating the whole person.

He began to carry out his own research. He isolated certain bacteria from the intestinal tract with which he prepared vaccines according to homeopathic principles. These vaccines proved remarkably helpful to people suffering from chronic diseases, and could be taken orally instead of injected (a method Bach particularly disliked). Remedies prepared from toxins such as viruses became known as the Bach nosodes, and are still used by many homeopaths today.

During his work Bach noticed that his patients tended to fall into distinct personality types, and those in a particular group frequently responded to the same treatment. Ahead of his time, he also recognized the link between stress, emotions and illness. Bach believed that the disturbing moods or feelings

different people experienced were a key cause of ill health. In *Heal Thyself*, a small booklet he wrote which sums up his philosophy of healing and the problems of orthodox medicine, Bach proposed that:

> The real primary diseases of man are such defects as pride, cruelty, hate, self-love, ignorance, instability and greed. Each of these defects will produce a conflict which must of necessity be reflected in the physical body, producing its own specific type of malady. (Bach 1996, p.12)

Correcting emotional factors, he reasoned, would go a long way towards increasing physical and mental vitality, which in turn would help to resolve any physical disease.

At the same time, Bach became interested in the idea of replacing vaccines based on bacteria, themselves the instigators of disease, with more wholesome remedies. He discovered these in the flowers growing in the fields and hedgerows. Bach was a sensitive soul who relied on his intuition for guidance. During a visit to Wales, he was drawn to two particular wild flowers, Impatiens and Mimulus. These flowers, he felt, emitted a special kind of energy or vibration which could exert a positive influence on certain negative states of mind.

In 1930 Bach decided to give up his lucrative London practice, and he spent the next six years living in several parts of rural England in the quest for a new floral healing system. Aware that personality affects the way we react to stress, the first remedies Bach looked for related to what he perceived to be the 12 key personality types (see Chapter 4). To him flowers had their own little personalities reminiscent of certain characteristics in us. The wistful Clematis reminded him of quiet, dreamy people who are wrapped up in their thoughts and fantasies, who as a result are prone to drowsiness, indifference, sensitivity to noise, poor concentration and difficulty recuperating from illness. As a remedy Clematis would lend support to people with these characteristics, reducing their susceptibility to such tendencies.

THE HISTORY OF HEALING FLOWERS

The colour, texture, flowering patterns and growth patterns of flowers told Bach something of their healing qualities. The sturdy Oak, for instance, suggested to him the type of strong, reliable, patient, dependable people who shoulder their burdens without complaining.

The next 26 flower remedies he looked for were intended to bring relief from different kinds of emotional discomfort and distress. Bach felt that they could deal with negative mind-states such as fear, apathy, loneliness and despair, which he believed were not truly a part of our nature but which we only succumbed to in difficult and trying times.

The flowers, Bach has said, have a particular quality which is an exact equivalent to the human emotion. For example, Wild Rose, a remedy for apathy and resignation, is a positive representation of this state. In other words, it replaces these negative feelings with dynamism and optimism.

For Bach the colours of flowers were also indicative of their remedial qualities. Blue flowers such as Cerato express receptive feelings, the red or yellow flowers are more dynamic, while green flowers such as Scleranthus are associated with balance. Remedies for fear have a dynamic colour reflecting their vibrant strength. Bach confirmed the effects of the various flowers by observing how each one affected his own emotional state. It is said that he would think himself into feeling a particular way, then search for remedies to help restore a sense of calm and contentment.

With a few exceptions such as Vine, Olive, Honeysuckle and Cerato, Bach's healing flowers can still be found growing wild in the fields and hedgerows of Oxfordshire. Almost half of them come from trees, while others (such as Gorse and Cerato) are from shrubs.

It was my good fortune to have grandparents who were at the leading edge of many pioneering healing modalities and were trained by the likes of Bach, Dr de la Warr, Montessori and others. My grandfather was well known for his form of X-ray vision, which was very useful as a diagnostic tool in his Harley Street osteopathic practice before the war (he helped set up the first school in London) and, which was rare in those days, for being a trained acupuncturist. My grandmother knew Dr Edward Bach very well and was in fact taught by him, and practised Bach Remedies and Radionics in Harley Street with my grandfather. She was also great friends with Nora Weeks, Bach's close friend and companion, whom I remember meeting with my grandmother when I was little. Apparently Nora pressed my grandmother that I should be taught all about the flower remedies, as she felt I would have a part to play in times to come.

In 1936 Bach passed away, satisfied that his work was complete. Nora was entrusted with and largely responsible for safeguarding and keeping his work alive. Until recently the flowers continued to be gathered from the Oxfordshire countryside, and prepared and bottled at Mount Vernon, as Bach himself had done, and each year hundreds of people from all corners of the world make their pilgrimage to Mount Vernon, to witness the place where Bach performed much of his pioneering work.

For many years Bach's Flower Remedies stood alone. Then in the mid-1970s, interest in the healing power of flowers was rekindled. Richard Katz was one of a few people in the forefront of this revitalization, establishing the Flower Essence Society in California. His aims were to research new flower essences and gather together those working with the essences so they could exchange ideas and information.

Others, too, have been inspired to research the healing qualities of locally growing flowers. From Alaska to Australia, the Mediterranean to Thailand, and Hawaii to the Himalayas, distinct remedies have been rediscovered in the flowers that are indigenous to each particular country or region. The Orchids of the Amazon, for instance, come from the exotic flowers that grow 100 feet up on the branches and treetops of the rainforests of Colombia.

These new essences come at a time when they are most needed, for the world has changed considerably in the last 70 years and is continuing to do so at an alarming rate. Many of the flowers address not only emotional problems but also aspire to more spiritual healing, as well as acting at the fundamental physical level, treating the whole person – mind, body and spirit.

CHAPTER TWO

ENERGY FIELDS

To understand how flower essences work, we have to become familiar with the idea that all living things are infused with energy, or life force. We cannot see or touch this energy but, like the air we breathe, it is essential to life. Most people living in the West find it hard to believe that there may be more to us than meets the eye. In other regions of the world, especially the Far East and Asia, this view is commonplace.

More than 5000 years ago, Indian holy men spoke of a universal energy. Known as *prana*, this energy is still seen as the basic constituent and source of all life. *Prana*, the breath of life, moves through all things and brings vitality to them. The same idea forms the basis of Taoism, the ancient Chinese philosophy which also emerged during the third millennium BC. It holds that the universe is a living organism infused and permeated with a rhythmic, vibrational energy called Qi. The concept of an energy pervading all things is not as mystical as it may seem. Modern physics is beginning to lend credence to what the ancient wise men supposed all those years ago. In the last century it has become outmoded to think of things as solid objects, as Newton and his colleagues in the late 17th and early 18th centuries suspected.

With the discovery of the atom, physicists felt they had found the fundamental building blocks of the universe. Yet as they delved deeper, they found that atoms are composed of even tinier particles which seem to be constantly on the move. Furthermore, the behaviour of things on this very tiny scale is very different to what one might expect. In 1905 Albert Einstein shattered the principles of the old Newtonian worldview when he published his theory of relativity. With this hypothesis came the idea that matter and energy are interchangeable. All particles can be created from energy, and matter is simply slowed-down or 'crystallized' energy.

A few years later another important discovery was made by Max Planck. He found that light and other forms of electromagnetic radiation are emitted in the form of energy packets which he called quanta. These light quanta, or energy packets, have been accepted as bona fide particles. Oddly, though, they also behave as if they were waves rather than individual particles.

The latest 'super-string' theories, which first came to light during the 1960s, now propose that these fundamental particles are not really particles at all. They are more like snippets of infinitely thin string. In 'string theories', what were previously thought of as pinpoints of light are now pictured as waves travelling down the string, like waves on a vibrating kite-string. This means that at the most basic level everything would appear to be shimmering, or moving in light waves all the time. What all this suggests is that our world of seemingly solid objects is composed of wave-like patterns and energy fields that constantly interact with one another. Indeed, some scientists view the universe as rather like a vast web of inseparable energy patterns.

In 1964 the physicist John S. Bell came up with the now well-known mathematical formula called Bell's Theorem. This supports the idea that subatomic particles are connected in some way, so that everything that happens to one particle affects all the others. The late David Bohm, Professor of Theoretical Physics at Birkbeck College, London, also came to the conclusion that the universe is an interconnected whole, after devoting 40 years of research into physics and philosophy. He would have received a Nobel Prize for his work had he not died unexpectedly in 1993.

In his book *Wholeness and the Implicate Order*, Bohm discusses the idea that, in reality, things are not separate and independent of each other; they only exist this way in our minds. We split things up and file them away in neat compartments to make the world around us more manageable. Seeing everything as being separate is purely an illusion which leads to endless conflict and confusion within ourselves and society as a whole. Not realizing this fragmentation is of our own making, humanity has always been driven by a quest for wholeness. Indeed the word 'health' derives from the word 'hale', originally an Anglo-Saxon word meaning whole.

This lends credibility to ancient philosophies which tell us that we cannot enjoy a sense of total wellbeing unless all facets of us – mind, body and spirit – are in balance. This in turn will come from living in harmony with nature. Should we slip out of this balanced state, nature possesses the remedies to make us whole again.

THE ESSENCE OF A FLOWER

Evidence to suggest that these energy fields do indeed exist came to light back in the 1940s. While investigating electrical phenomena, Harold Saxton Burr (Professor of Anatomy at Yale University Medical School) accidentally discovered energy fields around living plants and animals. He called these fields bioelectrical or electrodynamic L-fields – the fields of life. After discovering that the electrical fields around tiny seedlings resemble those of the adult plant, not of the original

seed, he suggested that the organization of a living thing, its pattern, is established by its electrodynamic field. Like a fingerprint, this electrical field is characteristic of a particular living thing and has a shaping influence on it, maintaining its established energetic 'status quo', or blueprint. Today, certain techniques can be used to reveal these fields. The most well-known is Kirlian photography, a form of high-frequency, high-voltage electro-photography which was developed by the Russian researcher Semyon Kirlian (see page 28 of colour plate). In very simple terms, Kirlian's photography captures the interference pattern which is set up when a high-frequency electrical charge interacts with the energy field of a living object. The pattern usually appears as streaks of light surrounding the outline of the object, be it a leaf or a hand.

Erik Pelham is pioneering the use of Kirlian photography to show that flower essences do indeed possess energy fields. Furthermore, he has discovered that the energetic patterns produced by different flower essences vary, often quite dramatically – lending support to the idea that each flower has its own personality or character. The first photograph Erik takes is of a cleansed quartz crystal. Having obtained his 'control', Erik then places a few drops of flower essence onto the crystal and makes a series of exposures. The individual energy pattern of the essence emerges, reflecting the unique qualities of that particular flower.

CAPTURING A FLOWER'S ENERGY

Flower essences are best described as a kind of 'liquid energy'. They literally encapsulate the energy pattern or vibration of the flower they come from. Since early times it has been believed that the early morning dew which settles on petals becomes infused with a flower's energy. The art of capturing this energy pattern so that it could be used therapeutically was perfected by Dr Bach (see Chapter 1). In the beginning Bach would collect morning dew from flowers, just as the peoples of ancient cultures did. He then noticed that the droplets taken from flowers that had been exposed to sunlight were more beneficial than those which formed on shaded flowers. Sunlight, he concluded, seemed to bring potency to the remedy. To his delight, Bach also discovered that by floating flowers in a bowl of pure spring water for several hours in the sunlight he could obtain powerful vibrational tinctures. The method he devised is remarkably simple and is still used by many people making flower essences today.

The sun method

Flowers for making essences are ideally picked very soon after they come into bloom. Freshly picked and undamaged flowers are floated in a glass bowl filled with spring water so that they cover the surface (see page 1 of colour plate). The bowl is then left out in the sunlight on a clear, cloudless day for three to four hours (or less if the petals show signs of fading). Bach believed that during this process a flower's energies were transferred to the water. Sunlight plays a role in charging the water with an energetic imprint of the flower's vibrational signature. The blooms are then lifted out with a twig and discarded. The energized liquid or 'essence' is then poured into bottles with an equal volume of brandy to form the flower stock. The brandy acts as a preservative which stabilizes and anchors the flower's energy.

The boiling method

A clean enamel saucepan is three-quarters filled with newly picked flowers and stems. These are covered with spring water and brought to the boil, uncovered. After simmering for 30 minutes the liquid is left to cool; when cold the essence is filtered. Again this liquid is bottled half-and-half with brandy. (For those who wish to try making their own remedies, these methods are described in greater detail in *The Healing Herbs of Edward Bach* by Julian and Martine Barnard – see Further Reading.) If possible, flowers destined for healing should be growing wild in places that are not often visited and are free from pollution. If they are taken from cultivated plants it is important they are tended with loving care and without the use of chemical pesticides or fertilizers.

New environmentally friendly ways of capturing a flower's energy are also coming to light. In India, Drs Atul and Pupa Shah have devised a technique which means they do not have to cut the flowers to make their Aditi Flower Essences (see page 280). And Andreas Korte has invented a crystal method which he uses to make his Amazonian Orchid, Rose, and Cactus essences (see page 112). Ever conscious that increasing demand for some of the rarer flowers may actually jeopardize their existence, many are turning to these and other alternative forms of extraction.

WATER HOLDS THE MEMORY

Water plays a vital role in making flower essences, for the energy is believed to imprint itself on the liquid. Do not expect to find any dissolved chemicals from the petals in the essence. All it contains is the flower's energy or signature. It may seem remarkable that energized water alone can possess healing properties, yet evidence to suggest this emerged in 1987 when a French immunobiologist called Dr Jacques Benveniste, working in laboratories just outside Paris, found that certain highly diluted substances can be as potent as vastly greater quantities of the same substance. Using a constant called the Avogadro number, Benveniste confirmed mathematically that it was impossible for water to retain a single molecule of the active antibody, immunoglobulin E. Despite this, the water set off a powerful reaction in the test tube. Somehow the water had retained the 'memory' or 'vibration' of the molecule.

The remarkable research conducted by Dr Masaru Emoto from Japan has also discovered that water is a mirror reflecting our mind; words, thoughts and emotions have a powerful effect on water which reacts by picking up and revealing, through water in its crystalline form, the different vibrational patterns to which it is exposed. When the imprinted water is frozen it is then possible to see and record the effect of the spoken word in the formation of beautiful crystals. (See plate page 2 for water crystal experiments by Dr Emoto as illustrated in his book *Messages from Water*.) This supports the efficacy of flower remedies as the water in which the flower is placed becomes imprinted with the vibrational qualities of that flower, and then has an easy entrance and absorption by the body, which is itself composed of a high proportion of water. So flower remedies have the power to erase negative disease or mental emotional patterns within the human organism, flooding the system with positive vibrations.

Gem or crystal essences are worth mentioning here, as they work in a similar 'vibrational' way to flower remedies and are prepared in much the same way. Flower and gem essences tend to complement each other and work well in combination. Like all living entities, we are also infused with energy; it permeates every part of our being and its abundance goes hand in hand with good health and vitality. This energy flows freely in newborn babies, but as we proceed on our journey through life it begins to wane for all kinds of reasons which we will discuss in Chapter 3.

The traditional medical systems of the Chinese, Japanese, Tibetans, Native Americans and Australian Aborigines all regard this energy as something tangible. As science has yet to validate this energy's existence, no one knows for sure what form it takes within us, yet for centuries healers have been working with energy systems described by ancient medical and esoteric teachings. As flower essences are believed to have a restorative effect on this energy, it is a good idea to know a little more about these different systems.

THE MERIDIAN SYSTEM

Traditional Chinese medicine views all matter as being infused with a subtle energy known as Qi, which manifests itself through vibration, circulation and waves of movement. This Qi flows along a network of channels called meridians, which spreads like an intricate web through the body. It may be likened to a second nervous system which forms a connection between the physical body and the subtler energy system surrounding it. It may also be perceived as an aura of light that may at times be colourful. According to the Chinese model, there are 12 pairs of meridians, each pair associated with a different organ system or function. The first reference to this energy network is found in the *Nei Ching*, or *Yellow Emperor's Classic of Internal Medicine*, written during the reign of the Emperor Huang Ti between 2697 and 2596 BC.

The concept of Qi continues to be very much alive today, and millions of people believe that good health and peace of mind rely on ensuring that this energy flows smoothly and evenly. Traditional Chinese medicine offers various ways to promote the movement of energy to preserve wellbeing and encourage spiritual development. The flowing movements of *Qigong* (pronounced 'cheegung') and *Taiji*, and the techniques of acupuncture and acupressure all use knowledge of the meridians to clear energy blockages and heal illness. All Qigong masters have the ability to diagnose illness at a distance by reading the subtle anatomy. According to Qigong master Zhixing Wang, any illness can be explained as an energy blockage in the body. Circulation and movements of the subtle energy can clear this blockage and, therefore, heal the illness.

But is there any scientific proof that such energy channels or meridians exist? More than 20 years ago Dr Hiroshi Motoyama, a researcher in Japan, devised a system of measuring the electrical characteristics of the 12 major meridians by attaching 28 electrodes to the 'entry points' on the skin for each of the meridians. It is known as the AMI machine (apparatus for measuring the functions of the meridians and corresponding internal organs). Using the AMI machine, Dr Motoyama studied over 5000 subjects and found strong correlations between meridians that are electrically out of balance and the presence of underlying disease in the associated organ.

A more recent study was carried out at the UCLA School of Medicine. It looked at the electrical conductivity of the distal lung acupuncture (meridian) point in 30 patients. X-ray examination had already shown that four members of the group had lung cancer, but the tester did not know which of the 30 these were. On the basis of the reading of the distal lung acupuncture point, the four patients were identified correctly.

THE CHAKRAS

Common to Eastern medical and mystical traditions is the idea that special centres known as 'chakras' play a vital role in moving energy around the body. There are seven major chakras which are inextricably linked to the meridian system.

The chakras may be regarded as 'transformers', simultaneously receiving, assimilating and transmitting energy. They are capable of gathering and holding various types of energy, and can also alter their vibration so this energy can be used for different purposes – for example, by bringing higher vibrations down to the physical plane. You could visualize the chakras as many-petalled, vibrantly coloured flowers which are attached by invisible threads to the spine. These 'petals', known as *nadis*, are woven into the nervous system and distribute the energy of each chakra into the physical body. The chakras are continuously opening to receive information about the state of the subtle bodies (see the Aura section below) and closing again, rather like a periwinkle which unfurls its petals when the sun shines.

The seven chakra centres govern the major glands of the endocrine system and influence both our physical and psychological health. The chakra associations differ slightly from East to West, which may help to explain why people from one culture can find it difficult to feel totally at ease in another. It should be noted that the definitions given below are based primarily on the Western chakra tradition.

Each chakra has its own 'pulse rate'. Some vibrate very quickly, others are slower, depending largely on the ways in which we use and regard our bodies. Indeed, it is said that each chakra has its own 'note'. If one chakra is not functioning properly it will affect those above and below it. Ideally the top centres should vibrate faster and more subtly than the lower ones, but this is not always the case and heavy vibrations can appear in all the centres.

First or root chakra

Situated at the base of the spine and associated with basic raw energy.

- Colour: red.

- Physical connections: large intestine, legs, feet, skeletal structure. Imbalance is linked to problems such as obesity, constipation, haemorrhoids, sciatica, arthritis, knee problems and poor circulation in the legs and extremities.

- Psychological influences: connecting with the earth (grounding), survival, letting go of emotional tension. Imbalance is linked to accident proneness, dependency, identity crisis and weak ego.

Second or hara chakra

Situated at the centre of the abdomen, just below the navel, and thought of as the seat of power and vitality.

- Colour: orange.

- Physical connections: ovaries, testicles, uterus, bladder, circulation. Imbalance is linked to low back trouble, infertility, reproductive problems, pre-menstrual syndrome, urinary problems and arthritis.

- Psychological influences: sexuality, creativity. Imbalance is linked to a weak personality, depression, hysteria and an inability to be sexually intimate.

Third or solar plexus chakra

Situated above the navel, this is the seat of the emotions.

- Colour: yellow.

- Physical connections: adrenal glands, solar plexus, spleen, pancreas and stomach. Imbalance is linked to nervous stomach, anorexia, diabetes and blood glucose problems, anaemia, allergies and obesity as well as liver, adrenal and spleen problems.

- Psychological influences: feeling empowered and being in control. Imbalance is linked to addictive and compulsive behaviour, excessive anger or fear, manic depression, sleep problems and all kinds of psychosomatic conditions.

Fourth or heart chakra

Situated in the centre of the chest, this is concerned with self-love and universal goodwill.

- Colour: green.

- Physical connections: heart, thymus gland, immune system, circulatory system, lungs and respiratory system. Imbalance is linked to heart and circulatory as well as lung and respiratory problems, high blood pressure, upper back troubles and childhood diseases.

- Psychological influences: understanding, compassion, unconditional love. Imbalance is linked to inner conflict, self-destructive tendencies, relationship problems and feelings of alienation and loneliness.

Fifth or throat chakra

Situated in the throat, this is the centre of trust.

- Colour: turquoise.

- Physical connections: thyroid, parathyroid, lymphatic system, immune system, neurological system. Imbalance is linked to teeth, ear, and neck and shoulder problems as well as to sore throats, bronchial problems and hearing and speech difficulties.

- Psychological influences: trust, expression, creativity and communication. Imbalance is linked to an inability to express oneself in words, poor memory, stuttering and doubt as to the sincerity of others.

Sixth or third eye chakra

Situated in the centre of the forehead and associated with perception, discernment and clairvoyance.

- Colour: indigo.

- Physical connections: the pituitary gland, left-brain hemisphere, central nervous system. Imbalance is linked to nervous upsets, eye and vision problems, headaches and sinusitis.

- Psychological influences: clarity and insight, interest in spiritual issues. Imbalance is linked to confusion, poor memory, inability to focus, paranoia, detachment from reality and, in severe cases, schizophrenia.

Seventh or crown chakra

Situated at the crown of the head, this is the seat of consciousness.

- Colour: white.

- Physical connections: pineal gland, right-brain hemisphere and the ancient mammalian brain. Imbalance is linked to migraine headaches, pituitary problems and epilepsy.

- Psychological influences: intuition, to be open and have faith; connection to higher energies or realms. Imbalance is linked to being gullible, having nightmares, having multiple personalities and being spiritually closed off.

For centuries mystics have talked about an ethereal body surrounding the physical one, which they refer to as the aura. It was first recorded by the Pythagoreans (circa 500 BC) as a luminous body. They believed that its light could produce a variety of effects in human organisms, including the cure of disease.

In the early 12th century two well-known scholars, Boirac and Liebeault, suggested that humans have an energy that can cause an interaction between two individuals even when they are some distance apart.

Count Wilhelm von Reichenbach spent 30 years during the 1800s experimenting with a field he named the 'odic' force, but it was not until 1911 that knowledge of the human energy field started to take shape. Using coloured screens and filters, Dr William Kilner, a medical doctor, described the aura as a glowing mist around the body which had three distinct zones. He found it differed considerably from person to person depending on age, sex, mental ability and health. Certain diseases showed as irregularities in the aura, which led Kilner to develop a system of diagnosis based on the colour, texture, volume and general appearance of this ethereal body. At around the same time Dr Wilhelm Reich, a humanist psychologist and pupil of Sigmund Freud, became interested in a universal energy he called 'orgone'. He studied the relationship between disturbances in the orgone flow within the human body and psychological and physical illness. He suggested that when strong feelings such as anger, frustration, sadness and even pleasure are not expressed, the energy that should have been released becomes locked in the body, thus sapping vitality.

During the mid-1900s Dr George de la Warr and Dr Ruth Drown invented new instruments to detect the subtle radiation being emitted from human tissues. Dr de la Warr was also responsible for developing Radionics, a system of detection, diagnosis and healing from a distance utilizing the human biological energy field.

Medical science now recognizes that the body does have a weak electromagnetic field which is generated by the activity of brain waves and nervous impulses. A group of scientists from the A.S. Popov Bioinformation Institute recently reported the finding that living organisms emit energy vibrations at a frequency of 300 to 2000 nanometers (nms). They called this energy field the bio-field or bioplasma.

No one knows for sure whether the aura, electromagnetic field and other forms of radiation emitted by the body are one and the same thing. It is more than likely that the human energy field is composed of many different vibrations. Based on their observations and other findings, researchers have created theoretical models of the aura and subtle bodies.

THE AURA

This is an invisible yet luminous kind of radiation which looks like a halo surrounding the physical body. From ancient times artists and mystics have 'seen' auras. Ancient Indian sculptures, Aboriginal rock paintings in Australia and Native American totem poles all show figures surrounded by light or with lines emanating from their bodies. Highly sensitive or 'psychic' people who claim they can see auras describe them as softly shimmering lights forming a misty outline around people, animals, plants and other objects.

Despite its mystical connotations, the aura has distinct parallels with the body's electromagnetic force-field. All life forms possess an aura. In humans it varies widely in size, density and colour. Its vibrancy and hue is said to depend upon the spiritual evolution of that person as well as his or her general health. Personality and emotions can also be glimpsed in the aura. Those whose auras have soft fringed edges are susceptible to the influence of others, while a hard, distinct outline may indicate a person with a defensive and hostile attitude resulting from deep insecurity.

The aura differs remarkably from the other energy fields known as the subtle bodies (see below) in that it is a general field of energy emanating from the physical form whereas the subtle bodies are fixed bands of energy at set distances from the body. The aura surrounds the person with an overall field of bio-magnetic energy which acts rather like a barometer of the body's physiological processes. Although we are not usually aware of it, the aura determines our first responses to people and situations. That sense of unease we feel when close to certain people may be the result of our aura literally clashing with theirs. It is a quicker and more accurate gauge than our more rational faculties. The aura affects overall balance in the system and is the direct result of the physical body's activities, whereas the function of the subtle bodies is much more specific.

THE SUBTLE BODIES

The seven subtle bodies are specialized bands of different types of energy at fixed distances from the physical body, rather like the rings of Saturn, creating a multi-halo impression. They are said to relate to the soul and its co-ordination on the physical level.

Each of these specific layers of energy emanating from the physical body via the chakras vibrates at a slightly different frequency and has its own specialized function. The layers differ in density, colour and appearance, and each is connected to a different chakra through which it exerts an influence over various psychological and physiological processes. It is helpful to imagine the 'Russian Doll effect': each body maintaining its own space but together creating a whole; each emanating from and attached to a particular chakra which in its turn acts as a porthole. As all the seven subtle bodies enter and leave the body through these chakras or portholes, the smooth flow of energetic information to maintain perfect harmony and balance throughout the whole system is essential.

It is useful to know a little about them in order to understand how the flower essences work their wonders.

Etheric body or etheric lining

Deriving from the base or root chakra, the etheric body is bluish-grey in colour. This is the first subtle body and lies between the physical and other subtle bodies, sustaining the dynamic equilibrium between them. This is one of its key functions.

The etheric body is the exact double, an energetic replica, of the denser visible physical body and contains a blueprint of all the organs. Whether leaving or entering the body, the life force always passes through the etheric body. The etheric forces are formative and creative, endowing matter with life, form and power. These same cosmic organizing energies are susceptible to control by the mind and will. The notion that a particular vibration makes a form out of disorganized matter is known as cymatics. Many experiments have shown that certain sounds can create patterns out of a random sprinkling of sand. The classic example is the word 'Om', which forms a kind of mandala. If the etheric body is imbalanced for whatever reason, any problems residing in the subtle anatomy (that is, in the aura and subtle bodies) can filter down and express themselves in the physical body, for the body is the medium through which all electromagnetic radiation and energies play.

The immunofluidium is an integral part of the etheric body. It is a sort of liquid energy which surrounds and nourishes all the cells in the physical body. It transports energy between the ethereal levels and the physical body, fuelling each cell with life force, or Qi. The immunofluidium flows freely and evenly through the body, maintaining and sustaining good health. When this liquid energy functions properly, genetic disease, viral and bacterial attacks may be kept at bay.

Emotional body

This band of energy is linked to the solar plexus and heart chakra. In appearance it is brighter than the etheric body, resembling multicoloured clouds in constant motion. It is closely aligned with the etheric body; together they balance the emotions. A strong sense of emotional security and stability at the psychological level is sustained when the emotional body is in balance. Negative emotions dim the emotional body's brilliance, whereas positive feelings of love and enjoyment enhance its colours and sparkle.

Mental body

This energy band is a vibrant shade of pale yellow, which varies in tone according to mental activity and is like the emotional body but brighter than the etheric. This mental energy enables people to think clearly and rationally. It contains the structure of our thoughts and ideas. Agitation in the mental body blocks the organs of elimination, especially the kidneys. Stress here results in the build-up of toxins in the physical body, which is often linked to allergies. Mental stress and tension also tend to become lodged in the muscular structure – many of us will be familiar with 'the tension headache' or with muscular pain (particularly in the neck and shoulders) when we are stressed.

Astral body

More intense but softly multicoloured like the emotional body, the astral body is connected to the solar plexus and heart chakras. It encapsulates the entire personality. When the astral body is in balance the individual is more likely to have an intuitive understanding of events and the flow of life. He or she may even glean insight into what lies ahead in the future. The astral body works to collate all past-life experiences, keeping this knowledge and information from spilling into our consciousness in a way that would disrupt our present incarnation. It can be visualized as a transparent shield which sifts and filters out karmic information and disruptive patterns acquired from past lives that reside in our subconscious.

Causal body

Crystal-clear and intensely blue in appearance, this layer is connected to the throat chakra. The causal body is the seat of our willpower. It facilitates the interaction of the individual with other people and events, allowing us to fulfil our personal destiny. It may be regarded as the gateway to higher consciousness. This body is responsible for organizing past-life information before it is released to the astral body when it is needed or appropriate.

Celestial or soul body

Vibrantly luminous and golden, this energy band is connected to the third eye (sixth chakra). It houses our spiritual essence and is, in a sense, the Higher Self which allows the soul to move freely through us. This energy band enters the body through the pineal gland.

Spiritual or illuminated body

This energy layer is a shimmering composition of pastel colours which is connected to the heart chakra. It represents a combination and fusion of the whole subtle anatomy with the physical body. Our basic energetic blueprint is housed within this subtle body.

Etheric envelope

This forms a sort of protective outer-coating around the subtle bodies, separating the subtle anatomy from the other energies around us.

Thermal body

In addition to the ethereal subtle bodies we possess a thermal body which can be likened to a heat source extending beyond the etheric body. The heat is generated by normal cell division and is influenced by our rate of metabolism. It is literally a by-product of physical activity.

These energy systems are considered separate entities for simplicity's sake, yet they are all interlinked and constantly interact with each other, functioning as an energetic whole. The meridians link up and pass through the organs of the body – it may help to picture the meridians as rivers of energy that are constantly on the move, flowing in and out of one another. There are a further eight energy channels (known as the extraordinary meridians) which hover between the etheric and physical bodies. They act as a sort of energy reservoir, borrowing points from the organ meridians yet forming their own pathways between the nervous and circulatory systems. These meridians relate strongly to our vitality and emotions/states of mind. Their prime function is to feed the main meridians with energy, Qi or life force. The most important extraordinary meridian travels straight up and down the centre of the body, connecting directly with the major chakras. As we have already seen, these in turn link up with the subtle bodies, and these seven subtle bodies enter and leave the body through the various chakras. The subtle energy system may be visualized as diaphanous layers held in place with thin membranes which separate yet allow them to diffuse into one another.

The aura has its own unique part to play; it is a reflection of the levels of our physical health and vitality. The more balanced and healthy you are, the greater your auric field.

This force field can radiate some three to four feet from the body, its energy infusing the whole subtle body systems. In ill health the aura shrinks back close to the body in an attempt to conserve vital energy.

This entire energy system is in a continuous state of motion. You might want to visualize the different energies as swirling mists of colour and light interacting with and receiving information from each other – a multilevelled interfusion; these energies are constantly interchanging, redistributing and rebalancing themselves.

ILLUMINATING THE ENERGIES

Scientists have yet to invent a device that confirms categorically the existence of these subtler energies, although many have turned their minds to it. However, some interesting energetic phenomena have been discovered using special techniques akin to Kirlian photography.

Harry Oldfield has dedicated 15 years of his life to illuminating the subtle energies. While working with Kirlian photography he found that sound and radio frequencies as well as light are emitted from an object. This inspired him to invent the electroscanning method (ESM) – a piece of equipment that surrounds an object or person with an electrical reference field which can be measured three-dimensionally around the body. He feels that fluctuations in this field could reflect what is happening on more subtle levels. For his own private research purposes Harry Oldfield has invented a piece of equipment which seems to make visible some interesting energy effects with light using computer technology. This is known as the PIP technique (Polycontrast Interference Photography).

Oldfield feels that the various swirls of colour he sees in and around the body relate in some way to the subtle energies and possibly the chakras. Over the years he has photographed the energies of literally hundreds of different people and he now feels he can detect the difference between vibrant energy fields belonging to the fit and healthy and the distorted fields which suggest the presence of or potential for illness. Oldfield uses his various detectors widely as a method of diagnosis to investigate the possibility of weakness, stress or disease in the energy field. On numerous occasions these methods have been verified by doctors using orthodox medical procedures such as X-rays and blood tests. Mr Oldfield insists, however, that his work is still in the research stage and has a long way to go before it can be accepted scientifically.

As we shall see in Chapter 8, flowers and their essences seem to interact with and influence the body's energy field in remarkable ways.

CHAPTER THREE

THE EFFECTS OF SHOCK, STRESS AND POLLUTION

Each person's whole energy system – aura, subtle bodies, chakras and meridians – forms a sort of personal 'blueprint' or 'body map'. We are all born with this energetic blueprint which, like a thumbprint, is quite unique and different from person to person, however subtly. This energetic pattern holds within it characteristics that endow us with the potential to be as perfect – physically, mentally, emotionally and spiritually – as we can possibly be.

When all the elements of your energy system are in balance you experience a deep sense of contentment and wellbeing. These are the times when life is joyful and everything feels comfortable. Think of those days when you wake up brimming with energy and looking forward to the day ahead. This abundant physical vitality goes hand in hand with a clear, focused mind. You are blessed with a sense of inner calm and cannot be ruffled by other people or the hustle and bustle of life. Deep down you feel safe and secure, as if cocooned from any danger lurking in the outside world, while at the same time totally involved in the here and now. These benefits come from knowing you are following a path or going in a direction that is right for you, one that will bring real purpose and meaning to your life.

For many of us such sensations are usually rare and fleeting. This is because the stresses and strains of living conspire to prevent us from growing to fulfil our potential to be perfect. However, we are all capable of feeling this way most of the time because we are blessed with an intelligence or Higher Self that is aware of this energetic blueprint and knows how to keep the entire energy network in order. In other words, we intuitively or instinctively know what is best for us.

Sadly, we do not always hear or heed the wisdom of this inner voice. In childhood it does not matter too much if our energy systems are thrown off-balance, for there is an abundance of energy or Qi which can be used to override any disturbance or misalignment. But there comes a point in time when this energy reserve is exhausted and the imbalance begins to become ingrained in the system.

The Higher Self knows when this is happening and sends us warning signals in the form of physical, emotional and psychological symptoms. Typical signs of an energy imbalance are tiredness, feelings of anxiety, irritability and depression, as well as a susceptibility to colds and other infections. If an imbalance is not corrected, it will become firmly entrenched in the energy system and the resulting symptoms will get worse with time. It is my opinion that disease shows itself in the physical body only after disturbances of energy flow have already become crystallized in the subtle structural patterns of the higher-frequency bodies.

I believe that nature holds a cure for every ill, and that the Higher Self will guide us towards certain plants, herbs and flowers that can restore balance in our energetic system. In Chapter 4 you will find out how to follow your intuition and choose a combination of flower essences that will displace the disharmony in your energy system.

Before looking more closely at how flower essences work their wonders, let us first look at ways in which our energy systems can be thrown out of kilter.

SHATTERING THE BALANCE

Shock and stress in their many guises have a devastating effect on the subtle energy system. You can visualize this sudden shock as a pebble being hurled into a tranquil pond, sending ripples or shock waves reverberating through the water or, in this case, the subtle anatomy. This 'pebble', then, can be seen as the root cause of any upset, while the ripples are the physical repercussions of shock. Unlike the pond, however, which becomes still once the pebble has dropped to the bottom, when shock makes an impact on our subtle energy systems the disruptive effects linger unless steps are taken to bring everything back into balance.

As a consequence of shock the subtle bodies are thrown out of alignment and end up becoming either too close or too far apart from one another. When the mental and emotional bodies are not properly aligned to the etheric, for example, we experience feelings of anxiety. When the mental and emotional bodies are too close together we become prone to feelings of frustration and unknown fears, and are unable to make clear-cut decisions. Sometimes the properties of the subtle bodies spill over into each other; this is known as the 'spillage effect'. When the mental body flows into the emotional one, mental lethargy and loss of confidence ensues. Any misalignment in the subtle bodies ultimately filters down to the physical body, where it triggers a range of symptoms depending on which part of the body is affected.

Shock can be divided into two categories: traumatic and long, slow shock.

Traumatic shock

We live in a world full of horrific events that are often too distressing even to think about. Some of these, such as natural disasters, unpredictable violence and the death of a loved one, are age-old. Others, such as car accidents and bomb blasts which can maim and kill, are relatively recent phenomena. At some time or other we are all likely to experience personally the shock of some traumatic event.

The worst kinds are invariably those that are sudden and unexpected because they take us unawares. As they are not part of our ordinary life, we are totally unprepared for them and they shake us to the very core of our being. The medical profession is only just beginning to appreciate the impact of such shock on our physical and psychological wellbeing. It has come to realize that such trauma gives rise to a range of symptoms resembling those experienced by shell-shocked war veterans. Symptoms can last a lifetime unless steps are taken to redress their far-reaching effects.

The so-called Post Traumatic Stress Disorder (PTSD) is now used to describe the aftermath of shock. The repercussions clearly permeate every level of our being. Physically, those suffering from traumatic shock feel exhausted and drained of energy. In time the tiredness may lift, but it invariably gives way to all kinds of minor ailments such as stomach upsets, stiff necks and so forth. As such symptoms appear some time after the event has taken place, they often seem to have no apparent cause. Little wonder, then, that those suffering from PTSD are often thought of as hypochondriacs.

Shock has a particularly potent influence on the mind. Concentration becomes difficult, thoughts are blurred and decisions about even everyday issues such as when to do the shopping can pose problems. Emotions are volatile and range from anger and irritability to depression and despair. Sufferers often overreact to events that would not normally upset them, and steer themselves away from any kind of pressure. They may even suffer from panic attacks. Confidence and self-esteem dwindle, making those suffering from shock less inclined to tackle new projects which they would previously have relished as a challenge.

On a spiritual level, many feel compelled to reassess their lives. In the worst cases doubts arise as to whether life is really worth living.

Long, slow shock

This is more insidious than traumatic shock, for we are often unaware of its existence and it becomes an integral part of our lives. Long, slow shock can start to take its toll even before we are born. Although safe inside the womb, the developing foetus will detect and react to its mother's stresses. Anxieties about her relationship with her partner and her fears and apprehension about motherhood can all be sensed by her unborn child.

In childhood we may experience stress when deprived of the right kind of love, attention and emotional nourishment. Ironically it can be equally stressful to be swamped by too much love (in the form of overprotectiveness or possessiveness). Parents who threaten to withhold their love unless they are obeyed also create a stressful environment for their offspring. In addition, children whose parents are always quarrelling can suffer the effects of long, slow shock, as will those whose mother or father has a drinking problem or an incapacitating illness. As this kind of stress goes unnoticed and is often present for prolonged periods of time, it becomes so familiar that it appears to be normal. We usually fail even to identify it as shock.

The effects of long, slow shock are cumulative, which means that by the time a person reaches adulthood it has produced the same disruptive effect on the subtle energy system as sudden trauma. Shock and stress set up an abrasive vibration which is at odds with the natural rhythm of the cells and forces them to 'dance to a different tune'. This ultimately affects the smooth and efficient functioning of all the organs and tissues. If left untreated, such distortion in the energy system ultimately manifests itself as a disease of the mind, body and spirit.

The medical profession now agrees that stress can indeed make us more susceptible to illness. This is the reason we often tend to catch cold or fall victim to an infection after a stressful event has taken place, or when we feel overly stressed at home or work. Some forward-thinking physicians believe that negative emotions such as anxiety, fear, anger, frustration and irritability play crucial roles in undermining the body's resistance to disease.

Researchers working in the relatively new field of psychoneuroimmunology (or PNI) are attempting to fathom the link between such negative emotions and various disease states. They suggest that psychological and emotional states undermine our resistance in the way that they interact with our nervous, endocrine and immune systems. Seen from an energetic perspective, shock has the effect of throwing the emotional and mental bodies out of alignment. They leak into each other and, in turn, spill into the etheric body. As a result of shock or stress the etheric body can no longer hold its boundaries and perform its job of defending the physical body from disturbance in the subtle bodies.

The etheric body is also closely affiliated with the nervous system, which in turn is closely bound to the immune system. This, then, is how mental and emotional disturbances act as immunosuppressants, weakening the body's natural defences and resistance to illness.

In cases of severe shock or trauma such as a bereavement or being violently attacked or wounded, the astral and etheric bodies are suddenly and dramatically thrown out of alignment. When this happens the aura breaks and holes appear. These gaps are potentially dangerous as the physical body is no longer fully protected and becomes vulnerable. It is essential to clear the effects of shock out of the system, for if the subtle bodies are misaligned, the Qi or life force that sustains us cannot filter through and replenish our physical body.

Years ahead of his time, Dr Edward Bach (creator of the Bach Flower Remedies) realized that psychological upsets can be a root cause of disease. Bach was also aware that shock and stress provoke emotional or mental distress by heightening imbalances in the personality. Someone who normally has a tendency towards impatience and who prefers to work at his or her own speed, for instance, will become increasingly irritable, impetuous and prone to outbursts of temper and nervous tension as a result of shock or stress.

Bach described and discovered flower remedies for 38 negative states of mind. These remedies aim to bring you back to a state of emotional equilibrium. In keeping with various ancient philosophies, Bach believed that peace of mind and physical wellbeing go hand in hand. In his book *Heal Thyself*, Bach wrote:

> We must steadfastly practise peace, imaging our minds as a lake ever to be kept calm, without waves or even ripples, to disturb its tranquillity and gradually develop this state of peace until no event, no circumstance, no other personality is able under any condition to ruffle the surface of that lake or raise within us any feelings of irritability, depression or doubt. (Bach 1996, p.53)

In this book's Encyclopedia of Flower Essences and Ailment Chart you will find essences helpful for almost every permutation of shock and stress, including the urban stress that comes of the loneliness, isolation and loss of identity many of us feel as cosy, tight-knit communities disappear and new technology and pollution insidiously change the very nature of our environment. In Chapter 5 you will also find excellent first-aid combinations to have to hand in case of sudden shocks and emergencies.

CHEMICAL POLLUTANTS

Clean water, fresh air and natural foods are essential for good health, yet slowly and insidiously they are being polluted by synthetic chemicals. Car emissions contain a noxious mixture of chemicals which irritate the lungs, trigger asthma attacks, exacerbate chest troubles and increase our vulnerability to respiratory infections. Carbon monoxide competes with oxygen in the blood and can, at high levels, suffocate the tissues. Breathlessness, dizziness, nausea, lethargy and faintness are typical symptoms. The situation is exacerbated during the summer months, for in the presence of strong sunlight the chemicals in exhaust fumes react to form ozone. At ground levels ozone creates smog that can cause eye irritations, headaches and breathing difficulties. It also damages plants.

Even indoors the air may be far from pure. Sealing buildings hermetically in order to conserve energy also encourages a build-up of irritant substances. While cigarette smoke is often the chief offender, chemicals given off by photocopying machines and carpets add to the load. Toxic gases may even evaporate from the adhesives and preservatives used in construction. Polluted air can cause headaches, difficulty concentrating, stinging eyes, sore throats and skin problems as well as lingering coughs and colds, in part because they create a grey etheric mucus-type substance which clogs up our energy system.

Chemicals in our food and water may come from industrial waste flushed into the seas and rivers, whereby they enter the food chain. Some of these synthetic chemicals, such as chlorinated organics, are extremely persistent. After entering the environment they accumulate in the food chain, sometimes building to high concentrations in certain animals. A typical example is PCBs (polychlorinated biphenyls), which are now banned but are still found in many foods, especially fish.

In addition to these long-lived chemicals, a huge number are also in daily use. Most commercially grown fruits, vegetables and cereals are liberally dowsed with at least one, but usually several, different chemicals as they grow and are kept in storage. Some crops may be sprayed with up to six different chemicals before they reach the supermarket shelves. Particularly worrying is the little-known 'cocktail' effect or combined activity of many different chemicals. Emerging evidence suggests that pesticides and PCBs may act as immunosuppressants, contributing to the incidence of allergies and viral infections.

On an energetic level, chemical pollutants cloud the subtle anatomy, preventing realignment and directly affecting the opening and closing of the chakras. If not cleared from the system they can damage these important energy centres.

Protecting yourself from chemical pollutants

- Vitamins A and E help the lungs and air passages to withstand smoke and chemical damage. Together with vitamin C and selenium they work as antioxidants, preventing pollutants from harming the body cells. Vitamin C also helps detoxify pesticide residues, while vitamins A and E protect the liver from chemical abuse and the B-complex vitamins increase efficiency of detoxification systems. The minerals calcium, magnesium and zinc also bolster resistance.

- Ionizers and air purifiers help to remove pollutant particles from the air and plants can help to diffuse office chemicals.

- Buy organically grown foods whenever possible. Alternatively, wash all fruit and vegetables in a mixture of filtered water and 1 tablespoon of cider vinegar.

- Cold-pressed vegetable oils such as sunflower, olive and safflower reduce the absorption of toxins and speed their elimination.

- Select free-range organic poultry, eggs and game whenever possible.

- Avoid eating organ meats, as chemicals and hormones can concentrate in an animal's liver and kidneys.

- Opt for spring water bottled in glass and invest in a water filter which will extract pesticide residues as well as nitrates and heavy metals from your tap water.

- Flower remedies to combat chemical pollution can be found in the Ailment Chart.

- A specific 'cleansing' recipe can be found in Chapter 5 on page 67.

ELECTROMAGNETIC POLLUTION

The Earth has its own electromagnetic field which pulses, like a heart, at 470 beats per minute or 7.83Hz (beats per second). These pulses are known as the Schumann waves after the German professor who discovered them in 1952. It is no coincidence that we have in our bodies a pulse that is approximately the same, in the electrical signals – the alpha and beta waves – sent out by our brains. It is thought that this natural electromagnetic pulse may have a role to play in maintaining and sustaining good health. It is well acknowledged that NASA fits its spacecraft with 7.83Hz oscillators to give its astronauts something to make them feel more comfortable – that is, it helps to regulate their sleeping/waking cycles.

Nowadays, however, the Earth's natural pulse is being swamped by other forms of electrically and magnetically generated fields. Electromagnetic radiation from overhead power cables and pylons, televisions, computers, VDUs and radio and satellite transmitters is filling the atmosphere with what is commonly known as electronic smog. It may literally blanket the natural signals needed for good health.

Those which are the greatest cause for concern are the so-called ELFs (extremely low frequencies) because they are so similar to those of our own bodies. Particularly strong electromagnetic fields generated by such frequencies may have the power to influence our brainwaves, resulting in various behavioural and physical problems.

Depression, anxiety, irritability, chronic tiredness, headaches, nausea, sweating and indigestion are among the wide range of symptoms that have been attributed to electromagnetic pollution. Offices in particular tend to be filled with a wealth of artificial fields, which may contribute to what is known as Sick Building Syndrome.

Electromagnetic radiation can also occur naturally due to geographic faults (also known as 'geopathic stress') or underground streams and rivers. Ley lines are believed to indicate places where the Earth's magnetic field is particularly potent. Such forms of radiation impinge on and affect our own electromagnetic force-field. X-rays, microwaves and even ultraviolet rays from the sun can distort the subtle bodies and, if powerful enough, can also alter the structure of DNA, the genetic material of our cells. The consequences of continual overexposure to such radiation may not show physically until 20 years after the event.

In his book, *Electromagnetic Fields of Life*, the Russian physicist, A.S. Presman of the Department of Biophysics at Moscow University, explains the detailed experiments he carried out in 1968 which led to his discovery that such radiation was linked to physical problems such as blood disorders, hypertension, heart attacks, sexual dysfunction, lack of energy and nervous exhaustion. Evidence is emerging that long-term exposure to emissions from VDUs, computers, word processors and television screens can cause chromosomal damage. Studies remain inconclusive and controversial, but some research has linked excessive VDU work with pregnancy problems including miscarriage, stillbirths and birth defects. Embryos are particularly vulnerable to electromagnetic radiation in the first trimester when the cells are rapidly dividing. During this incredible growth spurt, the subtle blueprint has a particularly important role to play in ensuring that everything runs smoothly. It is possible that harmful electromagnetic radiation

may damage the blueprint, with far-reaching consequences.

Protecting yourself from electromagnetic pollution

- Switch off electrical appliances when not in use.
- Prevent static build-up by filling your home or office with bowls of flowers, sprinkling water on all carpets and wearing natural materials such as cotton and silk instead of synthetics.
- Never wear rubber-soled shoes.
- Avoid being in the vicinity of pylons and overhead cables.
- Do not set up home in areas known to be affected by geopathic stress.

Flower remedies to combat electromagnetic pollution can be found in the Ailment Chart. Australian Electro Guard (FE Aus) is one suggested combination that works well (see study on electromagnetic radiation in Chapter 8).

SOCIAL POISONS

Many of us rely heavily on different kinds of props to boost our energy levels, steady or stupefy our nerves and generally help us to cope with our frantic pace of life. Alcohol, cigarettes and caffeine-laden drinks, however, only provide us with short-lived energy and, once the effects wear off, leave us feeling more depleted than before. These 'social poisons' also have dangerous side-effects.

Alcohol

Alcohol damages cells of the brain and nervous system, giving rise to a wide variety of symptoms ranging from lack of concentration, confusion, memory loss, insomnia or lethargy, to agitation, irritability and exhaustion. At an energetic level, alcohol loosens and misaligns the subtle anatomy. It has a particularly disruptive influence on the etheric and astral bodies, making them slip out of sympathy with each other, which is why self-control and willpower are weakened. Alcohol also gives rise to a murky, greenish-brown aura congested with a sticky, mucus-like substance.

Cigarettes

Cigarette smoke contains a cocktail of noxious chemical substances, many of which are known to be carcinogenic. The health hazards of smoking are well known, but the harm cigarettes cause the energy system is also significant. Smoke clouds and weakens the subtle anatomy, surrounding it with a fog which dulls and discolours the normally bright, vibrant hues of the aura. It also prevents the aura from cleansing itself. The etheric body is particularly affected by this grey mucus, which undermines the body's first line of defence.

Caffeine

Coffee and caffeine-rich foods and drinks stimulate the adrenal glands into producing adrenaline, a hormone normally secreted in times of stress which gives us a sudden rush of energy and mental focus. The effects do not last long, and when caffeine levels fall we invariably end up feeling as tired as before. Increasing caffeine intake acts as an additional stress, which produces feelings of anxiety, irritability and jumpiness. Excessive caffeine intake has also been linked to breast lumps in women.

From an energetic viewpoint, caffeine disturbs the flow of energy in the meridian system. This affects the etheric body, which in turn causes leakage in the emotional and mental bodies. An imbalance in these energies results in emotional instability and disruption to the nervous system. It also upsets the solar plexus chakra, the seat of emotional balance – and the effects then filter down to the stomach. Importantly, caffeine actually

prevents flower remedies from working by misaligning the subtle bodies.

Certain flower essences help to overcome addiction to these social props, while others counter their negative impact on the subtle energy systems (see the Encyclopedia, Ailment Chart and Chapter 5 of this book).

Social drugs

The chemical cocktails of recreational drugs, and the easy availability of cocaine, marijuana, etc., that are now so much part of society, are creating havoc with our systems, weakening the immunity and undermining the delicate balance of our physical, emotional and psychological health, causing co-dependence and toxicity in an environment already overloaded with pollution. To survive this toxic climate, we need to keep our bodies as healthy and clear as possible in order to be able to fulfil our potential destiny.

Here a combination of Blue China Orchid (Aus L) and the No. 24 Anti-Addiction remedy (Him A) or Detox Essence (FE Aus) would be helpful.

ILLNESS AND MEDICATION

Modern medicines may be essential when it comes to treating physical illness, and they undoubtedly do save lives. On the flip side of the coin, many also have undesirable side-effects. These vary from drug to drug, but they all have a generally disruptive influence on the energy systems. They tend to cloud the subtle anatomy and cause the subtle bodies to separate from one another; at the same time they prevent realignment. They also affect the chakras' function of regulating and dispersing energy – especially the throat chakra, which is particularly susceptible to drugs.

Steroids, for example, create congestion in the solar plexus and heart chakras, preventing the nervous and muscular systems from receiving energy or life force. Taken in conjunction with orthodox medication, flower essences gently help to buffer these undesirable effects. They can also be taken after a course of medication to realign the subtle bodies and generally rebalance the energy systems. More importantly, perhaps, flower essences actually allay the need for taking orthodox medication, for if taken soon enough they can help prevent disease from occurring in the first place.

Flower remedies may, for example, negate the need for antibiotics by boosting the body's natural immunity. They help by clearing away physical toxins as well as toxic thoughts, emotions and, last but not least, spiritual toxicity which pollutes the energy system. As a consequence the body's natural defence system is strengthened and becomes better able to repel viral and bacterial invasion.

At present there is increasing concern about the repercussions of using drugs such as antibiotics too frequently. It is well recognized that bacteria gradually adapt to any antibiotic, so in using these drugs too much they are made less useful for everyone. Yet in the United States sales of antibiotics have doubled since the mid-1980s, and seven out of ten Americans are prescribed these drugs when they seek treatment for common colds. Is it just coincidence that drug-resistant infections are also soaring?

Resistant germs are hard to treat and can spread through the community. They do not threaten us all equally. A healthy immune system repels most bacterial invaders regardless of their susceptibility to drugs. However, certain people such as the elderly and sick are more vulnerable, and when they contract such bacterial diseases they are harder to treat. While drug companies may see inventing new wonder antibiotics as the ultimate challenge, surely it is better to strengthen our natural immunity and encourage both doctors and patients to stop abusing the weapons we have? (For a recipe to help boost the immune system, see page 67.) An effective combination is Formula 38 from Him Adit range and Super Immunity from the Pacific Essences

Combinations and Dynamic Recovery from the Flower Essences of Australia range.

Physical injury

In cases where disease is already manifest and there is a need for surgery, it is good to know that flower essences can help to reduce the effects of such trauma and aid recuperation. When tissues are cut and injured during an operation or accident, the subtle energy system receives an almighty jolt. Wherever the physical damage occurs it is accompanied by a rupture in the etheric body print. This must be healed along with the tissues to ensure that the damaged area does not remain weak, vulnerable and prone to recurrent problems, for even when the scars have faded, the subtle bodies may still be misaligned.

Before undergoing any operation it is a good idea to take Bach's Rescue Remedy or Five Flower Remedy, or Flower Essences of Australia's Emergency Rescue Essence to ease the shock and trauma. As well as the shock of the operation, anaesthetics themselves also throw you into a state of suspension. This results in feelings of disorientation, unworldliness and dragging tiredness. (See page 68 for my recipe for clearing the after-effects of anaesthesia.)

INHERITING IMBALANCES IN THE SUBTLE ENERGY SYSTEM

It is important to clear away any imbalance in the subtle anatomy, otherwise it can become etched in the system and passed on to future generations. These inherited flaws in the energetic bodies are referred to as miasms.

The concept of miasms was originally introduced by Dr Samuel Hahnemann, the founder of homeopathy. He was puzzled to find that some patients failed to respond to treatment, while others who improved relapsed after only a short time. He looked at these 'difficult' cases and found a common 'blocking' factor in their personal or family history – such as the presence of certain diseases which have been passed on from one generation to another. He called these blocks 'miasms'.

We might visualize a miasm as a void or lack of life force. They are usually stored in the subtle bodies – especially the etheric, emotional, mental and, to a lesser extent, the astral body. Here miasms may lie dormant for long periods of time, only flaring up occasionally and leading to chronic or acute illnesses, trauma, stress and age-related conditions. A bad fall or emotional shock may easily allow them to filter down from the subtle bodies into the physical anatomy, resulting in the development of various symptoms. As we get older, our natural vitality diminishes, making it easier for miasms to emerge. This could help explain why we tend to become more prone to all kinds of disease as we age.

MIASMS

Flower essences help to remove miasms from the system. Once a remedy's life force filters down to the physical level, an immediate rebalancing and readjustment begins to take place. The essences release the miasm from the cells' genetic material and from the subtle bodies, so that it can be discharged from the system. It may take some time for these shifts to take place, so do not expect miracles to happen overnight.

Dr Hahnemann described three basic types of 'inherited' miasm (psora, syphilitic and sycosis) which he believed to be the underlying causes of chronic disease. Each predisposes a person to a particular range of health problems. Homeopaths have since added many more illness-causing miasms to this list, including tuberculosis, radiation and heavy metals.

Psora

Associated with suppressed skin disease, a psora miasm leads to imbalance in the rhythmic bodily functions and causes general mental and physical irritation. Typical symptoms

are tiredness, anxiety, sadness or depression as well as skin disorders, congestion in the tissues and bone structure deformities.

Syphilitic

Associated with suppressed syphilis, this miasm has a destructive effect on all the tissues, especially the bones. Cardiac and neurological symptoms are common. Those carrying this miasm are easily upset, sentimental, irritable and suspicious. This miasm may manifest as meningitis.

Sycosis

Associated with suppressed gonorrhoea, this miasm encourages congestion in the skin, the pelvic region, the joints and the digestive, respiratory and urinary tracts. It may cause fearfulness, nervousness and amorality.

Tuberculosis

This miasm may cause susceptibility to respiratory, circulatory, urinary and digestive problems, resulting, for example, in weight loss and poor circulation. Those carrying this miasm typically tend to be escapists who feel unable to make decisions or face life's realities. It may also manifest as mental illness and cancer.

MODERN MIASMS

Most homeopathic research into miasms was conducted in the 1800s and early 1900s, when infectious diseases such as tuberculosis and syphilis were prevalent. Today we are faced with new threats to our health, which derive from modern-day pollutants and are known as 'acquired miasms'.

Petrochemical

Springing from the major increase in petrol and chemical products, the problems this causes are fluid retention, diabetes, infertility, impotence, miscarriage, hair loss/greying hair, muscle degeneration, skin blemishes, or a metabolic imbalance resulting in the storage of fat in tissues. It also blocks assimilation of vitamin K, causing circulatory and endocrine disorders. Those affected find it difficult to resist stress and suffer from various types of psychosis, especially schizophrenia and autism. Leukemia, skin and lymph cancer can also occur.

Radiation

Associated with the massive increase in background radiation since the Second World War, this miasm primarily affects the skin, connective tissue, circulation and reproductive systems. Symptoms include premature ageing, slower cell division, loss of skin elasticity, rashes, lupus, skin cancer, anaemia, leukemia, arthritis, allergies, bacterial inflammations (especially in the brain), hair loss, hardening of the arteries, miscarriage, excessive bleeding in women and sterility or a drop in sperm count in men.

Heavy metals

Resulting from increased levels of toxic metals and chemicals such as lead, mercury, radium, arsenic, aluminium, fluoride and sulphuric acid, the symptoms of this miasm include allergies, fluid retention, an inability to assimilate calcium, viral inflammations and excessive hair loss.

Remedies to combat all these types of miasms can be found in the Ailment Chart on page 489. Lotus in particular is excellent as a general aid for miasms. The following Australian Essences are suggested for the following miasms:

- tuberculosis: Tall Mulla Mulla

- psora: Rough Bluebell

- sycosis: Bush Iris

- heavy metal and petrochemical: Wild Potato Bush

- radiation: Mulla Mulla.

PART II

ESSENCES IN
ACTION

CHAPTER FOUR

LEARNING TO CHOOSE AND PRESCRIBE FLOWER ESSENCES

No two people are identical. We may share similar physical characteristics, behavioural tendencies and personality traits but deep down each of us is unique. Our individuality determines the ways in which we cope with and react to any kind of stress in our lives.

Two people may exhibit typical symptoms associated with a frazzled nervous system. Each may be anxious, irritable, on edge and suffering from sleeping problems, indigestion and butterflies in the stomach, but each will be this way for entirely different reasons. One may be going through a marriage break-up while the other may be experiencing a conflict at work. Delve deeper and it will become clear that their problems arise from a certain personality trait or a particular behavioural pattern. For this reason it is essential to treat each person as a unique whole, rather than just addressing his or her symptoms or illness. The beauty of flower essences is that they help us to become aware of elements in our nature which are undermining our sense of wellbeing. They do not work on us, but with us. They bring our attention to any imbalance that exists within, in order to lend their energetic support so we can release it gently from our lives. In this way we can begin to take responsibility for our own health and happiness.

KNOW THYSELF

Whether you are a practitioner or just discovering flower essences, as you begin to use the flower remedies, you will be embarking on an exciting adventure of self-discovery which will enable you to understand yourself, and why you think and act in certain ways. As the remedies get to work your self-awareness will continue to grow, bringing with it a new freedom to do whatever you wish in life.

As a practitioner I've always felt it is important to get to know the energy and frequency of as many essences as possible, so as to understand their effects and healing power, so treating yourself goes a long way to achieving this.

In the Encyclopedia section you will see that there are literally hundreds of flower essences from all over the world to choose from. Each is associated with particular qualities or properties. The real art lies in selecting the essences that are best for you. To do this you need to devote some time to thinking about yourself. This may sound narcissistic, but it is an essential part of self-healing.

Reflecting on your own personality is a good starting point. Although this is as individual as your thumbprint, there are certain personality traits or tendencies which prevail in human nature. These characteristics have a strong influence on how you handle and react to stress.

BACH'S 12 PERSONALITY TYPES AND REMEDIES

Dr Edward Bach identified 12 key personality traits, and the first flowers he searched for related to these:

Fear

Terror

Mental torture or worry

Indifference or boredom

Doubt or discouragement

Indecision

Overenthusiasm

Discouragement

Weakness

Self-distrust

Overconcern

Pride or aloofness

Take Impatiens, for example. As its name suggests, this flower is for people whose outstanding characteristic is impatience. They tend to rush around and are critical of other people's shortcomings. As a result they are prone to irritability, nervous tension, overexertion and accidents.

In contrast, Clematis relates to quiet, dreamy, absent-minded people who are wrapped up in their own thoughts and fantasies. Their predominant characteristic is indifference. They tend to lack concentration and are susceptible to clumsiness and sleepiness.

Bach often saw human characteristics reflected in the plants themselves. In each flower family you will find remedies describing many permutations of the basic personality traits. Although some may seem very similar, if you read the descriptions carefully you will see there are subtle differences. You should look for flower essences whose qualities reflect the way in which you see yourself. The remedies will help to emphasize your positive characteristics while tempering negative tendencies which can lead you into trouble. It is important to remember that such tendencies are not fixed. With the help of flower essences we can alter certain aspects of our personality for the better.

A welcome side-effect of cultivating your better qualities and tempering the less attractive ones is that your relationships with others will be easier and more fulfilling. Many people seem to end up in partnerships that begin beautifully but then, when the magic has faded, become unworkable. When you become truer to yourself, you will automatically draw to you the sort of people who possess qualities you genuinely admire and find attractive. All relationships, be they intimate or purely platonic, will be fun and mutually satisfying.

While personality affects the way we handle other people and life in general, our constitution determines how resilient or susceptible we are to becoming ill. Constitution is best defined as temperament and state of health. It is your genetic inheritance which has been modified by experiences in life and the environment. While a strong constitution can withstand considerable pressure without flagging, a weaker one is more susceptible to illness.

If, for example, all your grandparents died of old age and your parents have been healthy all their lives; if your mother was healthy throughout her pregnancy (she didn't smoke, drink, etc.), if your parents' marriage was happy and your birth uneventful, you should be blessed with a strong constitution. If, on the other hand, your grandparents died at early ages of cancer or heart disease, one of your parents had tuberculosis as a child and the other suffered from asthma and eczema, then your chances of inheriting a weak constitution are far greater.

Take heart: you can still escape the worst of a poor inheritance if your parents were happily married, they took good care of their health and brought you up with plenty of love and a nourishing diet.

Similarly, you may have inherited a potentially strong constitution but if your parents were always arguing and your emotional needs were neglected, your susceptibility to illness will have increased. In any case, there is no reason to feel lumbered with a flimsy constitution. Flower essences can improve your resilience to every sort of illness in two ways. First, certain essences help to eliminate, at the vibrational level, the inherited genetic weaknesses known as miasms (see Chapter 3). Second, they can clear away the residual effects of any past traumas as well as the long, slow shock of, for instance, an unhappy childhood, which may have weakened your inherent constitution.

TAKING A CASE HISTORY

Making your own case history is a good way of finding out why you are not feeling as well as you could be. A thorough case history should take into account your personality, constitution, stress – both past and present – to help you to recognize any underlying patterns. You should list any physical symptoms and psychological problems you would like to treat. These are signs that your mind, body and spirit are out of balance, so it is important to write them all down, no matter how trivial some may seem. They are an expression of need, a call for help from your body.

In addition to noting any symptoms you have at present, it is important to consider your health as a child. Systems that are inherently weak often show up quite early in life. If you frequently caught colds, or suffered from sore throats or ear infections which were treated with antibiotics, your immune system is likely to be a weak area. An allergy to dust mites, pollens or certain foods is another tell-tale sign. Such immune system weakness does not go away of its own accord although your symptoms may shift to give you that impression.

When a weakness in one system exists, others will compensate for it. Over the years these systems may also begin to exhibit symptoms of upset because they have been overworked or overloaded. Adding stress of any kind may precipitate or exacerbate such symptoms because stress plays on any inherent weakness. If you are not sure what your symptoms are telling you, refer to Chapter 6 to discover which systems may not be functioning as well as they should.

YOUR OWN CASE HISTORY

Name	Date
Age	Date of birth
Occupation	Marital status
Children	

Medical history

Health problems of a) mother b) father

Illnesses running in the family

Your health as a child

Your health problems as an adult

Past operations, accidents, injuries

If you are a mother, how did you feel during your pregnancy?

Birth – was it trouble-free or difficult?

Personality traits

Write down as many different personality traits – good and bad – you can think of that best describe you. For example:

Are you impatient or easy going?

Do you prefer to be alone or crave the company of others?

Be honest and, if possible, ask someone whom you trust and respect to comment on your character assessment.

Lifestyle

Stress levels at home

Low (not noticeable)

Moderate (manageable)

High (struggling to cope)

Excessive (not coping)

Stress levels at work

Low (not noticeable)

Moderate (manageable)

High (struggling to cope)

Excessive (not coping)

Shock/trauma/loss

Past

Present

Assess your energy levels

Plentiful

Sufficient

Lacking

Totally drained

Best time of the day

Worst time of the day

Do you smoke?

Do you drink alcohol?

If so how often and how much?

Are you taking or have you recently taken prescribed medication?

Addictions

Alcohol

Tobacco

Coffee

Other

Sugar/sweet foods

Chocolate

Tea

Relationships (describe both good and bad points)

With your mother, father, spouse or partner, children

Present sense of wellbeing

Physical – do you suffer from recurring health problems?

If so list symptoms, for example: colds and flu (how often, seasonal or consistent throughout the year)

Headaches

Digestive problems

Poor circulation

Poor elimination

Sleeping difficulties

Breathing difficulties

Blood pressure (high or low?)

For women only – describe your menstrual cycle. Are your periods regular, do you experience any pain, premenstrual symptoms, mood swings, any other abnormalities?

Mental – do you have difficulty thinking clearly?

If so, list problems, for example:

Poor concentration

Mental fatigue

Forgetfulness

Mental chatter

Weak memory

Absent-mindedness

Learning difficulties

Emotional – do you feel emotionally calm and content?

If not, list your predominant feelings, for example:

Anger	Confusion
Lack of confidence	Depression
Irritability	Mood swings
Tearfulness	Fears

Spiritual – are you happy with and feel in control of your life?

If not, list reasons why, for example:

Feeling unfulfilled or empty

Not knowing which path to follow

Confusion about beliefs

Disillusionment with life and others

Wellbeing quiz

Give each subject a score of between 0 and 10.

0 = no problem 10 = serious problem

Stress	Trauma
Sleep	Health
Fear	Self-esteem
Thoughts	Emotions
Life changes	State of energy
Outside influences	Childhood
Motivation	Sexuality
Fulfilment	Crisis
Relationships	Other

CHOOSING FLOWER ESSENCES

By now you may be wondering how many different flower essences you are going to need to deal with your problems. Go through your personal case history again and underline those symptoms that stand out clearly and strongly. It is best to leave vague and unclear symptoms alone for the moment – you may refer to them later if you cannot make up your mind about which is the most appropriate remedy for you. If you are new to taking flower essences, begin with your psychological and physical symptoms before attempting to deal with any spiritual issues.

Chapter 6 discusses in some detail the different emotional and spiritual symptoms that can indicate the deeper cause of any imbalance or problem you may be experiencing. The Ailment Chart (Appendix 1), too, will show you at a glance which essences are indicated for a whole variety of physical, psychological and spiritual problems.

If, for instance, you are suffering from insomnia you will see ten essences listed in the Ailment Chart. Taking each one in turn, refer to the Encyclopedia section where you will find a fuller description of the essence. You may end up with just one or two that are best suited to your particular type of insomnia.

Using your intuition

Read the essence descriptions and determine which ones feel right for you. If you are not entirely sure, follow your intuition. Learn to recognize your instinctive 'yes' to some and 'no' to others. Usually certain essences will tend to catch your eye straight away. They are often flowers you naturally prefer. You may already have chosen them for your garden or they may be the kind you most often buy for your home. These may be the ones you will end up choosing for your combination.

Don't try choosing your essences when you are tired and confused. Come back to it when you are feeling more refreshed and relaxed. Taking a few drops of one of the Emergency or Rescue Remedies beforehand can help you calm down.

By pendulum

If you feel confident about using a pendulum you can dowse for your essences. Most people find they can become reasonably proficient with a little practice.

A pendulum can be anything from a ring to a quartz crystal on a thin chain or string. Its movements provide answers to the questions you choose to ask. To dowse, hold your pendulum between your thumb and forefinger so that it hangs downwards. Swing it gently back and forth. With practice you will find that when you concentrate or think 'yes' the pendulum will start to move in one direction. When you change this to a 'no' it will start to move in another, probably the opposite, direction. It may swing back and forth or in circles – there are no hard and fast rules.

Once you have your positive and negative responses when you ask your pendulum certain questions (such as 'Is this an appropriate essence for me at this time?') it should give you either a yes or no. If it is indecisive, test other essences and, in order not to be influenced by the bottle label, turn it away from you.

CREATING YOUR PERSONAL PRESCRIPTION

Ideally you should select no more than seven flower essences for your personal prescription. These should be the ones you feel will be most helpful at this particular time.

When purchasing a flower essence from any supplier you will be getting what is known as the Stock Essence. This is a concentrated form which will need to be diluted to the proper dosage level to make your personal prescription.

The self-healing process

Self-healing is invariably a slow and gradual process, so it is important to be patient. It may have taken many years for negative behavioural patterns or deeply ingrained emotional states to have become a part of your life, so you cannot expect them to vanish overnight. Similarly, physical problems do not appear without warning. Tiredness and

mood changes are early warning signs that our internal balance is disturbed, and other symptoms will follow if we do not take stock of our current situation.

Flower essences are not magic bullets – they are subtle remedies which act as catalysts for change. Don't be concerned if you become more aware of your physical or emotional symptoms when you start the course of treatment. This is natural and shows that the remedies have begun their conversation with the blueprint. My clients often report that a part of them (the Higher Self) is watching the whole process, making them more aware of what their symptoms are telling them.

Often a physical condition or emotional state will clear, only for a deeper emotion to surface. This particular emotion may be associated with an earlier stressful experience or trauma in your life. It is often important to retrace your steps, as if going back in time in order to release that emotion, before you can move forward. This is nothing to be alarmed about. You will not have to relive the emotional intensity or pain of the experience. It is more like being a passive observer who remains detached from what is happening.

Those using the flower essences for physical and psychological problems may find that as time goes on they are drawn to the more spiritually orientated remedies. It is rather like peeling back the petals of a rosebud until you finally get to the real source of your problems.

TIPS ON CHOOSING REMEDIES FOR OTHERS

Flower essences are wonderful remedies for babies, young children, animals and even plants because they are so gentle and free from harmful side-effects. They are incredibly effective – and you do not necessarily have to believe in them to reap their benefits! As babies and animals cannot say how they are feeling, you will have to use your intuition and read the signs to select the most appropriate flower essences. This is not difficult. After all, mothers instinctively know when their children are anxious, irritable, insecure, frustrated or angry.

For babies and young children you will find symptoms such as teething, restlessness, disturbed sleep, night terrors, temper tantrums and colic listed in the Ailment Chart (Appendix 1). Flower essences for these conditions are often best used individually. If you are making a combination, it is best to keep it simple – a mix of two or three flower essences is plenty. It is helpful, too, to have an all-purpose Emergency Rescue or Five Flower Remedy (see pages 173 and 217) on hand for minor accidents or traumas which end in tears, such as falling over or being given routine inoculations.

Pets and other animals can also benefit from being given flower essences, especially those that are deemed to be neurotic or aggressive. (See Pets and Animals section in the Encyclopedia.) It is worth bearing in mind that most animals are very sensitive to the emotional states of their owners, so if you are giving remedies to your cat, dog or horse, it may be a good idea to take some yourself as well.

Remedies for shock may be given to plants to aid their growth, reduce infection and minimize the shock of transplanting, pruning or any harm brought on by poor weather or accident.

Combinations

There are now some useful combinations available tailor-made in response to the challenges of today which can help when feeling too stressed even to think of choosing the right essence for yourself.

TAKING FLOWER REMEDIES

It is important to get into the habit of taking a remedy regularly to reap its full benefits. Take two to three drops in the morning (on rising) and in the evening (on retiring). At these times your mind is usually most relaxed and receptive to the essences. It may be a good idea to keep your chosen remedy beside your bed so you remember to take it as you wake up and before you go to sleep. Some people find it helpful to focus on the positive qualities of the essence and visualize their symptoms lifting as they take their remedy.

For severe cases you may need to take the remedy more frequently. In addition to your morning and evening dose, take another one at midday. If the symptoms become more intense or get worse – particularly those of a physical nature such as headaches or skin problems – double the number of drops you would normally take until they clear. Towards the end of the two-month treatment course you may find you need to take the essence less frequently. You may even forget to take it altogether, signifying that you no longer need that particular essence or combination of essences.

WAYS TO USE THE ESSENCES

These flower essences are vibrational remedies, so the best way to experience their effects is to surround yourself with them, both inside and out.

By mouth

The traditional way of taking flower essences (diluted to the dosage level) is to drop them under the tongue. Placing them under the tongue seems to enhance their absorption. This method also hearkens back to the way ancient healers would sip the dewdrops of flowers to cull their precious benefits. Try to avoid letting the dropper touch your mouth, as this tends to create bacterial growth in the essence.

The drops can also be added to drinks such as herbal teas, spring water and juices, but on no account to coffee or tea. You may dilute the remedies quite a bit. Rather like homeopathic remedies, flower essences are equally effective, if not more so, when they are very dilute.

On the skin

Flower essences can also be beneficial when gently rubbed onto the skin. The Petite Fleur therapeutic mists are useful here for spraying on the soft areas of the body. Good places to apply them are your forehead, lips, wrists, soles of the feet and palms of the hands.

This method is useful if someone is unable to take the essences by mouth. He or she may, for instance, be unconscious, in which case it may be helpful to give an emergency, first-aid essence to ease the state of shock (see page 175).

Another way to apply the flower essences is to add them, usually at Stock concentration, to compresses, body packs, creams, lotions, ointments and oils. To enhance the effectiveness of a relaxing massage, add a few drops of one or two of the soothing flower essences to your body oil. Good ones to try are Chamomile, Dandelion, Lavender (FES) or Yellow Ginger (Haii).

Another idea is to add a few drops to your favourite moisturizer or skin cream, one you use every day. Some flower essences are particularly helpful for revitalizing and rejuvenating tired, ageing skin (see page 482).

Bath therapy

You can create a remedy bath by adding a few drops of flower essence to your bath and soaking for up to 30 minutes. In these relaxing conditions the energy of the remedy is readily absorbed into the system. Choose one that is most appropriate to your needs at that particular time. After a fraught day at work you may benefit from an essence to clear your mind and promote relaxation – such as White Chestnut, Chamomile (FES) or Five Flower Rescue (Bach). If in need of a morning pick-me-up, it is best to choose an essence that helps counter lethargy (such as Morning Glory (FES; Haii)). A good way to enhance the benefits of the essences is to add a few handfuls of pure sea salt to the bath as it is running. For a curative night-time treatment, add five drops of your personal prescription to the bath. Stay in the water for 30 minutes.

Body splash/aura sprays

Splashing or spraying your body with flower essences (diluted with pure spring water) is an effective way of treating sensitive skin conditions such as eczema, cold sores, blisters, blemishes and surface grazes. Add seven drops of essence to a bowl of spring water and, if possible, leave out in the sun for a day. Splash the potentized flower water onto the part of your body needing treatment and allow it to dry naturally. Alternatively you could use an atomizer to spray the diluted essences onto your skin.

For burns, insect stings, animal bites or cuts where there is an element of shock or trauma combine a few drops of an emergency/first-aid combination with an appropriate flower essence (see pages 217 and 175). Spray night and morning, or more frequently for shock. There are a variety of aura sprays that various essence makers have produced for many eventualities such as clearing and protecting yourself from negative and discordant energies (see below to make up your own spray).

Another way to benefit from the essences is to spray your clothes and pillow cases before ironing them. For those who have sleeping problems such as insomnia or nightmares, it may be a good idea to place a few drops of an essence on your pillow before going to bed. This can be particularly helpful for babies and children who have a tendency to wake during the night because of nightmares.

Room spray

Spraying flower essences into the air is an excellent way to improve the atmosphere of any room. Add 4–5 drops to a 250ml plant spray filled with still spring water and spray the mixture around the room every couple of hours. Cleansing and protecting essences are beneficial for city environments as well as offices filled with cigarette smoke and chemicals given off by photocopiers and so forth (see page 489 of the Ailment Chart).

This method of using the flower essences is also recommended if you have a cold or influenza, as well as for breathing difficulties brought on by asthma or hay fever. An essence for boosting the immune system can help to protect you from infection if a bacterial or viral epidemic has broken out in your place of work. Some essences are particularly helpful for improving the general atmosphere (see pages 103–104).

STORING THE ESSENCES

It is important to remember that these remedies are pure energy. They are activated and will start to work on your energy system the moment the combination is made up and the spring water is added. Being 'vibrationally alive', they are highly susceptible to negative influences in the environment. Always store the essences in tinted glass dropper bottles to protect them from sunlight. Keep them away from any electrical or radiation-emitting appliance such as a television, radio or computer. Don't leave them on your dressing table or in your medicine cabinet next to prescribed medication, essential oils, perfume or herbs. If stored in these conditions the liquid may go cloudy, or a mucus-type substance or tiny specks of impurities may form. If this happens, throw it away.

The best place to keep your personal prescription is beside your bed, provided again it is not sharing a space with a clock-radio or other appliances!

CHAPTER FIVE

USEFUL REMEDIES TO START YOUR REPERTOIRE

Here are some ready-made recipes aimed as a starting point to build confidence about choosing flower essences to make your own personal prescription as well as for your family, friends or clients, and help with common ailments that we can encounter in ourselves and others as well as in our treatment rooms.

Note: all the recipes in this book are for your personal use. They are simplified versions of my professional recipes, which are also available directly from me (see Useful Addresses). Many flower essence producers have created some very successful combinations that are well worth taking. If any of the essences mentioned here are not available, please use those that seem appropriate.

MAKING UP A REMEDY

To make up a remedy you will need several standard 25–30ml dropper bottles (see Useful Addresses for suppliers), some spring water, a little brandy and some adhesive labels. It is a good idea to label each bottle with details such as name, the date you made the combination, a brief description of what this particular mix is for and the flower essences it contains.

- Rinse through a 25 or 30ml stopper bottle with spring water.

- For each recipe, put 2 drops of each of the essences listed into the bottle.

- Add 1" of brandy or vodka to the mix. This is used purely as a preservative. If you have a sensitivity to alcohol you may wish to use apple cider vinegar, vegetable glycerine or clear honey as a substitute for the brandy/vodka.

- Fill to the brim with spring water.

This is the course of treatment for the next two months. Two bottles of this mix will last about six weeks to two months. After a month it may be a good idea to stop taking the essence and review the condition. The emotional state, physical discomfort or other issue you were working on may have eased or even disappeared. If not, continue taking the combination until the course is completed. It is worth remembering that even when you have finished taking the remedy it will still be acting in your system for some time.

On regaining your balance there may be no need for further remedies for the time being. Alternatively you may become aware of another issue that is troubling you. In this case you will need to select appropriate remedies for your next prescription.

FIGHTING OFF DISEASE AND STRESS
Stress Buster

An excellent de-stressor for when you are feeling overstimulated and overwhelmed – in short, burnt out – by stressful situations and environments. Brings calmness, filtering out the stress from all situations. Restores balance and resilience. You can add 2 drops of Office Flower (Him A) to combat stressful office environments.

Black-Eyed Susan (FE Aus)

Crowea (FE Aus)

Pink Fairy Orchid (Aus L)

Macrocarpa (FE Aus)

Fairy Duster (DAl)

White Carnation (PF)

Energy Booster

A re-energizer and revitalizer for when you feel drained, tired or fatigued. Restores deep-seated vitality and helps you to learn to work with consistency to avoid becoming depleted either physically, emotionally or mentally. You can add 2 drops each of Bay (GM) and Vital Spark (Him E) for extra potency.

Banksia Robur (FE Aus)

Leafless Orchid (Aus L)

Cherry (Ma)

Forsythia (Hb)

Vanilla (PF)

Macrocarpa (FE Aus)

Environmental Protector

For those feeling overwhelmed and sensitive to a city environment, whose nerves are frazzled by the fast and frantic pace of life. For those living and working in crowded and polluted surroundings. Vulnerability to electromagnetic radiation from computers, fluorescent lights, pollution and other noxious substances often manifests as allergic reactions.

This combination boosts and protects the energetic system against all kinds of environmental hazards. Eases stress and allows you to remain calm, centred and grounded. Add 2 drops of Pink Fairy Orchid (Aus L) for extra potency.

Grass of Parnassus (Ask)

Yarrow (Ask, FES)

Dill (FES)

Indian Pink (FES)

Viridiflora (PF)

Radiation Cactus (AK)

T1 (AK)

Mulla Mulla (FE Aus)

Protection from Chemical Pollutants

This combination cleanses and detoxifies the system of environmental pollutants such as chemical residues and heavy metals, clearing vibrational debris and impurities from the body, mind and emotions. It also offers protection from pollution, rebuilds a suppressed immune system to alleviate allergic problems and guards against bacterial infections. Add 2 drops each of Star Tulip (FES) and Lily (PF) for extra potency. Portage Glacier Environmental Essence is available from Alaskan Flower Essences.

Portage Glacier (Ask)

Sweet Grass (Ask)

Fringed Violet (FE Aus)

Wild Potato Bush (FE Aus)

Lotus (FES)

Crossandra (PF)

Daylily (PF)

Immune Boost

Boosts immune resistance to all kinds of infections and speeds recovery. Restores balance to the immune system when it is overstressed or overworked; gives you greater mental control over your immune system. Builds resistance to auto-toxicity, enhances the body's natural defence network and invigorates the production of white blood cells and interferon to fight viral or bacterial attack and infection which has over-powered the system. Add 2 drops each of Knotted Marjoram and Snapdragon (PF) for extra potency.

K9 (AK)

Macrocarpa (FE Aus)

Silverlace (PF)

Gaillardia (PF)

Echinacea (Haii)

Infection Fighter

For helping to shake off viral infections such as colds and flu. Eases the chills and aching associated with the pre-influenza state. Helps fight off infection by clearing viruses out of the system. Especially beneficial for respiratory and throat infections as well as fevers. Add 2 drops each of Pansy (FES) and Korte (PHI) for extra potency.

Spinifex (FE Aus)

Thyme (PF)

Pansy (FES)

Babies' Breath (PF)

Nasturtium (Dv)

Drum Stick (Him A)

Echinacea (PF)

Onion (PF)

Anaesthetic Clearing Mix

Clears the effect of anaesthetic from the system. Acts as a tonic for a stressed nervous system and stimulates the cleansing of impurities and toxicity from the blood and lymphatic system. Releases the subtle anatomy from the shock and trauma of going through an operation. Enhances resistance to infection from bacteria and viruses, as immunity is weakened by an operation of any kind. Add 2 drops of Echinacea (PF) to boost immunity. To clear antibiotics from the system, use Coralroot (Spotted) (Peg).

Inner Cleansing Cactus (AK)

Bottlebrush (FE Aus)

Australian Smoke Bush (Aus L)

Wild Potato Bush (FE Aus)

Morning Glory (FES, Him A)

Red Carnation (PF)

Detox Essences (FE Aus)

White Hyacinth (PF)

HELP FOR SPECIFIC HEALTH PROBLEMS

Allergy Antidote

For hay fever, asthma and other allergic problems. Builds resistance to itching, watery eyes, runny nose and flu-type symptoms typical of an allergic reaction to grasses, pollens and so forth. Combats the breathing difficulties of asthma. Add 2 drops each of Sand Dollar (Pac) and Carrot (PF) for extra potency.

K9 (AK)

Lily (PF)

Grass Widow (Pac)

Eucalyptus (FES)

Lantana (PF)

Babies' Breath (PF)

Formulae 36 Immune Booster (Him A)

Sneeze Ease (Aus L)

Digestive Soother

For digestive upsets, nervous stomach, tension in the solar plexus, poor digestion, hyperacidity, ulcers and eating disorders. Calms the stomach, aids digestion, promotes enzyme activity and assimilation of nutrients. Add 2 drops each of California Pitcher Plant (FES) and Moss Rose (PF) for extra potency.

Paw Paw (FE Aus)

Salvia (AK)

Chamomile (Dv, FES)

Curry Leaf (Him A)

Crowea (FE Aus)

Orange Honeysuckle (Pac)

First Aid

For shock, trauma and accidents. Works on all levels – physical, mental and emotional – helping you to rebuild after shattering experiences. Clears grief, releases deeply held pain in the body after injury and trauma, restores the flow of energy and provides emotional stability in times of extreme stress.

Fireweed (Ask)

Waratah (FE Aus)

Cowkicks (Aus L)

Arnica (FES)

Ashoka Flower and Tree (Him A)

Pear (Ma)

Nootka Rose (Pac)

Grape Hyacinth (Pac)

Clare's Floral Clear Complexion Cream

To an organic aqueous cream base, which is available from most good health food stores, or Self Heal Cream (FES) add 3 drops each of these essential aromatherapy oils:

Chamomile

Jasmine

Rose

Plus 2 drops of each of the following flower essences:

Billy Goat Plum (FE Aus)

Lily (PF)

Aloe Vera (FES, AK)

Salvia (PF)

Sweet Annie (PF)

Headache and Migraine

For stress-related, tension-type headaches, migraines and the neuralgia associated with menstruation. Add 2 drops each of Black-Eyed Susan and She Oak (FE Aus) for extra potency.

Menzies Banksia (Aus L)

French Lavender (PF)

Mountain Devil (FE Aus)

Curry Flower (PF)

Plantain (Pac)

Mussel (Pac)

Narcissus (PF)

Insomnia

For insomnia and disturbed sleep. An excellent tranquilliser bringing deep harmonizing sleep. Refreshes and recharges your whole being with vitality. Eases hyperactivity, excessive worry and fears in the subconscious, restlessness and nightmares.

Macrocarpa (FE Aus)

Hibiscus (FO)

Valerian (Dv)

St John's Wort (FES)

Swallow Wort (Him A)

White Chestnut (Bach)

Jet Lag

For preventing and easing jet lag, typified by fatigue and feelings of disorientation. Protects you during air travel and realigns your system on all levels to reduce sensations of disorientation.

Mulla Mulla, Sundew, Bush Iris (FE Aus)

Thyme (GM)

Speedwell (Hb)

Premenstrual Relief

For premenstrual symptoms caused by hormonal imbalance. Eases over-emotional, agitated and irritable feelings, fluid retention and headaches. Aids absorption of iron, enhancing your strength and stamina during menstruation. Helps women to accept and accentuate their natural femininity. Add 2 drops of Cherokee Rose (PF) for extra potency. To tailor this mix for the menopause, add 2 drops each of Orange and Honeysuckle (Pac).

She Oak (FE Aus)

Macrazamia (Aus L)

Mala Mijer (DAD)

Pomegranate (FES)

Japanese Magnolia (PF)

Frangipani (FO)

SUBTLE BODY PROTECTION
Aura Protection and Repair Remedy

A combination that repairs and mends holes in the aura, strengthening, enhancing and protecting the auric field. Add 2 drops each of Vanilla (PF) and Pink Orchid (FO) for extra potency.

White Yarrow (AK)

Fringed Violet (FE Aus)

Angel of Protection Orchid (AK)

Subtle Body Harmonizer

A combination to clear blockages and discharge toxicity from the subtle bodies, bringing them all into correct alignment. Add 2 drops of Live Forever (GM) for extra potency.

Lotus (AK, FES)

Sweetgrass (Ask)

Swamp Onion (Peg)

Chakra Balance

Helps to rebalance and restore smooth functioning to all the chakras. Add 2 drops of Lilac (GM) and Hydrangea (Green) (Peg) for extra potency.

Lady's Slipper (Ask)

Sweetgale (Ask)

Lotus (Him A)

Viridiflora (PF)

Nootka Rose (Pac)

Note: as a general rule of thumb, flowers that are the same colour as a certain chakra will benefit that particular energy centre (see Chapter 2 for a list of the chakras and their associated colours). The effects will also spill over into those areas of the body linked with that chakra.

Meridian Rebalance

A potent remedy for clearing blockages in these energy channels, ensuring a smooth flow of Qi and generally rebalancing the entire meridian system. Add 2 drops each of Gladiola and Trumpet Vine Nepal (Peg) for extra potency.

Sitka Spruce Pollen (Ask)

Silver Maple (GM)

Northern Lady's Slipper (Ask)

Crowea (FEA)

Clearing Blockages (DL)

Immunofluidium

Strengthens, activates and binds the immuno-fluidium, improving the flow of nourishment to the cells. Aids in building immunity against bacterial infection by activating and stimulating the white blood corpuscles to detect and destroy viral and bacterial invaders. Add 2 drops each of Paw Paw (FEA) and Pokeweed (Peg) for extra potency.

Manzanita (FES)

Bells of Ireland (Peg)

ADDICTIONS
Anti-Addiction Remedy

This is a basic mix for the addictive personality facing and dealing with the reasons behind addiction.

Releases patterns of abuse present in the general consciousness, strengthens the will to fight and break free of addictive habits, and negates the need for stimulants. Detoxifies the system on all levels, especially focusing on the nervous system. Cleanses the aura and rehabilitates the whole energy system, leaving it refreshed and sparkling. Offers overall support in addiction therapy.

Add 2 drops of Tundra Twayblade (Ask) for extra potency.

Blue China Orchid (Aus L)

Morning Glory (AK, FES, Haii)

Nirjara (Him E)

Rose Damaceria Bifera (Peg)

Forsythia (Pac)

Bush Iris (FE Aus)

Withdrawal Remedy

This combination is for undoing the damage caused by heavy overuse of drugs. It repairs any deterioration in the nervous system, particularly that caused by morphine, counters 'spaced out' feelings, and encourages the letting go of habit patterns and lifestyles contributing to drug abuse, especially the tendency towards escapism. Mends holes in the aura resulting from drug abuse. Add 2 drops of Red Lily (FE Aus) for extra potency.

The basic Anti-Addiction Remedy (above) can be tailored towards specific addictions by adding 2 drops each of any or all of the following essences:

Pennyroyal (AK, FES)

Sundew (FE Aus)

Californian Poppy (FES)

Sagebush (FES)

Fringed Violet (FE Aus)

Give Up Smoking

Assists the will to give up smoking, providing emotional support. Re-oxygenates, repairs and improves the condition of the lungs after the long-term effects of smoke inhalation. You may add Drum Stick (Him A) and Babies' Breath (PF) for any congestion and breathing difficulties.

Add 2 drops of each essence to the basic Anti-Addiction Remedy.

Blue China Orchid (Aus L)

Nicotiana/Flowering Tobacco (FES)

Boronia + Bottlebrush (FE Aus)

Kicking Caffeine

Clears the effects of caffeine from the nervous system, alleviating any deterioration due to long-term use of caffeine. Strengthens and detoxifies the overall energetic pattern of the liver. Revitalizes willpower when you are tempted to indulge.

Add 2 drops of each essence to the basic Anti-Addiction Remedy.

Yellow Ginger (Haii)

Hibiscus (FO)

Alcohol Overuse

Helps to bring clearer insight into and understanding of the problems that lead to alcohol abuse. Cleanses the blood, protects the liver and kidneys and strengthens and repairs the etheric body, which can be damaged by alcohol's loosening effect on the subtle bodies.

If you are only suffering from a typical hangover after drinking too much in one sitting, a good essence to take is Soberup (Him E).

Add 2 drops of each essence to the basic Anti-Addiction Remedy.

Almond (Ma)

Pennyroyal (FES)

Angelica (FES)

Boab (FE Aus) for addictive family patterns passed on.

Note: Do not use extra alcohol or brandy; use glycerine as a base (see Suppliers under Useful Addresses).

FUN COMBINATIONS

Sassy Mix

A fun combination to help us women feel sexy, sassy and full of fun.

Orchid Queen (FO)

Frangipani (FO)

Lehur (Haii)

Pink Orchid (FO)

Little Rascal Mix

Try this combination to help your little rascal to calm, slow down, be less restless, more centred, reasonable, and to be able to listen and be co-operative.

Grape blossom (Ma)

Banana blossom (Ma)

Strawberry blossom (Ma)

Lettuce blossom (Ma)

Man Mix

To aid a feeling of courage, inner strength and empowerment as a man.

Sunflower (AK)

Banana (AK, FO)

Strength (Him E)

Tomato (Ma)

HAND-PICKING YOUR OWN ESSENCES

An ideal remedy can be created from the flowers growing in your own garden. Before picking and preparing the flowers it is important to feel still and calm, so if possible practise some form of meditation.

When searching for flowers in the garden choose those in full bloom with an intense, vibrant colour. Rinse a bowl with salt water, fill it with spring water and float the flowers in the bowl for 2–3 hours in the sunshine. After this time, or when the blooms have become limp, lift them from the liquid with a twig and return them to the soil. This is your flower essence, made from your immediate environment, and will help you to be more in tune with your surroundings and encourage your own balance and healing. To make the Mother Tincture use ½ flower essence and ½ brandy. To make the Stock Essence use ⅔ brandy and ⅓ spring water, then add 7 drops of Mother Tincture to every 25ml. To make Dosage Bottles use ¾ spring water and ¼ brandy, then add 7 drops of Stock Essence. Take 7 drops of this dosage essence morning and evening for two weeks.

CHAPTER SIX

TREATING COMMON AND COMPLEX CONDITIONS

Case Histories by Biological System

It is clear that flower essences are unique in their ability to restore and enhance a sense of total wellbeing in mind, body and spirit. Unlike most other remedies, flower essences act as catalysts to rebalance the body's vital energy. In doing so they provide the perfect antidote to stress-related upsets.

It is now also clear that stress in all its different guises disrupts and diminishes our natural life force. Feeling tired and depleted, for example, is a sure sign that the body's energies have been thrown out of kilter. Upsets at this level inevitably precede other kinds of niggling minor ills and may eventually lead to more serious conditions.

We may take a holiday to escape the stresses of life when we start to feel run-down. This temporarily recharges the batteries, but it will not get to the root of the problem. It is important that we redress the ingrained imbalance, which may originate and be linked to any shock or trauma that occurred many years ago.

Healers blessed with the ability to 'tap into' the body's energy may be able to bring all the systems back into balance. The problem with this is that we have to rely on someone else to rekindle our sense of wellbeing. The beauty of flower essences is that they have the power to evoke such changes. This means that you alone become responsible for inspiring your own happiness and good health.

To preserve an energetic equilibrium, we also have to become aware of those aspects of our personality and behaviour which are likely to upset the balance. Impatient people, for instance, who are easily irritated by the slowness or incompetence of others, merely agitate their own energy systems and always will – unless they find a way of tempering their impatience.

Many of these subtle remedies act on the mind, easing all kinds of emotional and mental turbulence. Feelings such as fear, guilt, anger, anxiety and irritability do not only detract from the pleasure of living; if left unchecked, they slowly and insidiously wear down the body's resistance to illness, leaving us vulnerable to all kinds of health problems. Negative, distracting emotions also cloud our vision making it difficult for us to see or understand our special role in life, so hindering any kind of spiritual development.

It should be stressed that flower essences are by no means cure-alls. They work best at nipping potential problems in the bud, so preventing illnesses from arising in the first place. However, these gentle remedies are also helpful at times when a more direct approach is required. Orthodox drugs, acting at the physical level, alleviate symptoms but do not give rise to a real sense of wellbeing. For example, tranquillizers may ease discomfort by distancing us from reality and dulling our reaction to stress, but they do not provide us with the tools we need for coping with and overcoming it.

For complete healing it is necessary to instil feelings of harmony and balance in mind, body and spirit. This is where flower essences come to the rescue.

The scale of remedies (see Table 6.1) shows the difference between the various forms of medicine available to us. The further up the scale you go, the more far-reaching are the benefits. Pharmaceutical drugs provoke profound physical changes, but they do not touch our emotional or spiritual wellbeing. In terms of our energy system, their effect can be likened to a sledgehammer, whose shattering impact can actually get in the way of complete healing.

In contrast, flower essences, and a new category, environmental and sound essences, act at the higher emotional, mental and spiritual levels before filtering into the body. When taken in conjunction with other forms of medicine, flower essences, environmental and sound essences enhance their benefits and at the same time clear away any unwanted side-effects provoked by the more physical or 'denser' types of medicine. These gentle remedies can be used successfully alongside prescribed drugs to speed recovery from accidents or operations and help you overcome all kinds of disease. They will also bring benefit to those who are trying to wean themselves off antidepressants, sleeping pills and other mood-elevating drugs.

Table 6.1 Scale of Remedies

Classification	Remedy/medicine	Mode of action/side-effects
Vibrational	Sound, light, environmental and flower essences	Acting at the subtle, emotional/psychological and spiritual energy levels filtering down to the physical – no toxic side-effects
Vibrational	Gems	Acting at the physical and subtle levels occasionally heightening symptoms – cleansing effect
Like with like	Homeopathy	Physical effect with reference to the emotional and psychological. Some side-effects and heightening of symptoms before they clear
Natural	Aromatherapy (essential oils)	Natural chemicals with gentle influence on physical system with emotional/psychological benefits
Natural	Herbal medicine	Natural chemicals with gentle physical effects
Synthetic	Pharmaceutical drugs	Basic physical level with toxic physical and subtle side-effects

HOW DO FLOWER ESSENCES WORK THEIR WONDERS?

In many healing traditions, our natural disposition is believed to be one of perfect health and happiness. Unfortunately, all kinds of shock and stress conspire to shift us from this state of grace. Given the right impetus, self-healing can be kicked into gear.

Flower essences act as catalysts in order to bring our energies back into balance so that we can begin to reach the potential for perfection which resides within our energetic blueprint. They have this capacity because they are able to vibrate at frequencies close to those of our own subtle energies. Vibrational flower essences are unique in their general effect of realigning and pulling the subtle anatomy back into order so the self-healing process can begin. They also act in a very specific way, by travelling to the area or areas most in need of attention.

The ideal combination of flower essences should be matched to your individual energetic blueprint. This sets up a sympathetic resonance, a dynamic conversation which constantly reminds the body of how it really should be. It is like sounding a chord that brings all the notes into perfect harmony.

The essence pathway

Flower essences appear to follow a particular pathway through our subtle anatomy. After a few drops are swallowed, the essence is taken up by the bloodstream before moving directly to the meridians, the energy channels which feed the life force or Qi into the body. The meridians form an energetic interface between the higher-frequency subtle bodies and the physical body. From here the essence's life force either enters the various chakras and subtle bodies or returns to the cells in the physical body.

Because of their ethereal nature, flower essences may at first be attracted to the subtle bodies. From here their beneficial vibrations may filter down into the physical body through the etheric body, chakras and the skin. However, a flower essence will also be instantly drawn to any place where vibrational imbalance exists. These areas act like a sponge, literally soaking up the essence's healing energy. Rebalancing occurs as toxicity, in the form of disharmonious frequencies, is flushed from the system. Flower remedies are particularly potent in inducing changes in the chakras and subtle bodies, although some also directly influence the physical body. The ultimate therapeutic action depends at which energetic level the being is out of balance.

These remedies also enhance the connection between spirit, mind and body. They facilitate the flow of information from the Higher Self or inner voice, which always knows what is best for us, so we are far less likely to fall victim to emotional and physical

problems in the first place. In other words, the remedies actually help to prevent the kind of problems that arise from ignoring what we instinctively know is right.

READING THE SIGNS: THE BODY PHYSICAL

For many people physical symptoms are the first sure sign that something is wrong. Seemingly minor problems such as headaches, stomach upsets or colds are the body's way of alerting you to the fact that you need to take steps to redress any imbalance. Such symptoms do not go away if they are ignored. They simply get worse and may spill into another system, giving rise to yet another source of physical discomfort. To make it easier to recognize the source of your symptoms we must now look at the distinctive systems of the body. It is important to bear in mind, however, that all these systems are interconnected and that each exerts a profound influence over the others.

The nervous system

The nervous system is rather like the body's telecommunication system because it is responsible for transmitting information around the body. It is composed of millions of tiny nerve cells called neurones which communicate with each other using weak electrical impulses. These cells are bundled together into fibres which spread, like branches, to form a vast and intricate network throughout the body. The main branch runs from the brain, which masterminds the whole system, down through the spine. The brain assesses all the information coming into the body via the senses, then decides what action to take. For this reason the nervous system plays a vital role in enabling us to respond and adapt to ever-changing environmental conditions. The nervous system is split into two parts, one we can control voluntarily (the voluntary system), and another which apparently functions below the level of consciousness (the autonomic system).

The autonomic system

The autonomic system has received a great deal of attention in recent years because of its link with stress. It is divided into two branches, the 'activating' sympathetic part and the 'pacifying' parasympathetic part. The sympathetic system comes into play when we need to handle emergencies or sudden changes. It gives rise to the so-called 'fight or flight' stress response characterized by a rush of energy, a racing heart and a feeling of alertness, changes caused by the secretion of the 'stress hormone', adrenaline. Once the stress has passed, the parasympathetic system should take over to calm all the systems down, but thanks to the pressures of life today we often get stuck in sympathetic mode. It now seems clear that our state of mind can influence the autonomic nervous system and that we can 'talk ourselves into' becoming more relaxed. Being the most reactive of all the systems, the nervous system is the first place where emotional upset takes its toll. From here it goes on to affect any system that is particularly weak and vulnerable.

Signs of nervous upset

- Increased heart rate; palpitations
- Rapid breathing
- Muscular tension
- Sweating, feeling flushed
- Disturbed digestion and a nervous 'knotted' stomach
- Irritability and edginess
- Restlessness
- Insomnia; lying awake worrying
- Aggressiveness
- Cravings for alcohol or nicotine
- Nervous habits such as nail-biting, foot-tapping or drumming repetitively with the fingers
- Loss of appetite or overeating
- Inability to relax
- Feelings of being totally unable to cope – nervous breakdown

CASE HISTORY: INSOMNIA

Rebecca, company director and self-confessed workaholic, was physically healthy but had suffered from insomnia for some time. She not only found it difficult to fall asleep, but also woke frequently during the night. By morning she was exhausted and felt she had not slept at all. She had also begun having slight premenstrual tension.

Some of the essences I prescribed:

- Star of Bethlehem (B) for long, slow shock, as it transpired that her drive to achieve stemmed from feeling unloved as a child. She had thus developed a strong desire to please and prove herself worthy of love.

- Five Corners (FE Aus), for her low self-esteem which had led to her desire to prove herself.

- Pomegranate (FES), which helped her as a woman deprived of the nurturing needed for a positive self-image.

- A combination of Elm (B), Indian Pink (FES), Chamomile and Valerian (Dev, PF), to combat her feeling of being overwhelmed by the pressure of work and its debilitating effect on her nervous system, resulting in her sleeping problems.

Rebecca soon began to relax and found she could pace herself better at work. She reported feeling uplifted and more confident, and told me she had slipped into a regular sleeping pattern. The premenstrual tension also improved.

Now she began to wonder what her real purpose was in life.

I prescribed:

- Silver Princess (FE Aus), to help her realize her inner direction and purpose.

- Zinnia (FES), to keep her from taking life so seriously.

- Pink Seaweed (Pac), to help her take stock before rushing into anything new.

- Positive Change (FO) and Fireweed Combo (Ask E) to integrate the change and help her to move in a new direction.

CASE HISTORY: ANOREXIA NERVOSA

Although women are more susceptible to anorexia than men, at the age of 25 John had the classic symptoms of this illness. He is a highly sensitive, gentle person whose problems began in childhood. John's mother was distant while his father's domineering, military style of discipline frightened him. John grew up feeling inadequate and reproached himself for not fulfilling his parents' expectations. He withdrew from life and his emotions, entering a fantasy world and following intellectual pursuits. The feelings of anxiety and inadequacy stayed with him, upsetting his nervous system and digestion, leading to severe weight loss over a period of time due to the need to control events by consciously starving himself.

I prescribed:

- Chamomile (FES) and Hau (Haii), for calming and restoring the nervous system.

- Indian Pink (FES) and Star of Bethlehem and Pine (B), to clear the long, slow shock of his repressed childhood and the guilt and self-blame he took from his parents.

- Scarlet Monkeyflower (FES), to release his repressed anger and frustration with his parents.

- Neem (Him A), to help him to feel safe with his emotions.

- Paw Paw (FE Aus) and Turquoise and Gold (AK), for anorexia and to facilitate absorption of vital nutrients.

While taking the remedies John lost the anorexic mindset and began to put on weight and felt happier and more able to be himself. He also began standing up to his father in a quiet but positive way.

The immune system

Like an army the immune system defends the body from invaders such as viruses, bacteria and other potentially harmful organisms. White cells, or leukocytes, act as soldiers and move freely around the body via the bloodstream to target the site of infection. The first battalion to arrive on the scene when something like a stomach bug enters the system is made up of granular leukocytes. These cells are armed with chemical weapons which immobilize and often destroy bacteria.

The rest of the army is broken down into two divisions of lymphocytes which are produced in the lymph glands and spleen. The T-lymphocytes are like the body's intelligence service, for they are concerned with recognizing foreign invaders. As well as viruses they regard implanted tissue as alien and prompt its rejection. The thymus gland, which orchestrates the functioning of the immune system, endows the T-cells with their discerning qualities. If the T-cells verify an invasion, the immune system is switched to 'red alert'. Some of the T-cells possess deadly weapons which they then put to use.

B-lymphocytes are also brought into play. These cells make antibodies which act as straitjackets, immobilizing the invader until it can be attacked. The B-cells have memories and can remember what type of antibody to make if they meet the same virus again. This means the invader can be dealt with more efficiently next time, and that any resulting symptoms will be mild. In the case of allergy, the B-cells start making a specific sort of antibody called immunoglobulin E (IgE). During the scuffle between antibody and invader, inflammatory chemicals such as histamine are released which cause the typical allergic symptoms such as a runny nose, watery eyes, etc.

The way the immune system functions is complex and is still not fully understood. However, we know that if overworked or sabotaged it may fail to know the difference between an enemy and something innocuous – or even between an enemy and the body's own tissues. In autoimmune diseases such as rheumatoid arthritis and myalgic encephalopathy (ME), it appears to turn on its own cells. Shock, long-standing stress, a poor diet and/or environmental pollutants appear to act as immunosuppressants. Some researchers have found that certain negative emotions such as grief and feelings of despair are particularly effective at disarming the immune system. In contrast, unconditional love seems to strengthen its reserves.

Signs of poor immunity

- Frequent colds, sore throats, swollen glands
- Recurrent bacterial and/or viral infections
- Allergies
- Aching joints and muscles
- Depression, irritability, anxiety, emotional upset
- Lank, greasy hair
- Dull, blotchy skin
- Watery eyes
- Itchy, streaming nose
- Bleeding gums
- An increase in the amount of time it takes cuts and grazes to heal
- Low or fluctuating energy levels – making it necessary to rely on stimulants such as coffee
- Dull headaches
- General lack of vitality

CASE HISTORY: FLU

Charlotte (a busy literary agent) had been laid low for a week with Asian flu, with the usual symptoms of fever, aching joints and a sore throat. Then the virus moved to her chest, giving rise to congestion and a debilitating cough. She was keen to avoid taking antibiotics, especially as the person who had passed the virus on to her had had the flu for eight weeks despite taking two courses of antibiotics.

I prescribed:

- Onion (PF) for clearing viruses.
- K9 (AK), a natural antibiotic.

- Formula 38 (Him A) to boost the immune system.
- Eucalyptus (FES) for the chesty cough.

Charlotte's recovery was speedy. Within a matter of days the flu symptoms and chestiness had cleared; she felt her healthy self again. Another good remedy is Coralroot (Spotted) (Peg), which helps to clear the effects of antibiotics from the system.

CASE HISTORY: HERPES VIRUS

Aged 32, Helen had first caught herpes from her boyfriend; after they'd broken up it continued to flare up for about five days in every month, making her feel depressed, unclean and unable to contemplate a long-term relationship.

She had a history of susceptibility to viral infections, having contracted scarlet fever and whooping cough when she was three, then glandular fever in her late teens.

I prescribed:

- Thyme (PF) and Spinifex (FE Aus), Marigold (PF), for fighting the herpes virus.
- Chamomile (FES) and Hau (Haii), for repairing and restoring the nervous system.
- Formula 38 (Him A) and K9 (AK), for boosting her immunity.
- Illyarrie (Aus L), to help her to realize she had the strength to cope.
- Billy Goat Plum (FE Aus), for her feelings of revulsion associated with having herpes.

After taking the course of treatment, Helen noticed that the recurrences were becoming less frequent; then they ceased completely and have not come back for more than two years.

CASE HISTORY: ME

Angela was 40 and had for the last three years been suffering from ME, which was getting progressively worse. She was exhausted and ached all over. She was confined to bed most of the time as she was unable to walk or stand for more than a few moments. Talking with her, I learned that as a child she had been pushed academically and told she was not clever enough to make the grade. She'd started taking drugs to evade reality, and had continued to use them heavily until her late thirties when she'd realized she needed professional help. However, the drugs had already taken a severe toll on her immune system and she had developed ME when at her lowest ebb, with no job, relationship or other form of support. She had been in and out of many relationships, all of them either unproductive or destructive.

I prescribed:

- Star of Bethlehem (B), for the long, slow shock of childhood and drug abuse.

- Morning Glory (AK, FES), to clear the toxic effects of drugs.

- Silverlace (PF), as an antiviral and immune booster.

- Comfrey (FES), to strengthen the nervous and muscular system.

- Dandelion (FES), to ease psychological tension stored in muscles.

- Dill (FES), to lift depression and to help her develop a healthier perspective on her emotional problems.

Angela reported that she was finding it easier to relax and felt less stressed. The burning aching in her body, especially in her legs, had eased and she was able to do simple (though previously impossible) daily tasks without getting exhausted. Now was the time for a follow-on prescription.

I prescribed:

- Formula 38 (Him A), to boost the immune system.

- Paw Paw (FE Aus), to encourage assimilation of vital nutrients.

- Tomato (Ma), to help her throw off the disease.

- Zinnia (AK, FES), to lift her outlook on life and inspire humour.

- First Aid Remedy (Him A), as an all-round booster.

Slowly but surely Angela grew stronger, reporting increased energy levels and an ability to be mentally detached from her problems. She has also overcome her dependency on addictive, destructive relationships. She continued to feel better each day and is now leading a happy productive life.

CASE HISTORY: ECZEMA

Charlie, aged three, had developed very bad eczema (linked to an allergy to dairy products). In addition, his birth had been traumatic and he appeared to be shy, fearful and apprehensive.

I prescribed:

- Arnica (FES) and Pear Blossom (Ma), for traumatic birth.

- Mimulus (B) and Pineapple (Ma), for shyness and timidity.

- Sweet Chestnut (B), for anxiety.

- Aspen (B), for apprehension.

- Aloe Vera (FES, AK) and Salvia (PF), for his skin condition.

- Formula 38 (Him A), to boost the immune system.

A month later the eczema began to clear and Charlie appeared to be more confident and less fearful. Before the end of the second course his eczema had completely disappeared; there has been no recurrence.

The lymphatic system

The lymphatic system is closely linked to the immune system because it plays a vital role in whisking away dead bacteria, disabled viruses and other debris from the tissues. Lymph itself is a colourless, faintly opalescent fluid which bathes the body cells, furnishing them with nutrients and cleansing them of wastes and other impurities. In this respect it is rather like blood. Lymph, however, is not pumped around the body by the heart. It flows freely, relying on full, rhythmic breathing along with the contraction and relaxation of major muscles in the body for its circulation.

The network of lymphatic vessels is intimately connected with the main circulatory system. Blood seeps from its own vessels into those of the lymphatic system where it is cleansed and reconditioned before returning again to the veins and arteries.

Each organ has its own lymph supply, and the system itself has its own organs. The spleen, thymus, tonsils, adenoids, appendix and Peyer's patch are all part of this complex purification system. So too are bundles of sinus tissue called lymph nodes. The main ones are found under the arms, in the neck, behind the knees and in the groin. They can be felt as small lumps beneath the skin. Inside these nodes, lymphocyte cells are busy detoxifying wastes by engulfing or destroying them. During an infection, the lymph nodes often swell and feel tender as battle gets underway within. Eating food laden with fats, sugars, salt, additives and preservatives, as well as drinking alcohol and coffee, tends to 'pollute' the lymphatic system. The lymph fluid draws liquids from the tissues to dilute these toxins, which is what makes you look puffy and feel waterlogged when there is a problem with your lymphatic system.

Signs of lymphatic disorder

- Puffiness
- Bags under the eyes
- Skin blemishes
- Cellulite
- Congestion
- Swollen, tender lymph glands

CASE HISTORY: SWOLLEN GLANDS

Sarah, a 27-year-old public relations officer, was distressed by the presence of painful boils under her armpits. She had been prescribed a course of antibiotics which had not helped. Her lymphatic system was sluggish, she tended to gain weight easily, felt nauseous after eating and suffered from poor circulation.

I prescribed:

- Chamomile (AK, FES) and Hibiscus (FO), for emotional stress and nervous conditions affecting the stomach.
- K9 (AK), Formula 38 (Him A) and Gaillardia (PF) for boosting the immune system.
- Wild Potato Bush (FE Aus), Yellow Ginger (Haii) and Vanilla Leaf (Pac), for clearing toxins from the blood and her whole

system, reducing lymphatic swelling and clearing the skin.

During the first week Sarah came out in a rash, which soon disappeared to be followed by a sore throat, which in turn cleared quickly along with the boils themselves. She felt wonderful. Not long afterwards she went out drinking to celebrate her birthday. That night her whole arm swelled up and the lumps reappeared. Sarah doubled her dosage and by morning both the swelling and the boils had gone.

The respiratory system

Oxygen is the vital spark that kindles the physical energy necessary for powering life processes. Many ancient traditions teach that air, not food, is responsible for vitality, for it facilitates the flow of life force. Breathing brings oxygen from the air into the lungs. Here the gas dissolves in the blood and is taken up by the complex iron-rich molecule, haemoglobin, present in the red cells or corpuscles. In this form oxygen is distributed to every cell in the body. The by-product of cell respiration, carbon dioxide, then combines with water in the red cells and is carried back to the lungs before being exhaled out into the atmosphere.

Full rhythmical breathing is best for the mind and body as it assures a continuous flow of oxygen to the cells and the swift removal of carbon dioxide. At rest, a typical man breathes around eight litres of air a minute – a woman somewhat less. If deprived of oxygen for as little as three minutes, brain cells die and the heart struggles to keep beating.

Although breathing happens automatically, normal breathing patterns are easily disrupted. Sudden temperature changes such as stepping outdoors on a frosty day or into a very hot sauna make us gasp and temporarily hold our breath. Everyday stresses also play havoc with breathing patterns, although we tend not to notice. When anxious, fearful, angry or frustrated our breathing becomes rapid and shallow, a phenomenon known as hyperventilation. Hyperventilation makes the heart pound, the head spin and the legs turn to jelly. Shallow breathing reduces the body's oxygen supply, leading to feelings of tiredness, lethargy and faintness as well as difficulty concentrating and frequent yawning.

Heavy air pollution also undermines our oxygen supply. Car exhaust fumes are rich in carbon monoxide, which competes with oxygen for haemoglobin in the blood. Other noxious chemicals include nitrogen oxides and hydrocarbons, which irritate the lungs and nasal passages – triggering asthma attacks, exacerbating chest troubles and increasing our vulnerability to chest infections and allergic rhinitis.

Signs of respiratory problems

- Shortness of breath

- Coughing

- Wheezing

- Frequent colds

- Hay fever and asthma

- Bronchitis

- Weakness and dizziness

- Anxiety

- Feelings of panic

CASE HISTORY: HAY FEVER

Michael, a businessman in his late forties in a stress-charged profession, had been suffering from hay fever since he was 12 years old. Each year, during the second week of June, symptoms of itchy eyes, sneezing and a streaming nose would begin and continue until the end of July, signifying a typical allergy to grass pollens. His normal treatment was to take antihistamines, although he had also unsuccessfully tried the inoculation method for several years.

I prescribed:

- Pink Fairy Orchid (Aus L), for feeling frenzied and overwhelmed by stress and the environment.

- Eucalyptus (FES) and Lantana (PF), for allergic reactions and hay fever.

- Gaillardia (PF) and Formula 38 (Him A), to boost immunity.

Michael began taking the combination a few months before the start of the hay fever season. That year he was symptom-free. He has repeated this treatment for three years, and to date his hay fever has not recurred.

CASE HISTORY: SINUSITIS

Rosemary's sinus problems began at the age of 24, following an infection she appeared to pick up in a public swimming pool. As a child she had frequent chest infections; she had contracted tuberculosis when she was 20 and it had left her with a weakness in the chest area. She had great difficulty shaking off winter colds and was very sensitive to cold winds and dust.

I prescribed:

- Formula 43 Sinus/Cold (Him A), to clear the nasal passages and sinuses.

- Drum Stick (Him A), for lung and bronchial conditions.

- Eucalyptus (FES) and Babies' Breath (PF), to help breathing.

- Echinacea (Haii), to boost the immune system.

- Tomato (Ma), to ease the hold this condition had on her system.

Her sinus condition has cleared and she is now able to breathe more easily. She reports feeling better than she has done in more than 20 years.

The circulatory system

The circulatory system is closely linked to the respiratory system, as one of its main functions is to transport oxygen-laden blood from the lungs to the tissues and return it again, this time carrying carbon dioxide. The heart is responsible for pumping an incredible five litres of blood around the body every minute. It starts beating when we are still in the womb, just a few weeks old, and continues to pulsate independently under the orchestration of its own inbuilt pacemaker for the rest of our lives. The heart was once believed to be the seat of emotion – not surprisingly, perhaps, for feelings such as anxiety, fear, anger, excitement and passion are felt here. Grief in particular seems to tear at the heart, hence the term 'broken-hearted'. This vital pump forces blood along highly elastic vessels which spread through the body becoming increasingly fine as they reach the extremities. Tiny blood capillaries feeding the skin surface may be just one cell thick. Blood itself contains a variety of cells including the haemoglobin-rich red blood corpuscles and the white lymphocytes. Along with oxygen, other nutrients absorbed from the digestive tract, hormones secreted by the glandular system and other chemicals are all circulated around the body in the blood. As blood comes into close contact with every part of the body, its composition is a particularly good reflection of what is happening at the cellular level.

A tendency towards good or bad circulation tends to be inherited, but it can also be influenced by lifestyle. Tension held in the muscles interferes with the swift flow of blood to certain parts of the body. Such deprived regions tend to feel cold. It is interesting to note that people who have experienced a great deal of trauma in childhood often tend to have poor circulation.

Signs of circulatory upset

- Sluggish circulation
- Cold hands and feet
- Chilblains in winter
- Irregular heart beat
- Palpitations
- Dizziness and feeling faint
- Blurred vision
- Nosebleeds
- Constant fatigue

CASE HISTORY: CIRCULATORY PROBLEMS

Anne, who runs a small family business, was 52 when she was diagnosed as suffering from nervous angina. She had flu-like symptoms all the time and experienced pins and needles as well as pains down her left side. Every 70 days she would get night-time palpitations lasting for 10 minutes. Anne woke frequently during the night in a sweat, her pulse racing. She was also suffering from water retention which caused her legs to swell, as well as cold hands and feet due to poor circulation. She had been taking several angina tablets a day to open the arteries, as well as tranquillizers to soothe her nerves.

I prescribed:

- Rose Quartz and Ruby (Gem), for childhood sadness, as her parents had argued all the time and she had always been trying to keep the peace. Her very repressive father made her angry, but she would not express this feeling.

- Bleeding Heart (Peg), for regulating blood pressure and circulation.

- Yellow Ginger (Haii), Wild Potato Bush (FE Aus) and Redwood (Peg), for cleansing the blood and strengthening the vessels.

- Saguaro (FES) to cleanse the lymphatic system and to ease fluid retention.

(**Please note**, gem and crystal essences are included in this edition; please see Section K of the Encyclopedia where they are described in full.)

After the first course of treatment Anne's circulation had improved, she had not felt the need to take a tranquilliser for a month and her angina pains had lifted. Five days after finishing the essences she experienced some discomfort and was given a repeat prescription. She has now come off the tranquillizers completely and is down to taking just one angina tablet a day.

The digestive system

The digestive system is responsible for extracting and absorbing essential nutrients from the foods we eat, as well as for disposing of wastes that would otherwise congest and clog up the system. Digestion begins in the mouth, where food is pulverized by chewing mixed with saliva which contains mild starch-digesting enzymes. It then passes to the stomach where digestion begins in earnest. Here food is mixed with a potent gastric juice rich in hydrochloric acid which creates an environment suitable for protein-digesting enzymes to carry out their task.

All kinds of emotional upset, from fear and frustration to anger and anxiety, upset the flow of gastric juice. While an oversecretion of acid gives rise to heartburn, undersecretion means food lingers in the stomach causing indigestion and feelings of heaviness.

On leaving the stomach, food passes into the small intestine, a long and convoluted tunnel where starches are broken down into sugars and digestion is completed. According to the traditions of Chinese medicine, emotions are processed in the digestive tract as well as foods. If sensations such as anger or fear are not properly dealt with, tension accumulates in this area, giving rise to symptoms such as stomach knots and colicky pains.

Everything we absorb into the bloodstream through the intestinal walls is passed on to the liver, a remarkable organ which emulsifies fats and changes sugar into glycogen so it can be stored away until it is needed. The liver also detoxifies any undesirable chemicals, such as alcohol and the food additives taken in with the vital nutrients. The liver functions best when we eat simply prepared, natural foods and keep regular eating and sleeping patterns; when overburdened with rich, fatty foods and impurities we feel nauseous and headachy, as if slightly hung-over. From an emotional viewpoint, the liver is affected by angry outbursts more than anything else.

Foods that have not been broken down for nutrients then enter the large intestine or colon, where any water is reabsorbed and wastes are gathered for elimination. Eating plenty of fibre-rich vegetables and foods helps to speed digestion and prevent wastes from stagnating in the bowel. Elimination is also carried out by two other organs in the body: the kidneys and the skin. The kidneys, like the liver, filter the blood to remove unwanted salts and noxious wastes. These are expelled in a diluted form as urine. The kidneys also play a vital role in maintaining the balance of body fluids by eliminating excess water and conserving it when in short supply.

Sweat glands in the skin secrete water that contains dissolved mineral salts and small quantities of other wastes through microscopic pores at the surface, helping to keep the body free of impurities. Wearing natural fibres such as cotton and wool allows the skin to breathe and perspire more freely than synthetics do.

Signs of digestive upset

- Indigestion/heartburn
- Bloating and wind
- Knots in the stomach
- Colicky cramps
- Diarrhoea
- Constipation
- Nutritional deficiencies
- Fluid retention
- Cystitis
- Blemished skin

CASE HISTORY: WIND AND BLOATING

Susan was experiencing abdominal discomfort due to bloating, wind and constipation which had become worse during her divorce from a husband who was both difficult and vindictive. During this period of intense emotional stress she had also started to react to city pollution, suffering hay fever-type symptoms.

Her childhood was traumatic. Susan had been brought up during the Second World War years by very strict parents who would not tolerate any show of emotion. She had suffered from constipation as a child and was allergic to dairy produce.

I prescribed:

For the past:

- Star of Bethlehem (B), for long, slow shock.
- Sweet Chestnut (B), for suppressed anxiety and not being able to express emotion.
- Mimulus (B), for timidity and fearfulness.
- Agrimony (B), for the British tendency to use a stiff upper lip as a protective mechanism.
- Vervain (B), for trying too hard to please and overexerting herself.

For the present:

- Chamomile (FES, AK) and Crowea (FE Aus), for stress that leads to a nervous stomach.
- Paw Paw, Wild Potato Bush (FE Aus) and Bamboo (PF), to cleanse the digestive system and ease wind, bloating and constipation.
- Eucalyptus (FES), to ease breathing and clear pollutants from the lungs.

Susan feels she has been able to clear the emotional upset of her childhood and present life. The wind and bloating have subsided, the constipation has cleared and her allergic reactions are less pronounced.

CASE HISTORY: GASTRIC ULCER

After three unsuccessful operations to treat an ulcer condition, Karen came to me for help. The ulcer flared up roughly every three months, causing her to wake in the night with severe pain under her ribcage. At these times she would feel cold, shivery and headachy, as if in a state of shock.

She was found to be allergic to milk and dairy products generally. Karen had also suffered long, slow shock as a child because her mother had never been there to nurture her and she was left to look after her younger brother most of the time. She had also been traumatized when her first child was stillborn. She had turned her fear and panic inward on herself.

I prescribed:

- Star of Bethlehem (B), for shock.
- Rock Rose (B), for fear and panic.
- Sweet Chestnut (B), for deep anguish and anxiety.

- Arnica (FES, AK), for suppressed shock which had turned inwards.
- Crowea (FE Aus), for continuous worry linked to stomach ulcers.
- Bamboo (PF), to soothe the stomach and colon.
- Pennyroyal (FES), to protect her from negativity.

Karen's ulcer seems to have been calmed, for she has not experienced any repeat attacks and is now sleeping peacefully through the night.

Diabetes

Another area for concern and on the rise is diabetes.

The pancreas is a very important but often overlooked organ and plays a vital role in diabetes, in that it helps with digestion and producing vital hormones, such as insulin.

- It produces insulin to help maintain the balance of glucose (sugar) in the body.
- It produces glucagon when the body needs to put more glucose in the blood to be used for energy.

The difference between glucagon and insulin is that insulin lowers your blood glucose by allowing the body to use the glucose in the blood for energy whereas glucagon raises blood glucose by causing the liver and muscles to release stored glucose quickly.

When the pancreas is functioning normally, the digestive system breaks down carbohydrates, fats and proteins, and nutrients to become smaller simpler molecules that can be readily absorbed into the bloodstream. One of these nutrients is glucose. As the concentration of glucose in the bloodstream rises, the pancreas receives a signal to release insulin which opens the door for glucose to enter the cell and eventually create the energy needed for the body to function.

Insulin resistance causes the pancreas to function abnormally which is when the cells stop responding to insulin, and the amount of glucose in the blood gets higher and higher, creating a diabetic situation. As long as there is too much glucose in the blood, and too little glucose in the cell, the pancreas will continue to produce insulin until the glucose level goes down. However, if the cells in the body have become insulin resistant, the amount of glucose in the blood will never go down. The pancreas will continue to try to lower glucose levels by producing more and more insulin. Eventually, it will wear out. Often this is the first cause of diabetes, of which there are two types.

In type 1 diabetes, the beta cells virtually stop producing insulin. Although a little insulin may still be produced, it is not enough to balance the glucose levels in the body. This is why insulin injections are needed.

In type 2 diabetes, the pancreas is not attacked by the immune system, but either produces less insulin than is needed, or the body is unable to use the insulin the pancreas does produce. The latter condition is called insulin resistance. An incorrect diet, stress or obesity can be major causes of insulin resistance.

CASE HISTORY: DIABETES

John, a 59-year-old chiropodist with a very busy and sometimes stressful practice, was shocked when during a routine check-up he was told his blood sugar levels were very elevated and verging on type 2 diabetes. He had a fairly healthy diet, so he couldn't quite understand why. He contacted me through a friend, who suggested Flower Essences of Australia Peach Flowered Tea Tree, which is for feeling nervy, unsettled, low or unstable blood sugar levels and is said to balance cravings and aid imbalances associated with the pancreas.

We started him on 7 drops morning and evening taken neat orally. After six weeks he returned to the doctors' for a diabetes test, and was delighted when he was informed that his tests were totally normal. I advised to keep on the remedy for a little while longer just to stabilize and consolidate the treatment.

The endocrine and reproductive systems

The endocrine system describes the body's so-called 'ductless glands', namely the pineal, pituitary, thyroid, parathyroid, adrenal, pancreas and thymus glands. They all secrete hormones – chemical 'messengers' which play a vital role in controlling and coordinating important processes such as metabolism and growth. Our behaviour and emotions are influenced to a degree by the hormones circulating in our bloodstream. Each gland and its hormones has a specific job to do. While some enable us to cope with changes in our environment, others orchestrate the rhythms that regulate our sleep and fertility patterns.

The pituitary is the gland which ensures that all the other glands work together in harmony. In spite of its epithet 'master gland', it in turn falls under the influence of the hypothalamus, a region of the brain that detects and responds to emotional upset. Stressful events, such as relationship problems and conflicts at work, can throw the entire endocrine system into turmoil. Is it any wonder that stress has such a disruptive effect on so many bodily processes? Hormones produced by the pituitary gland also control the activities of the reproductive organs in both men and women. Although not officially part of the endocrine system, they too produce hormones. Along with the other glands they are also responsive to emotional upset. Reproductive problems such as irregular periods are often one of the first signs that the whole endocrine system is under stress.

Sex drive is thought to be regulated by the hormone testosterone, which is produced in males by the testes and in females in smaller quantities by the adrenal glands. Male fertility is fairly consistent, which may explain why men tend to be less susceptible to emotional highs and lows. Female fertility, in contrast, is a cyclical affair marked by distinct fluctuations in the two predominantly feminine hormones, oestrogen and progesterone.

Hormonal changes may precipitate or enhance all kinds of feelings from irritability and anger to sadness and insecurity, which is the reason why all women suffer from premenstrual mood changes. It is only when stress is added that these emotions can spiral out of control.

A woman's ability to conceive or sustain a pregnancy can also be affected by stress-induced emotions. In instances where there is no biological reason for infertility, negative attitudes and beliefs may underlie problems with conception. A woman who has, for instance, grown up believing that being a parent is incredibly difficult – a view probably passed on to her by her own parents – may subconsciously fear starting a family. Pregnancy itself is a particularly emotional time, due to the hormonal upheavals that take place and because it raises all kinds of anxieties such as 'Will I love my baby?' and 'Am I ready to be a mother?' Emotional turbulence during this time may play a part in exacerbating symptoms such as morning sickness and feelings of exhaustion.

As the birth approaches it is natural to feel increasingly apprehensive and scared by the pain of labour, feelings that are sensed by the baby. Excessive fear at this time may encourage the baby to remain in a breech position. Interestingly, in India, flowers are thought to bring about mental and emotional balance during birth. During the early stages of labour, an Indian mother will bathe with water steeped in flowers.

Flower essences help to replace negative feelings such as fear and anxiety with a sense of excitement and anticipation.

Signs of endocrine upset

- Lack of sex drive or desire
- Premenstrual tension
- Absence of periods
- Irregular periods
- Period pains
- Infertility
- Mood swings in pregnancy
- Morning sickness
- Postnatal depression
- Menopausal problems
- Impotency in men

CASE HISTORY: THE PROBLEMS OF PREGNANCY

Mary had been married for eight years and although she was three months pregnant she had in the past experienced problems both conceiving and carrying a baby to full term. She had miscarried four years previously, had to have polyps removed from her uterus, then suffered another miscarriage two years later, in both instances at nine and a half weeks. She was very anxious about losing her baby, and her highly stressful job only made matters worse.

I prescribed:

- Star of Bethlehem (B), for past long, slow shock resulting from her parents' divorce when she was 14. It was very traumatic and set up a stress pattern which continued to affect her life.
- Hornbeam (B) for strength to cope.
- Chamomile (Dv, FES), to soothe the nerves and clear stress.
- Pomegranate (FES) and She Oak (FE Aus), to stabilize the baby and the whole reproductive area.
- Pear Blossom (Ma), to boost self-healing and buffer both mother and baby from any future stress or shock.

This combination was taken as a four-month course of treatment. At seven months Mary reported having had a trouble-free pregnancy and asked for more remedies for the last two months and for the birth itself.

I prescribed:

- A repeat of the Pomegranate (FES) and She Oak (FE Aus).
- Delph (AK) to help the baby through the birth process.

- Vanilla (PF) to act as a protective shield for mother and baby.

The birth was trouble-free; both mother and baby are thriving.

CASE HISTORY: MENOPAUSE

At 50, Jane began going through the menopause, suffering hot flushes and panic attacks. She had always suffered from premenstrual tension and depression around the time of her period. She was also finding her work as a counsellor highly stressful, as she tended to take her clients' emotional problems to heart.

I prescribed:

- She Oak (FE Aus), Pomegranate (FES), Orange Honeysuckle (Pac) for the reproductive area and hormonal balance.
- Candysticks (Pac), for releasing pelvic tension and to boost energy levels.
- Correa (FE Aus), for learning to accept her limitations in helping others.
- Pink Fairy Orchid (FE Aus), to filter out the emotional stress of those around her.

Jane felt all her menopausal symptoms ease, especially the hot flushes, and she had ceased having panic attacks. She now feels more like her normal self again.

CASE HISTORY: PREMENSTRUAL TENSION

For some time Sophie had been experiencing severe premenstrual tension. She generally felt exhausted and overwhelmed by stress due primarily to her two young children: one was not sleeping through the night and the other was having mild learning difficulties.

I prescribed:

- Star of Bethlehem (B), for past long, slow shock caused by the fact that her mother had not been very nurturing.
- Vervain (B), for overexertion brought on by trying too hard to please and achieve.
- Chamomile (FES), for sleep loss due to the effects of stress on her nervous system.

- Pomegranate (FES), for rebalancing the reproductive area.
- She Oak (FE Aus), for premenstrual hormonal imbalance and water retention.
- Noni (Haii), for awakening the maternal instincts of nurturing, caring and love so she could find it easier to cope with being a mother.
- Illyarrie (Aus L), for strength to overcome difficulties without feeling overwhelmed.
- Leafless Orchid (Aus L), to find energy from within to keep working without becoming physically depleted.
- Russian Kolokoltchik (Aus L Rus), to help conquer adverse conditions.
- First Aid Remedy (Him A), as an overall booster.

The month after Sophie started taking the prescription she did not have any premenstrual tension; the following month she experienced mild symptoms; since then she has been symptom-free and has felt much more balanced, with the energy to cope with a young family.

Endocrine balance using Australian flower essences

Pituitary: Yellow Cowslip Orchid

Pineal: Bush Iris

Hypothalamus: Bush Fuchsia

Thyroid: Old Man Banksia

Thymus: Illawarra Flame Tree

Pancreas: Peach-Flowered Tea-Tree

Adrenals: Macrocarpa

Ovaries: She Oak

Testes: Flannel Flower

The skeletal and muscular systems

The bones, joints, muscles and ligaments provide the body with structure, strength and suppleness. They work together, enabling us to move with ease and comfort. The spine is the linchpin of the skeletal system. It is made up of 24 drum-shaped vertebra separated by discs of fibrous tissue which act as shock absorbers. As babies our spines are relatively straight. Curves slowly develop as we spend more and more time upright. Its S-shape endows the spine with remarkable resilience to physical impact. Sadly this does not prevent us getting backache brought on by poor posture and emotional tension. Those who suffer from bad backs often tend to bear the troubles of the world on their shoulders and feel overwhelmed by responsibilities. As the archetypal providers and supporters, married men with families are the classic example. Joints form the connections between two or more adjacent parts of the skeleton; they are held together by ligaments, tough elastic fibres which allow the joints to bend to allow movement and flexibility. Inflammation of the joints, as in the case of arthritis, is traditionally thought to be caused by wear and tear or disease. However, all kinds of inflammatory chemicals, such as those produced during an allergic reaction, contribute to certain forms of arthritis.

Muscles move the joints and bones. There are 620 we can move of our own accord, plus many more involuntary ones in the heart, blood vessels, intestines and so on that we cannot control. Emotional tension is readily transmitted to the muscles. From early in life we often develop a habit of tensing certain muscles. Most people tend to raise their shoulders and tense the neck muscles when they feel threatened. We all develop our own ways of responding to stress. Repressed emotions, whether painful or pleasurable, are also stored in the muscles as tension, giving rise to a sort of 'muscular armour'. Such ingrained tensions not only limit our freedom of movement, they also stifle energy – which may explain why our natural vitality dwindles as we age.

Signs of upset

- Muscular aches

- Tension in the neck and shoulders

- Back aches and pains

- Slipped discs

- Stiff, sore joints

- Arthritis

- Rheumatism

- Poor posture

CASE HISTORY: HIP REPLACEMENT

Juliet was 48 when she discovered she needed to have a hip replacement. As the day for the operation approached she became increasingly fearful and was unable to eat.

I prescribed:

- Indian Pink (FES), Hau (Haii), Hibiscus (FO) and Chamomile (FES, AK), for stress affecting the nervous system and stomach.

- Star of Bethlehem (B), for shock brought on by any operation.

- Jasmine (PF), for healing the skeletal system.

- Russian Kolokoltchik (Aus L Rus), for courage and strength.

- Anaesthetic Clearing Blend to clear out anaesthetic from the system.

The operation was very successful and Juliet's recovery amazed her doctor. After just four weeks she reported no pain, bruising or swelling and could walk without crutches. She continued with the remedies to consolidate the treatment, adding Ohai-ali'i (Haii) to help knit and strengthen the bones and Comfrey to help repair and rebuild muscle tissue. A month later she completely regained her mobility and could even run upstairs.

CASE HISTORY: ARTHRITIS

Margaret developed extremely painful arthritis in her hands and knees. She was taking the usual combination of anti-inflammatory agents, painkillers and paracetamol. At the same time she was exhausted and was not absorbing nutrients properly from her food.

I prescribed:

- Yarrow (PF), for the inflammation.
- Zinnia (PF), for arthritis.
- Gold (AK, AK Gem, Him A), to aid the assimilation of nutrients.
- K9 and Formula 38 (Him A), for autoimmune problems.
- Morning Glory (Him A, FES) to clear the toxic effects of the medication she had been taking.

Margaret charted her condition from December to mid-May. For the first 20 days the pain continued, but the next day it started to ease. Five days later it had disappeared and has not recurred since.

She has more energy than before and, now able to kneel and squat without discomfort, she has resumed her passion for gardening.

THE MIND – THOUGHTS AND EMOTIONS

Nobody understands exactly how the mind functions. Our thoughts, feelings and emotions ultimately depend on our outlook on life. This in turn is linked to our personality and shaped by upbringing and personal experiences.

For simplicity's sake the mind is regarded as the seat of consciousness, intelligence, thought, reasoning, memory, imagination, creativity, emotions and instinctive drives. These functions take place within the brain, the most complex and highly developed structure that exists. The brain is composed of millions and millions of interconnecting nerve cells which pass snippets of information, in the form of chemical messages, from one to another.

Certain regions of the brain are associated with different functions. The most ancient reptilian region comprising the spinal cord, brain stem and midbrain controls our most basic survival and reproductive instincts. The next layer is the paleomammalian brain, also known as the limbic system. This is the control centre for emotions and states of mind such as fear, panic, pleasure and bliss. It is here that responses such as affection, sexual behaviour, altruistic impulses and even love originate. Bodily functions such as thirst, hunger, temperature and sexual drive are also regulated by this region.

The cerebral cortex is biologically the most recent region of the brain. It seems to have evolved once humans had overcome the basic function of survival and found time to sit around thinking, learning new skills, creating things and so forth. The cortex is where perception, memory, judgement and the intellect, something loosely defined as cognition, occurs.

The 'thinking' brain is responsible for mental activity. It is divided into two parts or hemispheres, the left and right, which deal with information in rather different ways. In modern Western society greater emphasis is placed on the logical, rational and analytical thinking which occurs in the left hemisphere. Recently we have begun to realize the importance of the right brain, which is concerned with creativity, inspiration and imagination. 'Whole brain thinking' is not only more effective, it also makes life seem richer.

Although the brain has a seemingly infinite capacity to store knowledge, in our information-orientated age there is a danger of mental overstimulation. By trying to make sense of it all, our minds become filled with swirling thoughts and an internal chatter which we cannot switch off. When mentally exhausted we cannot think clearly or concentrate properly, we become forgetful and find it hard to make decisions. When the mind is in turmoil, thinking is distorted and so too is the way we act or behave.

I remember once in a deep conversation with R.D. Lang (at a party no less!), the well-known psychoanalyst, that he pointed out that mental turmoil may also arise when something we are told or seems to be fact is at odds with what we instinctively know or sense. Suspicions of being deceived and lied to can, he claimed, torment us to the point of insanity.

Similarly, powerful emotions such as anger, fear and rage undermine our ability to think in a clear and rational manner. Emotions are part of our ancient inheritance and we probably share them in common with our distant ancestors. The psychologist Carl Jung referred to the 'collective unconscious' as being the hopes, fears and anxieties which all human beings hold in common.

It is natural and healthy for us to experience the whole gamut of emotions. However, certain ones such as anger and fear are seen as socially unacceptable, perhaps because they remind us of our primitive origins or just because they make us feel uncomfortable. We suppress them, learning from childhood that it is 'wrong' to lose our temper or break down in tears. Both Sigmund Freud and Carl Jung believed that repressed emotions do not go away; they stay in our psyche and crop up in our dreams. Without an outlet they become bottled up inside until the pressure becomes so intense that we may literally blow a fuse. Negative emotions will not do us much harm if they are fleeting. However, if they become part of our behavioural response they slowly and insidiously wreak havoc on the system.

We inherit many behavioural patterns from our parents. As young children we copy the way they react to situations and handle their emotions. We also acquire perceptions about ourselves, others and the world in general from them. Their attitudes and opinions undoubtedly influence the way we think of and view life. It is believed that all experiences, even those we cannot consciously remember from childhood, are stored in the subconscious mind. From here they exert an influence on our behaviour and on the way we react to other people and situations in our lives. This influence may be appropriate when we are growing up for it gives us a sense of structure and security. In later life, however, these inherited views and attitudes may no longer be helpful – can even be limiting – and their value to us has to be reassessed.

Thousands of years ago wise men realized we can only see things for what they really are when our minds are clear, still and free from cluttering thoughts. They developed meditative techniques for calming the mind and subduing the disruptive effects of our emotions. They also taught that, to be free of negative emotions, we have to find ways of turning seemingly negative situations into ones that can have a positive outcome. After all, what we think of as reality is really all in the mind.

Signs of mental and emotional upset

- Confusion

- Inability to think clearly

- Persistent unwanted thoughts

- Forgetfulness

- Inability to make decisions

- Poor concentration

- Feelings of being overwhelmed by emotions of all kinds

- Emotional outbursts

- Mood swings

- Feelings of being on an emotional roller coaster, out of control

CASE HISTORY: STRESS

Elizabeth, a self-styled company director, had built her own business into a growing concern. Despite being extremely successful in her career, she always found herself in relationships with men in which she felt abused. These played havoc with her self-esteem and were a continual source of worry. She felt confused, overwhelmed and unable to sleep properly. Her tumultuous emotional life was beginning to affect her work. She could not concentrate or make decisions and was in danger of ruining her business.

I prescribed:

- Paw Paw (FE Aus), for feeling overwhelmed and burdened by decisions.

- Scleranthus (B), to encourage decisiveness and belief in her own intuition.

- Stress/Tension (Him A), for general tension and nervous stress.

- Scarlet Monkeyflower (FES) and Relationship Combo (FE Aus), for her difficulties with relationships.

- She Oak (FE Aus), for bringing self-esteem by increasing sensuality and joy in femininity.

- Russian Kolokoltchik (Aus L Rus), to help her conquer adverse conditions.

Elizabeth recovered her strength and her sense of being centred. She spent some time on her own and began to feel more positive about herself, realizing that she did not need the sort of destructive relationships in which she was always trying hard to please someone else, but never succeeding. Later she was drawn to a man who was gentle, kind yet strong in his own way and who treated her with the respect she desired and deserved. Her business and her new relationship continue to flourish.

Spiritual harmony

Most people feel there must be more to us than merely mind and body. The dictionary defines spirit as the vital force, soul, the immortal part of us. It is not something that can be measured or analyzed by science. Nonetheless, this elusive part of us has a profound influence on our behaviour, beliefs and the kind of relationships we form. The spirit is the real person and is unique to each one of us, whereas the soul is viewed as that essential spark of creation that is part of the universal soul from which we all originate. This is what gives us being and existence, connects us to all living things.

Spiritual harmony is best described as an awareness of, a knowing of who you are, why you are here and what your particular purpose is in life. This brings a tremendous feeling of wellbeing, an abundance of vital energy and a real sense of security and belonging or being 'at home' in the world. Spiritual harmony manifests when your personality or ego is in touch with and works together with the deeper aspect of yourself, your soul.

At the same time you are still aware of a kind of spirituality that is indefinable. This is the highest form of existence which usually lies just on the edge of your consciousness. The spirit and soul seem to give us a great deal of freedom, but luckily if we stray too far from our true path, warning signals are sent out – which we ignore to our cost.

It is interesting that we begin life full of energy and sparkle. As children we often have a clear picture of what we wish to do with our lives, too. We may speculate that during those early years the ego/personality is more in touch with or in tune with the inner spirit/soul. As adults many of us end up in relationships, jobs or environments which leave us feeling empty, unfulfilled and craving something to make our lives more meaningful. From the spiritual point of view, we are lost.

More than 60 years ago Dr Edward Bach understood that physical disease is the direct outcome of emotional upset, which arises from a conflict between the soul/spirit and the mind/ego. He wrote:

> Man has a soul which is his real self – it ever guides, protects and encourages us, leading us always for our utmost advantage. The soul knows what environment and what circumstances will best enable us to develop virtues which we lack and wipe out all that is wrong in us. So long as our souls and personalities are in harmony, all is joy and peace, happiness and health. When our personalities are led astray from the path laid down by the soul, either by our own worldly desires or by the persuasion of others, a conflict arises. This conflict brings disease…which will never be eradicated except by spiritual and mental effort. (Bach 1996, p.6)

So we might view disease, whether physical, mental, emotional or spiritual, as the way our soul tries to attract our attention and make us realize that we are straying too far from our path, giving us the opportunity to take steps to regain our sense of inner harmony.

In difficult times, most people find themselves wondering why life seems so hard and full of suffering. One explanation is that we are here to learn certain lessons and can only do so by experience. Certain religions hold that the soul may incarnate over and over again into a succession of physical bodies to master lessons that can only be learned from a material existence. These lessons include how to give love without expecting anything in return and how to be compassionate.

The concept of reincarnation holds that life throws in our path a series of challenges that have to be met. As each situation arises we have to decide how we are going to deal with it. The choices we make constantly shape the rest of our lives. We create our own destiny. No two souls have ever walked an identical path; each chooses his or her own.

The notion of karma is part and parcel of a belief in reincarnation. What it basically suggests is that 'you reap what you sow'. In other words, what you have done and thought in the past are affecting you now. Similarly what you are doing and thinking now affects your future. We are creating our own good or bad karma all the time. If you are going through a time of pain and suffering, you may be paying off some past transgressions. If you are one of those lucky people who seems to be in the right place at the right time, you may be reaping the benefit of past good deeds. It is a sort of universal justice system.

If someone wrongs you it is best to forgive him or her, knowing that in due course justice will be done, if not in this lifetime then in the next. Any feelings of resentment, hatred, ill will or contempt will tie you to the person for whom you feel such antipathy. Eventually you will have to undo those karmic ties.

Philosophers and sages contemplating the meaning of humanity throughout the ages have come to the conclusion that our reason for being is to achieve purity of spirit and matter. It was once said by Rama Teph, a Second Dynasty Nubian Pharaoh, that man's special purpose is to have his head in Heaven but his feet firmly planted in the Earth. To be a complete human being we must be both spirit and matter, beautifully combined

together, each of us blending these two aspects in a unique way.

Sometimes we try so hard to find spiritual harmony that we literally get in our own way. The same problem occurs if we take this quest too seriously, over-complicating the whole process and missing the simplicity of it all. Life is best viewed as an adventure which enables the spirit to meet challenges, to rise above limitations, to grow in wisdom and vision. We don't need to take this spiritual quest too seriously – discovering our true nature can be fun. Life and this journey would be soulless without the essential element of humour. The art lies in taking life seriously in a non-serious way.

The beauty of succeeding is that it brings inner strength, a belief in your ability to achieve whatever you choose to do, a sense of purpose and a feeling of being in harmony with other people, with animals and the nature kingdom.

Signs of disharmony

- Feeling ill at ease with yourself and life

- Lack of fulfilment

- Feeling empty, insecure, alone

- Feeling that your life is not as you would like it to be

- Feeling out of control; needing to manipulate life and control others

- Lack of flexibility and adaptability with the environment

- No sense of direction or purpose

- Feeling spiritually impoverished

- Feeling disconnected from nature

CASE HISTORY: SHOCK

David was a wealthy businessman who suddenly lost all his money in a stock-market crash. He was shattered and traumatized. His life was falling apart, as money had given him his sense of security and he no longer saw any reason for living. His relationship with his wife began crumbling; he seemed paralysed, aimless, exhausted and at times suicidal. He turned to alcohol for comfort.

I prescribed:

- Emergency Rescue Essence (FE Aus), for shock.

- Fringed Violet and Waratah (FE Aus), for his black despair and suicidal feelings.

- Fireweed (Ask), to help him cope with and integrate the changes in his life.

- Gruss an Aachen (AK), for intense challenge and fears associated with this evolutionary process, to calm, stabilize and offer him support to move forward.

- Shooting Star (Ask), to understand his purpose in life.

- Strength (Him E), to have a clearer image of himself and his role in the future.

David stopped using alcohol as an emotional crutch. He became positive and dynamic, which made him feel empowered. He realized that money did not bring him happiness and that his purpose in life was to initiate more ethical projects linked to saving the environment via the world he knew best, that of business and high finance. He was then headhunted for a highly paid position to establish such ventures, enabling him to use money in a way that helped others. By his example he has instigated a change in consciousness and a realization in those he now works with that business can be both ethical and commercially viable.

CHAPTER SEVEN

USING FLOWER ESSENCES EFFECTIVELY IN PRACTICE

As practitioners, whether of complementary or orthodox medicine or both, we will find flower essences invaluable tools for helping others to help themselves. Like many natural remedies and therapies they are excellent for easing the ill effects of stress. Yet flower essences go further, highlighting the underlying patterns leading to emotional distress and its physical repercussions. They do so by cultivating self-awareness, helping others to see and understand the reasons why they are not feeling as well as they could be.

From the patient's or client's point of view it can be extremely beneficial to have someone with greater experience to help them become aware of their negative behavioural patterns and emotional responses, then guide them towards the most appropriate remedies.

As Dr Edward Bach pointed out over half a century ago:

> The physician of the future will have two great aims...firstly to assist the patient to a knowledge of himself and to point out to him the fundamental mistakes he may be making; the deficiencies of his character which he should remedy, and the defects in his nature which must be eradicated and replaced by the corresponding virtues.
>
> Secondly to administer remedies to help his physical body gain strength and to assist the mind to become calm, widen its outlook and strive towards perfection, thus bringing peace and harmony to the whole personality.

Such remedies exist in nature! (Bach 1996, p.39)

These remedies are, of course, the flower essences for which he is famed. Anyone prescribing these remedies needs to act as a finely tuned instrument, as a receptor, resonator and reflector for the patient. Clearly each practitioner will wish to evolve his or her own appropriate way of treating patients, and this will vary according to the actual needs of people coming for help. It is essential to be flexible, adaptable and creative in your approach to diagnosing and prescribing the flower essences. However, the following method can be used as a practical guide for those wishing to work with these remedies.

BUILDING UP A FLOWER ESSENCE REPERTOIRE

Ideally you should aim to have about 100 remedies at your fingertips. In order to choose the most useful ones it is important to familiarize yourself with the major flower essence families listed in the Encyclopedia section of this book. Slowly read through them all, placing a tick beside those that reflect the sort of problems you most frequently come across.

If you specialize in treating certain kinds of symptoms, such as women's problems, it will be useful to look at the Ailment Chart (Appendix 1); this will tell you at a glance which are the most appropriate remedies for each type of condition.

Even when you have composed your repertoire it is important to keep abreast of new additions to the flower essence families.

GIVING A DIAGNOSTIC SESSION

During the 25 years that I have been working with flower essences in a professional capacity, I have realized that straight discussion with the patient combined with a good working knowledge of the remedies does not always provide a clear enough picture of the more deep-seated problems involved. I have found that using a pendulum as a diagnostic tool helps me to be accurate in the selection of essences. The pendulum prevents the practitioner's opinions and ideas from impinging on the selection of essences, making the whole procedure far more objective. Almost without exception everyone can become proficient at using a pendulum with a little practice.

Before you begin a diagnosis, arrange the stock bottles of flower essence in neat, orderly rows before you so they are easily accessible. Then ask the client to place one finger on each test bottle in turn. Gently lay one hand over the client's to create a link with him or her. Holding the pendulum in the other hand, you will find that it begins to move one way or the other, giving a distinct 'yes' or 'no' the instant you make contact with the patient.

Pick out each of the chosen remedies from the batch of stock bottles and put them to one side. These are the essences the client has selected for him- or herself with assistance from you, acting as a mirror for or extension of the patient.

It is quite acceptable to have diagnosed up to 15–18 different essences. The real art then lies in making sense of what they can tell you about your patient.

I have found that each remedy is either for the client's past, present or future condition:

- The past – childhood and other early traumas.

- The present – immediate emerging emotions as well as the client's psychological and physical state at the moment of treatment.

- The future – protection from and prevention of certain mental and emotional states which have their roots in the past and present, and which could easily manifest as major blockages later on.

To find out how many drops of each essence are needed, use the pendulum again. Count slowly from one to three; the pendulum will indicate a 'yes' when the correct number is reached. The number of drops required will also tell you to which life phase that particular essence applies:

- Essences for the past – 3 drops of each.

- Essences for the present – 2 drops of each.

- Essences for the future –1 drop of each.

With experience you will begin to see that one remedy naturally follows on from and connects with the others. In this way you will begin to build up a picture of your patient, using the past as a starting point, progressing to current problems and ending with future issues. It is in relating and making the connection between each particular remedy that your insight and intuition will come into play.

CASE HISTORY

Emily was suffering from recurrent migraines and nervous stomach upsets. At the time she was working as a computer analyst in London and felt highly stressed.

During a diagnostic session the following essences were chosen for her:

For the past:

- Star of Bethlehem (B), for long, slow shock. Emily suggested that this related to childhood. She was always trying very hard to prove herself in order to please her authoritarian father, but never felt up to the mark.

- Vervain (B), for overriding the stress pattern set up in childhood. She had become forceful, highly strung and prone to exhausting herself through over-effort.

For the present:

- Indian Pink (FES), for stress from the environment.

- Chamomile (FES), for the effect of stress on the nervous system and stomach.

- Narcissus (PF), for stress resulting in migraine-type headaches.

- Illawarra Flame Tree (FE Aus), to cultivate self-approval, confidence and inner strength.

- Environmental Stress Remedy (Him A), to protect against radiation given out by her computer and contributing to her headaches.

For the future:

- Chicory (B), for countering feelings of self-pity which could impair her improvement.

Occasionally the pendulum will keep swinging, telling you that 4 drops of a particular essence are needed. This suggests stress stemming from a past life, a possible trauma that is spilling over into this lifetime and creating a blockage. This will need to be addressed before complete healing can take place. Past-life traumas are often responsible for irrational fears that do not stem from childhood. A fear of water, for instance, could indicate that the person died by drowning in a previous existence.

The essence in the 4-drop position could also pertain to the birth experience. It can also sometimes suggest a past-life overspill or carryover. If it was traumatic there may be a reluctance to be here, which may manifest itself as daydreaming, escaping to a fantasy world. Someone who was born with the umbilical cord wrapped around their neck may have a problem swallowing, or may dislike having anything close-fitting around his neck (such as a tie or polo-neck shirt).

What to say and what not to say

The whole reason for prescribing flower essences is to help patients become aware of their own stress patterns, enabling them to take back responsibility for their health and happiness. Handing back power to the individual is in fact the first stage of the self-healing process. It is therefore extremely important for you to inform and involve the client throughout the entire procedure.

You will need to give a brief description of what the essence is for, such as shock in the past. If the patient is relaxed and feels able to trust you, he or she will hopefully fill in the missing information by telling you the nature of the past trauma.

The Encyclopedia or Ailment Chart in this book can be used to discuss the descriptions of each essence with patients.

It is not a good idea to discuss issues such as reincarnation and past lives with clients during an initial consultation. If they already hold other beliefs they may feel uncomfortable with such concepts or react against them. Respect their views and you may find, in time, that they become more open-minded to these possibilities.

It is essential, however, that you give clients a brief description of the body's energy systems – the aura, chakras and subtle bodies, so they are able to understand how shock and stress affect the system (see Chapter 2).

Clients often ask me how long it will take to feel an effect and what to expect. I respond by letting them know that the remedies start to work at clearing the root of the problem at a very deep level and how soon they feel a change is dependent on how aware they are of their own processes. At times there can be a heightening of the emotional trauma or negative mental patterns from the past, but without the full impact of the original experiences, as it is cleared out of the system.

As remedies are excellent in speeding up the healing process it is good to reassure them that it will take less time to clear the stress pattern than it did to create the situation in the first place. In clearing the root of the problem the resulting physical manifestation is no longer being fed by the initial underlying cause.

Some of the qualities that develop when taking essences are:

- a growing awareness of the mind/body connection by feeling more in touch and caring towards their physical body

- reflective self-awareness, responsibility, moving out of victim mode into empowered choice

- the ability to respond and benefit from challenges, greater courage, strength and endurance

- vitality, enthusiasm and creativity enhanced

- harmonized relationships and a sense of being on their path in life.

COMBINING FLOWER ESSENCES WITH OTHER THERAPIES

Flower essences can be used in conjunction with both complementary and orthodox medicines because they are totally safe and free from any side-effects. They are a perfect complement to all kinds of natural healing therapies, particularly aromatherapy and acupressure, enhancing their effectiveness in relieving symptoms and speeding the rate of recovery.

Flower essences and aromatherapy

Flower essences and essential oils work particularly well together. As both belong to the plant world, they have a special affinity for one another. While essential oils are only extracted from aromatic plants, flower essences can be made from those with little or no perfume, which greatly enhances the range of flora you can work with.

Even when essential oils and flower essences do come from the same plant you will notice that their properties may be different – although there may be overlaps. This is because their vibrational qualities are not identical. Generally speaking, the vibration of flower essences is higher and more ethereal than that of essential oils. While essential oils tend to work primarily at a physical level, they can also have some psychological benefits. Flower essences, in contrast, concentrate their influence mainly on our thoughts and emotions, benefits which filter into the physical body. This means that a practitioner using essential oils can draw on a flower essence to provide a particular vibration that cannot be found in any of the essential oils. The converse is just as true. Used in combination the benefits of each become more profound and far-reaching.

When selecting flower essences to complement essential oils, always opt for those whose qualities are most relevant for that particular person. Whether they come from the same or completely different flowers or plants is irrelevant. Add a drop or two of the chosen flower essence to a massage oil. This will bring to the blend a vibrational quality that complements that of the essential oil, making the treatment more complete. The Petite Fleur range of essences blend especially well with essential oils due to the way they are made.

Floral acupressure

This is a budding form of therapy which is proving to be highly beneficial. Many find that improvements for all kinds of conditions occur faster and are more dramatic when appropriate flower essences are applied to certain acupuncture points on the skin.

Drs Vasudeva and Kadambii Barnao (Australian Living Flower Essences) and Drs Atul and Pupa Shah (Himalayan Aditi Flower Essences) have done pioneering work in this field. Their research is geared towards discovering which particular essences work best on key acupressure points. From their findings Drs Vasudeva and Kadambii Barnao have drawn up 'Floral Acu-maps' which can be obtained directly from the suppliers (see Useful Addresses).

I find that flower essences are particularly effective when used in combination with Shen Tao, thought by some to be the mother of acupuncture. This is a special kind of acupressure which differs from the traditional approach in that it accesses the extraordinary as well as the main meridians. The extraordinary meridians are seen as the reservoir, whereas the main meridians are seen as the rivers. They have a powerful influence on the whole subtle anatomy so the benefits they bring are emotional, mental and spiritual as well as physical. However, Shen Tao shares many key points with ordinary acupressure.

Useful acupressure points

The 'Hegu' or 'Hoku' acupoint is arguably the best pain-relieving point on the body. It is found on the back of the hand in the web between thumb and forefinger. In Shen Tao acupressure this point, known as 'Joining Valley', is also used for treating colds, constipation, laryngitis (sore throats), migraines and arthritis.

Good essences to use here are those that also have pain-relieving or relaxing qualities (see Ailment Chart, Appendix 1).

For headaches and other pains, Living Essences of Australia recommends either Dampiera (a mental and muscle relaxant) for dissolving rigidity in mind and body, or Menzies Banksia to help you to go with the pain rather than resist and so intensify it.

The 'Shenmen' acupoint on the ear is excellent for relieving stress and promoting relaxation. It can be found just inside the rim at the tip of the ear.

Suggested Living Essences of Australia

- Pink Fairy Orchid – good for stress from environmental factors such as noise.

- Hybrid Pink Fairy (Cowslip) Orchid – helps ease stress caused by oversensitivity to other people. Especially useful for easing premenstrual emotional and mental tension.

- Yellow Flag Flower – for when stress has taken all the sparkle out of life, making people dull and grim.

- Purple Flag Flower (Bush Iris) – releases stress which has been building up in the body. Acts as a valve for dispelling pressure.

In Shen Tao the 'Daling' point works wonders for calming the emotions. It can be found on the underside of your wrist, lying in the centre of the wrist crease. Use essences here that are appropriate for your particular emotional disturbance (see Ailment Chart).

For clearing the mind and lifting the spirit, one of the best points to work on is the 'Bai-hui' acupoint. Take a line from the top of each ear lobe and continue to the crown of the head. The Bai-hui point lies where these two lines meet.

Excellent essences to use here are Lotus (Him A) or Leafless Orchid (Aus L) to rebalance energy after excessive emotional or physical drain. Place a drop of either essence here every 15 minutes for an hour or so and you will find yourself revitalized.

In Shen Tao, working with the 'Shining Sea' point not only clears the mind but also helps to treat fluid retention, irregular periods and joint problems. It is found on the inner ankle directly behind the ankle bone.

Flower essences and nutritional support

Increasingly I have noticed with my clients a severe lack of nutritional assimilation and absorption. This stems not only from emotional and stress-related issues but also from the immune system being under so much strain from having to cope with the barrage of pollutants (both chemical and electromagnetic) with which it is faced.

The instances of intolerance have increased dramatically over the years not only due to foods as well as the chemical sprays on food, but also to the chemical cocktail that we put on our skin.

Unfortunately, even if the food is organic the soil is basically deficient in the essential minerals/vitamins and trace elements due to the overworking of the land and its lack of replenishment. These nutrients are of prime importance and are the elements that provide the vital sparks that ignite the correct functioning of our bodily systems as a whole.

This gap in the fulfilment of our fundamental needs became abundantly clear when testing for essences; Flower Essences of Australian's Paw Paw and Crowea would frequently be coupled together, indicating a lack of both absorption and assimilation.

The need to create a solid foundation by replenishing the nutritional reserve in the body seemed an obvious next step by allowing the flower essences to act faster and more efficiently within the body's system as well as building up the deeply depleted reserves. There is a large variety of vitamins and minerals on the market that make all sorts of wonderful claims, so why weren't my clients absorbing them? The answer became clear as it became apparent that the normal absorption of these tablets was only about 40 per cent. So I started my quest to find a liquid form of minerals/vitamins to do the job more efficiently, as a liquid would be more readily absorbed than tablets.

I came across an organic liquid mineral/vitamin with a unique delivery system that, when tested, acted really swiftly to replenish the area that normal tablets didn't seem to be able to reach. I noticed that this colloidal supplement called Maximol created a very rapid improvement in the absorption uptake as well as appearing to be suited energetically to work with the subtle energies of the flower essences. My conclusion was that Maximol significantly speeded up the essences' action

in the body and therefore the self-healing process. Only a small, almost homeopathic, amount is needed a day to effect a result, and together with the correct flower essences, which address the root of the problem, they create a formidable team with which to obtain optimum health and wellbeing.

In the quest to address the incidents of chronic and autoimmune conditions that presented at my clinic, I've found that the addition of glyconutrients ('sugars' for short), in the field of 'glycobiology', offers a wonderful opportunity to improve this situation, as does a more recent discovery of Laminine discussed further below.

Glyconutrients (sugars)

It has been discovered that eight essential sugar molecules are present in every cell of the human body. Whereas previously it was believed that carbohydrates/sugars are our fuel, and that protein/amino acids are our body's building blocks, it is now realized that the eight sugars are responsible for most of the cellular communication in our bodies. Basically these eight sugars provide the software to run the countless programs that our bodies need. If the right sugars are produced, the body maintains its extraordinary ability to heal and regenerate itself. Conversely, without them the cell-to-cell communication breaks down, resulting in the onset of many degenerative conditions that really should not have happened. The body also loses the ability to heal itself and begins to think there are problems where there are not. Here lies the cause of our autoimmune conditions – the body turns on itself. This is happening at an alarming rate.

Two of the eight essential sugars are found in the average diet. Until recently a healthy body was able to synthesize the remaining six from those basic two. Now the increasing toxic overload to which the body is subjected to, plus its daily exposure to free radicals, has seriously depleted our ability to produce these essential sugars for ourselves. As a result the body's defences begin to break down and chronic sickness, allergies and autoimmune diseases appear.

There is a large body of information beginning to emerge about this new science of glycobiology. I believe this to be important and essential. The product I offer to clients is from a natural plant source of eight of these glyconutrients. This is a broad spectrum and vital food supplement that I genuinely believe all of us should take. Almost everyone tested as needing these sugars has returned after three months feeling the benefits. They appear to benefit sufferers from allergies, loss of energy, autoimmune conditions or any chronic sickness, or those who simply are not as vibrant and resilient as usual.

After three to five months some of the changes people are recounting are extraordinary. Guy Burgs, healer and meditation teacher, has been using the sugars extensively in his healing practice with significant success. His mother was taken off HRT by her GP after only five weeks on the product. His diabetic sister-in-law showed reduced insulin requirements after only five days. My father, a natural sceptic, had only one functioning kidney working at 25 per cent, with dialysis being an almost inevitable next step. Five months ago, he was put on 1 tsp of the glyconutrient powder per day. At his most recent check-up, his rather astounded French consultants informed him that his kidney was now fully functioning and likely to outlive him! As he had taken nothing else but the sugars, it is clear that the body had healed itself!

Working in combination with flower essences I have found them to be mutually supportive, significantly speeding up the healing process. By shifting old ingrained patterns from the body consciousness, the cells get the message of wholeness and the rest of the body listens, and acts appropriately to clear the roots of ill health. Please see Useful Addresses for stockists.

A further supplement came to my attention.

Laminine

An all-natural revolutionary nutritional supplement, Laminine is simply a whole food and a form of a natural 'adaptogen' helping to create a state of balance and restoration, returning the body to its natural state of homeostasis and has been called 'the happy pill' due to its ability to reduce stress and increase the happy chemical, serotonin, creating an overall improved sense of wellbeing.

A unique formula provides essential proteins and all 22 amino acids needed to allow the body to manufacture more than 60,000 proteins. Amino acids contain the proper transport mechanisms that direct these nutritional building blocks to where our body needs them most. It also provides invaluable growth factors, specifically fibroblast growth factors which help the brain carry out directives to the body. It is a natural, synergistic superfood that contains most known vitamins, important trace minerals and eight essential amino acids sourced from land (sadly lacking in nutrients), sea and plant kingdoms, to re-awaken and nourish individual stem cells, so they potentially continue to repair, rejuvenate and bring the body into a healthy balance.

A Canadian researcher Dr John R. Davidson discovered a life-giving essence, fibroblast growth factors-extract (obtained from a fertilized avian egg on the ninth day, when its components are most potent), and theorized it would be helpful for his cancer patients. His research was virtually unknown and died with him, until almost 50 years later this research was revived by Norway's foremost expert on egg research, Dr Bjodne Eskeland.

Laminine sources the essential extracts of amino acids and nutrients from plant, marine and land, and helps the body to absorb all that it needs to repair itself by repairing the damaged cells, therefore improving all associated diseases. It aids sleep as well as boosting the body's energy levels, and also elevates mood in depression due to its effect on serotonin levels.

Some of the benefits include:

- more energy and stamina (mentally and physically)

- moderated stress response and maintain edhealthy cortisol levels

- regulated serotonin levels (eurotransmitter in the brain)

- reduced physical and mental stress and improved emotional balance

- deep calmness and relaxation

- more restful sleep promoted

- brain function and activity aided

- increased alertness and improved focus and memory

- faster post-workout recovery enjoyed

- improve dmuscle tone and strength

- enhanced sex drive

- fewer unhealthy cravings

- reduced signs of normal ageing

- collagen built for healthier skin

- shinier, thicker hair

- natural DHEA production stimulated

- overall sense of wellbeing improved.

Feedback from clients: A friend of mine, Christine Allen, a diagnostic reflexologist with a busy clinic in Northern Ireland, decided to give the Laminine a go, as like me she tries products out before she recommends them to her clients.

CHRISTINE'S STORY

When Christine was two years old, she was knocked down by a car which damaged her knee, which somewhat healed but not entirely, so that later on she needed a total knee replacement. The surgery wasn't that successful and she was left with a locked knee which she couldn't bend, nor could she walk without crutches. Painkillers only relieved the pain for up to three hours, and at night she swelled up, had pins-and-needles and not much sleep. She was ready to give anything a try and started on Laminine. For the first two months things seemed to intensify and she thought it was not working. I encouraged her to keep going as I felt it was what I call a 'burn off' and her empty reserve tank so to speak needed replenishing first. After another few weeks she suddenly had no pain and she started to attempt to walk without crutches. Gradually the weak muscles became stronger and the swelling disappeared, not to mention that the accompanying pains in her hips and back had also gone.

She was now walking freely without pain and without crutches, and no painkillers! She also forgot to mention that her carpal tunnel syndrome, gained from ten hours of reflexology per day, had disappeared too! She was also on Detox Essence and Woman's Balance (FE Aus) as well as a special blend from me to clear all the other levels of backlog.

She had a couple of weeks when she couldn't get the supply and the pains started to come back, but not as bad as before. (My feeling was that not all the repairing had been completed.) As soon as she was back on them the pain went and she is now down to one per day as a maintenance dose.

Needless to say, a lot of her clients are on the combination of flower essences and Laminine and their recovery is evident.

MY STORY

After taking Laminine for only a week, although being pretty healthy generally, I discovered my body was working better than ever. I felt as though my energy levels were the same as when I was 16 years old. Full of energy, joie de vivre, with more refreshed sleep, I experienced a sense of being more who I really am, and that anything is possible.

A month on and people are saying: 'Clare, you always look good but you seem to be looking younger and have an extra air of youth about you. Whatever you're doing or taking, I want it!'

Five months on, the reservoir of energy, the ability to sustain my focus and concentration levels for a long period of time has improved dramatically and the general feeling of wellbeing has been sustained.

I'm very impressed so I am recommending it to my Harley Street clients and seeing excellent results.

There are many more positive stories. For supply please see Useful Addresses.

Psychotherapy

Flower remedies are a valuable tool which support psychotherapy and speed up the healing process. Reaching beyond the verbal level, flower remedies are often described as a form of liquid therapy.

Flower essences and orthodox medicine

Many general practitioners realize that stress may be responsible for their patients' health problems, but feel powerless to help. While tranquillizers and other such drugs may help someone over a particularly bad patch, they do not provide the tools needed for dealing with stress. They tend to dull perception and subdue the stress response.

Tranquillizers also have less desirable side-effects and tend to be addictive; coming off them suddenly can give rise to frightening withdrawal symptoms. Flower essences can safely be given to patients to help them cope with their particular source of stress. Many open-minded general practitioners are now adding flower essences such as Star of Bethlehem (B) for general shock to their prescription list.

As a flower essence practitioner you may frequently see patients who want to wean themselves off tranquillizers, antidepressants and any other mood-altering drugs but are worried about withdrawal symptoms. Flower essences can help to free them from their dependency, ease any side-effects and clear the system of any imbalance that has been caused by long-term use of medicinal drugs.

PAST LIFE AND SOUL RETRIEVAL, PSYCHIC PROTECTION

Past-life and soul retrieval issues are usually treated by psychotherapy, hypnotherapy and shamanic healing practices.

Soul retrieval

In the case of soul retrieval, shock, trauma or long, slow stress such as wounding, abuse or rejection will have a powerful effect on the psyche, or soul, resulting in unbalanced beliefs and behavioural patterns. These states are often accompanied by feelings of emptiness or incompletion or lack of self-worth, so when one works with energy or vibrational medicine, it is possible to reclaim these parts of us that have separated for their own protection. It is not uncommon for children who have experienced trauma in childhood to have little or no memory of those years. In the case of shamanic healing ancient universal healing practices have been synthesized and adapted in a form appropriate to contemporary life. These modalities have proved highly effective in dissolving the traumas of past events and, in combination with precisely focused combination flower essences, have proved even more effective.

Past life

There are two ways of looking at this subject, symbolic and mythic, or a reality if one concedes that reincarnation is a possibility.

In the first case, the awareness of a troubling past-life memory may be a genetic or cellular memory, or early forgotten trauma which has become locked deep within the psyche. For some people, a hypnotherapy session may be effective in releasing the toxic energy pattern. For others, shamanic journeying can be a transformative experience. Here the client works with the practitioner to re-experience, heal and gain understanding of the past event. It is sometimes surprising when they may have been the offending party in a relationship, for example, and have been repeating the same personality fault in their current life. Equally, if the client has been the victim this tendency is also continued in their existing relationships with people and events.

Again, the flower remedies offer a profound support for these processes, helping to identify and pinpoint the root cause of the underlying imbalance. Dissolving the negative vibrational resonances makes it easier for the stress pattern to be released during the treatment, allowing the full force of the soul to be integrated into the personality. The flower remedies will stabilize and anchor the reclaimed soul energy to be integrated into the whole being. In the case of past-life healing, the remedies help to dissolve ancient inherited karmic patterns leaving the being free from previous attachments and influences.

Remedies for past-life healing

The following range of flower essences are particularly appropriate for and support shamanic processes.

From the Peter Aziz Shamanic Range and PHI Essences by Andreas Korte.

Past Life Orchid (AK) Assists us in opening the Akashic Records where hidden memories about our life experiences, past, present and future are stored. This essence can reveal deep-rooted causes for many emotional problems.

Release Cactus (AK) Helps us to release old negative patterns. It has a very deep effect as it reaches into the unconscious and even into our cellular awareness. It removes blockages and helps us to regenerate.

Shadow Cactus (AK) Has a releasing effect on the solar plexus; we become conscious of our inner processes and are able to overcome them and then move on. We say goodbye to our shadow and we learn to accept death and to live in total awareness.

Thorne Apple (HUB) A very initiating essence that should be taken with very clear motivation. Helps movement between different planes of consciousness. Breaks limitations in the mind. Seeing beyond life and death.

Yellow Archangel (HUB) For understanding and accepting the balance between light and dark. Puts one in touch with hidden realms, and helps one accept all that may be found in these planes.

Psychic protection

From an ordinary reality perspective, what is termed psychic protection could be the need for protection in what is perceived to be a hostile environment, for example an office environment in which there is a very negative atmosphere with a lot of backbiting and undermining. Most people are instantly aware of this the minute they walk into a room.

Realization is beginning to grow that the human body is not just a collection of solid systems and organs sealed within the skin, but a completely permeable organism, which the latest particle physics experts assure us is composed of pure energy, condensed and organized into different functions. This the ancient masters knew thousands of years ago as they were able to see energy. So this leaves us vulnerable to negative atmospheres or mental or emotional attack. We can also have our energy drained by certain people; this is of course generally completely unconscious. For example, how many of us have visited a hospital and come out completely drained?

There are many energy techniques to deal with this: acupuncture, visualization and various forms of vibrational healing of which flower remedies have proved to be one of the most effective. This works as a preventative by infusing the auric field with protective vibrational energy, or as a healing after a problem by dispelling any negative influences from the system.

Remedies for psychic protection

Angel of Protection Orchid (AK) Enhances communication with our guardian angels.

This essence acts as a protective shield; it is particularly recommended for sensitive people exposed to hostile surroundings who therefore urgently need protection.

Aura Cleansing Cactus (AK) Cleanses and protects the aura, especially on the astral level. For people with a too porous energy field who have problems establishing boundaries between themselves and others. Helps to free the aura from foreign influences.

Crab Apple (B) Cleanses and purifies. Overthrows old negative patterns to help us develop new positive priorities. Use in situations in which we fear being contaminated by others.

Cuckoo Pint (HUB) protects the spirit from invading entities, and quickly rebuilds vital energy when it has been lost. A great ally in soul retrieval.

Deadly Nightshade (HUB) Powerful third-eye stimulant and psychic purge. Clears psychic interference. To be used as a single dose when required.

Larkspur (HUB) Strengthens and clears the aura, particularly the psychic gate. A good protection remedy, it produces a vibration that casts out psychic parasites and external forces.

Lemon (AK) Cleansing and renewal. Removes old unwanted energies from the person.

MEDITATION: STILLING THE MIND AND ATTUNING TO THE ENERGY OF THE FLOWERS

In order to tune into the vibration of flowers and sense their subtle energies it is important to have some ability to still the mind in order to be able to receive the nuances that the flowers' message brings.

Meditation is practised in many philosophies, but to most of us it is associated with the Lord Buddha and has its roots in an ancient Brahmarual tradition born of Hinduism. In this tradition belief in rebirth, and its teachings (dharma) that Sansara (human suffering) can be transcended through individually working for liberation to the state beyond, known as Nirvana, is at the heart of this worldview.

Sacred texts and teachings were written which focused on understanding the mysteries of the universe, the interconnected continuum of life, man's relationship to the Divine, and of meditation as the discipline and concentration of the mind needed in order to achieve self-realization.

In Buddhism, 'attainment' through a form of sitting meditation is the bedrock of its philosophy. The Buddha, known as the awakened one, liberated himself through meditation, and it was his search for truth that led him to attain enlightenment. So when meditating one is tapping into an ancient and sacred lineage.

Gifted modern teachers such as Guy Burgs have benefited from this lineage and have been taught by significant living masters from Burma and Bali. He is known for his penetrating insight into the body/mind connection and its role in the disease process. Burgs purports that the first goal of meditation is to develop a harmonious and balanced mind by strengthening our mental capacity in preparation for higher concentration and meditation.

By working on developing awareness of the cellular and subtle anatomy systems and ensuring the base of the mind is strong, the body is able to provide support to shift stored dysfunctional energy that blocks accessing the high state of mindfulness. In this way a good foundation of energetic support is built in order to progress. Burgs talks of listening to the sound of the heart because it knows only truth and has a higher intelligence that can give the answer to all life's challenges, and suggests that through meditation, if you are able to quiet the mind, learn to listen and hear the silence of the heart you will find the answers already there.

When tuning into the subtle qualities of the flower essence it is helpful to have an experience of quieting the mind to be able to listen with the heart, as the flower's energy often connects with the chakra system, especially directly with the heart chakra, and communication begins from this point. This is beautifully illustrated by SSK in the plate section where she shows a colour impression of how she experiences the process of attunement and communication with Orchids. This is how she receives the information and makes The Dancing Light Orchid Essences.

According to Burgs, the following flower essences will facilitate the meditation processes.

Blue Dragon (Him E) Enhances single-mindedness. Pierces straight into the heart of any matter. Excellent for meditation.

Lotus (Him A) A spiritual elixir and aid to meditation. Calms the mind and improves concentration. Gently releases negative emotions, correcting imbalances. Aligns and balances the chakras by releasing, adding and directing energies to them. Clears the entire system of toxins. Balances, cleanses and strengthens the aura.

Red Lily (FE Aus) The sacred Lotus embodying Aboriginal spirituality. For day-dreamers who are vacant and accident-prone. Balances spiritual and earthly aspects, enabling you to be grounded and practical while evolving spiritually.

White Nymph Waterlily (Aus L) is for uncovering your deepest spiritual core. Brings tranquillity for reaching into the soul and using your Higher Self to integrate and respond to life from a universal rather than personal perspective. Helpful for spiritual practices such as meditation.

For meditation courses with Burgs see Useful Addresses.

HELPING YOURSELF

As a practitioner it is easy to be affected by the problems of others. If steps are not taken to protect your own emotional wellbeing, you could start to feel energetically drained. With this in mind I have composed a special 'practitioner mix' for boosting energy levels and safeguarding against exhaustion:

Delph (AK)

Fringed Violet (FE Aus)

Leafless Orchid (Aus L)

Lotus (AK, Him A)

Healing (Him E)

Use 2 drops of each essence.

CHAPTER EIGHT

RESEARCH IN FLOWER ESSENCE TREATMENTS

PROVING THE ESSENCES WORK

Some people argue that flower essences act as placebos, in other words that they make us feel better simply because we believe they are doing us good.

This does not explain, however, the numerous incidences in which flower essences have brought benefits to animals, babies and young children, who obviously do not know that what they are being given is 'supposed to' bring relief.

To test the placebo argument scientifically, Michael Weisglas, PhD conducted a double-blind test on the Bach Flower Remedies in 1979. Neither he nor his subjects (who were suffering from depression) knew beforehand who had received and taken the remedies and who took the placebos. Results showed that those who were given the remedy mix reported experiencing a feeling of wellbeing, growth and self-understanding and acceptance, a better sense of humour and increased creativity, while those who took the placebo reported no significant change. Dr Weisglas concluded that the effect of the remedies does not depend on the belief or faith of the user.

For at least 15 years I have conducted my own investigations into many flower essences. I have recently tested all the Bach remedies, the Orchids of the Amazon and most of the Californian remedies, as well as many others. During my teaching courses I typically give one particular anonymous remedy to ten people and ask each one to describe its properties. Without fail their descriptions of the essence, its qualities and place of action are accurate.

At their clinic in Delhi, Drs Atul and Pupa Shah (Aditi Himalayan Essences) combine flower essences with other natural therapies such as homeopathy, acupuncture, aromatherapy and crystal therapy. They claim great success in treating all kinds of problems including mental retardation, the problems of childhood, tumours, infertility and pregnancy problems, arthritis and any condition related to stress and tension such as irritable bowel syndrome, insomnia and hypertension. They have also found that flower essences work extremely well in conquering addictions. To prevent their own expectations from getting in the way of their assessments, the Shahs often ask other doctors to assess the improvements in their patients' conditions.

A STUDY ON RADIATION WITH AUSTRALIAN FLOWER ELECTRO ESSENCE

It is notable to mention that there is continued serious concern about the rising levels of radiation and the effect on mankind, and many have been researching into finding solutions to this modern problem as well as other health concerns that are present in our society today. Andrea Korte with his T1 made at Chernobyl, site of the nuclear disaster, that absorbs radiation and the Australian Electro combination essence were both designed in response to those particularly vulnerable to radiation and especially to target the increase in exposure to radioactivity and electromagnetic radiation. This combination and other ranges have practical day-to-day implications, for instance whilst using mobile phones or working on computers.

It seems especially important to use it for our children when they are on their mobiles, chatting and texting, or on computers emailing their friends. Children, whilst they are still in the process of development, are particularly affected by electromagnetic radiation.

In terms of large-scale exposure to radiation, one only needs to remember Chernobyl and the fact that, 20 years on, the fallout from this disaster is continuing to affect millions of people as it spreads further throughout the food chain and water systems. Especially vulnerable were those countries in its direct path or in the vicinity of the winds that carried the fallout from that fateful day of nuclear power plant meltdown.

The republic of Belarus is one such place where the children are now heavily contaminated with high levels of accumulated radioactivity as a direct result of the Chernobyl accident. Australian Bush Flower Essence Company have been donating Electro Essence to the medical team in Belarus for The Radiation Rescue Program as part of their health rehabilitation programme. This specialist team of medical and health professionals takes care of these children on a physical, emotional and psychological level, using many rehabilitation modalities. Recently the team has begun to utilize complementary therapies, and the medical team has discovered the treatment to be the most effective to date as it reduced the radiation levels by 25.3 per cent.

Then they tested Electro Essence on the same children and the results were amazing! The Electro reduced the radiation by 43 per cent in comparison with the control group which had only a 3.5 per cent reduction.

These dramatic results were achieved after only two weeks on a dosage of 4 drops twice a day as opposed to the usual 7-drop dosage. Encouraged by these positive results the Belarus medical team is continuing to administer Electro to the children to find out just what the combination is capable of!

One of the ancillary effects of the Electro has been in treating the condition known as neurocirculatory dystonia syndrome. Its symptoms of fainting, headaches, heart palpitations, feeling as if the heart has stopped were very common when these children physically exerted themselves. However, there was a marked reduction in these symptoms when the children started to take Electro Essence, something that Ian attributed to the action of Waratah in Electro.

The other special ingredients in this combination are Mulla Mulla, which has the ability to address electromagnetic radiation, and Bush Fuchsia, which helps to protect and correct any imbalance that radiation causes. A further blend of Paw Paw, Fringed Violet and Crowea is included to help with blocking the absorption and storage of radiation in the body and helps to expel any already stored so as to keep the body's energy intact and the neurological systems functioning normally.

Generally Electro Essence is used to reduce electrical radiation emitted by meter boxes, overhead power lines, fluorescent lights and electrical equipment, especially televisions and mobile phones. It is useful in radiation therapy where it helps normal healthy cells withstand the radiation and recover after therapy. It has also been useful to negate Earth radiation, found where ley lines cross and in houses where underground streams run.

Carrying a bottle of Electro or T1 (AK) offers protection from absorbing radiation from phones and computers for at least 6–9 months, at which point it then needs to be replaced with a fresh bottle. It is advisable to back this up with a 7-drop dosage at the end of the day, especially if the use has been excessive.

WOMEN'S PROBLEMS

The rising incidents of hormonal imbalance in women is another area of concern. It may be due to stress as well as being caused by the amount of hormones present in our drinking water due to the increased use of the pill.

These factors can upset a woman's delicate balance, and result in PMT, irregular periods, hot flushes, menopausal problems, weight gain and most worryingly, infertility. Ian White as well as others have been working with the flower essence from She Oak and its benefit on the 25 per cent of infertility cases due to unknown causes. He has successfully addressed the infertility that stems from deep emotional causes, and he suggests, from his naturopathic stance, that dehydration of the uterus is one of the causes of infertility. He has discovered, something that the Aboriginal women seem to know instinctively, that She Oak is a tissue rehydrator which will correct the lack of hydration whilst simultaneously balancing the hormonal levels, regulating the cycle and the oestrogen/progesterone levels, which greatly enhances fertility and the ability to conceive. When working with She Oak, Ian and other flower essences practitioners had a 75 per cent success rate, and one Sydney doctor had a success rate of more than 90 per cent!

She Oak is one of the ingredients of Woman Essence and Woman Balance Combination which is designed to harmonize hormonal imbalances, menstrual cramps, PMT, irregular menstruation and weight gain, and has proved to be very good at alleviating hot flushes and the general discomfort of menopause.

In hospitals in Brazil and Switzerland, She Oak and Woman Essence are being successfully used as an alternative to hormone replacement therapy without the increased risk of breast and cervical cancer.

Flower essences are so safe to use that it is one system of complementary medicine that can be given throughout pregnancy without fear of contraindications; in fact they are a tremendous support right from conception through to birth.

She Oak is not the only essence being used successfully in hospitals. Waratah essence has had great success in Brazilian hospitals when used by cardiologists treating heart imbalances, ventricular failure and mitral valve insufficiency. It has also arrested the development of the condition of glaucoma, and in some cases it has even reversed it.

With kind permission of Ian White.

CANCER STUDY USING PETITE FLEUR RANGE

According to Dr Judy Griffin, who has taught in hospitals, hospices and cancer support groups for the last 20 years, research with the Petite Fleur essences has provided some of the most powerful transformations with cancer, in particular Lilac flower essences, which she found released self-healing.

According to Judy's observations and deep understanding of the nature of the disease, cancer occurs on a subtle level, originating from a suppression of emotions and desires, when thought and feeling are suppressed in order to conform to the rules of society, and no alternative expression is substituted. When the emotions attempt to express themselves spontaneously, the intellect puts a block on them by a judgement call; this prevents dispersion of the natural expression of emotion which turns back in on itself. This negative energy collects in the chakras and expresses itself through an immune response, usually in an area of inherited or weakened immunity. As this energy becomes concentrated, abnormal tissue growth may occur forming tumours. However, if the immune system is strong it will respond correctly by surrounding the area with an inflammatory response, attempting to protect it, so cutting off the negative energy feeding it.

The remedies appear to stimulate the electromagnetic charge that normally triggers the helper cells to replace killer cells, and produce new healthy tissue growth. The success in reversing this situation lies in understanding the underlying suppression pattern and how it is expressed through the personality; this is where Petite Fleur Essences can help.

Suggestions for use from Judy in certain situations are as follows:

Blue Danube Aster To enhance antibody production and the power of encouragement.

Bouquet of Harmony Protection.

Christmas Cactus To reinforce strength and focus on what is right.

Dill To overcome the ego and fear of death.

French Lavender To appreciate every blessing and release the need for something very strong to 'kill' cancer.

Gaillardia To enhance macrophage bombardment of foreign matter, and determination.

Iberis Candytuft For self-healing and regeneration.

Indian Paintbrush For a success consciousness.

Lilac To release suppressed energy and let go of past hurts.

Old Blush Stamina.

Rose Campion For an inherited or predisposition for an illness.

Wandering Jew To overcome discouragement.

To any of these add from the following list for specific cancers:

Bone cancer Crossandra, White Rose and Sunflower, then African Violet, Borage and Viridflora.

Brain and neurological cancer Stock, Echinacea, Verbena, then Iris, Azalea and Sweet Annie.

Breast cancer Chamomile, Pansy, Zinnia and Lemongrass, then India Hawthorn, Crepe Myrtle, Wisteria.

Colon cancer Garden Mum, Poppy, Periwinkle and Bougainvillea, then Black Mushroom, Dandelion and Rosemary.

Kidney/prostate cancer Combine Marigold, Meadow Sage and Lilac, then Red Carnation, Pansy and Bachelor's Button.

Leukemia (and bone marrow cancer) Jasmine, Dianthus, Red Malva, then Yarrow, Wandering Jew and Anemone.

Liver cancer Pink Geranium, Chamomile and Silver Moon, then Abate Anger, Bougainvillea and Wisteria. Add White Petunia for gallbladder.

Lung cancer Babies' Breath, Spike Lavender and Thyme, then Poppy, Lantana and Morning Glory.

Lymphomas Soapwort, Salad Burnet and Tansy, then Lobelia, Cinnamon Basil and Curry.

Ovarian or testicular cancer Japanese Magnolia, Marigold, Ligustrum, then Self-Image, White Hyacinth and Bluebonnet.

Pancreatic cancer Primrose, Moss Rose, Mexican Hat, then Mexican Bush Sage, Bouquet of Harmony and Yarrow.

Sarcomas from HIV Silver Lace, Aquilegia Columbine, Lilac and Marigold.

Stomach cancer Peppermint, Bamboo, Snapdragon, then Amaryllis, Lily and Magnolia.

Uterine cancer Lilac, Marigold, Carrot and Ranunculus, then Madame Louise Levique, Marie Pavie, Marquis Bocella.

To help block metastasis and re-entry of cancerous cells Tansy, Lobelia and Snapdragon, then Dill, Yarrow and Wild Oats.

With kind permission of Dr Judy Griffin.

Another area of research involves observing the changes in the body's energy field after a patient has taken different essences. I asked Harry Oldfield to use his electro-scanning machine (which in effect photographs the aura) in an attempt to see what happened when certain flowers and their essences were introduced into my energy field. Looking at Figures 1 and 2 (see page 29 of colour plate) it seems clear that flower essences indeed have a measurable effect. This surely paves the way for further research into this field of investigation.

THE EFFECT OF DELPH ESSENCES ON BRAIN WAVE PATTERNS

In the area of the flower essence research academy, there are several scientists and physicians investigating the bio-information of flower essences. We have scientific support with regard to effect of essences from, among others, Dr Garcia from Geneva with opto-crystallography research and Günter Haffelder with his electroencephalograph (EEG) research to capture brain activity (in collaboration with various experts in the fields of biology, education, psychology, medicine and information technology).

Some fascinating research into the effect of essences on brain activity has been carried out on Andreas Korte Delph Essences by academic and medical doctors. The study was carried out by Dr Garcia (opto-crystallographic research) and Mr Haffelder (EEG research). The EEG monitors the brain's electrical activity (oscillations per second: hertz) when someone is exposed to different stimuli. It is divided into four frequency ranges or bands:

- the Waking state, BETA
- relaxed concentration, ALPHA
- full relaxation and dreams, THETA
- Deep Sleep state, DELTA.

In his Institute for Communication and Brain Research in Stuttgart, for the past 20 years, Günter Haffelder has further developed EEG measuring techniques for the study and analysis of brain waves. He is able to decompose (i.e. split into parts) the signals recorded by the EEG into their individual vibration components using sophisticated techniques of spectral analysis.

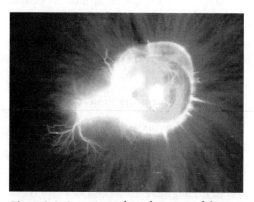

Figure 8.1: One way to show the power of the essences is with Kirlian photography. Every essence shows its own energy structure. This is Kirlian photography of Aggression Orchid.
With kind permission of Andreas Korte.

As a result, he is able to detect very subtle changes in brain wave vibration due to external stimuli, and identify the specific brain structures that are affected. He does this with the aid of a chronospectrogram, a 3D visualization of brain activity depicting the interplay of the individual brain wave vibrations, divided by the right and left hemispheres, and how they change over time. This procedure is analogous to recording an orchestral performance and analysing it to produce a musical score; different instruments (brain structures) can then be identified by their characteristic frequency range, and one can look at the effect that the conductor (external stimulus) has on the music.

Using this precise method, holding a bottle of Delph Essences in the hand was proved to be enough to change the individual brain wave patterns (see page 29 of plate section). This demonstrates that a change of consciousness can occur simply by holding a bottle of essence or flower remedy. This is something that highly tuned individuals are already fully aware of but it is refreshing to note that there are pioneers willing to explore, and find ways of recording, these subtleties.

Chapter NINE

THE EVOLUTION OF THERAPY WITH ESSENCES

Andreas Korte

It is my great pleasure to introduce you to Andreas Korte, who is a truly uniquely gifted pioneer and expert in the field of vibrational remedies and medicine.

Andreas Korte is a researcher and specialist in the field of essences. Brought up in a small village by a forest near Lake Constance in Germany, he has always believed in the flower devas. He regards Orchids as queens of the plant kingdom, feeling that they have an exceptionally high vibrational rate and are responsible for creating a link between the cosmos, ourselves and the Earth. The Orchids often take the form or shape of angels and appear to have human features.

Andreas has invented a gentle, ecological method of preparing essences so that the flowers are not harmed in any way. This involves cleaning and preparing one half of a quartz geode (a naturally occurring stone containing crystals split into two semi-spherical halves) and filling it with natural spring water. He then carefully places the geode into the energetic field of the blossoms and leaves it in the sun for a length of time (which differs from flower to flower). The special crystal formation of the geode acts to focus and capture the energy of the flowers.

Co-author of *Orchids, Gemstones and Their Healing Energies*, Andreas is currently involved in research projects in Europe, Africa and South America. With the Delph Essences (see page 110) he has conducted research into their effectiveness with water activation, illustrated in his book *Dolphins and Whales* and in Chapter 8.

He has developed a unique method which involves light and multilevelled use of all his essences called Light Treatment, as well as creating combinations which address the mind/body and spirit.

Andreas has a unique take on the evolution of therapy with essences and here I will let him elaborate.

ESSENCES AND THEIR LEVELS OF DEVELOPMENT

The biological origin of an essence (i.e. where it is grown or formed, whether it is of a plant, flower, mushroom, gem or environmental origin, etc.) provides us with an indication of how and in what way each of the essences acts on the human being. We distinguish the following essence groups according to various biological levels.

Gem essences: the root to Earth

Essences that are made from the Earth's physical environment are designed to root you to the Earth: the essences of gems, semiprecious stones and crystals are already well-known and used by many. They are the highest and purest manifestation of the mineral kingdom and, with some exceptions, share a similar effect on the body, such as grounding and balancing the physical energy. (*I have included a section on gems and their essences in Section K of the Encyclopedia.*)

Mushroom essences: the door to the subconscious

The next level to minerals are the plant and fungi kingdoms, which also include mushrooms. What is generally known about mushrooms is that they simply are the carrier of spores, but they are far more complex. The Mushroom is in actual fact the mycelium, the fibrous network that grows underground and is hidden from view. As an essence the Mushroom acts on aspects that we are not ready to see and which lie dormant deep in our subconscious. They also act on the body by effect on physical processes. Like the Mushroom itself, which is seen for a brief period in autumn, these aspects can remain hidden inside ourselves.

In this respect it is interesting to note that lichens also have a special place and part to play. Lichens are a result of a combination of a species of algae and species of fungus functioning together as symbiotic organisms. Some lichens are real survivors and are capable of growing where other species can't survive, for example, on bare rock or colonizing on solidified lava. Essences of lichens reinforce our vital Qi and our strength to survive.

Flower essences: provide emotional balance

All flowering plants share the same characteristic that they are connected to the land and gain sustenance through their roots, so are united with the Earth's physical environment.

Most of the flowers' active energy is found above the surface. So it makes sense that flowers' essence effect would be felt more in the vibrational environment that is above the Earth, while still maintaining its connection to the Earth's inner environment.

In us humans the flower's essence has an emotional compensating effect (according to each individual orientation) in the astral and ethereal environment of the body. The development of a person is shown through his feelings and emotions; that is why flower essences are important for the personality's developmental processes. They can help to release and clear fears and blocked emotions resulting in the continuation of personal development.

Orchid essences: spiritual development

Orchid essences are a specialty and represent the culmination of creation in the plant kingdom. They are the last development of evolution in the plant kingdom. The orchids belong to a 'new era' of plants. They have become so specialized in the search of light that in the extreme they are said to 'climb up' trees. Similar to the epiphyte plants group, together with the *tillandsias* and the *bromeliads*, their roots are no longer fixed to the land, but to the trees. It is interesting to observe that they always live in a symbiotic relationship with a mushroom that makes use of the tree organic material (for example, old leaves and cortical substrate) which it puts at the disposal of the plant. Nevertheless, the Orchids are, by nature, the queens of the air and they feed chiefly off water and sunlight (cosmic energy). The implication for us is that the Orchid flower's essence transmits to us cosmic light and enhances our ability to open our conscience to higher knowledge.

THE ORIGINAL CRYSTAL METHOD OF PREPARING ESSENCES

In my personal evolution as producer of flower essences, I sought to discover an alternative method to the traditional classical production method already in place, that is, the solar and cooking preparations, in order to obtain the mother tincture. The fact that such methods required cutting and removing the blossom from its plant has always seemed a contradiction to me, and caused pain to the plant. The healthier the flower is, the better will be its quality and ability to heal people. For that reason, I designed the crystal production method, which consists of taking the information from the flower in a similar way to taking a photograph. Just as in photography a light-sensitive film captures a given image, the crystal transmits the vibrations of the flowers directly into the water that acts as a liquid medium that captures its energetic vibrational image. This dispenses with the need to pick the plants, leaving each and every plant absolutely intact and with no damage caused, therefore conserving all the healing qualities inherent in its bloom. The essences prepared this way are of a high vibrational quality.

ESSENCES: USAGE

Essences can be used both internally and externally. Their effect can be perceived as soon as they are in contact with the person's auric field. For this reason, it is enough to apply the essence externally to any one of the 12 cutaneous regions or on the corresponding chakra. Adding it to the bath water can also have the desired effect. In external application of the essence, it can be mixed with ointments and dermatological creams (between 7 and 9 drops). Generally, the essence is applied twice a day (morning and afternoon), using about 2 to 4 drops each time, or directly on the cutaneous region or chakra. In cases of emergency, the frequency of use should be increased to intervals of five minutes.

When the application is internal the essence is diluted. It is very important here to understand that the effect does not depend on the quantity, but with the frequency of application. Generally, the dilution should be administered three times a day with 5 drops

of essence each time. In a 30ml bottle put a third part of high-quality cognac or brandy and two thirds with spring water; to this add 7 droplets of the essence. Close it and shake it; this action allows the information of the essence to be transferred to the water. Alcohol is only used for preservation purposes; for a child, cider vinegar or vegetable glycerin is used instead. It can also be diluted in water, but here the recommended quantities for the dilution will be smaller, due to the short longevity period, and it should be consumed in a few days.

ESSENCE COMBINATIONS AND THEIR CONSERVATION

As each case is unique, different essences can be combined. The essences used will depend entirely on the needs of the person. There are methods of diagnoses to help verify which are the essences needed. However, if after testing there are several different essences to be used at different intervals and/or frequency, it is recommended to administer the essences separately. The best place to keep the essences is a wood cabinet, far away from direct sunlight and from electromagnetic fields.

TESTING FOR THE ESSENCES

When choosing an essence, whether for yourself or others, the choice should not be by intellectual means alone. The first principle before making a choice is to be free of any preconceived ideas and approach with the intuitive mind.

Flowers and gem cards: usage

There are essence cards for most traditional essences: flower (Bach), gems or Orchids. Place the cards in front of you, concentrate on your problem and choose the illustration (or illustrations) to which you are attracted and compare it with the description of the flower.

Using the pendulum

See pages 61–62.

Diagnosis by muscle testing

Another method of diagnosis is the muscle testing or Applied Kinesiology as applied in physiotherapy. Muscle testing corresponds to and registers the biological feedback from the body and was developed by Dr George Goodheart in the United States. It is a reliable method with which to choose essences for others. However, this test needs a certain amount of sensitivity and use of intuition in order to read the muscular reactions which often can be barely noticeable. It takes practice to use this method with confidence.

1. The person to be tested should be standing (wristwatch having been removed). The left arm hangs down loosely; the right is extended at 90 degrees and parallel to the floor.

2. Stand in front of the person. Put your right hand on their left shoulder for stability and the left hand on the wrist of the extended arm.

3. Explain that you will push the extended arm indicating the direction of the movement (usually down).

4. Return to the initial position and explain that when you reattempt to push the arm downward they are to resist the pressure.

5. So the subject is not taken by surprise say, 'hold' before pushing the arm slowly and evenly downwards.

Note: Muscle testing is not a test of strength, but more about feeling the muscle's tension. Only enough pressure to feel the resistance is required, so it is quite subtle! The test person should expend just enough energy required to resist downward movement when the tester gently pushes the arm down. Initially this is difficult, so the test should be repeated several times to be sure.

With practice you will be able to recognize the differences in the body's varying reactions. A weak muscle response suggests the body is saying that it does not agree, 'no' in other words. If the muscle appears to test 'strong', the body is indicating that it agrees and is saying 'yes'.

With the box of flower essences in front of you test which essence is the one that is needed.

Place the chosen essence in the person's left hand and ask: Is this the essence that is needed right now? (The question can also be asked in the mind.) Repeat the muscle testing and continue in this way until you have tested several essences.

This is also the way to determine how many different essences are needed, how frequently and how long they should be administered. Here the subject should ask: Do I need two (three, four, etc.) essences? After each question, carry out the muscle testing until you are sure how many essences the subject needs. Similarly determine the individual dosage and length of treatment.

Diagnosis through pulse testing

This testing method originates from Chinese medicine and is a kind of diagnosis skill that needs practice and requires a strongly developed sensitivity in the fingertips. Despite this, it is a very reliable method of diagnosis. As if it has an interior pendulum, our body reacts to different substances when in contact with them. This way the body's reactions to different essences can be verified.

1. In general, the pulse is always taken on the inside of the wrist with the thumb extended, where either one or traditionally three fingers are placed (the index, the middle or the ring finger are recommended, as the thumb already has a pulse so is not to be used).

2. Take the person's hand, placing your finger(s) on his or her wrist pulse while holding the test essence in the other

hand and slowly introduce it to the person's body by degrees. As soon as the essences come into contact with the astral body (about 40cm of distance from the subject's physical body) you will be able to detect a brief reaction which shows up as a disturbance of the pulse rhythm: it won't speed up or slow, but rather you will perceive it as *enlivened* and *intensified.*

3. Continue moving the essence closer, about 15 or 20cm from the subject's body, where you will detect some brief and intense pulsating. At this point, contact is made with the energetic body and the pulsating will normalize as the essence almost touches the subject's physical body. You should be able to perceive a change in the pulse. Now that the physical body is in contact with the essence the pulse will normalize again. Once the body has integrated the essence's energy, the pulse is stabilized.

4. As a test, try with a harmful substance, that is, a toxin. The body will react violently, accelerating the pulse, a clear indication that 'it doesn't want it'. When the toxin is removed, the pulse *will* calm down again.

When you test for flower essences, you will note that the body's reactions are positive. That is to say, the body accepts the energies as a positive force. The pulse will calm down as soon as the essence remains on the skin for a while. Once the pulse goes back to normal, withdraw the essence from the energetic and the astral body, then count the pulse beat, until it weakens. When the pulse is stronger, the body is saying: 'Why do you take the essence away? I want the energy.' As the result can vary by at most two beats, count the beats and then make a control test. If you detect more than seven beats in the subject until normalization, you can deduce that, for the moment, it is the correct essence for that person. Try it with different essences and you will check how well the body knows what is best for it or what energy it needs urgently.

NUMBER OF ESSENCES USED IN DILUTION

When using Korte essences I would like to recommend, if you are just starting to explore using essences, mixing the minimum number together (for example, two to three). This is due to the fact that each essence has its own unique effect and influence on particular levels. If you mix many essences that address specific imbalances, the final result is an unbalancing effect. It is best to address any imbalances sequentially, and take into account their influence on the personality. Orchid essences generally should not be mixed with other essences because of their potent, varied and powerful energy fluctuations.

CHAKRAS: ENERGY REGULATING CENTRES; SECONDARY CHAKRAS

NB, here is extra information from Andreas to complement Chapter 2 on the chakra system.

Chakras are part of our body's subtle energy centres. We already are aware we have seven main chakras or energy centres; a plus is the additional chakras in the hands and feet and the so-called higher chakras.

Secondary chakras: hands

Situated in the centre of palms of the hands, they regulate the energy exchange with the outside. The energy colour associated is white.

Properties: Harmony, receiving information and energy exchange, clarity, externalization of energy.

Changes of energy flow: Externalizing insufficient capacity, poor blood circulation in hands, and lack of sensitivity.

Secondary chakras: feet

These are found in the soles of the feet; they connect the body and all chakras to the Earth. Their associated energy colour is black.

Properties: Union with the Earth, balance, endurance, stability.

Changes of energy flow: Escape from the world, neglect of bodily needs, disharmony, and discomfort in the legs.

Upper/higher chakras

During our youth, we accumulate experience in the energy centres found in and above the head. The upper chakras connect us with our creative abilities of which we are not yet aware, with our Higher Self and also the divine consciousness. At this moment in our evolution, we are more aware of our energy centres, and are able to utilize their qualities just when we need it in order to cope with the challenges and new forms of energy that we are now experiencing on the planet. Orchid essences have a strong vibrational effect on the higher chakras.

The **eighth chakra** is connected with the right brain, where intuitive thinking resides. At this point, located above the seventh chakra, the soul is united with the Monad (Greek for 'unity').

The **ninth chakra** corresponds to the third-eye chakra and the left brain that is responsible for logical thinking.

The **tenth chakra** is assigned to a superior quality of creativity.

The **eleventh chakra** is the centre that remains attached to each and every one of the cell nuclei of our physical body.

The **twelth chakra** represents direct union with the divine source.

The Orchids, which grow as epiphytes, are linked to the higher chakras through their effect. Thus, they promote and enhance contact between people and the Earth with the cosmos and the different areas of the invisible world of angels. They could be defined as the highest development level of plant evolution.

THE RAINFOREST

This area of the Amazon is the largest and the oldest rainforest on our planet, and hosts an infinite variety of life forms. Whether we allow ourselves to glide on a boat in one of the Amazon's many meandering tributaries or walk through and explore the deep lush green native forest we immediately notice the immense variety and abundance of insects, plants and animals closely packed together that have made the jungle their home. This great variety of species has also been documented in a research project carried out by the University of Bogota (Colombia). Just on the trunk of a single giant tree of the Amazon forest you can find countless species of insects, as many as in England and Ireland put together.

No matter where one is in the forest, one will feel the intensity of life that surrounds one. The warble of the iridescent and colourful birds combines with the shrieks of the monkeys and the buzz of the insects. Here, everything blends together to orchestrate a magnificent concert of the sounds of nature in front of a lush green backdrop. The tree trunks, the lianas and the aerial roots characterize and give shape and form to the image.

No matter where you look, you will discover new life forms: mushrooms of every dimension and magnificent colours imaginable, multicoloured birds, paradisiacal butterflies and animals. The tropical forest is characterized by two special features: first by its division into three distinct levels, each with its own living community and relationship between its life forms; and, second, the way in which each life form is nourished. The level closest to the ground is where we find poor lighting and is the dark zone. This landscape is formed by the large anchoring and wader roots of the trees, shrubs and small palms. At the next level, we find the tallest bushes and trees that are 5 to 20m high. Here you'll find insects and animals completely different to that of the lower level. There are also many more flowers at this level. The third level is at about 25 to 35m high consisting of the canopy of the rainforest, the area that lets the light in. At this height we find a great diversity of really incredible species. Many of the mammals, birds and amphibians that live here never touch the forest floor. At the topmost of the branches of these giant trees, which plant their roots on a thin humus layer of only 8cm, bloom the Orchids, which, along with other epiphytic plants, lead an independent life from the tree. They grow as queens of the air facing the sun and the stars.

Tropical rainforest

The imposing giant trees of the forest grow on a comparatively thin layer of humus of about 8cm thick. As opposed to the trees that absorb the nutrients from the soil through the roots, in the rainforest nourishment comes from above. Falling leaves and animal droppings are broken down by millions of insects and fungi that live in the humus in a very short time and reabsorbed by the tree through its roots.

Depending on the composition of the soil and on the speed of the river, its waters are clear and light or dark and muddy. In this river, there are about 4000 different species of fish.

Amazon natives have a beautiful and wise ancient saying about the four brothers, which is as follows:

Human beings will never dominate the Amazon.

Here reign the four brothers, jungle, river, rain and Earth.

If one dies, all of them die, and with them the Amazon dies too.

If you destroy the jungle, the rain will cease, the land will crumble and the river will dry.

If the rain does not come, the jungle will disappear, the land will dry and the river will dry.

If the land is bare, the forest will die, the rain will not fall again and the river will dry up.

If the river is no longer flowing, the jungle will die, it will not rain and the Earth will become rock.

These brothers are of divine origin. At the beginning, the Amazon was also considered a 'deity temple' on the planet (where the plant spirits and other beings reside). Amazon natives have always known this; that is why they respect their land, as well as the four brothers and sisters, because their hearts were filled with humility.

These days, arrogance and confusion have led us to a critical situation. On the other hand, human communities are becoming more global; that is to say, there are increasingly close contacts between its members, whether through direct contact, or indirectly through the word, the image or trade relations. We are on the threshold to a united world. With regards to survival, however, we are at the edge of a precipice.

Nevertheless, neither reason nor the muses have abandoned us completely. The new task for humanity is the conservation of nature. This will be a peaceful crusade, one that will change both our spirit and our worldview. It will also help us to change our production processes, our way of trading and, of course, our habits of consumption, in order to be healthy and happy in a natural way.

Human culture will begin again to find the essence of the divine in nature. The rediscovery of contemplation, the return to revelation and inner experience of the eternal and infinite: this is the true liberation of human nature.

Antonio Villa-Lopera,
General Director of Forestry and Wildlife
Amacayacu National Park (Parque Nacional de Amacayacu), Colombia, 1991

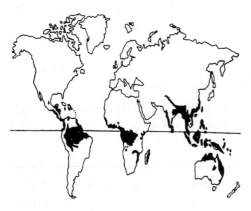

Figure 9.1: Rainforests.

Adapted from BUND.
Wolfgang Fremuth: Tropische Regenwilder.
BUNDfakten Bundfür Umwelt und Naturschutz
Deutschland e. V (BUND), 1990

THE AMAZON RIVER

The Amazon River flows through the South American continent over 5000 kilometres parallel to the Equator. Its water surface covers about 7,000,000 square kilometres. With its branches and tributaries it looks like an immense tree of life that connects the two hemispheres of the planet.

THE CENTRE OF THE EARTH

Observing the shape of the human body, we notice that it consists of two mirror images, the axis of which is a line running along the spine. If we compare the energy structure of man we will see that our seven chakras are also arranged on this line.

If now we observe Planet Earth's structure, we will notice this same division into two halves. From the Equator, representing the planet's axis, the different climatic zones, savannahs, steppes, etc., extend North as well as South. Again there is the importance of the central axis as energy centre. Together with important natural deposits of precious stones and species-rich coral reefs in the oceans, in the rainforests along the Equator we find the

greatest riches of species of animals, insects and plants. It is here where Orchids live, epiphytes representing the higher level in the evolution of plants.

ORCHIDS AND THEIR ESSENCES

In Europe, including the Mediterranean basin, we can find a total of 264 different species of Orchids. In the tropical rainforests exists an unbelievable abundance. Orchids belong to the youngest variety of plants in the evolution of the plant kingdom. With around 25,000 to 35,000 different species identified throughout the world, Orchids have developed the most perfect form of expression. This extends to imitate shapes of insect, organs and symbols. Especially noticeable are those Orchids that even take on the shape of angels.

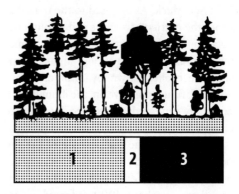

Figure 9.2: Temperate zones.
1. *Earth*
2. *Dead plants*
3. *Live plants*

Due to the cold winters, only a portion of the waste (leaves, etc.) becomes minerals. Only a substance partially transformed – the terrestrial substrate – meets with the function of food reserves.

Adapted from BUND.

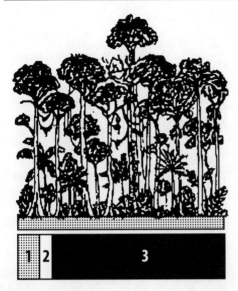

Figure 9.3: Rainforest.
1. *Earth*
2. *Dead plants*
3. *Live plants*

The organic waste decomposes quickly. The forest soil retains only a small amount of it. About 90 per cent of the food reserves is accumulated among the alive vegetation.

Adapted from BUND.

This magnificent pictorial language, with its exuberance of forms and colours, points to the highest energy specialization of Orchids.

Orchids of Europe and the Mediterranean region are, like other plants and flowers, rooted to the Earth and thus directly united to it. Therefore, their energy effect is directly related to the human body; that is to say, they address our seven chakras and they show their action especially in the astral body. The Orchids of the Amazon, due to the light conditions, have evolved in such a way that many species no longer have their roots in the ground; instead they serve to attach themselves as guests to the crown of the trees in the upper level of the jungle. Here, at a height of about 25 or 35m, they lead a life independent of the tree, like other epiphytes.

What does it mean that these plants are no longer in direct contact with the ground? On the energy level, it means that their effects are focused on the area of the emotional and ethereal body. Just as they grow at the top of the trees, which energetically represent the astral body, so their effect begins there and then will go far beyond. As described in the Chakras section, pages 115–6, they are related to the higher chakras, or to the information level.

Orchid essences as a group represent the highest level of energy among the flower essences. As already mentioned, Orchids no longer have any direct contact with the Earth. From the point of view of energy, they live above the astral body which is represented by the tree. Orchids vibrate on the level of angels establishing the link cosmos–individual–Earth. They put us in contact with the various cosmic levels of the angels' love and they permit us to transmit this experience to the Earth, thus helping to heal us and the planet.

It is no coincidence that exactly at the beginning of Age of Aquarius our attention is drawn to Orchid essences. Just as there is an increasing number of people who develop spiritually, there will be increasingly more people who will be attracted to Orchid essences, which will accelerate this evolution as the action of individual Orchid essences is highly vibrational, and each flower has a gem assigned for grounding.

It is best to use a gem essence first, then work on the emotional level with flowers, and only work with Orchid essences after the first two. If new to Orchid essences please *never* mix Orchid essences together and at first use the essence separately.

For Andreas's full range of essences, see section A 'Africa and the Amazon' in Part III.

PART III

ENCYCLOPEDIA OF FLOWER ESSENCES

INTRODUCTION

This Encyclopedia section is a compilation of flower essences from all around the world. Each floral family offers a wide variety of different essences, many of which are made from flowers that grow locally or are indigenous to a particular country.

You will notice that the properties of one type of flower, for instance Chamomile, may vary slightly according to the family to which it belongs. Just as wines from different regions have their own distinct characteristics, so have flowers. The same rose growing wild in the hedgerows of Britain may have slightly different qualities to that found several thousand miles away in New Zealand, due to differences in habitat, climate and so forth. The description of each flower essence also depends on the interpretations of the person who discovered and originally prepared it.

The essences listed address a broad spectrum of physical, emotional, mental as well as spiritual issues. You may wonder why it is important to have so many different essences at hand, but once you begin to use the remedies this will become clear. As your awareness expands, there will be times when you find that you need remedies of an increasingly refined or higher vibration.

FLOWER ESSENCE FAMILIES
A. Africa and the Amazon

PHI Essences by Andreas Korte (AK)

Amazonian Shamanic Sacred Tree Essences (AmT)

Spirit of Makasutu Essences (West Africa, Gambia) (SME)

B. Australia, Japan and Thailand

Flower Essences of Australia (FE Aus)

Living Essences of Australia and the Life Academy (Aus L)

Japanese Essences (Aus LJ)

Flowers of the Orient (FO)

C. New Zealand

First Light Flower Essences of New Zealand (NZ)

D. Europe

Bach Flower Remedies (B)

Bailey Flower Essences (Bal)

Findhorn Flower Essences of Scotland (F)

Harebell Remedies (Hb)

Green Man Tree Essences (GM)

Sun Essences (Sun)

Wildflower Essences of England (WF)

Habundia Shamanic Flower Essences (HUB)

Channel Island Flower Essences (Chi)

Deva Flower Elixirs (Dv)

Mediterranean Essences (Med)

Bloesem Remedies Nederland (Blos)

Russian Essences (Aus L Rus)

E. India

Himalayan Aditi Flower Essences (Him A)

Himalayan Flower Enhancers (Him E)

F. USA, South America and Canada

Alaskan Flower and Environmental Essences (Ask)

Dancing Light Orchid Essences (DL)

Desert Alchemy Flower Essences (DAl)

Flower Essence Society (FES)

Spirit in Nature/Master's Flower Essences (Ma)

Green Hope Farm Flower Essences (GH)

Hawaiian Gaia Flower Essences (Haii)

Pacific Essences of Canada (Pac)

Pegasus Essences (Peg)

Petite Fleur Essences (PF)

Star Peruvian Essences (Peru)

Butterfly Essences (Bfy)

G. Shamanic Essences

Habundia Flower Essences (HUB) (See Europe)

Jaguar Calling Essences (Jag)

H. Essences for Babies and Children

Spirit in Nature/Master's Flower Essences for Mother and Child (Ma)

Bloesem Flower Essences and the Children Vortex (Blos)

I. Essences for Pets and Animals

Spirit in Nature/Master's Flower Essences for Pets (Ma)

Sun Essences for Animals (Sun)

Dancing Light Happy Pet (DL)

Star Peruvian Essences (Peru)

Bloesem Remedies Nederland (Blos)

J. Environmental and Sound Essences

Alaskan Environmental Essences (Ask E)

Sound Wave Essences (SW)

K. Crystal and Gem Essences

Andreas Korte PHI Gem and Crystal Essences (AKGem)

Pacific Gem Essences of Canada (Pac G)

Findhorn Gem Essences (FH Gem)

A.

AFRICA AND THE AMAZON

The Amazon is home to a vast number of different species of flowering plants. In Colombia, for example, more than 4000 species of orchid can be found, many of which live 25–35m (80–115ft) up in the trees. Here, at the top of the tropical rainforests, they obtain sufficient light to support their existence. Their roots have adapted to anchor them to the branches so they have no direct contact with the Earth. The continent of Africa has many regions of total wilderness and is also home to many unusual flowering plants, as well as many that have yet to be discovered. It was the promise of such untapped potential that attracted Andreas Korte to these subtropical regions in his quest for new and unique flower essences. The names of some of the flowers from which he prepares his essences are protected because they are so rare – to these he gives only code letters/numbers.

PHI ESSENCES BY ANDREAS KORTE (AK)

Orchids of the Amazon

Aggression Orchid (*Acineta superba*)
Essence effect: Frees and transforms blockages in lower root chakra. Releases blocked, basic energy, sexuality, impulsiveness and aggression. This powerful essence should be used sparingly and with conscious positive intent. If any feelings regarding sexuality are not expressed or when aggression and anger isn't transformed, this creates blockages in the root chakra resulting in lack of vitality, weakness

and abdominal disorders. Supports the process that helps to discover vitality as a true 'act of liberation' for the personality. Stimulation of the first chakra can lead to an increase of the Kundalini energy. This is a very powerful essence and should only be used once it has been tested and administered after expert analysis. It directs the energy of the root chakra to the higher chakras; therefore it is important that these are opened so that the energy can flow properly. This Orchid serves to reset chakras and the flow of energy between them and helps to experience new spiritual knowledge and to integrate into daily life.
Affirmation: I accept my feelings and I transform my aggression.
Corresponding gem essence: Elestial Crystal.

Amazon (*Preparation of the Amazon River*)
Essence effect: Brings us into contact with the powerful energy of the Amazon, which awakens the understanding of our planet and of every being inhabiting it. For loosening energetic blockages; pain that causes muscle tension often has its origin in negative situations or negative feelings, especially in the back. Strengthens the ability to develop more 'support' to deal with stressful situations calmly. Eliminates most physical blocks. It can be applied directly on the outer ear with two cotton swabs. The 'triangular fossa' is stimulated with the tip of the cotton swab. The 'triangular fossa' represents the energy of the backbone. So, the call of the essence is transmitted with energy through the nervous system and

the vital energy is set in motion. Brings free-flowing energy, helps us to be in touch with the centre of the Earth and aware of other dimensions relying on the Earth's protection and helps develop understanding and comprehension of the planet.

Affirmation: I am in touch with the centre of the Earth and I let my energy flow freely.

Corresponding gem essence: Aquamarine.

Angel Orchid (*Epidendrum secundum*)

Essence effect: For opening up to higher states of consciousness. Brings lightness, stepping up the vibrational rate in order to open us to the higher levels of consciousness in a safe manner and allow communication with our spirit guide (guardian angel). In order to ascend to higher levels of consciousness, a lighter and faster body vibration is also required. Blocked emotions that have so far prevented us from achieving or from experiencing higher levels of consciousness can be cleared. Communication improves, it enables us to hear clearly everything said and experienced and prompts the expansion of our consciousness upwards, until we are in contact with the level of the angels, giving us the ability to reach out and communicate with the angels.

Affirmation: I'm light and I join the angels.

Corresponding gem essence: Blue Tourmaline (indigolite).

Angel of Protection Orchid (*Miltonia phalaenopsis*)

Essence effect: For fragile, sensitive people who need shelter from hostility and harsh environments. Provides a protective umbrella or shield around them to deal with the hostile unfriendly environment to which they feel exposed. When sensibilities and vulnerabilities create weakness, as well as agitation and irritability, it reinforces our self-confidence to quickly identify and deal with attacks. Creates the kind of mental strength and stability that exerts a positive influence so we feel safe enough to open to higher vibrations. Deepens our inner knowledge and improves our communication with our spirit guides and

guardian angel making it easier for us to get help from the spiritual world.

Affirmation: My guardian angel guides me and protects me and I trust him.

Corresponding gem essence: Black Tourmaline (chorlo).

Channelling Orchid (*Oncidium incurvum*)

Essence effect: For increasing direct contact and communication with your spirit guide or our original source, universal being and to listen to the 'inner voice'. Allows channelling – the receiving and passing on of messages transmitted through us. The work of a medium requires not only cooperation with spirit and soul but also our body and when the messages flow through it requires a great amount of energy and vitality. Unless able to replenish themselves it can leave a medium worn out emotionally and physically exhausted. Helps to clear the residue of emotional toxicity, to recover and regenerate physically as well as emotionally. In order to perform the work of mediation of spiritual messages, energy and clarity is needed.

Links to all 12 chakra and to the Divine Source and stimulates the direct contact with our spiritual guides so then you are able to obtain messages and to share them.

Affirmation: Light is in me. I listen to my inner voice.

Corresponding gem essence: Diamond.

Chocolate Orchid (*Stanhopea wardii*)

Essence effect: For those who need to open themselves to more pleasure, who take spirituality too seriously to continue our journey in life with joy. Freedom from self-imposed limits and structures and spiritual limitations allows you to walk the path of joy. An incorrect perception produces spirituality with a stubborn exaggerated seriousness which creates a tendency towards bitterness. The Orchid with its 'sweetening' vibrations helps us to leave the 'valley of tears and difficulties' and to enjoy the best of life; this 'sweetness of life' can also be experienced on the spiritual level. Appropriate for macrobiotic people who think that everything should be exact, are very strict with themselves and often have a sad and dry face. When painful emotions are released, what follows is the disappearance of negative restrictive structures of thought, which allows us to feel and express our emotions with more spontaneous happiness. We will feel that we are taken care of in a marvellous way, that we are guided and that we are granted the 'permission' to love enjoying life (not to suffer it).

Affirmation: I love myself. I enjoy myself here and now.

Corresponding gem essence: Citrine.

Color Orchid (*Oncidium lanceanum*)

Essence effect: For those who have a tendency to be sad and think life is grey and hopeless. Helps you to recognize that your thoughts determine perceptions (we are what we think, because the way we think determines our experiences) and guide our life's direction. Releases dark thoughts, conflicts, disappointment, sadness, lack of love, feelings of desolation, allowing the recognition that our thoughts determine the colour of our life. Kicks in the body's self-healing process, cleaning and releasing our heart and mind of sadness, etc. When feeling well in our body we recognize that our body is the 'temple' of our spirit and soul and to have a positive opinion of life opens us to life and love for this life.

Affirmation: I recognize the love that the Earth gives me. I let the rainbow of my joy and feelings glow.

Corresponding gem essence: Topaz.

Coordination Orchid (*Cymbidium lowianum*)

Essence effect: Connects with chakra 11, the centre of organization and coordination. Opens us to deep cellular consciousness on the physical level, thereby initiating the self-healing process. Each cell nucleus is in contact with this chakra and, therefore, also with the cosmos.

This essence has great energy that can be intensely perceived in the heart and in the frontal lobe of the brain. Healing information can flow through the heart chakra

and provide support for the body's healing process. The exchange with the cellular consciousness makes it easier to separate the illness from a predisposition to an illness and allow contact with a diseased organ to discover an appropriate form of healing.

Affirmation: My conscience is printed in each and every cell of my body. I heal myself.

Corresponding gem essence: Watermelon Tourmaline.

Deva Orchid (*Epidendrum prismatocarpum*)

Essence effect: For opening up to experience communication with the natural elemental energy: the devas or the spirits of flowers and trees, the mineral kingdom and the spirits of water. Brings integration with the natural environment and an opening up to healing from nature, by dissolving the walls that separate us from nature; we can receive consolation, motivation, reinforcement or advice from the unseen world. Perceiving the higher dimensions more easily enables us to discover the 'treasure' of nature. The flow of energy between the individual and nature reinvigorates direct relationship with the plant, mineral kingdom and the elements as well as with the devas, the fairies and the sylphs and helps transfer this into our reality.

Special features: Deva Orchid stimulates the plant's growth. Add a few drops of the essence in the water to irrigate the plant or to spray the plant in a spritz.

Affirmation: I open my heart to the flower's message.

Corresponding gem essence: Amazonite.

Fülhorn Cattleya (*Cattleya warscewiczii*)

Essence effect: For experiencing infinite, 'universal' love, horn of plenty, giving without restriction. Brings the ability to give and receive this love freely. Brings abundance into our lives. Has a harmonizing effect on the body, and stimulates the energy in the feet. When we focus on and are paralyzed by the fear of competition and sense of lack, this helps us to understand we can have abundant material wealth as well as unlimited cosmic wealth and love. The 'horn of plenty' can fill

us with positive energy, which will turn into positive vibrations. When we understand that true security and stability is based on the wisdom of love of the Universe and Earth we can accept the gifts that the Universe offers us.
Affirmation: The love of the universe flows through me to the Earth.
Corresponding gem essence: Hematites.

Fun Orchid (*Vanda tricolor*)
Essence effect: For laughter, harmony and love of life. Increases humour and zest for life. Allows you to see life's problems and idiosyncrasies from a different and wider perspective. Aids depressive sad people, with repressed emotions, long-term disappointment, emotional wounds creating blockages. It lifts mood and re-awakens the child within and allows us to radiate calmness and tranquillity inside out. When increasing our sense of humour we can analyze a situation from a higher level and look at our earthly discords with greater clarity and serenity, release blockages that prevent us from going ahead, and face the tasks in a more relaxed way. Often recommended for children. The flower angels are saying 'Look at the grumpy person you've become'. This spiritual presence injects renewed vigour so we can elevate ourselves and discover the authentic joy of living we had hoped for.
Affirmation: My vital happiness makes me light. I laugh with the angels.
Corresponding gem essence: Olivine (peridot, chrysolite).

Heart Orchid (*Laeliocattleya* hybrid)
Essence effect: Helps us see with the heart. Strengthens the heart and solar plexus. (Any disharmony can be reflected in digestive disorders.) For raising self-centredness to the heart level, linking the solar plexus energy with the qualities of the heart. The welfare of others will move to the first place and an expansion of consciousness will take place. Harmonizes and balances the emotional body. Transforms ego-centred love to pure spiritual love, to experience inner peace and relaxation. With this essence we learn to transform

selfish emotions in love and actions that are in harmony with the spiritual world and the divine plan.
Affirmation: I open my heart to infinite love.
Corresponding gem essence: Rose Quartz.

Higher Self Orchid (*Laeliocattleya anceps clara*)
Essence effect: For communication and self-knowledge. Connects you to your Higher Self and increases your capacity to act as a messenger of the spiritual world. Enhances channelling abilities by learning to listen to our inner voice, and gain confidence in the guide of the Higher Self as an infallible counsellor. When harassed by multiple emotions, we're unable to connect with our Higher Self to be guided by its wider perspective. It reinforces clear vision and picture of personal situations. With the opening of the higher chakras, through them we perceive and receive the cosmic energy and let cosmic love flow.
Affirmation: I am the expression of my Higher Self. I am open and I enlarge my vision.
Corresponding gem essence: Rock Crystal.

Inspiration Orchid (*Cattleya trianae*)
Essence effect: For inner inspiration, stimulates and cleanses the Higher Chakras especially the third eye. Helps you get in touch with higher spiritual levels, bringing inspiration that can be used creatively. Helps fulfil our dreams. Dissolves tension and stress that disrupts inspiration, artistic activity and motivation making it impossible for us to implement our ideas and plans. Enables artistic work to be carried out quickly and with greater freedom of expression, increases the power of accomplishment and the creative spiritual force. Also helps us to contact our spiritual guides, to accept their message, to understand it and translate it onto the physical plane. We learn to live and work in harmony and in constant communication with the spiritual world.
Affirmation: I join myself to divine love and I receive it.
Corresponding gem essence: Moonstone.

Special features: This Orchid essence was part of a national program in Colombia, and was given to prisoners, children with learning difficulties and to victims of terrorist attacks.

Love Orchid (*Oncidium abortivum*)

Essence effect: For opening the heart chakra. Allows energy and love to flow freely. Eliminates the negative emotions that up to now have prevented us from being whole hearted, causing a 'hardening' of the heart. Opens the heart, awakes and allows love and cosmic energy to be utilized for healing and compassion. For those pursuing energy or personal growth therapy and for healers to incorporate it into their work to improve their channels of the healing.

Affirmation: I let love flow through me. I heal myself and others.

Corresponding gem essence: Pink Tourmaline.

Past Life Orchid (*Paphiopedilum harrysianum*)

Essence effect: For enhancing self-knowledge, understanding and inspiration. Facilitates access to past-life stream of consciousness, where every memory and all knowledge resides – 'the Akashic Records' – to retrieve lost skills, meanings and stored knowledge. This essence can help reveal deep-rooted causes for many emotional problems, inexplicable reoccurring physical problems, diseases that plague us or accidents, or painful situations that are repeated. Encourages one to explore further through meditation or reincarnation therapy to find and eliminate the root cause whether it is related to karma or events in a previous reincarnation. Past Life Orchid Essence helps us to descend the depths of our 'kingdom of shadows' to bring clarity and detect what is hiding behind suffering. It evokes our past lives memories to self-investigate in order to get in touch with our original knowledge and work on the issues.

Affirmation: Knowledge is within me and it shows me the way.

Corresponding gem essence: Smoky Quartz.

Psyche/Soul Orchid (*Paphiopedilum insigne*)

Essence effect: For knowledge of life. Allows access to the depths of our subconscious in order to discover the reason for our existence. For when our direction is unclear, and we have reached a point of crisis and questioning: Who am I? What is my task in life? Where does my path take me? This encourages self-analysis and self-awareness so as to be able to identify and recognize our life's purpose, integrate and put it into practice and to be recognized as members of a more extensive divine plan. A complementary essence for psychotherapy.

Affirmation: I recognize my vital task and I know that I am part of the Divine Plan.

Corresponding gem essence: Amethyst.

Sun Orchid (*Epidendrum chioneum*)

Essence effect: For balance and harmony. The third chakra. Connects us directly with the energy of the sun by opening and harmonizing the solar plexus and rebalancing the ego. Disharmony in the solar plexus area can manifest into various intestinal dysfunctions. When we learn to be 'right people', and fight selfish feelings and not act only according to our needs, our ego is again in harmony with the cosmic laws; being free from selfish demands enables us to be a part of the cosmic plan once more. In this spiritual process we will be strengthened by uniting with the sun's energy.

Affirmation: The sun is in me. The cosmos and I are one.

Corresponding gem essence: Rutilated Quartz.

Venus Orchid (*Anguloa clowesii*)

Essence effect: Venus and the moon. For developing the positive qualities of patience, understanding, tenderness, love and listening skills. Stimulates the female (yin) receptive energy promoting these qualities. Enhances our womanly attractiveness. One of its most appropriate applications is to redefine the 'tough guy' that we carry within, developing our tender side that is often masked behind hardness and insensitivity. A deep pleasant relaxation ensues, helping to leave behind the hardness of the day, revealing our true vulnerability. Physical areas it influences are the abdominals, solar plexus and the heart. Venus Orchid encourages opening to the qualities of feminine energy, and as we develop the female part of our personality there is a vital treasure of abundance waiting for us, enabling us to radiate all this loving energy.

Special features: Venus Orchid cream is very smooth; it has a harmonizing action and it revitalizes the skin.

Affirmation: I accept my femininity. I am sweetness and love.

Corresponding gem essence: Emerald.

Victoria Regia (*Victoria amazonica*)
Essence effect: For explosive energy and transformation. Acting on the first chakra, it brings a powerful release of natural energy, or kundalini. Liberates from deeply held fears of life survival. Through the emotional release, it eliminates past obstructions giving the strength and ability to take a new road. Supports the transformation process of dying and death itself. For facilitating the release of the soul from the body, rub a few drops of the essence between your hands and gently massage the person passing over. The overall vibration of the body is increased, becoming more sensitive to the spiritual process.

Affirmation: My energy flows fast and easily. I trust and I let things happen.

Corresponding gem essence: Ruby.

Rose essences: queen of the flowers

Since before Roman times, the Rose was appreciated and venerated for its beautiful flower and exquisite perfume. It has developed into the most incredible variety of shapes, colours and fragrances. The spectrum goes from the simple and elegant wild roses with their traditional soft colours and intense smell, to the modern brightly coloured hybrids, which are the result of cross-breeding several species of roses.

A native of Persia, it migrated to India, and since the Crusades many varieties of Rose can be found in Europe. It has a long tradition and is known as 'the Queen of Flowers'. The Rose is the Lotus flower of the West and it symbolizes the flower of love and is the emblem of inner development that leads to perfection. The quality of this perfection is shown in the combination of shapes, colours and perfumes of the Rose and all engender a positive healing effect simply by looking at them.

The Rose is the subject of many legends, myths and stories – for example, a young Persian girl told me the following anecdote in a market: 'When at home there was something wrong with Grandma; she was upset and the atmosphere was charged. Grandfather quietly placed a posy of roses under her pillow. Shortly after, everything returned to normal.' This is one of the many signs that roses act at the heart level.

Rose energy and its effect

In ancient times, people talked about the Rose in relationship to the human heart: as it opens the heart and engenders happiness in your life. The aroma of the Rose causes tensions and fears to fade, assuaging worry and heartache. The Rose is the flower that accompanies one through life welcoming newborns, until after death, symbolizing the transition to the other world. The Rose and the human being are united by the strong bond of love, which is why the Rose is the symbol of love, from blossoms of young love to that of mature love and also symbolizing past love. The rose seals the promise of love between two people.

As a healing plant, it is of great importance and is a balancing force in disharmony of the body and soul. It has a positive invigorating influence on cardiac activity, as well as a relaxing and reinforcing action on the nerves. Said to reduce inflammation, especially in the female organs, and has a stimulating effect on fertility. Used as an essential oil it can help to overcome insomnia. Its pleasant fragrance purifies the atmosphere and, as in ancient times, many natural remedies contain rose oil.

Cinnamon Rose (*Rosa majalis*)
Essence effect: Enables us not to lose faith when darkness has set in. Gives us hope when we can see no way out of present troubles. Opens us to new possibilities. Helps us heal our emotional wounds and returns our optimism in a positive future, awakening the joy of living when all seems dark. The self-healing comes into play when despair, doubt, grief and loneliness can lead to future physical disorders. Regain hope we will see beauty in day-to-day life. Useful for healing the doubts, grief, emotional wounds, worries and solitude that lead to mental breakdowns or in addictions to drugs, alcohol or prescribed medicine. Invaluable during addictions therapy to eliminate emotional emptiness or coldness. Good for claustrophobia. A new spiritual force gives us wings to escape from this dark.
Affirmation: My yearning for love finds its fullness.

Green Rose (*Rosa chinensis viridiflora*)
Essence effect: Anti-stress Rose which alleviates the negative effects of too much pressure and stress, and has a liberating effect on the heart chakra. The relaxation of nerves restores inner calm and detachment. The release of tensions and elimination of blockages widens our perspective by renewing the heart (fourth chakra). It stimulates the joy of communication and contact with others. Helps to integrate spiritual change in our life, which also has a positive effect on our creativity and motivation.
Affirmation: I open my heart and my spirit to the flow of things and I enjoy my progress.

Japanese Rose (*Rosa roxburghii*)
Essence effect: Provides modesty and humility in love. Good when high expectations of others, such as perfectionism, impatience and despair, are due to feelings of injustice and internal despair. Allows us to show our 'thorns' only when necessary and clear old patterns of behaviour (greed, selfishness,

self-overestimation, bitterness, cynicism, etc.). Teaches us modesty and humility and an understanding that love is the essence of life whilst helping develop hope for love in life. As we practise restraint, we learn to use our thorns only when necessary. It stimulates our willingness to reflect on ourselves, helping to develop new energy in our hearts that we will convey to others warmth, kindness, sympathy, affection and openness. The freedom from negative feelings establishes a new base for our perceptions and reinvigorates the power of hope, opening up the spiritual road of confidence, satisfaction, patience and moderation.
Affirmation: I let hope enter in my heart and I transmit this force as love.

Provence Rose (*Rosa centifolia*)
Essence effect: Connects heart and mind, thereby helping us resolve (apparent) conflicts and contradictions between our thoughts and our emotions, our hearts and mind. Helps those who only consider love intellectually, who seek to 'explain' it instead of feeling or experiencing it. On the other hand, this Rose can also help us face reality instead of being ruled solely by our emotions. Both can lead to the exhaustion of the body. Allows us to contemplate our circumstances in the light of love from a higher plane. In this way, our words and gestures will acquire a new quality of love and integration that will allow a deeper connection with other people.
Affirmation: My spirit and my senses come together, and my heart beats full of love.

Queen of Denmark Rose (*Rosa alba*)
Essence effect: Relieves emotional distress and tension when we feel hurt and injured. Helps us to pull out the 'thorns' from our heart and alleviates past wounds, grief and disappointments, so we are free to go beyond the experiences which are part of life's destiny. By working on the emotions we are able to recover our balance, liberating the spirit. Revival of love in our heart becomes a very deep spiritual experience, infusing our personality with new love and affection, the energy of

which radiates extensively over the world, returning to us in the shape of positive reaction.
Affirmation: I let my love unfold and grow. I accept with an open heart the love from others.

Sarah Van Fleet Rose (*Rosa rugosa*)
Essence effect: Opens the heart (fourth chakra) profoundly so we can experience sweetness of love at its deepest levels, the kind of unconditional love that gives without expecting anything in return. For a childlike, cheerful heart. During pregnancy and after childbirth it helps the mother connect spiritually with her newborn. Lack of motherly love causes loneliness and feelings of sadness, not only in young children but also in adults. Unfulfilled longing of maternal love creates a negative imprint on the spirit. The essence provides feelings of self-nourishment, inner peace, protection and internal heat. The stomach and the heart will be warmed so you can feel a vital force within. It develops loving and caring qualities towards others as well as towards yourself. This essence allows us to feel the love and protection of a transcendental mother, and there is no longer the need to confine ourselves to seek love in our relationships, but we will perceive love from a higher level and in our inner depths.
Affirmation: I feel love in all its magnitude and serenity, living inside me.

Souvenir de Philemon Cochet Rose (*Rosa rugosa*)
Essence effect: True love requires a unity of mind, body and soul. This Rose helps establish that link, connecting the different energy levels. Heart and mind merge and the heart and spirit are united by the vibrations of love so that love embraces our entire being. Opens the door to higher vibrations, and has a purifying effect on the spirit. This invaluable experience of fusion among the body, spirit and soul with love and cosmos gives the capacity to perceive oneself in union with the wholeness and give space and distance to day-to-day problems by reflecting on them from this new viewpoint. A couple's relationship

can achieve a new quality of spiritual union of body, mind and soul and a more universal spiritual love.
Affirmation: My body, my spirit and my soul melt in love with the cosmos.

Spring Gold Rose (*Rosa spinosissima*)
Essence effect: Has a harmonizing effect on the solar plexus and unites it to the heart chakra. Clears negative thoughts and self-loathing. Allows us to accept ourselves as we are and to embrace a profound state of love. Restores the energies of the solar plexus (third chakra) and ties them to the heart (fourth chakra), thereby allowing us to accept who we are calmly and dispassionately. This positive sense of self-worth encourages the ability to achieve self-fulfilment. Enables us to open our heart without becoming too emotionally involved. It permits us both mental clarity and warm feelings. Particularly indicated for those people who can only think of themselves, and during pregnancy, this essence helps to accept the physical changes that occur in childbirth and develop deep love for the child. Encourages acting with mental clarity, and a manifestation of our personal strength. Develops access to a greater spiritual potential and clarity that gives rise to a powerful spiritual energy and inner wisdom in order to transfer them into everyday life.
Affirmation: I love myself the way I am and I achieve my self-fulfilment.

Tibetan White Rose (*Rosa moyesii*)
Essence effect: Helps our love for ourselves to grow stronger. Has a grounding, rooting effect. Reinforces our sense of strength, self-confidence, inner joy and zest for life, and allows us to accept ourselves as we are. When our body is invigorated it awakens our forces of self-healing and establishing emotional ties with other people. The union with the Earth and our environment brings healing from Mother Earth and we can enjoy the lightness of being while remaining firmly anchored to the source of strength, the Earth. This opens us up to higher knowledge that provides us with a very intense mental force

that encourages our spiritual and creative force which we can live and integrate into daily life.

Affirmation: I live the nature around me and through me, and I love myself in this union.

Wild Rose (*Rosa × pruhoniciana*)
Essence effect: Integrates the energies that flow through us. Opens us to experience a love that embraces all of creation and teaches us to return this love to the Earth. In a world full of obstacles and contradictions, this Rose allows us to remain steadfast and true to our own convictions. It helps us to reconnect with nature and develop a new zest for life. Restores inner stability and power when previously nervousness, fear of life, lack of energy, dissatisfaction and insecurity had prevailed, especially when those nervous reactions had disturbed our constitutional Qi. In a world full of contradictions this essence helps us to establish a union between our heart and the Earth and feel a love for life. The improvement of our spiritual capacity of integration will consequently produce clearer decision-making, and we will be able to set and pursue goals with greater firmness. There is a huge underlying force behind this integration, which not only awakens a renewed love for life, but for existence and the whole of Creation.

Affirmation: I am centred and I join my heart with Mother Earth.

Essences of wild plants

Almond Tree (*Prunus amygdalus*)
Essence effect: Helps us accept and make sense of each stage of life so we can enjoy and develop ourselves more fully and mature with ease. As we recognize that all is relative, we accept the impermanence of material things and lose our fear of the natural ageing process. A positive tonic and rejuvenates the whole body, good for lack of nutrition and encourages a healthier diet and support when fasting. For growth imbalances in children. Balances hyperactivity and oversensitivity. In adolescents, during puberty, encourages self-control and assuages inner turmoil. Mentally clears repetitive thoughts and feelings, is restorative so a state of balanced, inner harmony and spiritual guidance is reached.

Affirmation: I am aware of the meaning of the phases of my life, I accept them and I let myself be driven by the flow of life.

Arnica (*Arnica montana*)
Essence effect: A basic first-aid essence in emergency situations, for any kind of injury, even emotional shock. In the same way that the plant extract is used in herbal medicine to treat external wounds, the delicate Arnica essence stimulates the self-healing processes in the etheric body plane. Also heals emotional wounds. For re-establishing the connection to the Higher Self, enabling the body, spirit and soul to recover the energy balance especially after anaesthetics, drug addiction or shock. It smooths the way so that we can feel whole again and restore our union with the Higher Self.

Affirmation: I search for myself and for my balance.

Basil (*Ocimum basilicum*)
Essence effect: Links and harmonizes all the energy centres helping to experience and value each level of being. Strengthens the root chakra. Helps the digestion and offsets the trend to have the sensation of being full up, gas and nausea. Recommended for nursing mothers. Basil essence stimulates the ability to eliminate conflicts in social relationships and to replace them with feelings. People who suffer from sexual dysfunctions often feel attracted by this essence. Helps overcome the fear of sexuality and it is indicated to establish a link between sexuality and spirituality. Useful to compensate feelings when sexuality and spirituality are perceived as separate entities.

Affirmation: I integrate my sexual needs with my spiritual life, and live with inner harmony.

Bistort (*Polygonum bistorta*)

Essence effect: For those whose mind wanders and is scattered when trying to concentrate and focus. Helps to remain centred and fully present for the task at hand. It promotes mental stability. For when emotional wounds are so deep, a feeling of disorientation and alienation creates that basic desire to look after oneself. Beneficial for digestive disorders. For those who feel that they are in the 'wrong place' or 'the wrong body', a 'control' essence allows a total cleaning of the body and soul, and removes old poisons that date back to the past, that have taken control of our lives and sapped energy and vitality. Gives greater self-perception and clarity and a renewed empowered feeling about ourselves and our body and translates that into our lives.

Affirmation: I find myself and take a central position in my life.

Blackberry (*Rubus fruticosus*)

Essence effect: For those who have problems initiating projects. Lack of get-up-and-go, weakness, lethargy, laziness, procrastination and sadness. Stimulates initiative and strengthens the will. Helps us to gather positive energy and reinforces it, enabling us to realize our creative power and to execute personal projects and follow them through with enthusiasm.

Acts as a catalyst on our spirit to overcome apathy and spiritual distraction. Renews perseverance and contact with our Higher Self to ask for direction on objectives and how we can achieve them, so we can act in ways that are in harmony with the Creation Plan and to shape our ideas with clarity. It is also recommended for schoolchildren.

Affirmation: I group my thoughts and capacities, and I carry out my plans until the end.

Bleeding Heart (*Dicentra spectabilis*)

Essence effect: For all affairs of the heart. Useful in all kinds of heart disease. A regenerative and energetic balm for the heart chakra. Offers support to those who have lost someone dear, or when a relationship ends. Allows acceptance of what life brings and consolation when disappointed by creating distance from painful situations to leave behind painful spiritual experiences and reach a state of freedom and harmony. For insecure characters who depend on their relationship/partner or other relationship for internal security, any overidentification with feelings of jealousy, mistrust, possessive behaviour, sarcasm and fear of abandonment will dissipate. Painful and sudden separations, or loss of a loved one (separation or death), causing heartache will be released. Brings freedom of thought increasing the ability to decide independently about one's life. Feelings that a burden for our hearts are a burden for our soul. True source of love is in the freedom that lies in the ability to allow loved ones to be free whether they are dead or temporarily separated. It allows us to establish a spiritual union without binding them to us.

Affirmation: I open myself to the richness of free love.

Borage (*Borago officinalis*)

Essence effect: Gives power and courage to confront exhausting emotional situations, helps us to proceed in life with optimism and rediscover joy in our hearts. Promotes the regeneration of the heart chakra after emotional wounds and deep sadness. Contributes to an overall strengthening of the body and stability. This essence helps us find the way out when we feel defeated or heavy when in sorrow, grief and pain. People who feel 'overwhelmed' by life are often attracted by this essence. With it, you may find more lightness, joy and confidence. The motivation to return to get something spiritual.

Affirmation: I live with fullness my inner joy and I am filled with courage, hope and renewed serenity.

Buttercup (*Ranunculus acris*)

Essence effect: Helps us realize our full potential when we lack self-esteem and are shy and reserved. Reinforces our self-confidence and to have no fear to say no when we encounter high expectations by others, particularly parents or teachers or dominant representations of them. Helps develop inner greatness, a sense of self-worth and to be independent, by not letting others run our lives. Provides energy support, straightens the spine and corrects posture of the shoulders. It helps to have a better image of ourselves and to be in harmony and organize our life mentally, experience spiritual freedom and define the path that we need to follow to carry out our desires and goals.

Affirmation: I find myself, I feel my energy and I enjoy my independence.

Callalily (*Zantedeschia aethiopica*)

Essence effect: Restores the yin and yang balance in the lower chakras (first and the second chakra). Helps us to learn to accept and integrate the male and female aspects of ourselves, and reach a balance between active and received energy. Any dilemma about sexual identity can create a great emotional overload. Encourages us to clarify our sexual identity. Enhances self-worth, connection to the Earth and creativity.

Affirmation: I admit my sexuality and accept myself as I am.

Chamomile (*Matricaria chamomilla*)

Essence effect: For the overstressed, when feeling too much is being expected. Especially for those who are easily worked up, irritable and have a short temper, and have difficulty calming down again. Excitable, the nerves, physical disorders, internal tensions, the stomach in particular. Reduces tension, relaxes, soothes and calms, allowing objectivity and emotional space in order to regain strength, sense of peace and serenity so we are careful with our words and use them wisely. Combine with Dill essence for children exposed to irritation, when travelling or having to assimilate new life situations. Very practical assistance for sensitive and hyperactive children. A source of balance which prevents strong mood swings and extreme emotional reactions. Helps nervous children to sleep and any adults who suffer from insomnia. By discovering our calm, it will allow us detachment from everything external. Immersed in this serenity, we can listen to our intuition and hear our inner voice clearly which is intensified during meditation.

Affirmation: I am cautious and I react with serenity.

Corn (*Zea mays*)

Essence effect: Ideal for town-dwellers who are stressed and have lost their inner balance, may suffer from lack of concentration, obsessions, nightmares, lack of relationship with the environment and are searching for contact with the Earth. Brings back life's natural rhythms. Promotes connection with the Earth, and harmony with the rhythm of nature, balances and grounds by keeping our feet on the ground in order to reclaim our true inner self. Encourages a desire to seek open spaces, to relaxation by taking a walk in nature where intense emotions and conflicts can seem irrelevant and exaggerated when confronted by the greatness of nature. Allows us to generate a new spiritual space and the possibility of organizing our life in another way. Also indicated for the daydreamers who walk in the clouds.

Affirmation: I connect to the Earth and I find myself again.

Courgette (*Cucurbita pepo*)

Essence effect: Strengthens the second chakra, clearing any tensions, anger and frustration, opens to growth and creativity and the patience to let things mature. For integrating femininity and beneficial for balancing the hormones during a woman's time of month. Brings harmony during pregnancy, enhancing and promoting bonding and communication between mother-to-be and the unborn child. As we learn to accept the waiting game it allows us to be in contact with our Higher Self. Gives new impetus and motivation, to birthing a new business idea or other venture.

Affirmation: I allow life to mature with patience and I let events happen.

Daisy (*Bellis perennis*)

Essence effect: For integrating many different thoughts, and understanding the whole picture. Ideal for children and adults during the learning process. Helps make it easier to take in and analyze new information. Eliminates stress, unrest, dissatisfaction and overload of information. Recommended for children with sleep disorders.

Affirmation: I am ready to continue my life.

Dandelion (*Taraxacum officinale*)

Essence effect: For reducing stress and tension generated by emotional conflicts. Loosens emotional tensions, especially those manifesting in stiffness and pain in the muscles. For those who need to have everything under control, with self-imposed restrictions, and personal limitations creating tightening and bitterness. Spirit needs freedom to move and when it follows a 'single track', it becomes stiff and suffers a great deal of stress. Helps open up to life restoring a feeling of lightness, faith and wisdom and achieving new higher spiritual dimension. Effective addition to massage oils, and complements the work of massage therapists, physiotherapists and osteopaths.

Affirmation: My body relaxes; I break all my spiritual chains and dedicate my life to my genuine needs.

Dill (*Anethum graveolens*)

Essence effect: Ideal for children of which too much is expected; facing changes, travelling or visiting unfamiliar places. Enables those with a fast and intense pace of life, who experience nervousness, disorientation and anger to digest, process and integrate seemingly overwhelming impressions, experiences and information. Helps to keep calm situations of high demand and diversity, for example, work situations that demand concentration and serenity, exams or professional challenges. We can then access our inner strength, increase receptivity and learn to live an open life and to link only to those experiences that are good for us.

Affirmation: I am ready to have new experiences and to process my impressions.

Forget-Me-Not (*Myosotis sylvatica*)

Essence effect: Stimulates the subconscious and promotes positive dreaming. Opens up inner communication and creates connections with loved ones. Helps us to integrate memories of those still alive and remember those who are no longer here. Helps in dealing with painful, chronic or health problems passed on down from parents and grandparents. When a memory is triggered in the subconscious, we are able to identify and eliminate the problem from our path. Contact with the dead can be of great help when we have any pending issue with them, such as the fears and negative energies which would otherwise prevent us from moving forward. The accumulated tensions in dreams are dissolved, leaving us free from their influence. With a more objective perspective of our life certainty we can forge forward with our destiny.

Affirmation: I am able to remember myself, shadows faded by the light and I feel free.

German Garlic (*Allium angulosum*)

Essence effect: Calms and soothes all forms of fear. Releases the energies locked up by fear, fear of the future, insecurity, fear of acting thereby strengthening our entire system: body, spirit and soul. Teaches us to remain more consistent and calm and develop greater serenity in fearful situations. Helps in stressful situations. Revitalizing and gives protection against all fears that affect the physical body. Stimulates our capacity to digest what life serves up on both physical and emotional levels. Teaches how through meditation and other methods of expanding consciousness we can discover the origin of fears and work to overcome them. Initiates a purifying process that breaks the chains of fear and stimulates the willpower as well as the metabolism. Also an antidote to psychic attack.

Affirmation: I am protected and invulnerable to all dangers.

Iris (*Iris germanica*)

Essence effect: For accessing and developing creative potential and connection to inner artistic inspiration. Helps us when feeling blocked and internal tensions of anger against oneself, despair, frustration, weakness and negative emotions. For those who feel spiritually empty, breathes new life and energy in our etheric body by enhancing a 'renaissance' and regeneration. Connects with the higher self, and enables us to receive creative inspirations from high dimensions and to integrate them into life. Unblocks the creativity of those in the artistic professions such as advertising designers and graphic artists, inspiring them to incorporate new ideas.

Affirmation: I tap into the source of my creativity and talent, and immerse myself in the creative flow of ideas and inspiration.

Lavender (*Lavandula officinalis*)
Essence effect: Mitigates irritability, and calms the mind when agitated or emotionally upset. Its balancing effect restores inner peace and clears and harmonizes our inner thoughts. Helps us reconnect with our spiritual self and integrate experiences into daily life. Has a purifying effect on the physical body and the motor system. Teaches us to reconcile the spiritual level with the material one and, in this way, you can discover new ways of thinking. Also especially useful for providing energy support during exams.

Affirmation: I find the source of peace within.

Lotus (*Nelumbo nucifera*)
Essence effect: Considered the universal flower which promotes clarity, this includes spiritual clarity and openness at all levels. Aids self-discovery (through meditation, yoga, psychotherapy). Stimulates the self-healing process and brings to light old dormant experiences in order to clear them out of the system. Opens and harmonizes all chakras, stimulates the crown chakra gateway to higher energies and establishes communication with the Higher Chakras in order to enlighten and to guide all the other aspects of our personality which restores spirituality and accelerates spiritual growth.

Affirmation: I live day to day from a place of meditation.

Mistletoe (*Viscum album*)
Essence effect: For help with going through a radical process of change. Aids transformation on both the physical and psychological levels. Any insecurity, fear, depression, feeling of dizziness is helped as well as being a support to debilitating and complex diseases, and also eliminating emotional disorders during illness. Energy tonic. It strengthens our will to live and gives us renewed fortification to participate in our self-healing process. Spiritually integrates our crucial life changes with the universal plan.

Affirmation: I stand on the threshold of change and I surrender with full trust to the transformation process.

Morning Glory (*Ipomea purpurea*)
Essence effect: Supports withdrawal and rehabilitation. Helps us become conscious of our bad habits, shortcomings, negative living habits and addictions. Excellent soothing of the symptoms of physical restlessness, constant turmoil, high level of nervousness, restlessness and insomnia. Also displays of nervous habits such as nail biting, teeth grinding and habits of dependency. Helps to be aware of self-destructive trends and that all changes begin in the mind. With its purifying qualities new energy is found to put our lives in order. Life will seem brighter, as changes release vitality and we can let go of addiction and a new creative forecast appears for our life. A fresh overview gives us the opportunity to start again in a creative way.

Affirmation: I discover my creativity.

Mullein (*Verbascum thapsus*)
Essence effect: Strengthens our connection to our inner guidance, helps us listen to our inner voice and conscience. When issues of abandonment have created a great need for love, understanding, care and patience, it encourages finding this within to become more independent from the others. Aids in the ability to be true to ourselves, gives a healthy sense of perspective, especially in teamwork, allows us to develop ourselves and gives energy to be able to launch projects, arouses

enthusiasm for our goals and feeds our perseverance to achieve them. As confidence grows in our decision-making ability to make decisions that are in line with the spirit, soul and body and the path we chose to follow in life we achieve a sense of self-fulfilment.

Affirmation: I feel I am more at one with the group and I can integrate my experiences for the benefit of other people.

Passion Flower (*Passiflora bryonioides*)
Essence effect: For raising energy levels so that we can face life's difficult challenges more successfully, helps overcome painful periods resulting from serious diseases, unfavourable diagnosis or after an operation. Also helps overcome phases of depression, for example, the sudden loss of work, a partner, or the empty nest syndrome. Allows stepping back and seeing things from a new perspective and distance from the causes of our pain. Develops a belief in change for the better, internal support and security and the ability to recognize the challenge as an opportunity for growth and to have control over our fate. When reducing our sense of personal involvement when problems threaten to overwhelm us the tension is softened and we are open to receive positive energy. The intense and harmonizing effect soothes and brings new strength to our soul and aids processes of physical recovery. In this higher state of consciousness we can observe any traumatic situations in life with a sharper, more spiritual outlook, and adopt a fresh new positive approach to life.
Affirmation: I let my soul be guided.

Pink Yarrow (*Achillea millefolium*)
Essence effect: For those who are too easily influenced by the emotions, statements or opinions of others, helps them worry less, be independent, protects those who catch every illness going, protects the heart and emotions and strengthens and protects the energy system against external attacks. Indicated for children (nursery school, etc.) and useful in times of transformation (pregnancy, separation or death). Therapists who have a tendency to absorb their patients' problems find

this effective for protection. Highly recommended as energy protection for those with jobs and work that involves contact with the electromagnetic vibrations of computers or other electronic equipment; a bottle of the essence in front of the computer creates a positive energy field. The lack of concentration or memory disorders that have their origin in contact with electromagnetic flows will improve. Any situations where one is highly receptive to negative vibrations will experience a dispersal of negativity, complete protection and a regeneration of body, spirit and soul.
Affirmation: Flooded with energy, my body, my spirit and my soul will regenerate.

Red Clover (*Trifolium pratense*)
Essence effect: An emergency essence for panic and fear; helps you maintain inner calm and self-control even in extreme emergency situations or in the midst of mass hysteria. Helps to remain centred and focused in serious crisis and panic situations whilst others are panicking around you, preventing the bodily automatic response and reactions occurring that are results of states of fear or panic. Aid in emotional crises, for example, conflicts in the workplace, serious or incurable diseases, violence, and massive states or advertising that cause mass fear and hysteria. Helps keep a cool head and returns us to a place of peace and inner quiet, to act in a clear and thoughtful way, overcoming fear (panic of crowds) to take control of the situation. Connects us to our Higher Self to gain perspective and tap into intuition about what is the best course of action even in serious situations.
Affirmation: I live in a state of total calm, my thoughts are clear and actions confident and assured.

Red Lily (*Lilium bulbiferum*)
Essence effect: For achieving the correct attitude towards sexuality. Connects the second and fourth chakras, brings self-understanding and helps to direct sexual energy towards the heart. Promotes a positive, loving attitude towards intimacy, helps young overcome the fear of the first sexual experience. Balances

hyperactive children to concentrate better. Activates creative forces, helping overcome considerable obstacles that prevent movement towards goals. Teaches us to develop creative ideas in a constructive way and to reinforce the spiritual readiness to give and receive energy in a new way, so life is infused with a cosmic fullness.

For healers who work in the therapeutic field, sets up a large flow of warm energy into the hands, directing strength and love through the hands in hands-on healing. During radiation therapy, or after it, protects and strengthens the body's energetic defence levels. The feeling of physical weakness fades as it benefits the whole body.
Affirmation: I project my life full of energy and enthusiasm.

Rosebay Willowherb (*Epilobium angustifolium*)
Essence effect: Restoring energy after a shock, trauma and any accident when there has been physical damage. (Interesting to note: this plant grows in places where the Earth has suffered a shock.) Aids in emotional wounds, after a separation, abuse, torture or wounds acquired through war. Past trauma will fade and areas of injury be restored to eliminate the related trauma. Dissolves negative thoughts and memories, especially any experiences that are related to a tough situation. Free from the negative energy and pains, the essence restores the natural energy flow of the soul, and leaves the door open for further development and reorientation. We learn that even after the worst experiences our inner flower can be reopened. Brings the connection between body, spirit and soul more closely together.
Affirmation: Old wounds heal and I plan my future.

Rosemary (*Rosmarinus officinalis*)
Essence effect: Strengthens brain function, enhancing mental concentration and alertness. For forgetfulness. Helps us to live in the present. Helps us to be more aware and conscious of who we are and what is happening in our lives. More physical awareness helps

to maintain a good relationship with it. General tonic for those who have poor circulation, cold hands and feet, tend to run away from life's difficulties, are easily distracted by external elements, daydreaming, find it difficult to come back after meditation, and fail to integrate their spiritual experiences in the daily living. Its essence encourages structure, spiritual awareness and it nourishes thought, giving grounding and stability. Anchors the soul on the Earth and highly recommended to help newborns to get a good start in life.
Affirmation: My body, my spirit and my soul are alert and I develop myself with grace and awareness.

Sage (*Salvia officinalis*)
Essence effect: Purifying. Cleanses and purifies us at the energetic level. Restores our inner rhythm, especially if suffering from jet lag. Allows us to integrate travel experiences more easily and promotes awakening of consciousness. The purifying effect on the energetic level helps to restore our body clock, balancing the effect of time changes. Stimulates the digestive processes and is good for protection in times of fasting. Recommended for those who lean too much towards spirituality or, conversely, too many materialistic and selfish tendencies. Here it neutralizes the feelings of selfishness and materialism and associated feelings of envy, jealousy, etc. The whole body benefits from the harmonizing effect of this flower. With harmony between inner and outer, the higher meaning of the events of our lives can be discovered, resulting in new thought patterns arising that will give a new direction to our lives.
Affirmation: The external and internal worlds work in harmony with each other.

St John's Wort (*Hypericum perforatum*)
Essence effect: Strengthens the emotional body's defences so that we regain a natural healthy sense of optimism that allows us to think more clearly. Recommended for those suffering from deep-rooted fears and nightmares ('childhood' fears, fear of darkness, sleeping alone, the unknown, strangers, situations, places and unknown fears). Increases

our ability to confront conscious or unconscious fears that have created a state of anxiety. Has a calming, clarifying and grounding effect. For those very spiritually open, with intense spiritual experiences, and vulnerable to negative influences. Creates a powerful energy protection so that the negative vibrations cannot affect us. Acts like an inner light that illuminates the dark and increases belief in the protection of Divine Guidance.

Affirmation: The light of summer gives me warmth and strength. Fears dissipate and joy lights up my world.

Scarlet Pimpernel (*Anagallis arvensis*)

Essence effect: Brings spiritual consciousness into everyday life. Through this we experience compassion, self-confidence and are able to integrate into groups. Has a positive effect on health, a general tonic and calming influence on the whole body that has highly beneficial results. Helps discover the warmth of our feelings and transmit them. People who lean towards coldness, cynicism and reserve can use this essence and observe its excellent results. Allows us to remain open, to express our feelings, and solve mental problems that are due to closing off at the spiritual level or narrow mindedness.

Affirmation: I communicate through the heat of my heart and I realize that, when I express my feelings honestly, others understand me better.

Self-Heal (*Prunella vulgaris*)

Essence effect: Stimulates the body's self-healing powers, especially on the cellular level. Strengthens our will to be healthy and listen to our internal doctor. Promotes a sense of wellbeing and is especially effective when used in a cream. Self-heal essence can be applied when the feelings of weakness, loss of forces, hopelessness or guilt feelings do not allow physical or spiritual recovery. Helps us to activate our energies of self-healing and stimulates the courage to be healthy for ourselves.

Affirmation: I let go of disease and I am healthy.

Sunflower (*Helianthus annuus*)

Essence effect: Helps rebuild self-confidence and encourages personal responsibility by harmonizing the energies of the solar plexus. For those in conflict situations with the father figure, both natural and archetypal, or the idea of fatherhood. Problems with low self-esteem. Conflicts with authority father figures can manifest as imbalances in the spine and posture. Recommended for use in osteopathy and chiropractic fields, especially related to conflicts with the parents and lack of support. Clears tensions and blockages, stabilizes energy, feeling free to develop and strengthen our individuality which can show externally to create a better posture. Also indicated for children who grow up without a father or whose father, for example, spends time away from home as it strengthens self-awareness and encourages responsibility.

Affirmation: I feel empowered as I break all my chains.

Valerian (*Valeriana officinalis*)

Essence effect: Calms the body, soul and spirit, allowing sleep and restoration of vital energies when stress or pain has led to insomnia, nervousness or inadequate rest and encourages the realization that the body and soul are both tired. Recommended when under major stress and strain, and has a calming effect; a greater spiritual clarity is generated. Inner peace makes us more receptive, stimulates the astral body and relationship between the etheric body and the astral to be in harmony. As a result of relaxing all nervous tensions and gaining a higher perspective on life's stresses, astral activity is softened and calmed, promoting deep sleep. Valerian is a plant that induces cosmic experiences in the earthly world.

Affirmation: Deep peace fills me as I release all my worries and concerns.

Violet (*Viola hirta*)

Essence effect: For people who feel lonely or isolated in a group. Feeling ignored often leaves behind a trail of painful feelings of loneliness and disappointment, feelings of anxiety, shyness, unsteadiness, weakness and insecurity, which can manifest in instability of the spine, and a mindset of avoidance. Helps maintain self-identity while increasing openness so you can interact with others better. Develops inner warmth, trust and confidence and helps us remember the past more easily. Helps us realize our importance within the Plan of Creation leading us gently towards our own personal greatness. Through meditation, spiritual experiences can reveal the meaning of our life and provide the energy and motivation to put aside our reserved, insecure personality and live truly in accordance with our life's purpose.

Affirmation: I am an important link in the chain of life and my ultimate goal is to discover its meaning.

White Paradise Lily (*Paradisea liliastrum*)

Essence effect: Reawakens divine-consciousness and higher realms. Opens the crown (seventh) chakra establishing our link to Higher Self and fills the body with white light. Aid for meditation and strengthens inner awareness and sense of belonging to 'All that Is'. Assists in fasting or changing eating habits, releasing impurities, negative feelings, old upsets, accumulated anger or disappointment. In breaking free of old patterns of thought a new page can be turned in our lives. Ideal for meditation, because it gives support to the knowledge of being an integral part of everything and an awareness of our inner Christ. This essence expands our angle of vision and it can promote the ability to see auras.

Affirmation: God's love guides and leads me.

Wild Carrot (*Daucus carota*)

Essence effect: Strengthens both inner and outer visual acuity. Stimulates the sixth chakra. Good for eye strain, also a tonic that brings energy to the spine. Its calming effect opens us to inner visions so it is an ideal essence for creative visualization or dreams in order to gain a deeper level of spiritual understanding. A source of spiritual clarity throwing a new light on a situation allowing us to eliminate negative patterns and has a calming effect on the soul.

Affirmation: I see with clarity and I free myself from the distortion of negative thoughts.

White Yarrow (*Achillea millefolium*)

Essence effect: For sensitive people exposed to negative environmental influences. It strengthens the light of aura protecting us from negative influences, when disturbed by inner stress or harmful effects from the environment such as negative radiation as electromagnetic pollution (computer), air pollution, and presence of strong electromagnetic fields, for example, Earth radiation. Increases and strengthens our personal protection when we are exposed, reinforcing our protective energy shield, when especially vulnerable to getting sick, the extra sensitivity of pregnancy, in changing situations and life crises. Also meditation or during sleep, when at risk of absorbing vibrations. This essence intensifies our aura in such a way that it becomes protective armour in any situation and against any influence.

Affirmation: I have a total protection and this allows me to get rid of any negative influence.

Special feature: White Yarrow is one of the ingredients of the spray to the aura.

Zinnia (*Zinnia elegans*)

Essence effect: Helps those who take life too seriously to lighten up. Stimulates childlike humour in spite of the difficulties. Helps us relax and loosen up emotionally, easing any physical tensions which allows the body to recover its flexibility and encourages a positive forward movement. 'Laughter is the best medicine.' Many problems are the product of our own seriousness and we can leave behind the mentally outdated and restrictive mindset and develop a new optimistic way of thinking. Spirituality doesn't have to be a solemn undertaking but a journey of joy and humour.

Affirmation: I feel the power of joy in me and I enjoy a cheerful disposition free from worries.

Wild plant extension

Canary Islands Pine (*Pinus canariensis*)
Essence effect: Helps free us from deep feelings of shame and guilt. Protects us from the negative thought projections of others and helps us to 'breathe deeply'.

Coltsfoot (*Tussilago farfara*)
Essence effect: Enables us to resist harsh physical or emotional environments by strengthening our inner forces. Provides hope and power to endure in the face of obstacles.

Cone Flower (*Echinacea purpurea*)
Essence effect: Has a releasing and detoxifying effect on the emotional body, stimulating its defences and dissolving pent-up emotional burdens that have been carried too long. Thus relieved, we get back into life's flow. This essence smooths the way to restoring emotional health.

Evening Primrose (*Oenothera biennis*)
Essence effect: Shines a light into the darkness of our deepest fears. Soothes and calms our emotions so we regain the sense that we are safe and protected.

Eyebright (*Euphrasia officinalis*)
Essence effect: Sharpens our ability to see clearly, both physically and inwardly. This essence helps us act rationally during emotional crises and also consoles us in times of grief.

Hawthorn (*Crataegus oxyacantha*)
Essence effect: Resolves deep feelings of sorrow or grief, bringing serenity and permitting our inner inspiration to flow again. Helps us let go of the past.

Lemon (*Citrus limon*)
Essence effect: Cleanses us at all levels, bringing new clarity and feelings of wellbeing. Helps 'restore the soul'.

Maidenhair Tree (*Ginkgo biloba*)
Essence effect: Enables us to resist harsh physical or emotional environments by strengthening our inner forces. Provides hope and the power to endure in the face of obstacles.

Nettle (*Urtica dioica*)
Essence effect: Takes the 'sting' out of conflicts within a group. Helps individuals living or working together to present different points of view without provoking hurt feelings.

Paprika Pepper (*Capsicum annuum*)
Essence effect: Sharpens all our senses and sensory perceptions. This essence strengthens our energy level.

Pennyroyal (*Mentha pulegium*)
Essence effect: Protects us against external disturbances on the mental level. Replenishes us with new energy after a shock so that we can make a fresh start.

Periwinkle (*Vinca minor*)
Essence effect: Has a calming and balancing effect. It strengthens the nervous system so that we remain calm and centred, even in very stressful situations. Promotes 'nerves of steel'.

Petunia (*Petunia Hybrid*)
Essence effect: Helps use mental energy accurately. Promotes our ability to focus our thoughts and achieve both clarity and acuity.

Pot Marigold (*Calendula officinalis*)
Essence effect: Helps us recognize and accept our different emotional states. This essence enables us to remain centred and to release energy blocks caused by shock or trauma.

Primrose (*Primula veris*)
Essence effect: Loosens energy blockages at key points so that our creative powers begin to flow smoothly again.

Snapdragon (*Antirrhinum majus*)
Essence effect: Promotes our ability to 'strike the right tone' when expressing our opinion by harmonizing the fifth (throat or larynx) chakra so that we express ourselves appropriately and even elegantly.

Sorrel (*Rumex acetosa*)
Essence effect: This essence is a survival artist among plants because it grows even in extremely polluted environments. Likewise, this essence strengthens our life force and endurance capabilities.

Turk's Cap Lily (*Lilium martagon*)
Essence effect: Releases emotional blockages that were formed in childhood when we couldn't defend ourselves against abuse or bullying. This essence frees us from uncertainty about our own abilities and restores our self-confidence.

Wild Garlic (*Allium angulosum*)
Essence effect: Stimulates our capacity to digest what life serves up on both physical and emotional levels. Enables us to release burdens and emotional blockages so we can enjoy life again. Helps us remain more consistent and calm in stressful situations.

Carnivorous plants

Butterwort (*Alpenfettkraut / Grassette des Alpes*)
Cleanses us at all energy levels, thereby removing those emotional poisons that result from negative thought patterns or excessive criticism and self-doubt. When burdened by negative thoughts, this essence helps us extract their harmful energy from both body and aura.

Sundew (*Rossolis filiforme*)
Helps free us from old negative karmic patterns by bringing past experiences back into consciousness so we can release them with love and understanding. This helps raise our overall energy vibration.

Venus Fly (*Venus Fliegenfalle*)
When we feel trapped in a situation and cannot see any way out, this essence helps us develop a broader perspective so that we recognize the relativity of our circumstances. Helps us solve what appear to be insoluble problems.

African and Canary Island essences

This legendary continent is home to an incredible abundance of flowering plants in different climatic zones ranging from the Sahara through to tropical forests. As our research advanced, we quickly realized the importance of this unique vegetation for the development of flower essences nowadays.

Geographically the Canary Islands belong to Africa. The vegetation in this archipelago, along with Madeira, the Azores and the Cape Verde Islands, is a treasure trove of the plant world. Many of these were endemic (i.e. occurring naturally on a specific area) until the arrival of the ice age where they then could also be found in large parts of southern Europe and northern Africa. Laurel forests are the exception.

Within the limits of its shores the Canary Islands have many different climatic zones, and from the dunes, leaping ravines, pine forests and laurel forests to the top of canyons are host to an amazing variety of plant.

Aloe (*Aloe striata*)
Essence effect: Restores life energies in cases of exhaustion and our inner balance and life force when we are spent. Aloe essence helps to recover when the capacity concentration is low, there are memory problems, and when the speed of thought is decelerated. This type of exhaustion carries the inherent danger of no longer listening to your own intuition or your Higher Self so you are limited to just 'function'. It brings back our life energy, especially when we have spent much of our igneous energy reserves (i.e. energy to act, energy to go after our goals, energy to do our tasks) and the tiredness has 'governed' our emotional bar which is now at its lowest point. Stimulates the energy balance of the heart chakra and regenerates our body enabling it to regain strength. There is also the danger that you close yourself to any spiritual experience, thus taking the risk of darkening the light of your own body. So regeneration comes to (re)open ourselves to spiritual experiences.
Affirmation: I can feel how the energy grows inside me and I nourished myself in my strength.

Artemisia (*Artemisia arvensis*)
Essence effect: Regenerates and energizes our life force energy when it has been depleted

after a lengthy strenuous illness or a long period of emotional distress. Helps us recover from exhaustion or deep emotional wounds. In case of psychic attack it stimulates the energetic protection of the body used as an energic reinforcement. The tests that life imposes on us can make us face many feelings that often appear to be insurmountable. Gives us courage when a complicated illness obliges us to face an exhausting and arduous therapy. A deep understanding of the networks that make up life is encouraged and thus provides the individual the capacity to consider and recognize disease or setbacks as part of destiny and a learning opportunity that we must internalize to face and overcome these complex phases.

Affirmation: The confidence in my energy grows within me.

Banana (*Musa paradisiaca L. 'nana'*)

Essence effect: Strengthens yang energies (masculine, active force). Helps restore and reinforce male sexual potency especially when hindered by the fear of failure, the pressure at work or different worries. Helps those people who have difficulties with the second chakra and problems with expressing their feelings to their partner. Also helps overachiever personalities express their true feelings openly so they may set more realistic goals in life with confidence and determination. Banana essence revitalizes our male energy and it induces a greater driving force and self-awareness. This means that thoughts of impotency, hopelessness, insecurity and fears vanish and they are replaced by a spiritual driving force. Integration of the right and left brain hemispheres (rational side with the creative) occurs and this balance of our masculine and feminine energy enriches spiritual experience.

Affirmation: I take care of my male energy and I accept myself in all my energy.

Bird of Paradise (*Strelitzia reginae*)

Essence effect: Helps us discover our true 'inner beauty', regardless of outward appearances. Teaches us to learn to accept ourselves as we are and to follow our inner vision unerringly.

As we pursue our goals and begin to radiate light from within, an unattractive body will no longer be considered as such. The overall good vibration of the person will compensate for the lack of beauty and a real exterior transformation can take place as there is an understanding of true beauty and love for oneself; the features are relaxed, the eyes shine again, it is easier to become slim. Reaffirms our spiritual guidance, and a clear vision during meditation. Through the spiritual receptivity, we will notice that our creativity is increased and that we have the courage to follow unusual paths.

Affirmation: I live consciously my inner beauty and I let it flow.

Canary Island Bell Flower (*Canarina canariensis*)

Essence effect: Helps integrate the yin (feminine, receptive) side of one's nature. Provides confidence and security in difficult situations, moments of 'hesitation' and helps us to develop, admit and demonstrate tender feelings. Support to the body to breathe with more ease and relaxation. Any feelings of fury, rage and aggressiveness will experience a transformation through this essence, which will soften our nature. In puberty, especially, when the female part (yin) of the sexuality needs to be integrated, so tenderness can be experienced and expressed in everyday life and then this energy can be translated into ideas and projects. As we radiate a spiritual energy, all acts of kindness and tenderness will help others to overcome 'hiding their feelings'.

Affirmation: Tenderness fills me and I open the door to it. Thus, I find confidence in myself and in my life.

Cape Leadwort (*Plumbago auriculata*)

Essence effect: Helps set us free from the past, bringing serenity to composure when we must reflect and address old problems. Its grounding effect allows us to step back and disengage from what's going on around us so we can 'let bygones be bygones'. Beneficial at the energy level, for losing weight, which can be especially good for those who despite a regime find it hard to get slim. Works on the throat chakra and has been introduced with success as a complement to speech therapy treatments. For the overcommitted who find it hard just to let things happen. They get highly emotional and upset when things do not happen as expected and it awakens the ability to let events take their course. Stimulates appreciation of ourselves, gives us integrity and an acquired knowledge through meditation that liberates us and allow us to move forward.

Affirmation: I get rid of past problems and I leave the door open to the flow of events. Here is where the strength to be myself lies.

Coconut Palm (*Cocos nucifera*)
Essence effect: Helps us accept our inner sensitivity while recognizing the need for external protection. Especially for those extremely sensitive people who need to develop clear boundaries, and a 'resistant' shell around them while maintaining personal harmony and sensitivity. It helps us be aware that the skin is both a protective barrier of the inner life and an organ that allows us to be in contact with the environment. Helps deal with all those elements that come to us from outside that cause skin reactions, for self-loathing, aversion, fear of allergies. Breastfeeding mothers can benefit from the protective effects of this essence. It also helps homosexuals to accept their orientations. Auric protection is very important for spiritual development, particularly those sensitive to negative vibrations, and helps eradicate energy intrusions so that they are able to tap into and process superior knowledge (e.g. messages from the spiritual world).

Affirmation: I have a complete protection and I can perceive as my spirit grows.

Blue Gum (*Eucalyptus globulus*)
Essence effect: Releases and opens us emotionally so that we can accept life for what it is, adopting an attitude of 'live and let live'. Refreshing effect on the throat and chest area and releases the lungs of tension and it allows us to breathe normally again, providing a sensation of expansion and relaxation. Internal tensions that can arise from oppressed feelings can physically externalize in headaches. It promotes our ability to express our emotions and talk about them freely, making everything flow and encouraging deeper communication between people. This spontaneous liberation from old patterns and feeling of freedom will guide us to be more receptive to the development of our consciousness, so organize our lives with greater serenity.

Affirmation: I am free and I can unfold my whole being.

Geranium (*Geranium perforatum*)
Essence effect: When everyday life seems dull and grey, this essence brings out our light and restores inner joy and zest for life. Releases negative emotional bonds and adds colour to our life.

When we have been receiving hard knocks in life and remain trapped in our emotions, and doubt, discouragement and desperation overwhelms us, this essence can help us to overcome such emotions, giving us renewed energy to be able to find our way back to our road and see the light at the end of the tunnel. Develops a new spiritual energy that will allow us to organize our lives rationally and therefore we can lead a simpler life, just the way we would like. Being open to spirit can give us our first 'lessons' in spirituality. This can be especially helpful when one is still full of disbelief and questions one's perceptions. A new spiritual strength and sense of joy develop.

Affirmation: My life is light that I turn into joy.

Chinese Hibiscus (*Hibiscus rosa sinensis*)
Essence effect: Helps us integrate the yin (feminine, receptive) side of ourselves allowing it to vibrate within our being once more and lets us show our more tender side and the depth of our feelings. Establishes strong connection and renews a women's contact with the power and richness of her femininity and sexuality. Anyone with body disorder (dysmorphia) caused by an oppressed femininity will accept their womanness, where the root

could be in unsatisfactory relationships making them feel undesirable. It could also lead to frigidity or be a suppressed desire to bear children. Recovers self-esteem and feeling attractive, enriching energy, stimulates our intuition creating new ideas within ourselves.

Affirmation: I enjoy my femininity and sexuality, in addition to my creative ideas.

K9 (the name of this flower is protected)

Essence effect: For the immune system. Strengthens and reinforces our 'life force' – the body's natural defence system – on all levels. Antiviral effect. Still being researched. We can energetically dispel the fear of getting an infection (we will discover that fear is an energy predator that unnecessarily harms our immune system) and therefore we can increase our vital energy. Also, during the course of serious diseases, a feeling of resignation can develop and the feeling that 'nothing makes sense any more' and the situation cannot be changed. Allows us to be courageous, reinforces us and provides positive thoughts contributing to self-healing; with a renewed desire to live, our immune resistance will increase. Brings back the energy to be receptive to positive life and move forward to reach our goals. It unifies the energy of the body and the spirit so our soul can contribute to our self-healing process.

Affirmation: My immunologic capacity grows acting inside me. I am strong and stable.

Recommended combinations: K9 + RQ7 (the seven rescue remedies). These essences should not be absent from any domestic kit.

Milk Thistle (*Sonchus acaulis*)

Essence effect: A great ally in stormy times, relaxes and dissolves tensions at all different levels. Helps us gather thoughts calmly so we don't overreact emotionally, useful when overcome by hysteria or violent episodes. Highly effective when combined with massage oils. It stimulates our ability to eliminate scattered thoughts and to bring our thoughts together, concentrate, feel guided in moments of retrospect and meditation in order to reorientate and find new answers to our inner

emptiness so as to be able to live as a single spiritual unity.

Affirmation: I free myself of inner and outer discordant energy, and I find calm in my inner space.

Petticoat Daffodil (*Narcissus tazetta*)

Essence effect: Allows us to see the 'light at the end of the tunnel' when we feel surrounded by darkness and may have given up hope, in despair with a heart numb with heaviness, sorrow and pessimism (especially indicated for adults as well as to children after sexual abuse and violence). Opens the door to spring once more and helps us to regain self-confidence and radiate happiness, optimism and joy of living; in this way we open to spirit as well.

Affirmation: I enjoy my inner 'sun' and I see that it dissipates the darkness and illuminates myself with its healing rays.

Poinsettia (*Euphorbia pulcherrima*)

Essence effect: A 'feeling essence'. Brings the energies of the heart and throat closer together so that we may express what we truly feel inside. Helps us to talk freely about our feelings to others. Provides courage to express feelings especially for those who have difficulty expressing their feelings, for example, young people, teenagers who are dissatisfied with themselves or their environment. Provides positive mental support clarifying the mind when negative feelings have 'wrapped our soul in the dark' and paralyzed our full development. We will have courage to recognize our mistakes and, if necessary, to apologize. As our spirit will be free of 'darkness', our heart chakra will be opened and we will be able to develop our spirituality.

Affirmation: I can clearly express my feelings and I feel free.

Swiss Cheese Plant (*Monstera deliciosa*)

Essence effect: Strengthens, integrates and balances yang (active) energy and male potency. Helps us accept our yang (masculine) side. Leads to the source of our energy helping us find our place in life. It stimulates considerably men's vital energy and is a positive support in the treatment of male sexual problems. A driving force in putting our lives in order when a feeling of helplessness, hopelessness and a lack of confidence, etc., invades us. Helps connect with our inner wisdom and live our own truth. Also useful for women, so that they accept, integrate and balance their own male energy. Mental processes are clarified so that we are free from the spiralling of thoughts. Indicated for opening up spiritually and developing oneself through spiritual challenges, and carrying the wisdom of the lessons into the reality of everyday life.

Affirmation: I am in the source of my energy and I live my truth.

Tree Heath (*Erica arborea*)

Essence effect: Reduces emotional dependency on others and helps establish one's own independence and self-acceptance. For those who tend to live life through others. Tree Heath essence helps to overcome an exaggerated need of self-importance, attention seeking which has its origins in fear of being alone, insecurity and lack of confidence. It conveys real self-confidence and it helps the person find the inner peace to accept himself as he is. Indicated for children who feel the need to boast and for adults who play one-upmanship (my car is the more beautiful, fastest, better, etc.). Simulates a state of great sense of tranquillity and harmony. The spiritual experience of this essence can be summarized in the following sentence: 'My contribution may be small, but it is important for the whole.'

Affirmation: I gained independence from the opinion of others and I find myself within me.

Touch-Me-Not (*Acacia*)

Essence effect: Improves our relationship with others and helps us to be conscious of our energy. It will guide us to discover our inner riches and inner light. Overcomes the fear of starting afresh, due to deeply held and rooted emotions, eliminates the fear of being in contact with others. Helps reinforce the ability to face situations and find the necessary strength to make important changes in life

and experience a new joy of living. Stimulates the body's natural self-healing processes with skin disorders; it has a relaxing effect and contributes to maintaining the skin smoothness. In meditation helps in opening the crown chakra allowing the union with the spiritual level. The light of the spiritual world will enlighten our soul.

Affirmation: I let the light burst into me, bringing peace, transformation and healing.

Viper's (Common) Bugloss (*Echium vulgare*)

Essence effect: Works as a 'softener' and 'opener'. Enables us to discover that humour and friendliness take us further than a grim sense of duty or discipline. For those who have been interested in the exercise of power and leadership patterns focused on success and are prey to their own sense of obligations, preventing them from knowing other aspects of their lives. Teaches to learn to 'nourish' our thoughts, to move forward easily with love and kindness. Develops warm-hearted side and teaches that a smile can often open doors. Emotional values will be considerably enriched and we will learn to discover and to be receptive to the spiritual consciousness and move closer to our spirituality and make it part of everyday life.

Affirmation: Laughter opens my heart and connects me to other people's hearts.

White Leaved Rockrose (*Cistus albidus*)

Essence effect: Strengthens our inner resolve so that we remain centred and can open up and take part in a group with clarity, being able to express thoughts and ideas and aware that personal contribution is important and necessary in a group whilst being able to remain faithful to your own ideas. Good support for a teamwork development. Assists those who lack assertiveness or 'backbone'. On the energy level, it stimulates and contributes to stability of the second chakra. Very effective in helping to overcome different female pains.

Affirmation: I express my experiences and I am one more within the group.

European Orchids

Cephalanthera (*Cephalanthera rubra*)
Essence effect: Helps maintain our focus on the task at hand, if problems develop. It creates a spiritual structure in our mind and strengthens our concentration.

Epipactis (*Epipactis helleborine*)
Essence effect: Allows us to dive deep within ourselves in order to bring hidden inner aspects of our personality to the surface, so we can accept them with love. Facilitates access to the subconscious.

Neottia (*Neottia nidus-avis*)
Essence effect: Brings suppressed feelings to the surface so they can be transformed in a loving fashion. Removes unjustified emotional fears that we are being wrongly treated or betrayed.

Orchis (*Orchis mascula*)
Essence effect: By keeping our feet firmly on the ground, this Orchid essence permits us to soar to new spiritual heights in our mind. It assists astral travel while keeping us solidly grounded.

Platanthera (*Platanthera chlorantha*)
Essence effect: Helps us see clearly what is spiritually right for us when we must make difficult decisions; a powerful spiritual cleansing agent.

Cacti and succulent plants: courageous artists of survival

Cacti are known for their hardiness in extreme climates; their ability to survive with little water and their prickles suggest both their defensive and protective properties. These essences are drawn from plants that are found mainly in South America and Africa.

There is no doubt that cacti are excellent representatives of succulent plants, as these fleshy plants store water. Aeons ago as climatic conditions worsened on the planet and the presence of water was gradually reduced, the first cacti appeared in Ancient South America. Especially in those places where the impact of the sun was strongest, some plants began to collect water in their thick stems to overcome periods of severe drought. At first, they differed little from other plants, but eventually they developed the qualities that would make them a new category of succulent plants. The cacti evolution took place, increasing their degree of succulence, with some the leaves becoming needle-shaped, and others their stem length being reduced by becoming more rounded, until both elements reached the shape we know today.

The body language of cacti

With their thorny appearance the cacti seem to be saying: 'Warning, stay away: do not get too close; I know how to defend myself.' This is their plant signature and symbolizes the protection of life. They live and flourish in places where no other plant would be able to exist and endure extreme environments setting themselves up as real artists of survival. This feature is clearly demonstrated by some cactus flowers that have an aggressive looking interior: a protective armour of thorns. Cacti store large amounts of liquid; their juicy flesh, generously swollen with water, is the elixir of life to birds and insects. The cactus essence helps reinforce our defensive capacity, dissipates the fears of lack in times of shortage keeping a sense of hope to survive in critical periods, and 'to flourish'. Cacti and succulent plants provide warmth and a lightness to the heart allowing it to open.

A note regarding the names of the cactus essences: Many cacti have only a Latin American name, which turns out to be incomprehensible. In this case I have named these essences by their principal energetic healing quality. Many of the cacti family are night blooming and then only once a year, so some changes are inevitable.

Aura-cleansing Cactus (*Cleistoicactus strausii*), South America
Essence effect: For cleansing, protection and regeneration of the aura, especially clears the astral body of energetic parasites and helps

those people whose auric field is too open and affected by various different external energies. To cleanse and protect those who have problems defining their boundaries. When our auric field is disturbed, our mental energy also suffers from a lack of strength, concentration problems, forgetfulness, daydreaming and unexplained feelings, and mood changes. This essence can significantly eradicate intrusion from strong personalities that affect our auric field initiating spiritual purification.

Affirmation: I am free and I can start breathing again. I am surrounded by protection and security.

Beauty Cactus (*Echinocereus scheeri*), Mexico
Essence effect: Helps us to discover the inner beauty of our hearts. Helps us to find an equilibrium, nurtures modesty, humility and hope when confronted with dissatisfaction, frustration, fury, doubts, self-hatred, contempt, with our body and about appearance but equally feelings of vanity, pride, arrogance, when overattached to external looks and who therefore have forgotten the values of modesty, humility and patience. Develops the natural warmth of the heart, helps us to develop our inner potentials and true inner beauty, harmonizing the inner and outer. You can open your heart and, with each beam of love that emanates from us, our features will be softened and our smile will be widened.
Affirmation: My inner joy makes me beautiful and it radiates from my heart for all to see.

Blueberry Cactus (*Myrtillocactus geometrizans*), USA
Essence effect: Helps us to develop our own potential. On the one hand it aids by helping us to set healthy boundaries and protect the heart chakra, and on the other hand, it encourages us to realize and accept that who we are is good and unlimited in potential. Repression of potential and if a passion for life is suffocated it can be reflected in many bodily disorders. When we are in distress this can cause stresses in facial gestures and we can develop deep wrinkles. Overcoming self-recriminations and personal dissatisfaction

and a discovery and use of our own potential as well as the desire to enjoy life awakens our reserves of mental energy. With this essence, we develop the ability to improve planning, structure and fulfilment of our potential. Thus, we can better develop our true selves and our work and then we will feel greater satisfaction. Spiritually the body, spirit and soul are in harmony.

Affirmation: I accept my potential with happiness and I am able to show it. I enjoy this experience and life. Satisfaction comes when we identify our mission (the meaning of life) and walk on our path.

Earth Star Cactus (*Stapelia desmetiana*), South America
Essence effect: Powerfully cleanses and stimulates the first chakra, connecting it directly with a feeling of rooting to Mother Earth. Clears and releases bottled-up negative emotions and poisons, of the body strengthens the role of the eliminatory organs and it acts on the masculine energy (Yang), strengthens our sense of self, and grounds. Base chakra is balanced with the heart chakra and we feel free and light again. With its invigorating energy, this essence can be an energy help for women during pregnancy.
Affirmation: I feel the Earth and its force, which reinforces my heart and makes me free of every negative feeling.

Formation Cactus (*Mammillaria rubrograndis*), Mexico
Essence effect: Provides protection and stability at all levels, from the cellular to the mental. Stimulates the inner life force and helps to eliminate the burden of internal negative energies. Has a protective effect on the organs and internal processes, stimulates the removal of negative energy out of the body. This is observed externally as tired looking skin. The revitalizing effect acts positively on the surrounding tissues and organs. Also can be used to cleanse polluted areas around us. It reinforces and revitalizes the environments that are negatively affected. Spiritual consciousness is opened up on all levels of our being,

introducing a new rhythm of life, and healing energy that is stabilized at a higher level.

Affirmation: Love and stability are inside me and they release me from every burden.

Golden Barrel Cactus (*Echinocactus grusonii*), Mexico

Essence effect: For protection and being centred. When we have been exposed to many different external influences and disruptions, creating hesitation, insecurity and nervousness, it helps regain balance. It is particularly indicated for those in a leadership position and who have many external contacts. This essence helps us stay calm in the swirl of emotion, stand firmly and be centred again. Protects us from environmental influences, and helps one to focus on the essential. Good for those whose work brings them into contact with people and spirituality acting from our own balance.

Affirmation: I am balanced and I stay firmly with my feet on the ground.

Grounding Opuntia (*Opuntia dejecta*), Cuba

Essence effect: Activates the first chakra, stimulating rooting and deep interior tranquillity and stability. It helps us find calm, be ourselves with a stronger sense of connection to the Earth. For protection. Stimulates our life force, our capacity for action while giving greater stability and assisting us in defending our boundaries. By recognizing where and what blockages affect us negatively in the mental and emotional plane it creates a liberating energy. From this new healthier spiritual base, we will be able to develop new clearer positive mental structures.

Affirmation: I identify and I eliminate my blockages and, in this way, I feel my energy and my freedom growing within me.

Here and Now Cactus (*Hylocereus undatus*), Mexico and Central America

Essence effect: Helps us to accept and love being incarnated; to be here. When we do not feel comfortable in our body, when there are some health issues that, somehow, do not quite 'add up' to us, helps us develop a sense of body 'comfort'. Stimulates contact with Mother Earth, opens us to an awareness of her love. Brings awareness of her light bodies. Helps when we evade reality, and guides us toward reconnection with our lives and gives it form and shape for our body, mind and our soul to be here and now.

Affirmation: I perceive myself intensively; I feel the energy of my body, the clarity of my spirit and the love of my soul.

Inside-Outside Cactus (*Pilosocereus pachycladus*), Brazil

Essence effect: At the energetic level to protect and regenerate the skin. Expands and opens us up on the surface levels of our consciousness, including the cellular levels of our physical boundaries, that is, the skin; stimulates the exchange between the interior and the outside through our skin and makes us aware of the 'inside' and 'outside' of our being. Helps to contribute to the self-healing of certain skin conditions on the energy level as well to identify the causes of the skin reaction providing support during the phases of elimination of the negative suppressed feelings or intense emotion reactions.

Affirmation: I see my skin as the mediator between the inside and the outside and I find my balance.

Inner Cleansing Cactus (*Cleistocactus ritteri*), Bolivia

Essence effect: Stimulates positive inner processes and helps us to digest all the impressions to which we are exposed. It promotes both cleansing and renewal of our innermost processes.

Beneficial effect on the digestive tract and calmly eliminates from the spiritual level our adherence to old behaviour patterns that can manifest in the body, for example, as constipation. This essence can also be administered during puberty as an energy protector. Creates a protective aura around the head and therefore can be particularly useful to people who often have to 'keep their head up'. Opens to new experiences, and a new consciousness by being released from old patterns.

Affirmation: I purify myself and my body of everything that affects it negatively.

Inspiration Cactus (*Echinopsis oxygona*), South America

Essence effect: Stimulates the third eye, and has a deep cleansing and expansive effect on our state of mind. It protects us against disturbing thoughts and negative influences, dispelling negative thoughts about oneself, which lead to self-destructive tendencies and otherwise might appear in various body disorders. It helps people to accept themselves just as they are and it encourages self-love thereby allowing us to develop a clear sense of our own purpose and inner direction. Supports separation and detachment processes, especially for girls and women who have not freed themselves from their father's image and constantly compare their partner with the father or, conversely, of boys in relation to the mother. Encourages independence, enabling us to explore our own path. Also helpful in facilitating the farewell and detachment process not only for those who are on their deathbed but also those who remain.

Affirmation: My energy of thought is clear and I am conscious of my independence in the course of my life.

Joyful Cactus (*Opuntia cardiosperma*), Paraguay

Essence effect: Works on the heart chakra and on the solar plexus chakra. Brings joy back to our lives, especially when suffering great emotional burdens, for example, sadness, separation, illness, at those difficult moments when life seems a heavy burden. Restores a sense of optimism, security and self-confidence and a wider perspective when we need to look beyond immediate problems and have faith in life and it awakens in us a new joy of living. This essence connects us to the child within ourselves, and Aborigines used this cactus for women in labour, and it is said to harmonize the skin's functions.

Affirmation: I leave behind sadness and I face life full of light and love. I rediscover the feeling of joy.

Radiation Protection Cactus (*Cereus peruvianus*), Peru

Essence effect: Offers strong protection against all kinds of radiation (electromagnetic pollution from computers, electrical equipment, contaminant fog, ozone) and negative influences and better guard against it. Likewise, encourages conscious awareness of our own negative thoughts and being able to transform them, as well as recognize and neutralize the negative thoughts and desires of others. Helps us to develop our full potential, including our intellectual potential. Useful for solar protection and stimulates the skin's natural protective ability.

Affirmation: I have full protection and I am positive.

Release Cactus (*Ceropegia fusca*), Canary Islands

Essence effect: Helps us to recognize and accept our shadow sides. This essence is profound in its effect, reaching the level of cellular consciousness and unconsciousness, dissolving old blockages, which allows the body to realize the trauma of the psyche's old wounds, aiding cellular regeneration, allowing us to renew ourselves and develop our self-confidence and our inner strength. This plant's segmented stem resembles the backbone and awakening the vital energy that emanates from the base chakra and helps us to continue to stand up tall and straight in life. Endows spiritual strength to persevere and reach our goal. We will be able to identify and to dissolve any spiritual blockages caused by ourselves or others. Promotes complete relaxation and stimulates intense experiences during meditation.

Affirmation: Everything flows and I am strong, immersed in the flow of life.

Self-Esteem Cactus (*Ferocactus schwarzii*), Mexico

Essence effect: Emanates an indestructible force and reinforces self-confidence and provides energy support for our body's immune system. It reinvigorates it on the energetic level which has benefits for the body as a whole.

Detoxifies the body's energy and can be a good complement to fasting cures. Creates a stable basis for co-operation and mutual assistance; when becoming involved with a group, enjoyment of the spiritual exchange develops with the ability to trust in others and compassion with those close to us and sympathy for all living things. Introduces a new sense of spiritual growth in our lives. People of solitary habits can greatly benefit from this essence.

Affirmation: I know who I am and what I can give to the others. I give the freedom to 'myself' that I had once suppressed and open myself to life and people. I accept my virtues as well as my weaknesses.

Life Force Cactus (*Orbea variegata*), South Africa

Essence effect: Works to protect and regenerate the skin. Our overall vibration will be increased which will remove and free us from energy parasites that sap our vital energy and create a protective barrier against possible further attacks. Helps us to be aware of what is 'inside' and what is 'outside' our being so we can shed old limits and boundaries, thereby allowing us to grow. Establishes the contact with the Earth. Protects those who have lost energy through blood loss (via surgery, or donation.) Metaphysical processes, such as astral travel, should not be underestimated as such processes could be the ones in which you may suffer the 'attack' of energy parasites. This essence allows us to have our own protection barrier and so we can strongly radiate our vital energy and its intangible protection against the aggression of other beings. Many sensitive people can be absorbed by 'energy parasites' for years, unaware; sometimes they lack the strength to protect themselves.

Affirmation: I access my vital force, I radiate it and I have an invincible protection around me.

Love Cactus (*Seticereus icosagonus*), north of Ecuador and Peru

Essence effect: Has a strong effect on the second chakra (creativity), and helps us become conscious of our creative powers at all levels. It helps us to discover how to achieve a balance between work and play and how to maintain integrity when dealing with others. Allows us to be more conscious of our sexual energy, providing stability and energy protection. It supports a positive experience through complete union through the connection of the second chakra with the fourth chakra (sacral with the heart chakra). Teaches us to give when we receive, and to receive when we give and achieve a perfect balance in our relationship with the others. On the spiritual level, we will be in constant contact with our Higher Self.

Affirmation: I enjoy love, my creativity and my happiness. My life is sunshine.

Noble Heart Cactus (*Stenocereus marginatus*), Mexico

Essence effect: Promotes better physical posture, reinforcing the spinal column, and also an awareness of our upright nature. Helps us to open and expand the heart chakra, developing sincerity and integrity, and receive happiness and love. Acts positively on any problem derived from stress, pressure, worries, fears, sorrows. Useful for cold-hearted people; through hurt they play the 'tough guy' as it helps them to thaw the ice block. With this essence, a change in inner attitude which makes us start again, the love and protection of this essence will guide our spiritual development.

Affirmation: I straightened up and, through a change in my inner attitude, I open my heart.

Queen of the Night Cactus (*Selenicereus grandiflorus*), the Caribbean

Essence effect: Acts on the third chakra, brings light and hope when we are overly afraid, worried or sorrowful. Helps purify our thoughts and clear our mind as we recognize which parts of our being feel very dark when we are confronted with a tide of emotions.

Affirmation: 'The rays of the sun expel the night; they deprive darkness of its treacherous power' (Mozart).

This essence is a guiding light in the valley of shadows and it can show us a renewed spark of hope as a result of its purifying energy. Helps those people who live in spiritual darkness and is a great ally for those who would like to find God within themselves.

Affirmation: I feel a deep purification and I step from darkness to the divine light.

Shadow Cactus (*Caralluma russeliana*), East Africa

Essence effect: Has a releasing effect on the solar plexus; we become conscious of our inner processes and are able to overcome them and move on. For mental or emotional problems that arise in this area and that may be reflected in physical disorders, when overloaded by conflicts, deep emotional wounds, negative thoughts, etc., this essence restores harmony. We say goodbye to our shadow, learn to accept death as a precursor of life (we cannot be without dying first) and to discover yourself to be once and again in this circle to accept death of the past and live in total awareness.

Affirmation: I accept death and I am reborn into a new being.

Mushrooms: release of energy at the physical level

Mushroom essences combine very easily with flower essences. While closely related to plants, they lack chloropyll and are classified as fungi, a separate biological kingdom. The mushroom is the mycelium, the fibrous network that grows underground, and is dependent on existing organic substances. In this environment, they perform their vital functions (e.g. decomposition and the use of leaves and bark) and will also pass these to other plants. There are three main types of mushrooms:

1. Purely de-constructive mushrooms. They can be linked to our body's digestive activities.

2. The second class, which is more extensive and interesting, is composed of the mushrooms that live in symbiosis (co-existence) with the roots of trees. The majority of known edible mushrooms are found within this group. They constitute the mutually advantageous link between trees and mushrooms.

3. The parasitic mushrooms. These fungi inhabit living trees or other living beings. Through injury, for example, damage to the bark, the fungus spores enter the host triggering an infection that will spread throughout the organism. Similarly, the essences of this group are closely linked to situations arising from parasitic problems, for example, fungi invasions, etc.

Mushroom essences are perfectly suited to match or complement flower essences. In these combinations, flower essences act on the emotional body, while mushroom essences carry these changes to the physical level, integrating the energy absorbed into the cells. As mushroom essences can have a very strong effect they need to be tested before use. They enter deep into our subconscious revealing deeply buried issues. Timing is all important when taking mushroom essences; the individual personality needs to be mature enough to cope with confrontation of deep issues and be able to process the information that is released.

In practice, the combination of flower essences and mushroom essences has proved to be useful. Flower essences act at the consciousness level, while mushroom essences act at the subconscious one, enhancing the effects of the flower essence, say Slippery Jack with Pine.

As some of the mushrooms are difficult to find (especially the ones coming from the Amazon region), so we reserve the right to introduce modifications.

Amethyst Deceiver (*Laccaria amethystina*)
Essence effect: A strong effect on the third eye (sixth chakra) supports internal change as well as the transformation processes, eliminates

negative perceptions, bringing to light personal problems that may cause blockages and emotional poisons. Useful in times of change so that spiritual problems are not reflected in physical discomfort. Breaks old mental patterns and repressed emotions that cause damage and limit our mental energy. Releases spiritual blockages and allows one to be free to pursue new spiritual paths.

Affirmation: I recognize that I was poisoned and I get rid of such poison. So, I experience an unlimited liberation which I enjoy.

Slippery Jack (*Suillus luteus*)

Essence effect: Helps us to be aware of deeply rooted feelings such as shame or guilt, and frees us from blockages caused by negative feelings. Those who are dominated by these emotions and carry physical pain associated with feelings of shame or guilt often feel attracted by this essence. Aids conflicts between mother and child and contributes to the final resolution including those on the physical level. Dissipates associated mental blockages and self-imposed restrictions and so understanding there is no guilt but learning processes. Freed we can open ourselves to higher planes of consciousness so experience a new spiritual freedom.

Affirmation: I free myself of the feelings of shame and guilt and I breathe a free life.

Common Puffball (*Lycoperdon perlatum*)

Essence effect: Affects the fontanel and, therefore, the seventh chakra. Affords contact with higher levels of consciousness. Helps a deeper understanding of illness or physical limitations and to place less credence on the restrictions that a disease imposes on us and to find inner peace enabling us to stay calm and balanced. Helps to distance oneself from the environment and to define some clear boundaries. Enables us to keep a cool head, be mentally focused without being distracted and helps to improve the ability to assess situations better.

Affirmation: My free spirit can rise.

Fly Agaric (*Amanita muscaria*)

Essence effect: Works on the sixth chakra upwards and purifies perception. Cleanses the toxic information of psychotropic drugs especially when they have negative effects on the body. Eliminates these by expelling the negative information on the energic level. Purifies emotional intensity emotions that are evoked from reliving negative images and experiences.

Fly Agaric essence should only be used when mentally stable and the physical body has been stabilized. Strengthens the intuitive voice; a lighter feeling will be experienced. Of great help in gaining access to other dimensions, ties with the material reality will loosen and an experience of the cosmic dimension of the whole self occurs.

Affirmation: I purify my body, spirit and soul from all the negative influences and I am flooded with light and energy.

Grey Coral Fungus (*Clavulina cinerea*)

Essence effect: Has a stimulating effect on the nervous system and thought processes. Helps us to achieve a new dimension of perception when negative emotions dominate our consciousness and quickly translate into tangible physical problems. Aids recognition and clarity about conflicts, allowing more mental energy to find solutions and therefore freedom from physical problems and the energy to deal with reactions of the nervous system. Through harmonizing the interaction between intellect and intuition, we can listen to our inner voice which is helpful in planning our lives and defining new goals. Establishes a new spiritual and physical order allowing a wider and greater perspective and connection to higher dimensions. We will be aware that it is possible to find God in this balance.

Affirmation: Light and clarity shine within me as I follow my inner voice.

Horn of Plenty (*Craterellus cornucopioides*)

Essence effect: Acts strongly on the first chakra, and binds us closely to the Earth and to our deepest-dark physical aspect. Called the 'Halo of Hades' as it reveals the darkest side of ourselves, helping to integrate it. As we enter our depths and darkness, we recognize and experience our own light and great personal power. Allows us to determine the origin of and eliminate physical problems. In the same way that the Earth inhales and exhales through the funnel, our energy blockages will find release through the respiratory cycle – a useful complement to breath therapy or re-birthing. Used to treat and dissipate fears, included childhood fears, redirecting this energy towards creativity, in order to further develop our creative and mental energy. Giving an abundance of vital energy as well as more strength to carry out our plans. A mushroom of transformation and with Dolphin essence an aid during pregnancy, and in labour can relieve childbirth pains.

Affirmation: I accept my dark side and I expel all the energy blockages in order to be able to feel the light of life.

Hercules Mace (*Clavariadelphus pistillaris*)
Essence effect: This essence unites with the upper chakras (from the eighth chakra above) offering a better perspective of life as we are able to experience ourselves from this higher perspective. Promotes mental energy, useful in periods of confusion providing energy support. In times of helplessness and feeling of being worn-out, stimulates trust in creative energy and the ability to direct our energy correctly. It permits us to place great confidence in the Creator and it establishes a union between this energy and the vital energy of the first chakra; both provide a renewed inner strength for healing. The blueprint of our life plan exists in the higher chakras, which we will now be able to visualize enabling us to act in harmony with the creative process.

Affirmation: I can see myself from a higher viewpoint and I am able to discern what suits me at all times.

Clustered Tough Shank (*Collybia confluens*)
Essence effect: Acts on our 'spiritual antennae' making us more sensitive on all energy levels. Curiously enough the hair acts as 'physical antennae', informing us of any external negative influence. We also perceive physical reactions with greater sensitivity, for example, when the body suggests that we need to rest. As our awareness of the feelings of others is sharpened we will be able to handle our emotions better, and face negativity and dissipate it. Clarifies our mental state, and in this way our mental development can be improved and intensified (for example, planning). Our 'antennae' are not restricted to the mental realm but also open to new spiritual perceptions. Intensifies perception of the higher spiritual dimensions and our soul is free and receptive to information and transfers this into our daily lives.

Affirmation: My soul and my senses are open and I perceive the most subtle of information.

Trumpet Funnel Cap (*Clitocybe geotropa*)
Essence effect: Dissipates energy imbalances and blockages of the first and second chakras. Enhances our basic vitality and supports the removal of toxins, also frees us from emotional toxicity and adds vitality to our emotional body. Strengthens areas of physical and spiritual weakness. Beneficial for fungal diseases. The essence works on the physical level, frees toxic information and provides support to our brain and, at the same time, helps to develop a new mental strength. Through freeing our physical body of malfunctions, and mental and emotional blockages, our spiritual energy can then receive a new impulse and a new spiritual experience can lead to a discovery of the meaning of our life.

Affirmation: I am purified and I receive new vital energy.

Aleuria (*Aleuria aurantia*)
Essence effect: Helps us find a balance between matter and spirit, while regulating both either a strong or weak attachment to material things. Both excessive and insufficient attachment to matter can cause bodily discomfort. In the first case, inertia or fear of the new can paralyze us. In the second, we long for support, strength and nurturing, and feel dizzy and become nervous if it is lacking, etc. In both cases, the essence helps us to have

a physical feeling of harmony and stability. Good for regulating the sense of numbness and absent-mindedness, and to find a harmonious balance. It has a two-way effect and is applicable for those clinging to spirituality at the expense of their physical needs as well as those who ignore spirit and focus on the physical at the expense of their spirituality. Supports the spiritual development; those who have paid little attention to their spirituality will become more sensitive to it, and for those who are extremely sensitive to spiritual experiences it enables them to test whether spiritual goals are realistically achievable and for both translates their spirituality into everyday life.

Affirmation: I find the balance between Heaven and Earth.

Parasol (*Macrolepiota procera*)

Essence effect: Helps us to recognize, accept, unfold and develop our personal potential. We can recognize our true greatness and accept it. Good for parental conflicts, affected by the diseases or negative behavioural patterns of their mother or father which blocks their personal development. Identifies potential patterns of transference and eliminates them. Consequently, this essence has a highly liberating effect on the emotions that may have been repressed for years and sets them free. With this freedom from imposed external influences or restrictions we can open the way to our own spirituality.

Affirmation: I am conscious of my great potential and am able to take advantage of it.

Velvet Shank (*Flammulina velutipes*)

Essence effect: Transmits a freshness to our thought patterns and releases old ties and helps to rid ourselves of outdated repetitive structures. On the physical level, helpful for overcoming long-standing illnesses, aids the regeneration process and encourages healthy thoughts rather than thoughts of illness. It is revitalizing and promotes wellbeing and the understanding and release of deeply rooted past emotions allowing new positive feelings to emerge. The wellbeing and health of body,

spirit and soul begin with how you think and freedom from thought patterns, allowing our thoughts to be led in a new direction to open our spirituality.

Affirmation: I feel a lightness and freshness inside me, and leave old patterns of thought behind as a new life opens up before me.

Many-Zoned Polypore (*Coriolus versicolor*)

Essence effect: Increases our capacity of self-knowledge, protects us from external influences and energetically protects us in moments of crisis and change which can leave traces on the body. The strong protective effect of this essence helps people who are susceptible to infections or energy-sapping parasites and to ward off unhealthy outside influences.

Through its invigorating energy, it helps during difficult times and to resolve physical problems. Helps to reinforce perception of self and awareness of our inner energy reserves leading to freedom from crisis situations. When overshadowed by worries and fears, this essence can help us to create a new mental goal in life and pursue it. Energy parasites can consume our strength and prevent spiritual experiences. It enables us to recognize these influences and to eliminate them and regain an intense self-awareness.

Affirmation: I perceive myself, I am conscious of myself, and I feel sure again.

Summer Cep (*Boletus reticulatus*)

Essence effect: Connects us to the Earth's energy and builds an energy protection for the entire body. Physically, acts as an energetic protection for the entire organism, especially helpful when there is risk of infection. Good for protection during travel. People who feel emotionally vulnerable and are looking for safety will find support using this essence. Inner strength and the eradication of weakening emotions develops. A strong emotional connection with the Earth means we can immerse ourselves in its powerful energy. The essence predisposes us to live in communion with the Earth, so we can open ourselves to the Earth's message and develop a strong bond with our planet.

Affirmation: I feel the energy of the Earth and I form a strong bond with it.

Lichen (*Caloplaca flavescens*)
Essence effect: Helps to redefine the contact to the outside world. Promotes healthy skin which is the organ linking us to the outside world. Physically balances the skin and supports the self-healing processes especially with skin problems. It furthers our ability to identify and to eliminate their cause. It also dissolves physical tension. Skin problems often have a deeply rooted emotional cause. Lichen essence helps us to be aware of these emotions and work on them. It is an energetic aid to lead us step by step to create the harmony that our skin needs. The skin is the point of contact with the outside and when disturbed an allergic reaction can occur. Lichen helps define a new mental understanding. With this essence we can reflect on and eradicate those experiences that have led to skin problems. We can get rid of old patterns and build a protective energy field around ourselves.
Affirmation: I release myself from the shadows of the past and I leave behind skin problems.

Vesuvius Snow Lichen (*Stereocaulon vesuvianum*)
Essence effect: Transmits energy to start anew after a tragic event and stimulates the will to move forward one step at a time. During difficult stages of life, many physical problems that result from psychological weakness can adversely affect us. Helps to find inner strength to overcome physical problems of psychological origin. When difficult events in life cause radical changes on all levels, this essence provides new hope, courage and the strength and will to start anew, move forward and mentally prepares us to reach our goals. Life changes require great energy which we will find at the spiritual level and be able to understand situations and to make sense of everything, including Creation. Finding inner peace that will bring strength and guidance in life.

Affirmation: I am at the beginning and recognize my new sense of direction in my life.

Violet Rötelritterling (*Lepista Irina*)
Essence effect: Purifies the energy flow between the chakras. The fifth, sixth and seventh chakras promote access to the third eye (sixth chakra) and to clarity and intuition. The energy flow is anchored at cellular level. Any blockages or restricted flow of energy in the chakras can create physical problems. Repressed feelings can result in an energy blockage of the 2nd chakra though all other chakras can also be affected as they are interrelated. The essence will help us to identify and eradicate negative emotions. This essence stimulates energy flow in the chakras and balances different energy levels and this restored energy flow will provide an energetic protection of the physical body. Blockages of the fifth, sixth and seventh chakras limit our mental energy. By reactivating the energy flow it creates space for new experiences and is the basis for spiritual experiences.
Affirmation: Clarity resides in me and I am open to my energy flow.

Toothed Jelly Fungus (*Pseudohydnum gelatinosum*)
Essence effect: Stimulates concentration, stability and equilibrium. On the physical level, it helps to conserve rather than dissipate strength. Energetically strengthens our cell structures, especially the solar plexus, enabling us to act with renewed vitality. Those who are easily swayed, full of doubts and insecurity, can experience a new stability and become centred, are better able to resist distractions, and make better use of their energy. Helps focus and thoughts will become clear and disciplined and we will be fully conscious of our energy.
Affirmation: I sense my renewed energy and I can focus on my goals.

Fungus Amazonas No. 1 (*Cordyceps*)
Essence effect: Supports and purifies the second chakra, encourages the elimination of emotional toxins that have settled in the body.

Acts particularly on the kidneys, although the whole organism benefits from its vibrations. This essence allows us to get rid of all emotional toxins usually caused by very old emotions.

Stimulates the elimination of these toxins from all levels of our being. Emotional toxins can weaken our mental energy, causing a spiral of negative thoughts. This essence helps us to overcome the 'thought toxin' and create a new mental plan. Establishes a connection between the heart and kidneys, encouraging our spiritual willingness to open ourselves to others. We are ready for interactive spiritual experiences and experience God in others.

Affirmation: Free of emotional toxins, I open myself to other people and to Divine Love.

Porling-Fungus Amazonas No. 2 (*Pycnoporus sanguineus*)

Essence effect: It connects the first chakra to the Earth and exerts a strong stimulating effect on the feet. The rooting quality of the essence creates a feeling of general stability and security while increasing energy awareness. Those who have a strong emotional dependence on others and depend on others' opinions and perceptions can find their own spiritual truth and will discover their capacity to be independent. Emotional ties will be loosened and clear thought and life planning is encouraged and we will be directors of our own life. Also stabilizes consciousness and helps in any tendencies to schizophrenia.

Affirmation: I am connected to the Earth's energy and I sense how it transmits an inner stability.

Special essences

Anti-radiation Essence T1 Essence (made at Chernobyl in Russia) The singularity of this essence is that it acts in the opposite way from all other energy essences we have researched. Instead of radiating energy, T1 essence soaks up surplus energy, thereby restoring the organism's energy balance in cases of overexposure or stimulation.

Our research has led us to conclude that this essence can be used positively in the following situations: in cases of field lines pollution (high-tension electricity); after X-ray treatments; and in cases of overexposure to electromagnetic nuclear radiation. T1 and Delph (see Dolphin and Whale essences) together is a powerful combination used to clear radiation in the subtle energy field.

Teide – Volcano Essence This is an environmental essence that was produced on the 'Teide', a 3716 metre-high volcano on the island of Tenerife. This essence brings our consciousness down to the deepest cellular level. We can then experience our consciousness in the smallest building blocks of matter. It also brings us the experience of both the universal microcosm and macrocosm forces – subject to alterations, that is, changes.

Essence skin creams

The range of essence skin creams (with the exception of Amazon and RQ7 First Aid Cream) can be personalized by adding a few drops of your own prescription mix (see page 64) or other specially selected flower essences. Each cream uses avocado and wheat-germ oil as part of their base.

Amazon Skin Cream Recommended for massaging into areas of the body when the energy flow is stifled or energetically blocked. For treatment of the back, apply directly on the fossa triangularis of the auricle (the indent at the front and top of the ear).

Delph Skin Cream An energetically strong cream that helps open the heart chakra. It activates and purifies the skin.

Lotus Skin Cream Restores energetic harmony and balance to the skin through its relaxing properties. Based on the Lotus flower, considered to be the universal flower of peace and harmony.

RQ7 First Aid Cream Contains seven different flower essences. Apply externally in acute emergencies such as shock, and injury to the skin such as cuts and bruising. It also energizes and stimulates and relieves exhaustion or deep fatigue.

Self-heal Skin Cream Stimulates self-healing for irritated or chafed skin. Ideal for using as an aftershave balm.

Venus Orchid Skin Cream Deeply relaxing preparation for the face and body which enhances the gentle side of one's nature and softness of the skin. Recommended for sensitive skin.

Korte energy balancers

The energy balancers herald a multilevelled approach to combining essences. Andreas has created a synergistic blend of all the vibrational octaves that his range of essences operate on from mushrooms on the ground level to the higher vibrations of the Orchids at the top level.

Forever Young Energy Essence Gives us the feeling of permanent inner youth. Helps us to let go of the fear of ageing. Provides an energetic revitalization of our body – reconnecting with the mind and spirit. Lets our inner beauty shine through.

Heart/Emotional Energy Balancer Heightens and grows our qualities of the heart. Teaches us to give unconditional love without disempowering ourselves. Supports and nurtures the emotional body. Gives us the wonderful feeling that we are lovable beings.

Jet Lag/Sleep Energy Balancer Balances sleep and rest times. Helps us to regenerate energetically. Supports us during travelling through different time zones.

Joyful Sexuality Essence Heightens our emotions and awareness of those beautiful special moments. Helps us to enjoy sensuality with more love and creativity.

Connects the experience of body with mind and spirit. Recommended in combination with the Women or Men Energy Balancer Essence.

Men Energy Balancer Strengthens the male energy (yang). Creates balance when men are too achievement-oriented. Helps us to connect with their true inner nature. Aids men to be truly empowered and succeed in manifesting that empowerment in their lives.

Protection Energy Balancer Strengthens our protection shield for the emotional body. Gives us the feeling of distance and protection. Increases our feeling of trust and that we are always protected. Enables our growth into our true power as a unique being.

Purification Energy Balancer A deep purifying cleanser, helpful for those times when we feel internally clogged or unclean. Clears energetic blocks and toxins from the subtle body. Gives us the feeling of inner and outer purification and a fresh clear perspective.

Regeneration Energy Balancer Revitalizes us when we feel lethargic or weak. Unleashes new energy and power. Gives us the feeling of inner stability and strength. Helps balance our mind, body and spirit in an energetic unity.

Stress Energy Balancer Nurtures us with a sense of calm when we feel we want to explode. Guides us to develop more distance and perspective. Assists in protection of ourselves. Allows us to give more time to ourselves and accept the good things in life.

Women Energy Balancer Increases the female energy (yin). Empowers women to accept their feminine side with joy. Heals emotional pressures; provides emotional stability when we need it. An energetic aid during pregnancy.

Dolphin and whale essences

This section describes Andreas's amazing encounters and work with dolphins and whales.

Water activation: A powerful dream called me to make the Delph essence. In it I journeyed to the islands off Brazil where I made the essence, and there experienced the unique communication with the dolphins and their desire to help us. I have been conducting energetic healing of the waterways with Delph and co-authored a book on dolphins, *Dolphins and Whales.*

Delph (*Tursiops truncatus*) Delph® (Dolphin) is an extraordinary essence that re-energizes and cleanses the whole chakra system and subtle bodies. Produced with the conscious help of free, sea-dwelling dolphins, it has the amazing ability to work on all our chakras at once, stimulating and harmonizing our entire being. The dolphins' message is one of unconditional love. It is said that dolphins are the guardians of the ancient wisdom and secrets. Like a personal encounter with wild dolphins in the ocean, this essence opens our heart chakra so that we experience life's unity and the interrelatedness of all living things. Delph has a powerful cleansing effect both on our physical body, which is over 80 per cent water, and spiritually. It is also used in 'water activation' for the cleansing and activation of rivers, lakes and seas polluted by industrial or agricultural waste. Recommended for childbirth to ease the trauma of coming into the world. Helps babies to be peaceful and serene.

The Pink Amazonian Dolphin (*Sotalia fluviatilis*) Connects us with the heart of Planet Earth giving us a deep inter-connection with our soul which calms and raises the consciousness.

Whale (*Globicephala melas*) This powerful essence should only be used after one has worked with Delph® (dolphin essence). Please, always test it first! Whales are the keepers of knowledge. They are quite serious but in a loving, fatherly way. Their essence throws our heart chakra wide open so that we can connect deeply with all life forms on Earth. This experience, which can be overwhelming for the unprepared, reminds us of our role as caretakers of this planet and our need to live up to our real purpose for being here.

Aura sprays

Due to the destruction of the ozone layer, we are exposed to radiation that is becoming stronger. We know that this harmful radiation reaches the ethereal body, known as the aura, before it touches our skin. Damage to the physical body only arises after the aura's protective shield has already been considerably weakened. Therefore, PHI has developed an aura spray for strengthening our natural protective shield. It combines gem-energy essences, which absorb harmful radiation and cleanse the aura, with flower and Orchid energy essences, which deflect radiation away from the body.

RQ 7 (Emergency Spray) PHI has also created a pleasant flower-essence combination emergency remedy for external use, in spray form. When under stress or in situations that cause shock, spray RQ 7 several times around your aura or even directly onto the skin.

Delph-Spray The pleasant and cleansing effect of Delph® is now also available in spray form. It is helpful for cleansing energetically polluted rooms (offices, treatment rooms, conference rooms, etc.). Delph® creates a better energetic and cleansed atmosphere and promotes the opening of the heart chakra. It is also recommended for use during air travel.

New developments in methods of flower essence use

Andreas has a vision for integrating the consciousness of nature into our world and its importance of the infinite balance of nature; how vital it is at this moment on the Earth for us to recognize this, and to find a way to become more in harmony with the healing gifts nature has to offer the world – not only on a personal level, but healing the environment, as well as our social and health structures.

Andreas has devised a pyramid of healing, developed from his vibrational range of essences, which include:

- **crystals** – are in and of the Earth; they store vital knowledge and information. Work on our structure and overall energy.

- **mushroom essences** – grow close to the Earth and deal with our negativity. Related to the lower chakras.

- **flower essences** – growing from the Earth, reaching upwards. Related to the middle chakras.

- **Orchid essences** – growing 'in the air'. Related to the head/crown and higher chakras.

- **Delph essence** – all-encompassing energy of love and compassion.

A combination of these essences has extraordinary power to cleanse and rebalance the physical being and is part of the 'Korte light treatment'.

The future of vibrational therapy

Our research has led us to continue developing essence therapy and move beyond the traditional methods. We find an interrelationship between essences, light and colour therapy, the transference of light, colour and vibration.

States of disharmony or disease can be perceived first as misinformation in the subtle body. Here, the essences' energy frequencies can restore the cohesion of body, mind and soul. The methods of transferring the light, colour and vibration directly allow us

to work on the different levels of the energy body, as well as apply other essences.

With this method the intention is that every therapist and doctor can use essences, as they are applicable in any kind of practice.

It is hoped that in the future, there will be many treatment centres using vibration therapy.

Find information online at: www.health-houses.com.

AMAZONIAN SHAMANIC SACRED TREE ESSENCES (AMT)

I had the pleasure of meeting Mimi when she contacted me in Harley Street and sought my advice about flower essences and how to bring them to the attention of the general public. Knowing my passion for the Amazon she presented me with some bottles with handwritten labels with mother tincture of Amazonian tree essences which she had recently made in the Peruvian jungle. I have found them to be truly profound in their effect over the last two years of using them in my Harley Street practice. To my delight I discovered that since then she has developed the essences into a beautifully presented range. Here is her story:

While working as a nurse in England, Mimi Buttacavoli experienced an inescapable calling to visit South America, a journey which lasted seven years. Whilst working as a volunteer nurse in Lima, Peru, Mimi saw that many locals were using plants for healing and talking about shamans. These traditional medicine men sparked her interest and she went in search of knowledge of other healing modalities. By the time she had completed a course in alternative therapies and studied herbalism in the mountains of Bolivia, Mimi had a profound desire to go deeper into the relationship between plants, healing and the spirit world. For the next five years she lived in the Peruvian jungle, where she undertook a very disciplined and rigorous apprenticeship with master shamans. A deep psychic connection with the spirits of the forest was established and at the end of this time she was given the title of *Maestra*. Her desire to share the wisdom and transformational power of the Amazon inspired Mimi to create Sacred Tree Essences. She now makes sprays and essences from the sacred teacher trees, and paints her visions of their healing energies. She feels honoured to have learnt these ancient traditions and to be able to share these wonderful gifts.

Sacred tree essences

Shamans in the Amazon jungle have been working with sacred trees for thousands of years. They use their voice as a gateway to the spirit world. They use *icaros*, medicine songs, to perform all their healing work. They learn the icaros directly through the spirits and also have them passed down through their shamanic ancestors. All of the essences are made using sacred teacher trees of the Peruvian forest. Each essence has been blessed with its own song calling the spirits of the trees and asking them to share their divine wisdom and mystical healing energy.

Ayahuma The head medicine spirit of this tree is a giant. It helps to recover from emotional shocks and release past traumas. The essence enables us to connect to the strength, support and protection of the Ayahuma tree. The colour of this tree's energetic medicine is orange, representing its beautiful and therapeutic flowers. This colour is warm and revitalizing.

Bobinsana The head medicine spirit of this tree is a grandfather spirit who wields a spiritual staff of strength and protection. This essence is used to bring peace and tranquillity by calming the heart and mind. The colour of Bobinsana's energetic medicine is deep pink, representing the tree's beautiful and therapeutic flowers. This colour is vibrant and nurturing.

Camalonga This essence is made from the seeds of the Camalonga tree. It is a teacher plant that works in the dreamtime. Connect to this tree to stimulate lucid and vivid dreaming. The colour of Camalonga's energetic medicine is light blue, representative of sky, water, spaciousness and expansiveness. This colour is cool and calm.

Capirona Capirona has a very light energy that can brighten dark moods. Connect to this tree to help combat negative energies from other people or the environment. The essence can make your energetic body slippery, like the bark of this tree, so that negative energies slide off. The colour of Capirona's energetic medicine is lime green, representing the tree's distinctive bark. This colour is refreshing and invigorating.

Chuchuhuasi The head medicine spirits are doctor spirits, who work on realigning the energetic centres of the body. The colour of this essence's energetic medicine is red, representing physical life force and vitality. This colour is energizing and vibrant.

Cielo Ayahuasca The head medicine spirit of this vine is Papa Tua, a grandfather spirit. The essence is made using Cielo (Heaven) Ayahuasca, which has the ability to create spiritual ascension. It is used for cleansing and purification, opening the way to change and new beginnings. The colour of this essence's energetic medicine is multicoloured, representing the plant's ability to work through the entire energetic system and etheric layers.

Cumaceba The energy of this tree is light and uplifting. Connect with this tree to open your heart centre and bring a sense of happiness and wellbeing. The colour of Cumaceba's energetic medicine is pink, symbolizing love and the inner child. This colour is gentle and playful.

Huaira Caspi This tree's energy is light and airy. Connect to this essence to bring freshness to the mind, clearing negative thought loops. The colour of Huaira

Caspi's energetic medicine is green, representing the tree's ability to balance the heart and mind. This colour is peaceful and relaxing.

Lupuna Blanca Lupuna is one of the biggest trees in the Amazon. It stands tall and proud. Connect to this tree to bring you strength, courage, expansion and self-esteem. Its energy is light and very grounding. The colour of this essence's energetic medicine is turquoise, representing the expansion of Lupuna from the Earth, reaching the skies. This colour is calm, serene and uplifting.

Punga Amarilla The head medicine spirit of this tree is a yellow anaconda. The snake's energy is agile and perceptive. This essence can be used for extracting negative energies from the body. Connect to this tree for cleansing and protection. The colour of Punga's energetic medicine is yellow, representative of this tree's name and the snake's markings. This colour is inspiring and illuminating.

Remo Caspi The head medicine spirits of this tree are native warriors. This essence helps to move dense negative energies and break cyclical patterns of behaviour, as well as allowing us to connect to our personal power and inner strength. The colour of Remo Caspi's energetic medicine is a deep red, representing the tree's earthy and grounding nature. This colour is rich and nourishing.

Shiwawaku This tree is used to transmute negative energies. Connect to this essence to move through obstacles and transform. The colour of Shiwawaku's energetic medicine is purple, representing psychic intuition and transformation. This colour is spiritual and creative.

Tortuga The head medicine spirit is a giant land tortoise. This essence can help those who lead a fast-paced lifestyle to find balance in their lives, keeping them centred, calm and productive. The colour of Tortuga's energetic medicine is bronze, symbolizing the protective nature of the tortoise shell. This colour is unifying and earthy.

Uchu Sanango The head medicine spirit is Abuelo Sanango, a grandfather spirit. This tree provides energetic protection in the form of steel armour. Connect to this tree for inner truth, clarity and spiritual development. The colour of this essence's energetic medicine is magenta, representing mysticism and spirituality. This colour is revitalizing and spontaneous.

Una de Gato The head medicine spirit is a black jaguar that removes blocked energies from the body. The jaguar's energy is fearless, focused and determined. Connect with this tree for purification, inner security and confidence. The colour of Una de Gato's energetic medicine is indigo blue, representing the jaguar's regalness. This colour is intense and electric.

Amazonian shamanic sacred tree sprays

All our aura and space sprays are made by master shaman Mimi, using tree essences from the Amazon jungle. The essences have been infused with sacred songs and combined with essential oils. Each spray has been prepared in a traditional shamanic way, awakening the spirits of the trees and oils, unlocking their mystical healing powers.

Calming Mist Connect to the stillness and tranquillity of the Amazonian trees. Allow the tree spirits to bring a calming force to your energetic field. Amazonian tree essences: Lupuna Blanca, Shiwawaku and Huaira Caspi. Palmarosa and Lavender essential oils are added to bring a peaceful and relaxing energy.

Cleansing Mist Invite the Amazonian tree spirits to cleanse away negative thoughts and feelings from your auric field and environment. Amazonian tree essences:

Ayahuasca, Remo Caspi and Una de Gato. Juniper, Melissa (UK) and Lemon essential oils are added for extra cleansing and a revitalizing renewal of energy.

Ceremonial Mist Gently mist your aura and space when participating in or creating a ceremonial space. Connect to two powerful teacher trees of the Amazon for spiritual guidance and protection. Amazonian tree essences: Ayahuasca and Uchu Sanango. Frankincense and Camphor essential oils are added to increase spiritual receptivity, connection and protection.

Confidence Mist Connect to the strength and support of the Amazonian trees. Allow them to help you find your inner strength and confidence. Amazonian tree essences: Lupuna Blanca, Remo Caspi and Una de Gato. Vertiver, Bay and Bergamot essential oils are added for confidence and empowerment.

Energizing Mist Connect to the restoring energies of the Amazonian trees. Amazonian tree essences: Chuchuhuasi and Uchu Sanango. Melissa (UK), Ginger and Black Pepper essential oils are added to bring an uplifting, revitalizing and invigorating energy.

Grounding Mist Connect to the energy of the grounding trees of the Amazon. Allow these trees to firmly root you to the Earth. Amazonian tree essences: Remo Caspi, Ayahuma and Lupuna Blanca. Vertiver, Amyris and Cinnamon essential oils are added to bring a warm, supportive and earthy energy.

Guiding Mist Receive guidance from two powerful teacher trees of the Amazon and share their divine wisdom. Amazonian tree essences: Uchu Sanango and Ayahuasca. Frankincense, Cypress and Holy Basil essential oils are added to increase spiritual receptivity, connection, focus and clarity.

Her Sensuality Mist Connect to the aphrodisiac trees of the Amazon and heighten your feminine sensuality. Amazonian tree essences: Chuchuhuasi and Cumaceba. Ylang Ylang, Rose Geranium, Vanilla, Ginger and Petitgrain essential oils are added to increase playfulness, femininity and sensuality.

His Sensuality Mist Connect to the aphrodisiac trees of the Amazon and heighten your masculine life force energy. Amazonian tree essences: Chuchuhuasi, Cumaceba and Huacapurana. Patchouli, Petitgrain, Amyris, Vanilla, Black Pepper and Clove essential oils are added to increase sensuality, energy and vitality.

Inner Clarity Mist Connect you to your inner truth. Allow the Amazonian tree spirits to help you find your inner clarity and wisdom. Amazonian tree essences: Ayahuasca and Uchu Sanango. Myrrh and Frankincense essential oils are added to increase awareness of your higher self, enhance meditative states and elevate your spirit.

Mind Clearing Mist Invite the Amazonian tree spirits to calm and clear the mind. Amazonian tree essences: Huaira Caspi and Bobinsana. Peppermint and Eucalyptus essential oils are added to bring mental clarity, focus and a cool refreshing energy.

Peaceful Sleep Mist Connect to the supportive and protective energies of the Amazonian trees. Allow them to help you let go, unwind and relax. Amazonian tree essences: Ayahuma and Shiwawaku. Clary Sage, Vertiver and Neroli light essential oils are added for their soothing, sedating and sleep-inducing energies.

Protection Mist Invite the Amazonian guardian tree spirits to create a field of protection around your energetic body and space. Amazonian tree essences: Capirona, Punga Amarilla and Una de Gato. Star of Anise and Camphor oils are added to bring extra energ.

Shining Heart Mist Connect to the universal love flowing through your heart. Allow the Amazonian tree spirits to strengthen your connection to your heart centre. Amazonian tree essences: Cumaceba, Shiwawaku and Bobinsana. Rosewood and Rose Geranium oils are added to open your heart chakra and elevate your spirit.

Uplifting Mist Uplift your spirit and connect to the light energy of the Amazonian trees. Amazonian tree essences: Capirona and Cumaceba. Rose Geranium and Benzoin essential oils are added to bring an uplifting, soothing and positive energy.

Inner Clarity Mist Gently mist your aura and space to connect you to your inner truth. Allow the Amazonian tree spirits to help you find your inner clarity and wisdom. Amazonian tree essences: Ayahuasca and Uchu Sanango. Myrrh and Frankincense essential oils are added to increase awareness of your higher self, enhance meditative states and elevate your spirit.

Grounding Mist Gently mist your aura and space to connect to the energy of the grounding trees of the Amazon. Allow these trees to firmly root you to the Earth. Amazonian tree essences: Remo Caspi, Ayahuma and Lupuna Blanca. Vertiver, Amyris and Cinnamon essential oils are added to bring a warm, supportive and earthy energy.

Guiding Mist Gently mist your aura and space to receive guidance from two powerful teacher trees of the Amazon and share their divine wisdom. Amazonian tree essences: Uchu Sanango and Ayahuasca. Frankincense, Cypress and Holy Basil essential oils are added to increase spiritual receptivity, connection, focus and clarity.

SPIRIT OF MAKASUTU ESSENCES (WEST AFRICA, GAMBIA) (SME)

Created mainly in Gambia (with a few also in Jamaica and Florida), a tiny, gentle country in West Africa, which, although poor in material wealth, is rich and strong in spirit. The Spirit of Makasutu essences were the inspiration of Sheila Balgobin, an African American, who discovered her passion for flower essences when she found herself drawn to two flowers, a Pink Oleander and a Prickly Pear, while on holiday with her husband in the Gambia, West Africa. A natural healer as a child she instinctively massaged her relatives and pets and was drawn to flowers and plants. Always happiest walking outdoors, her earliest memory is of tending the Morning Glories with her mother, which were growing in a window box on her fire escape in New York City.

When she returned home from Africa she bought both mother tinctures back with her, not quite sure what they were for. A chance encounter with a sad, old and very nervous dog gave the answer. Remembering the essences Sheila sprinkled some Prickly Pear on the dog's muzzle and paws, which he licked off, sneezed, stopped trembling and flopped down to sleep! The reaction was so instant that those around shook their heads in amazement. It was clear Prickly Pear is helpful for pets who didn't like being left alone or had been abandoned creating nervousness and anxiety.

Sheila's range grew to 38 essences, and she named them 'Spirit of Makasutu', in honour of the sacred Gambian forest. The name 'Makasutu' comes from the Mandinka language: Maka = Holy (= Mecca) + Sutu = Forest. The first 30 essences of the range were created after her visit to the sacred Gambian forest of Makasutu. The remaining eight essences are made from flowers growing in Jamaica (the Xaymaca Sun Essences) and the Flores del So(u)l Essences range was made from flowers found in Florida. The essences are preserved with a natural non-alcohol preservative called Red Shiso, a Japanese mint (*Perilla frutescens*) which is documented as being 1000 times stronger at preserving than synthetic food preservatives. It also has a pleasant taste, so is good for adults, children and animals and for those who can't tolerate alcohol.

Also an aromatherapist, teacher, crystal healer and psychotherapist, Sheila specializes in addictions, bereavement, spirituality and multicultural issues.

Spirit of Makasutu essences

Ackee Renders palatable situations which are 'hard to swallow'; reduces irritation; sweetens one's outlook on life.

Amazon Lily Spiritualization of intimate relationships.

American Tulip Tree Encourages the ability to see the sweet side of life.

Angel's Trumpet Spiritual growth; mental clarity; aids absentmindedness and helps to ground daydreamers; for people in healing professions; purity of thought; insight into one's path in life.

Baobab Strength in adversity; grounding – for those who 'live in their heads', perseverance.

Ben Tree Clears the aura of negative energy.

Birds of Bakau Balances energy at all levels.

Bougainvillea Eases transition.

Calabash Addresses emotional factors behind menopausal symptoms; improves the ability to 'listen with the heart'.

Coconut Palm Generosity; encourages feelings of physical wellbeing.

Corn Poppy Enhances functioning of the third eye; engenders clarity of thought and decisive action.

Coyote Mint Enjoyment of food; calming; enhances intuition; intellectual pursuits; opens the third eye; detached analysis/understanding of situations; clarity of purpose.

Crocodiles of Katchikally Helps remove creative blocks at all levels; strength combined with gentleness.

Devil's Trumpet Shamanic healing; psychic vision; vision quests.

Dutchman's Pipe 'Digestion' of trapped/blocked emotions; expression and release of hidden feelings.

Ethiopian Apple Loving and gentle speech.

Hawaiian Bell Public speaking; addresses rigidity/frigidity in communication; softens an abrupt/brusque manner.

Jaboticaba Recognizes and releases deep hurt held within; renewal of inner joy; unburdening of the soul.

Jasmine Helps to reconnect to and recognize one's own and others' divinity; helps those too grounded in day-to-day reality.

Mango Renders palatable situations which are 'hard to swallow'; reduces irritation; sweetens one's outlook on life.

Mimosa Restful sleep; relaxation; eases 'frazzled' feelings.

Ocean Awareness of one's natural body rhythms; emotional balance; adjustment to change.

Oil Palm Encourages the desire to eat; encourages a sense of security.

Orange Enjoyment of life; raises low mood; calming.

Orange Jasmine Energizes the aura.

Pink Oleander Agitation; worry; meditation/stillness; letting go and letting God.

Pomegranate Enhances intuition; harmonizes/balances feminine energy at all levels; engenders change at a deep level.

Prickly Pear Feelings of being 'boxed in'; boundary setting; gently, but firmly holding one's ground; calms impatience/prickly manner.

Red Hibiscus Intimacy issues; creativity; low energy.

Samambaia Opens and expands the heart chakra.

Saw Palmetto Protection; increases sense of self-preservation; helps address feelings of vulnerability.

Sea Grape Assists in recovery from emotional or mental burn; encourages self-nurture.

White Frangipani Opens and aligns all chakras.

Yellow Frangipani flower Lightens emotional heaviness; spiritual growth.

Yellow Hibiscus Feeling 'down'; cheerfulness – see the bright side and a positive self image.

Yellow Oleander Loosens 'knots' in the stomach.

Yellow Trumpetbush Express oneself in a loving way; encourages forgiveness.

B.

AUSTRALIA, JAPAN AND THAILAND

Australia was once part of the southern land-mass known as Gondwanaland. The land has a powerful and vibrant energy that has not been weakened by civilization, war or pollution. Some of the oldest and most spectacular flowering plants in the world can be found growing in the wilderness of the Australian outback. They bloom prolifically throughout the year and draw upon and reflect the power, strength and vitality of this extraordinary region.

The native Aborigines are custodians of an ancient natural system of medicine and have long acknowledged the power of the flower kingdom and have been using flowers to heal emotional imbalance and physical injuries for more than 10,000 years.

It was these Aboriginal peoples who understood how to draw upon the vibrant healing powers of the flowers around them and were one of the first to lay claim to this unique system of medicine.

They discovered the therapeutic value of flower essences as effective emotional healers and are considered the grandfathers of the art, just as Dr Edward Bach who is responsible for their rediscovery and wide use today is considered the Father.

Both recognized and understood that the root of many health imbalances lay in emotional and physical build-up of shock and stress and that once in balance the body was able to heal itself.

The main focus of Australian remedies is to bring out and cultivate the positive qualities present in everyone. The Waratah, one of the Aboriginals' most sacred flowers, is unique to Australia. It comes from one of the oldest plant groups in the world whose origins date back 60 million years to Antarctica. Steeped in Aboriginal dreamtime legends that have been passed down from generation to generation, the Waratah is known by its Aboriginal name meaning beautiful. It has a magnificent red bloom comprising many individual flowers which are tightly packed together.

The Waratah is a survival remedy. It embodies the Australian bush-dweller's qualities of adaptability and the ability to cope with all sorts of emergencies and many believe that in the years to come there will be major economic, social, physical and spiritual upheavals which will take us by surprise. The Waratah will help by aiding people to find the courage and strength they need to cope with such change.

Due to the power of the land some interesting flower essence lines have developed over the last few years, some of which I have actively supported and brought to general attention in the UK as well as worldwide.

The Australian Living, Australian Bush, Australian Living WildFlower (Love Remedies) and the Flower Essences of Australia all have similarities as well as their own uniqueness.

Here it is interesting to note that Ian White of the Australian Bush essences has researched and conducted studies into the use of the combinations he has created, especially Electro, which is designed for reduction of radiation (see p.100); and also studies on a combination for hormonal imbalance in women.

FLOWER ESSENCES OF AUSTRALIA (FE AUS)

Angelsword (*Lobelia gibbosa*) Lack of protection, vulnerability, exposed to negative influences, spiritual and energy protection rebuilding the whole energy field. Allows access to gifts from past lifetimes.

Banksia Robur For low energy levels, burnout after setbacks, for those who are normally dynamic but are experiencing a temporary loss of drive. Renews energy and enthusiasm.

Bauhinia (*Lysiphyllum cunninghamii*) For thinking outside the box, for difficulties with change, resistance and inflexibility. Encourages an open and flexible mind.

Billy Goat Plum (*Planchonia careya*) For those uncomfortable with physicality, repulsion, sexual guilt. Encourages an ease with and enjoyment of all that is physical. Good for skin conditions such as eczema, psoriasis, herpes and thrush.

Black-Eyed Susan (*Tetratheca ericifolia*) A remedy for stress. For those always on the go, rushing, constantly striving and impatient. Slows you down, enabling you to turn inward, be still and enjoy inner peace. Balances the adrenal glands.

Blackboy Grass Tree (*Xanthorrhoea preisii*) For feeling flat and cut off spiritually. Supports heightened spiritual awareness and interconnectedness, the meditative mind, the spiritual warrior, Useful for the adolescence stage and the insecurity around puberty as well as adults emotionally stuck through trauma at this time.

Boab (*Adansonia gregorii*) Supports releasing inherited attitudes, family thought patterns and states of mind allowing mental freedom by clearing negative thoughts and mindsets.

Boronia (*Boronia ledifolia*) Obsessive thinking that is difficult to move out of, deep sadness and heartache. Clarity and thinking outside the box enables a fresh start in order to move on.

Bottlebrush (*Callistemon linearis*) For those going through and overwhelmed by major changes. Support for all significant life transitions from birth to death. Clears stuck energy, letting go of old thought patterns and supports the ability to cope calmly with change. Said also to help with pregnancy, bonding and the vulnerability of new mothers.

Bush Fuchsia (*Epacris longiflora*) Lack of trust in following intuition. Supports left-right brain balance, clarity of thought, creative expression and courage to speak in public. Has been used for resolving learning difficulties, for example, dyslexia, etc.

Bush Gardenia (*Gardenia megasperma*) For those caught up in their own world and affairs, taking for granted and being oblivious of those close to them. For stale or failing relationships. Brings passion and renewed interest in a partner; improves communication.

Bush Iris (*Patersonia longifolia*) Acceptance and understanding of the transitory nature of life, encourages spiritual awareness and growth, has been used to aid elimination of blocked kidney Qi.

Christmas Bell (*Blandfordia nobilis*) This remedy assists one with manifestation of dreams into reality. Eliminates belief in lack and undeservedness and promotes openness to fresh perceptions on life.

Crowea (*Crowea saligna*) The worry essence. For individuals who experience anxiety and stress felt in the stomach and muscular tissue. Supports feeling in balance, calm and centred, renewing vitality.

Dagger Hakea (*Hakea teretifolia*) For build-up of and backlog of resentment. Aids in dissolving and letting go of personal bitterness and deeply held resentments. Brings forgiveness enabling feelings to be expressed without residue from the past.

Five Corners (*Styphelia laeta*) Self-dislike developing into low self-esteem and self-effacing behaviour, feeling invisible and colourless. Celebration and appreciation of and confidence in one's inner worth and beauty.

Flannel Flower (*Actinotus helianthi*) For distrusting of intimacy, and therefore wary of physical contact. Has been useful for agoraphobics. Supports openness, emotional trust and being nurtured by physical expressions of tenderness and sensuality.

Fringed Violet (*Thysanotus tuberosus*) For shock and trauma. Auric and energetic protection and auric rebuild after damage as a result of shock and trauma, provides a protective shield. Creates psychic protection field for those who have allowed energy and vitality to be drained by other people as well as environmental factors such as electromagnetic radiation. Speeds up slow recuperation removing the effects of recent and old trauma, realigns the subtle bodies and energy system as a whole.

Green Spider Orchid (*Caladenia dilatata*) For those disturbed by phobias, dark thoughts, nightmares. Encourages positivity and a deeper insight and non-identification with negativity, and a receptivity and brighter outlook on life.

Grey Spider Flower (*Grevillea buxifolia*) For those who can be caught in extreme fears and night terrors, psychic attack and phenomena. Especially good for sensitive and vulnerable children who are too open to negative external influences. Restores a deep faith in the goodness and sweetness of life and brings internal courage, faith and calmness.

Isopogon (*Isopogon anethifolius*) For learning from repeating the same mistakes and finding oneself in similar situations due to inattention, lack of focus or stubbornness. Good for poor memory and an inability to learn from past experience. Keeps one's attention in the present moment allowing the ability to 'get in one's own gap' and catch the repeated habitual responses before they take the same old route. This affords a conscious change in direction so a fresh more positive road is taken, correcting the mistake therefore effecting a different outcome. Aids learning from past experiences, and a retrieval of forgotten skills and past lives memories and lessons.

Jacaranda (*Mimosifolia*) For tail-chasing, scattered due to overwhelm and being uncentred. A tendency to be always rushing around and accident prone. Focused, centred and decisive follow through, quick thinking and a clear mind.

Kangaroo Paw (*Anigozanthos manglesii*) Difficulty in relating due to self-absorption. Encourages being content, relaxed and comfortable with company. Helpful for those who are socially inexperienced or shy, also for teenagers who can go through a period of being clumsy, gauche and insensitive to the needs of others. Encourages social awareness, sensitivity, relaxation in company.

Little Flannel Flower (*Actinotus minor*) Overly serious, especially when a child having to grow up before time has lost the joy of living. Supports and restores sense of playfulness, spontaneity and *joie-de-vivre*.

Macrocarpa (*Eucalyptus macrocarpa*) For those who are drained, tired, worn out or totally exhausted. Pick-me-up, after burn-out, supports recovery after illness, inadequate immune resistance and setbacks. Aids bounce back, restoring energy, adrenal gland strength and vitality.

Mountain Devil (*Lambertia formosa*) Helps dissolve outward aggression, anger outbursts that hide fear and insecurity and grudge bearing. Supports inner security, forgiveness and an unconditional spirit.

Mulla Mulla (*Ptilotus atripicifolius*) For difficulty with any form of heat, fear of agitation, clammy and feeling overheated. Useful in the hot flushes of menopause, night sweats and any heat in the liver and blood. Used in Traditional Chinese Medicine. Supports balance and feeling cool.

Old Man Banksia (*Banksia serrata*) The Aboriginals considered this a symbol of female spirituality. For sluggishness, thyroid imbalance (over or under), low energy, tendency to weight gain. Balances and supports core energy that brings the spark back.

Paw Paw (*Carica papaya*) Unresolved problems, lack of integration, overwhelm that creates lack of absorption and assimilation, poor digestion. Aids assimilation, more efficient absorption of essential nutrients and integration of problems solved with clarity from a higher more altruistic perspective.

Peach-Flowered Tea-Tree (*Leptospermum squarrosum*) Feeling nervy, unsettled, mood swings, low or unstable blood sugar levels. Balances cravings, said to aid imbalances associated with the pancreas. When overly worried about state of health, aids preoccupations, stabilizes and calms.

Pink Mulla Mulla (*Ptilotus exaltatus*) Dissolves old wounds, deep hurt and defensiveness, enabling the ability to forgive and trust to be restored once more.

Red Grevillea (*Grevillea speciosa*) Negatively affected by criticism, emotionally blocked and stuck and disempowered. Cultivates independence from others' opinions and criticisms and feeling empowered and moving on.

Lotus or Red Lily (*Nelumbo nucifera*) A flower that the Aboriginals also held most sacred as they felt it embodied their spirituality. For those who can be ungrounded, dreamers prone to accidents. Balances spirit with matter, grounding and evolving spiritually in a practical way. Said to be useful in autism and for counteracting the damaging effects of drugs.

Rough Bluebell (*Trichodesma zeylanicum*) Defensiveness, using manipulation and revenge to hide deep hurt. Can use cutting or snide remarks in order to be in control. Supports resolution of pain, encouraging compassion and gentleness in interaction with others.

She Oak (*Casuarina glauca*) Female essence, balance for women on all levels, hormonally at all stages of a woman's reproductive life, has been used in menstrual problems, premenstrual tension (PMT), fluid retention as well as menopause symptoms and is also a support to be emotionally open to conception and reproduction.

Southern Cross (*Xanthosia rotundifolia*) For a positive abundant mindset and personal empowerment, letting go of past negativity, and hard done by, emotionally impoverished and complaining and victim mentality supporting empowerment.

Spinifex (*Triodia* sp.) Used for skin conditions such as herpes, chlamydia and surface cuts or grazes. Heals by helping you realize the emotional issues involved that are behind the physical manifestation. Can be applied topically added in a cream base.

Sturt Desert Pea (*Clianthus formosus*) Releasing past emotional wounds and trauma, grief and deep-seated sadness, supporting a fresh start and emotional ease.

Sturt Desert Rose (*Gossypium sturtianum*) Held back by past regrets and guilt, compromising self-esteem. Supports integrity, and the courage to let go of regret and remorse.

Tall Mulla Mulla (*Ptilotus exaltatus*) Apprehensive, shy and uneasy in company. Encourages relaxed confidence with social interaction. Supports the Qi of the lungs.

Turkey Bush (*Calytrix exstipulata*) Frustration due to blocked creative expression. Supports focus and confidence to tap into and renew creative expression and inspiration.

Waratah (*Telopea speciosissima*) Survival and strengthening essence, dark night of the soul, depression, deep despair. Supports courage, optimism, hope that all is not lost, inner strength and tenacity and clear vision.

White Spider Orchid (*Caladenia logicauda*) Overwhelmed by sadness of life creating nervousness and anxiety. Encourages energy and spiritual protection for oversensitivity of the gentle soul and a wider more philosophical worldview.

Wild Potato Bush (*Solanum quadriloculatum*) Overloaded and weighed down, emotional toxicity, feeling physically burdened and overloaded. Supports cleansing mentally, emotionally and physically, ability to move through life with more ease.

Yellow Cowslip Orchid (*Caladenia flava*) Releases a judgemental attitude with others as well as self-criticism, and giving one's self a hard time; encourages a compassionate overview, and less judgemental behaviour.

Essences in preparation (check with distributor to see when available)

Alpine Mint Bush, Bluebell, Bush Gardenia, Dog Rose, Dog Rose of the Wild Forces, Freshwater Mangrove, Gymea Lily, Hibertia, Illawarra Flame Tree, Kapoc Bush, Mint Bush, Monga Waratah, Philotheca, Pink Flannel Flower, Red Helmet Orchid, Red Suva Frangipani, Silver Princess, Slender Rice Flower, Sundew, Sunshine Wattle, Sydney Rose, Tall Yellow Top, Wedding Bush, Wisteria plus a few more new essences.

Combination essences

Calm & Relax Emotional and mental calm after times of stress, worry and panic.
Indicated for: Feeling stressed, wound up, nervy, worried, overextended and panicky.
Promotes: Calmness of mind and emotions, ability to relax deeply and be stress and care free.
Contains: Black-Eyed Susan, Bush Fuchsia, Crowea, Jacaranda, Little Flannel Flower, Paw Paw, Bottlebrush, Old Man Banksia.

Confidence Boost Confidence and courage after bouts of self-doubt, lack of worth and self-esteem.
Indicated for: Low self-esteem and not feeling good enough leading to lack of confidence.
Promotes: Self-assurance, self-worth, courage to dare to speak one's truth and go for it!
Contains: Boab, Southern Cross, Sturt Desert Rose, White Spider Orchid, Five Corners, Flannel Flower, Turkey Bush, Tall Mulla.

Detox Essence Clearing mind/body and emotions of toxicity and sluggishness associated with headaches and weight issues.
Indicated for: Feeling heavy, toxic and sluggish in the organs of elimination: lymph, liver, circulation that may contribute to headaches and weight issues. Beneficial for toxic emotions past and present and weight issues with an emotional context.
Promotes: Cleansing the system, clearing mental overload and emotional toxicity, lightens the load and helpful for feeling clear and generally cleansed on all levels.

Has been used for: A spring clean for physical body, heavy metal toxicity, chemotherapy, imbalance in any organ of elimination, mind and body to clear toxic waste, constipation, acne, eczema and other skin conditions as well as bad breath and headaches.

Contains: Wild Potato Bush, Bottlebrush, Dagger Hakea, Bauhinia, Bush Iris, Peach-Flowered Tea-Tree, Fringed Violet.

Dynamic Recovery Energy boost for exhaustion particularly after stress and illness.

Indicated for: Tiredness, exhaustion and low adrenal energy with an inability to get going again, poor recuperation after ill health.

Promotes: Dynamic recovery, balances the whole system, may be supportive as a pick-me-up and extra energy boost after exhaustion and illness.

Contains: Banksia Robur, Macrocarpa, Black-Eyed Susan, Crowea, Old Man Banksia, Yellow Cowslip Orchid.

Electroguard Clear and protect against build-up of adverse electromagnetic energy.

Indicated for: The negative effect on the system of the build-up of electromagnetic toxicity from computers, mobile phones, TVs, microwaves and any other equipment.

Promotes: Clearing and provides protection whilst working with electromagnetic equipment, allowing the body's system and energy field to be clear and in balance.

Has been used for: Feeling drained, flat and sensitive due to overload from radiation emitted by meter boxes, overhead power lines, etc., and during radiotherapy treatment.

Contains: Fringed Violet, Crowea, Paw Paw, Waratah, Mulla Mulla, Wild Potato Bush, Bush Fuchsia, White Spider Orchid.

Emergency Rescue Inner strength and fortitude to cope with crisis and emergency with courage and calm.

Indicated for: All emergency and crisis situations, shock, trauma and the inability to cope effectively in extreme situations.

Promotes: Clearing shock and trauma, galvanizes forces for dealing with courage in a crisis and extreme situations that can throw one off balance.

Contains: Crowea, Fringed Violet, Grey Spider Flower, Waratah, Sturt Desert Pea, Sturt Desert Rose, Red Grevillea.

Intimacy Renews interest, passion and bonding, for fear of intimacy, trauma or abuse.

Indicated for: Inhibitions, trauma, fear of intimacy, feeling uncomfortable in one's skin. Difficulty associated with invasion of personal space.

Promotes: Renewed interest, passion, sensuality, bonding, aids in dissolving abuse and trauma. Encourages acceptance and feeling at ease with our physical body and physicality.

Contains: Billy Goat Plum, Sturt Desert Rose, Fringed Violet, Little Flannel Flower, Rough Bluebell, Mountain Devil.

Learning and Focus Assists mental focus, aiding concentration, learning and ability to follow through.

Indicated for: Lack of focus, mental fog with poor memory, mentally overwhelmed with low attention span with the inability to follow through.

Promotes: Enhanced concentration, mental acumen, absorption and learning as well as keeping attention in the present moment so as to be able to observe and catch repeating patterns, learn from past mistakes, make a different choice and move on.

Has been used for: stuttering, Attention Deficit Disorder and Attention Deficit Hyperactivity Disorder, right and left hemispheres imbalances, procrastination, study pursuits that require intense focus, and problem-solving, improving higher self-awareness and access to past knowledge and experiences.

Contains: Bush Fuchsia, Isopogan, Jacaranda, Boronia, Paw Paw, Peach-Flowered Tea-Tree.

Positivity Positive and abundant thinking, a fresh view after a negative cloud.
Indicated for: Falling into the same old patterns, a negative mindset and self-sabotage which keeps one stuck in repeated unhealthy situations.
Promotes: Positive and abundant thoughts, thinking outside the box, enhancing the possibility to make a change and attract self-affirming situations and abundance into one's life.
Contains: Boab, Turkey Bush, Christmas Bell, Bauhinia, Southern Cross, Wild Potato Bush, Little Flannel flower, Banksia Robur.

Relate-Well Unhealthy relationship patterns, encourages heartfelt direct communication.
Indicated for: Relationship issues, resolves emotional hurt and pain, negative patterns, lack of communication, or feeling isolated in a relationship.
Promotes: Direct communication, breaks unhealthy patterns, dissolving fears associated with speaking truth within relationships, helps maintain integrity in all interactions, plus a healthy relationship with oneself.
Contains: Pink Mulla Mulla, Boab, Flannel Flower, Kangaroo Paw, Mountain Devil, Flannel Flower, Green Spider Orchid, Dagger Hakea, Rough Bluebell.

Travel-Well Helps with adaption to time zones, feeling balanced and refreshed after jet lag, travel sickness or water retention.
Indicated for: All forms of travel, by air, road or sea. Helpful for travel sickness, water retention, dehydration, jet lag, sleeplessness and feeling drained and tired.
Promotes: Easy and comfortable travel, adaptation to time zones, enables arriving at one's destination in balance and feeling refreshed.

Contains: Bush Fuchsia, Crowea, Bush Iris, Wild Potato Bush, Paw Paw, Tall Mulla Mulla, She Oak, Bottlebrush Banksia Robur.

Woman Balance Balances emotions associated with hormonal conditions, PMT, mood swings and menopausal symptoms, bloating and hot flushes.
Indicated for: Hormonal imbalance, PMT, mood swings, menopause, hot flushes.
Promotes: Feeling in balance with hormonal conditions, irregularity, PMT, bloating, menopausal symptoms.
Has been used for irregular menstruation, candida, hot flushes, weight gain, sluggishness, feeling disheartened and weary. Also skin problems, mood swings, hypoglycaemia and for women feeling overwhelmed by pregnancy.
Contains: She Oak, Peach-Flowered Tea-Tree, Old Man Banksia, Mulla Mulla, Bottlebrush, Bush Fuchsia, Billy Goat Plum, Crowea, Dagger Hakea, Wild Potato Bush.

Calm & Relax, Emergency Rescue, Dynamic Recovery and Detox Essence also are available in a 15ml pocket handbag-size oral spritz.

Here Calm & Relax can be useful to have to hand for feelings of overriding stress and panic, Emergency Rescue for a quick spritz in the mouth to alleviate any shock situation, and Dynamic Recovery for when you need that extra boost when you have to be up to the mark and energy levels are running on empty, and I always take Detox with me before and after the dentist to clear the anaesthetic out of my system.

Kits
Detox Kit

The Detox Kit contains three flower essence combinations which are designed to work together to complement each other. They are beneficial when the need to spring-clean the system is in mind, at any time of the year. These combinations can be used together or individually at different times depending on the need.

Detox Essence Clears the system, mind/body and emotions of toxicity and sluggishness, mental overload, weight issues with emotional context, lightens the load and is helpful for feeling clear and generally cleansed on all levels.
Contains: Wild Potato Bush, Bottlebrush, Dagger Hakea, Bauhinia, Bush Iris, Peach-Flowered Tea-Tree, Fringed Violet.

Electroguard Clearing and protection. The daily build-up of electromagnetic toxicity from computers, mobile phones and other electromagnetic equipment can have negative effects on the system. Clears build-up allowing the body's system and energy field to be refreshed and in balance.
Contains: Fringed Violet, Crowea, Paw Paw, Waratah, Mulla Mulla, Wild Potato Bush, Bush Fuchsia.

Dynamic Recovery While detoxing it is important to keep the system in balance. Supportive as a pick me up and extra energy boost after feeling stressed, tired and low.
Contains: Banksia Robur, Macrocarpa, Black-Eyed Susan, Crowea, Old Man Banksia, Yellow Cowslip Orchid.

Suggested use: Detox Essence can be used as a baseline essence by taking 7 drops orally in the morning and again in the evening. It is beneficial to take 7 drops of Electroguard in the evening so that the system can be cleared of electromagnetic toxicity during the night, followed by 7 drops of Dynamic Recovery first thing in the morning to keep the energy system in balance while going through the detox process.

Emergency Rescue Kit

The Emergency Rescue Kit contains three flower essence combinations which are designed to work together to complement each other. They are particularly useful as a first-aid flower essence kit when challenging

situations occur. These essences can be used together or individually at different times depending on the need.

Emergency Rescue Galvanizes forces to deal with shock, crisis, and trauma. Supports inner strength to cope with emergency situations with courage and calm.
Contains: Crowea, Fringed Violet, Grey Spider Flower, Waratah, Sturt Desert Pea, Sturt Desert Rose, Red Grevillea.

Calm & Relax Supports calmness of mind and emotions especially after feeling stressed, nervy, worried, over-extended, panicky or so wound up that sleep is impossible.
Contains: Black-Eyed Susan, Bush Fuchsia, Crowea, Jacaranda, Little Flannel Flower, Paw Paw, Bottlebrush, Old Man Banksia.

Dynamic Recovery Encourages energy conservation especially after tiredness, exhaustion, low adrenal energy with an inability to get going again. Supports recuperation after ill health.
Contains: Banksia Robur, Macrocarpa, Black-Eyed Susan, Crowea, Old Man Banksia, Yellow Cowslip Orchid.

Suggested use: The essences in the Emergency Kit are designed to be used frequently. Emergency Rescue especially should be taken, 7 drops orally, every 15 minutes to half an hour in acute situations and then continued as often as required. Calm & Relax is supportive taken frequently in panic and nervous stress situations or at night for simply being too wound up to sleep. Dynamic Recovery should be taken, 7 drops orally, as often as needed when one is stretched beyond the point of exhaustion and energy reserves are needed to meet challenges.

Inner Beauty Kit

The Inner Beauty Kit contains three flower essence combinations which are designed to work together to complement each other. They are designed to support a feeling of confidence and positivity and encourage a feeling of empowerment in being a woman. These combinations can be used together or individually at different times depending on the need.

Woman Balance Supports feeling emotionally balanced and gives a sense of ease with one's inner woman and an appreciation of one's inner beauty.
Contains: She Oak, Peach-Flowered Tea-Tree, Old Man Banksia, Mulla Mulla, Bottlebrush, Bush Fuchsia, Billy Goat Plum, Crowea, Dagger Hakea, Wild Potato Bush.

Positivity Supports change, allowing old patterns, a negative mindset and self-sabotage which keeps one stuck in repeated unhealthy situations to fall away and creates a positive spin about one's self as a happy, healthy and beautiful woman.
Contains: Boab, Turkey Bush, Christmas Bell, Bauhinia, Southern Cross, Wild Potato Bush, Little Flannel Flower, Banksia Robur.

Confidence Boost Provides the inner support for a positive self-assured image and the confidence to be the woman that one truly is.
Contains: Boab, Southern Cross, Sturt Desert Rose, White Spider Orchid, Five Corners, Flannel Flower, Turkey Bush, Tall Mulla Mulla.

Suggested use: Woman Balance can be taken as a baseline essence by taking 7 drops orally in the morning and again in the evening. It is then beneficial to take 7 drops of Positivity essence in the evening so that it can work on negative mindsets during the night, following it by 7 drops of Confidence Boost first thing in the morning so one is ready to step out into our day ready as a confident positive woman.

Woman Balance Kit

The Woman Kit contains three flower essence combinations which are designed to work together to complement each other. They are tailor-made with women in mind. These combinations can be used together or individually at different times depending on the need.

Woman Balance Supports feeling emotionally balanced when experiencing hormonal conditions, PMT, mood swings and menopausal symptoms, bloating and hot flushes.
Contains: She Oak, Peach-Flowered Tea-Tree, Old Man Banksia, Mulla Mulla, Bottlebrush, Bush Fuchsia, Billy Goat Plum, Crowea, Dagger Hakea, Wild Potato Bush.

Detox Essence Beneficial for clearing a negative self-image and past toxic emotions about oneself as a woman which can result in weight issues.
Contains: Wild Potato Bush, Bottlebrush, Dagger Hakea, Bauhinia, Bush Iris, Peach-Flowered Tea-Tree, Fringed Violet.

Dynamic Recovery Gives a woman that much-needed boost in times when extra demands are made on her energy. A balanced endocrine system is one of the keys to good health.
Contains: Banksia Robur, Macrocarpa, Black-Eyed Susan, Crowea, Old Man Banksia, Yellow Cowslip Orchid.

Suggested use: Woman Balance can be used as a baseline essence by taking 7 drops orally in the morning and again in the evening. It is then beneficial to take 7 drops of Detox Essence in the evening so that it can work on the system during the night, followed by 7 drops of Dynamic Recovery first thing in the morning to set one up for the day.

Travel Well Kit

The Travel Kit contains a flower essence combination and a flower essence floral hydrating mist which are designed to work together and complement each other. They are specifically formulated to be supportive in allowing arrival at one's destination refreshed and stress free.

Travel-well Essence Supportive for all forms of travel, by air, road or sea, making for easy and comfortable travel. Helpful for travel sickness, water retention, dehydration, jet lag, sleeplessness and feeling drained and tired. Aids adaptation to time zones and enables arriving at one's destination in balance and feeling refreshed.

Contains: She Oak, Peach-Flowered Tea-Tree, Old Man Banksia, Mulla Mulla, Bottlebrush, Bush Fuchsia, Billy Goat Plum, Crowea, Dagger Hakea, Wild Potato Bush.

Travel-refresh Spritz A hydrating flower essence, Lemon Myrtle and Rose water mist designed to create a sense of ease and take the stress out of the travel process. Moisturising and replenishing, this mist is refreshing and uplifting during long-haul flights and other forms of travel when maintaining your energy and personal space is important to feeling comfortable and at ease during travel.

Contains: Crowea, Bush Iris, Wild Potato Bush, Paw Paw, Tall Mulla Mulla, She Oak, Bottlebrush, Banksia Robur, Fringed Violet flower essences with organic Lemon Myrtle oil and floral water and organic Rose Otto floral water.

Calming and de-stressing, Lemon Myrtle is the most antiseptic, antiviral and antifungal of the Australian essential oils and is helpful with many common ailments.

Suggested use: Taking 7 drops of Travel-well morning and evening one week before and during travel, and for one week on return, is supportive in alleviating the negative effects of travel. The Travel-refresh mist comes in a useful 25ml handbag/pocket size. Misting your face, neck and around you frequently not only keeps your skin moist and hydrated during flight, train and car travel, but helps to keep your personal space fresh and clear.

Flower Essences of Australia spritzers

Flower Essences of Australia's spritzers have been formulated with a base of pure botanicals, and exquisite aromatic essential oils organically grown and harvested in Australia to create and encourage positive healing environments. The Flower Essences of Australia have been blended within a deeply nourishing rehydrating and moisturizing protective environment whilst the gentle yet profound qualities of the flower essences care for your mind and emotions. They can be used any time there is a need to create a safe healing environment, at home, at work, while travelling and with any other situations.

Lemon Myrtle is the main organic essential floral oil ingredient in both spritzers and compared to the normal lemon's citral content of 3–10 per cent, it contains a higher percentage of 90–98 per cent citral.

It is a wonderful mood lifter! Calming and destressing, it is the most antiseptic, antiviral and antifungal of the Australian essential oils (more powerful than Tea Tree) and is helpful with colds, flu, chest congestion, irritable digestive disorders, wind, skin conditions and as an air purifier.

It has long been used as a bushfood and herbal spice for cooking, in herbal teas, and as a natural flavouring in drinks and medicines, but Lemon Myrtle is increasingly popular as one of Australia's 'new' essential oils with powerful bioactive properties.

Clear & Protect spritz Clears negative emotionally charged areas and toxicity from the environment as well as protecting against build-up of adverse electromagnetic energy, leaving spaces clear and fresh and re-energized. Spritz around the body and spaces as needed.

Contains: Flower Essences of Australia: Fringed Violet, Boab, Crowea, Blackboy, Paw Paw, Bush Fuchsia, Black-Eyed Susan, Banksia Robur, Wild Potato Bush.

Organic essential oils: Australian Sandalwood, Bergamot, Lavender, Mandarin, Cyprus Blue, Lemon Myrtle, and Kunzea, purified water, ECOCERT organic alcohol.

Travel-refresh Spritz

A hydrating flower essence, organic Lemon Myrtle and Rose water mist designed to create a sense of ease and take the stress out of the travel process.

Moisturizing and replenishing, this mist is refreshing and uplifting during long-haul flights and other forms of travel when maintaining your energy and personal space is important to feeling comfortable and at ease during travel. It enables a person to arrive at their destination feeling refreshed, in-balance and ready to go. Also the antibacterial qualities of Lemon Myrtle come fully into their own here as during a flight is often the time when we can pick up a cold or flu virus due to the recirculation of air.

Contains: Flower Essences of Australia: Crowea, Bush Iris, Wild Potato Bush, Paw Paw, Tall Mulla Mulla, She-Oak, Bottlebrush, Banksia Robur, Fringed Violet. Organic Lemon Myrtle oil and floral water, organic Rose Otto floral water.

LIVING ESSENCES OF AUSTRALIA AND THE LIFE ACADEMY (Aus L)

The Living Essences of Australia are mostly made from flowers that grow in the southwestern region of Australia, called the Wildflower State, an area known for its prolific and unique flora. They have been developed by pioneers Vasudeva and Kadambii Barnao who have been conducting far-reaching research into mind-body medicine and the evolution of consciousness for the past 28 years.

The medical results they have been able to achieve through the application of their flower essences have been so successful that their qualifications in holistic counselling and mind-body medicine and flower essence therapy are now recognized by the Australian

Government and are equivalent in professional standing to the highest naturopathic and homeopathic qualifications.

Their education programme teaches unique techniques for the application of flower essences along with an in-depth pragmatic understanding of the metaphysical world and the place a human being has within it. With the utilization of this knowledge and the application of these techniques the student is able to go beyond using psychological profiling as the primary tool for the diagnosing and prescribing of flower essences.

By combining the metaphysics of yogic science and traditional Chinese medicine with modern-day science, a deep knowledge of the inner and outer nature of a human being is understood. Upon this foundation, practical, effective diagnostic and treatment techniques are taught that take into account the mind and body of an individual along with their unique evolutionary journey, or, to put it another way, their unique life path.

After moving to Australia from New Zealand, Vasudeva began his pioneering research into the native flowers of Australia in 1977. In 1982 Vasudeva and his wife Kadambii started working together, setting up the Australasian Flower Essence Academy and the Living Essences Clinic in Perth, Western Australia. Together they have made and researched more than 200 flower essences and developed the Microvita range of creams and lotions for the relief of pain, arthritis, hypertension, stress and lethargy which are now used in hospitals on a professional basis and by orthodox practitioners (see page 186). In 1994 this led to the Barnaos being invited to create the first university flower essence course in Perth, WA. Kadambii's work from 1985 with an Aboriginal community brought her into contact with an elder who had been entrusted with the secrets of native folk-healing. He still used the traditional flower sauna, one of the oldest-known forms of flower essence therapy dating back at least 10,000 years. They also initiated research into the benefits of combining flower essences with the ancient Chinese art of acupuncture/acupressure to strengthen the potency of both modes of healing. Their findings led to the creation of some of the world's first Floral Acu-maps, which pinpoint specific flowers for specific acupuncture points. This therapy is proving highly effective in the treatment of pain and stress. In addition, they have pioneered many new flower essence diagnostic techniques such as Baihui diagnosis, Field of Flowers technique and Flower Photography Diagnosis, all of which are taught internationally through their academy's correspondence course and lecture tours.

They researched further and created the Japanese Flower Essences as well as the Combination Living Helpers.

The Barnaos feel the future in health is mind-body flower essences. Flower essences work by unlocking the inner wisdom innate within every human being. Faulty attitudes, with the consequent negative reactions to life situations, can cause physical disease, unpleasant mental states and are obstructive in the fulfilment of our desired goals.

The singles

Antiseptic Bush (*Calocephalus ass. Multiflorus*) For cleansing oneself from negative influences in the environment which may have built up over some time. Maintains inner sanctity when living among negative or harmful aspects or people.

Balga Blackboy (*Xanthorrhoea preissii*) For those who are unaware that their personal desires and goals can create emotional or environmental catastrophes. Brings an awareness of the impact your desires may have on others, so that you understand and do not resent any natural obstacles placed in your path. For the maturation of the masculine principle.

Black Kangaroo Paw (*Macropidia fuliginosa*) For those unable to forgive parents for

controlling them in the past. Replaces hate and resentment with love and forgiveness.

Blue Leschenaultia (*Leschenaultia biloba*) For those who can be emotional and physical 'Scrooges', self-sufficient, unmoved by the needs of others. Breaks down the walls of selfish isolation, allowing you to see the needs of others and learn to share with them.

Brachycome (*Multifida dilitata*) For lack of empathy, intellectual arrogance, overcriticism and contempt of others. Encourages appreciation of people for who they are, not how intelligent they seem.

Brown Boronia (*Boronia megastigma*) For an overactive mind, working excessively without rest in an attempt to solve pressing problems yet being unable to find adequate solutions. Brings patience and acceptance so you do not worry unnecessarily about things you cannot change, as well as the realization that the journey of life will deliver solutions.

Cape Bluebell (*Wahlenbergia capensis*) For those who have a chip on their shoulder and can be negative, displaying hatred and malice. Confers the ability to let go of the past and be loving and empathetic.

Catspaw (*Anigozanthos humilis*) For depression, sadness and anger caused by the insincerity and selfishness of others. For families and close-knit groups with undefined problems. Helps you to drop expectations of fairness while refusing to let others take advantage, so that they too can learn fairness. Promotes mutual consideration.

Christmas Tree (Kanya) (*Nuytsia floribunda*) For those times when duties and everyday pressures cause you to become distant and avoid your share of the load, causing resentment among others. Helps you to meet your responsibilities and reap the rewards of consistency and shared goals. Brings inner contentment which enhances your enjoyment of your family or group.

Correa (*Correa pulchella*) For those who are too hard on themselves. Teaches acceptance of our limitations and shortcomings without regret. Enables us to see how we make mistakes unintentionally, and helps us to do better next time.

Cowkicks (*Stylidium schoenoides*) For the unsuspecting optimist who is devastated by an unexpected crisis and trauma, making him or her the depleted, hopeless victim of circumstance. Helps you to rebuild and pull the pieces back together after a shattering experience to create a wiser perspective.

Dampiera (*Dampiera linearis*) For those who are fearful and unable to relax, blowing all situations out of proportion. Allows you to let go and be open, to let things happen in different ways and allow people their own style.

Fringed Lily Twiner (*Caladenia falcata*) For those who blame others for their misery when thwarted. Also for spoiled children and manipulative parents who can be vengeful and brooding. Allows you to see that selfishness lies at the root of misery. Teaches you to turn your focus away from yourself, and stimulates love.

Fuchsia Grevillea (*Grevillea bipinnatifida*) For those who tend to be two-faced. Brings the realization that hidden negativity is destructive, as well as a release from smugness, anger and a dislike of being exposed.

Fuchsia Gum (*Eucalyptus forrestiana*) For claustrophobia, both physical and emotional. Prevents feelings of panic in confined spaces.

Geraldton Wax (*Chamelaucium uncinatum*) For those who feel trapped and resentful, who feel they are under someone else's thumb (for example, a parent who always tries to appease a demanding child). Helps

you to become strong enough not to be pressured against your will or influenced by the desires of others.

Goddess Grasstree (*Kingia argenta*) For maturation of the female principle (in both men and women). Brings inner strength, nurturing, sensitivity and loving wisdom that is not emotionally dependent. Releases the female aspect into society.

Golden Waitsia (*Waitsia aurea*) For those who worry about details as well as those needing to accept their present imperfect state of health and wellbeing while convalescing from illness or trauma. Reignites spontaneity and carefree feelings, healing all aspects of the anxiety that is caused by perfectionism.

Green Rose (*Rosa chinensis viridiflora*) For people intolerant of advice when needing to break through a problem, becoming agitated when challenged by new ideas – and stagnating in their isolation. Maintains progressiveness, helping you to embrace new thoughts and ideas, not to stagnate, become negative or blame others for your situation.

Grevillea Golden Glory (*Grevillea tenuiloba*) For those whose trusting, open, relaxed nature has been abused, creating within them an uneasy feeling about the motives of others. Rekindles a sense of trust and confidence to allow other people into your life, and not to expect or worry about being judged.

Happy Wanderer (*Hardenbergia comptoniana*) For those who doubt their abilities and need others for security and support, either emotionally, mentally or physically. Helps you stand on your own feet, knowing you are strong enough to do things by yourself. Clears insecurity.

Hops Bush (*Dodonaea* sp.) For those who cannot sleep or relax due to frenetic energy. Earths excessive, scattered energy, re-establishing a natural and healthy flow which feeds your need for activity without overstimulating you. Brings inner mental and physical peace, restoring your control over life and a balanced state of rest and activity.

Illyarrie (*Eucalyptus erythrocorys*) For those who have been badly hurt and suppress the memory. Allows you to realize that you have the strength to face and deal with any pain, that it is never as bad as you fear and it will not overwhelm you. Useful in past-life therapy to uncover forgotten experiences affecting the present.

Macrozamia (*Macrozamia reidlei*) For balancing basic flows of yin and yang. Balances sexual energy to free blockages brought about by bad experiences such as rape or incest. Heals and restores all aspects of the male/female – releases blockages, corrects underdevelopment and adjusts hormonal fluctuations.

Many-Headed Dryandra (*Dryandra polycephala*) For those seen as irresponsible or 'fly-by-night', displaying erratic behaviour and panic. Brings composure and strength. Helps you to confront and deal with life's problems rather than running away from them.

Mauve Melaleuca (*Melaleuca thymifolia*) For the emotional idealist who has been hurt and is sad. Also for the unloved spouse, parent or child. Eases despondence about an uncaring world. Allows you to find fulfilment within and tap into the source of eternal love.

Menzies Banksia (*Banksia menziesii*) For clearing the fear that history will repeat itself, in the form of past experiences of hurt and rejection. Also for psychic paralysis. Allows you to let go of past pain, move on through present pain with courage, and have no fear of new experiences.

One-Sided Bottlebrush (*Calothamnus myrticae*) For those who are over-burdened and depressed, caught up in themselves, complaining about their workload. Brings the realization that others also have burdens to bear and keeps you from getting caught up in the 'poor me' syndrome.

Orange Leschenaultia (*Leschenaultia formosus*) For true survivors, tough-skinned people who have become insensitive and lack compassion. Encourages benevolence and caring and puts you in touch with the softer qualities of life.

Orange Spiked Pea Flower (*Daviesia divaricata*) For those who feel undermined by what others say, feeling angered to the point of violence. Helps you to let words spoken by others pass over you and not destroy your poise. Promotes self-expression.

Pale Sundew (*Drosera pallida*) For unscrupulous people who use people and situations for their own benefit, such as the business shark or ambitious politician. Brings the realization that being manipulative and predatory is senseless and destructive. Increases repulsion to wrong-doing. The essence is conscience.

Parakeelya (*Calandrinia polyandra*) For quiet, passive people who become the unappreciated workhorse in the family, business or community; for deep-seated loneliness and pain that comes of feeling used and uncared for. Helps you to stand up and be respected so you become the inspired worker who can enjoy belonging to the group. For self-esteem and assertiveness.

Pincushion Hakea (*Hakea laurina*) For those who feel their beliefs may be threatened or their logic undermined by new ideas, such as scientists and religious people. Allows you to be open to new ideas, not to fear the views of others, to relax and be more accepting without compromising your own ethics.

Pink Everlasting Straw Flower (*Helipterum roseum*) For those who perceive others' feelings but cannot respond to them emotionally due to feeling 'dry' and depleted.

Renews springs of love and joy. Helpful for teachers and care-givers.

Pink Fountain Triggerplant (*Stylidium bulbiferum*) For those losing their inner vital force which keeps us alive, either by a slow draining on the physical level or a rupture in the subtle bodies. Reignites the vital flame and restores its dynamism.

Pink Impatiens (*Impatiens* sp.) For the idealist, the moralist who compromises through struggling to maintain his or her standards. Helps you to retain ideals and standards no matter the obstacles, to have determination and creativity to carry on without compromising.

Pink Trumpet Flower (*Gladiolus caryophyllaceus*) For those who find it difficult to maintain their sense of purpose, who get lost during a thought process or activity. Brings clarity and focus. Harnesses inner strength of purpose and directs it towards important goals. Encourages achievement through new mental directness.

Pixie Mop (*Petrophile linearis*) For sensitive, emotionally needy people who have become hard because they feel let down. Brings the realization that forgiving those who let you down frees your heart, so that you can help others as you would hope to be helped yourself.

Purple Eremophila (*Eremophila scoparia*) Very helpful during relationship upsets. Helps you to gain and maintain serene objectivity amidst very personal issues of the heart, without compromising your richness of feeling and sensitivity towards loved ones.

Purple Flag Flower (*Patersonia occidentalis*) For those who push themselves to their stress threshold, making them feel extremely anxious and unable to relax. Brings healing relaxation of mind and body. Helps you to unwind, releasing built-up pressure and tension.

Purple Nymph Waterlily (*Nymphaea violacea*) Helps those wishing to share their treasures with others but finding themselves holding back. Brings selfless service, while making sure you are not caught in emotional traps in your dealings with others.

Purple and Red Kangaroo Paw (*Anigozanthos manglesii*) For clearing negativity and non-constructive criticism, such as blaming others all the time. Encourages you to do something positive and constructive.

Queensland Bottlebrush (*Callistemon polandii*) For clearing a conflict of desires and unsettled behaviour. Allows us the freedom to be ourselves, to know that people and experiences come and go; we do not have to be isolated from them to stay safe.

Red Feather Flower (*Verticordia mitchelliana*) For the laziness and dishonesty that can arise in those who feel life owes them a living. Teaches that it is better to give than to receive; that we should not exploit the goodness of others or feel resentful when they feel they have given enough; to rely on our own energy and resources; to be there for others.

Red and Green Kangaroo Paw (*Anigozanthos manglesii*) For being in touch with the here and now, and realizing that those close to you are a priority. Encourages sensitivity and patience; brings joy.

Red Leschenaultia (*Leschenaultia formosa*) For those who feel contemptuous of weaker people, are harsh, lacking in sensitivity. Turns harshness and lack of empathy into sensitivity. Helps you to become caring and considerate towards those weaker than yourself.

Ribbon Pea (*Brachysema aphylla*) For those who feel a sense of nameless dread, but don't understand why. Helps you to rise above the fear and foreboding that prevents you from having a positive attitude and real direction for a fulfilling life. Heals the panicky fear of annihilation.

Rose Cone Flower (*Isopogon formosus*) For those who feel frazzled and touchy, have difficulty coping, are easily disturbed, want to be alone, need space and peace (such as the parents of babies or young children). Helps you to discover peace amidst the storm, releasing tension so you can enjoy being around others.

Silver Princess Gum (*Eucalyptus caesia*) For those who lose interest or give up easily, displaying rebellious and frustrated behaviour. Teaches you to persevere when things are not working out, to keep caring and not rebel – thereby overcoming obstacles and achieving your goals.

Snakebush (*Hemiandra pungens*) For those who give but are motivated by the need to be loved. For people emotionally unsettled and frustrated in love. Helps you to learn to be self-contained and to care for others without seeking anything in return, so easing disillusionment and anxiety.

Snake Vine (*Hibbertia scandens*) For victims of destructive gossip or character assassination. Also helpful during relationship break-ups, when bitter feelings can undermine your self-confidence. Replenishes confidence and appreciation for your own achievements when others are sowing the seeds of negativity and doubt.

Southern Cross (*Xanthosia rotundifolia*) For those with comfortable lifestyles who feel bewildered when life deals them a sudden blow and they have to struggle for survival. Brings a realization of how life is for others and how, one day, it could be for you.

Star of Bethlehem (Australasian) (*Calectasia cyanea*) For resignation, frustration and lack of initiative due to a feeling that there is no hope of improvement. Brings the realization that there is always hope; helping you to see all the solutions life can offer, and to know that you can find happiness

by breaking through problems with creativity.

Urchin Dryandra (*Dryandra praemorsa*) For those who feel downtrodden, the underdog in unequal relationships. Encourages you to rise above the feelings of inferiority stemming from ill-treatment by others.

Ursinia (*Ursinia anthemoides*) For idealists who are cynical, critical and frustrated with being part of a group or organization. Allows the bright-eyed enthusiast to see the reality of group dynamics and still retain his or her idealism. Fosters co-operation and productiveness to ensure healthy progress and growth despite problems with selfish members of the group.

Veronica (*Caladenia* sp.) For isolation and alienation stemming from the feeling that you go unnoticed and are misunderstood. Teaches you to relate to others differently, and not to dwell on loneliness and the belief that no one understands you.

Violet Butterfly (*Stylidium maitlandianum*) For those feeling emotionally shattered during and after relationship traumas such as break-ups. Calms flaring sensitivities and emotional pain, speeds emotional recovery, heals the damage and allows you to get on with the rest of your life.

Western Australian Smokebush (*Conospermum stoechadis*) For those feeling pressurized to achieve when they have no desire to, resulting in loss of mental control, nervousness, anxiety, fearfulness and severe stress. In extreme cases, fear of going mad. Promotes mental stability; reconnects mind and body and reintegrates the subtle with the physical aspects. Helpful for concentration, faintness after anaesthesia – promotes quick recovery.

White Eremophila (*Eremophila scoparia*) For developing a broad perspective when messy situations threaten to drag you down. Brings clarity to complexities and difficulties. Helps maintain your equipoise, consistency and direction in life.

White Nymph Waterlily (*Nymphaea violacea*) For uncovering your deepest spiritual core. Brings tranquillity for reaching into the soul and using your Higher Self to integrate and respond to life from a universal rather than personal perspective. Helpful for spiritual practices such as meditation.

Wild Violet (*Hybathus calycinus*) For pessimists and worriers who are apprehensive, depressed, complaining and single-minded. Balances caution with the willingness to be carefree and optimistic, to take a chance on happiness.

Woolly Banksia (*Banksia hookeriana*) For those who are losing heart when the struggle seems too much. Rekindles the desire to go ahead with ideals and goals, to face new aspirations without fear of inevitable failure. Helpful during long, tiring, seemingly pointless phases in the journey to reach your higher ambition.

Woolly Smokebush (*Conospermum incurvum*) Helpful for maintaining forward progress without getting distracted. Offers perspective and humility. Helps you avoid the traps of glamour and self-importance, so that you look at life objectively.

Yellow Boronia (*Megastigma lutea*) For an overactive mind, scattered thinking, those who are easily distracted. Helps you to remain calm and centred so the mind can be focused and follow thoughts through.

Yellow Coneflower (*Megastigma lutea*) For a sense of inferiority and lack of self-esteem. Brings acceptance of inner worth and freedom from the need to seek recognition from others. Prevents situations arising in which you are used.

Yellow Flag Flower (*Patersonia xanthina*) For those stressed by daily chores, who feel unable to cope with the trying events in life. Brings calmness and brightness during times of stress, to help you to find the fortitude to handle all situations without making life one long, difficult grind.

Yellow and Green Kangaroo Paw (*Anigozanthos manglesii*) For the perfectionist, hard task master, uncompromising parent or boss who is supercritical and intolerant. Teaches tolerance, the value of mistakes and the importance of being non-judgemental and patient with imperfections.

Yellow Leschenaultia (*Leschenaultia formosus*) For those who always know better – teachers, parents, teenagers who dismiss out of hand the views of others. Helps you to become open to others, to listen, be patient and tolerant.

Australian Orchids

Blue China Orchid (Caladenia gemmata) For addictions of one sort or another, the inability to control yourself, feeling overwhelmed or unfulfilled, lack of willpower. Breaks the spell of addiction, strengthens the will, and helps you to take back control of yourself. Brings the realization that you no longer need a crutch.

Cowslip Orchid (*Macropidia fuliginosa*) For those with a superiority complex, who crave recognition and overrate their own importance, use arrogant, pompous behaviour and are negative and contemptuous to those who do not acknowledge them. Helps to deflate egos and to reveal the value of interacting with and enjoying people from all walks of life.

Fringed Mantis Orchid (*Caladenia falcata*) For the destructive, psychic predator, or the busybody with an unhealthy curiosity and no conscience. Brings conscience into one's activities; curbs unhealthy curiosity about the affairs of others. Confers the realization that you should only use information for benevolent reasons.

Hybrid Pink Fairy/Cowslip Orchid (*Caladenia* sp.) For those who take others' attitudes too personally, feeling unfairly persecuted or threatened; for oversensitivity, paranoia, tearfulness over small matters. Enables one to get on with life without being concerned with others' reactions. Generates contentment, inner tranquillity and self-contained positivity. Also helpful for PMS and the sensitivity of pregnancy.

Leafless Orchid (*Praecoxanthus aphylla*) For those who feel bogged down – such as the uninspired therapist who is drained, tired and lacking vitality. Promotes attention to central not peripheral needs in yourself and others. Allows you to find the energy deep within to keep positive and active in your work for others without becoming depleted and tired, mentally and physically.

Pink Fairy Orchid (*Caladenia latifolia*) For those who feel panicky due to circumstances, creating mental instability and the feeling of being overwhelmed by the environment. Filters the stress of environmental situations which can cause feelings of panic and being overwhelmed. Calms the inner core and helps to lessen oversensitivity to the environment.

Purple Enamel Orchid (*Elythranthera brunonis*) For those who begin a task feeling unmotivated and useless, then behave like workaholics to prove themselves. Maintains a consistent and healthily balanced energy input – not too much, not too little and not all at once – to gain an equilibrium between rest and work.

Rabbit Orchid (*Leptoceras menziesii*) For those who tend to be superficial and insincere – socialites. Bestows sincerity and straightforwardness, not shallowness and emptiness. Provides the ability to see the rewards of meaningful, honest relationships. Helps you to find your true self.

Red Beak Orchid – Burnout Orchid (*Lypercanthos nigricans*) For the frustrated housewife or husband, lethargic employee, lazy student or truant. Resolves the clash between desire and responsibility that often causes a sense of burden and mental paralysis. Counters lethargy, rebelliousness, boredom and depression.

Shy Blue Orchid (*Cyanicula amplexans*) For those dedicated to the path of light. Gives a sense of protection and dynamism where powerlessness had prevailed. Focuses spiritual energies that dispel negative forces in the environment.

Wallflower Donkey Orchid (*Diuris magnifica*) For those who feel they are the victim of circumstances, becoming vengeful, cynical, empty and disillusioned. Allows 'letting go' rather than feeling the sickness of revenge. Allows you to take responsibility for making life positive so that you do not live with a chip on your shoulder.

White Spider Orchid (*Caladenia patersonii*) For spiritual, humanitarian people such as volunteer workers with a tendency to introversion, sadness, hypersensitivity, and anguish deep in their souls. Brings love and caring without devastation at the insensitivity and suffering of others. Allows you to empathize while not being brought down by the world.

Combinations

Crisis Relief For times of shock and trauma. This essence combination is designed for times of crisis, when one finds it hard to cope with sudden events which impact negatively on one's vital force and nervous system.
Contains: Cowkicks, Red Beak Orchid, Donkey Orchid, White Spider Orchid, Southern Cross.

Essence of Clarity Brings calm focus and a centring of mental energy. This essence combination reflects internal causes for difficulties in concentration and meditation: lack of yang energy which encourages setting and achieving goals, scattered mental energy, inability to centralize energy, difficulty in focusing and carrying through an activity to its completion.

Contains: Balga, Yellow Boronia, Leafless Orchid, Pink Trumpet.

Essence of Creativity For opening up to expanded thought. This essence combination reflects internal causes for blocked creativity: being resigned to a lack of options and creative solutions, needing more flexibility, needing openness to learning, difficulty in focusing and carrying through an activity to its completion, being caught up in minute details.

Contains: Star of Bethlehem, Dampiera, Yellow Leschenaultia, Pink Trumpet, Golden Waitsia.

Essence of Emotions in Balance Relieves emotional churning and re-affirms one's quiet centre. This essence combination reflects internal causes for highly emotional states. The need for more clarity and an objective, balanced perspective, and the need for greater resiliency in dealing with relationship upsets calmly and realistically.

Contains: White Nymph Waterlily, Goddess Grasstree, Purple Eremophila.

Essence of Energy Revitalizing, energizing and rebuilds vigour. This essence combination reflects internal causes for lack of energy: inner conflict between desires and responsibilities, the aftermath of shattering experiences, and loss of energy that can occur due to expectation of further painful experiences.

Contains: Red Beak Orchid, Cowkicks, Menzies Banksia.

Essence of Positivity Brightens outlook and rebuilds the capacity for joy. This essence combination reflects internal causes for lack of positivity: being caught up in minute details, the tendency to be pessimistic, becoming glum and negative when stressed with feelings of inevitable failure because of past experiences.

Contains: Golden Waitsia, Wild Violet, Yellow Flag Flower, Woolly Banksia.

Essence of Relaxation Releases feelings of rising pressure and calms scattered frenetic energy. This essence combination reflects internal causes for the inability to relax: needing more clarity and an objective balanced perspective. Aids with stress and irritability due to little quiet or private space. For worry, feelings of rising pressure and states of frenetic scattered energy.

Contains: White Nymph and Purple Nymph Waterlily, Rosecone Flower, Brown Boronia, Purple Flag Flower, Hops Bush.

Microvita creams

The Microvita creams in the Living Essences of Australia range contain specially selected flower essences derived from the flora of the natural pristine landscapes, in combination, cold-pressed and essential oils in an aqueous cream base. These creams and lotions are designed to relieve stressed states of mind associated with physical discomfort, and to bring long-term benefits.

Medical science now recognizes that stress and negative states of mind can alter body chemistry and create physical disease. For instance, recent medical studies prove that depression is a greater cause of heart disease than smoking. Researchers found that in depressed people the blood platelets became stickier, clogging arteries and veins. Depressed people lose hope, they view life from a negative perspective, lacking optimism and positivity. Quality of life is dependent on a healthy mind and body.

Arthritis Cream Designed to alleviate arthritic pain. Relief should occur within four to eight weeks.

Body Bliss A body lotion that reduces stress and promotes a feeling of wellbeing and relaxation. Use for conditions where a calming effect would be beneficial, for example, the temporary relief of tension pain and insomnia, and to ease anxiety which causes the tightening of the lungs, apply the lotion to the chest, back and neck.

Body Sports Provides an excellent massage medium and has an invigorating effect. A body lotion which is useful for the temporary relief of soft tissue injury and pain. For general muscle pain, energy loss, cramping, sunburn, stiffness, menstrual discomfort, bruising, sports preparation and invigoration.

De-Stress Moisturizer A moisturizing cream with stress-relieving qualities. Using this moisturizer daily can help to ease tension and allow body and mind to relax, as well as improving skin lustre and appearance. For stressed-out adults, fretting babies, overactive children. For anxiety, depression, sleeplessness, devitalized skin.

Pain Cream Concentrate for pain, bruising, cramping. Also used for menstrual or birth cramps. Has invigorating effect. Pain Cream is like a first-aid kit in a bottle for muscular aches and pains and many other conditions where pain and discomfort are a problem. It can be helpful for the temporary relief of the symptoms of pulled muscles, minor sprains and bruising, back and neck pain, headaches, sinus pain, sunburn and insect bites and itches.

Skin Rejuvenation Moisturizer For wrinkled, devitalized skin and stress-related lines. Brings back the vital energy to your face, which is where stress first shows.

JAPANESE ESSENCES (Aus LJ): FOR THE 21ST CENTURY

Japan conjures up a vision of wild cherry blossoms displaying drifts of delicate white and pink blossom in the spring, and snow-capped mountain peaks, the most sacred place in the Japanese universe.

The evolution of Japanese flowers takes us back tens of thousands of years to the distribution of the Magnolia and Mahonia, an ancient species of plants older than mankind; the Magnolia especially has been discovered in fossil deposits some five million years old. The study of these plants is a key factor in the hypothesis that North America and eastern Asia were once a continuous landmass.

The Japanese, with their profound affinity with nature and deep love of flowers, have been cultivating the Rose, Magnolia and Chrysanthemum for up to 1500 years. The Cherry is so much loved and held sacred that in the spring flower festival of Hanami, the Japanese have special celebrations of flower-viewing parties, held under the blossoming trees in the temples' shrines, in honour of the Cherry's vitality. The Japanese marvel at the way the trees burst into bloom, then suddenly, at the height of their magnificence, all the petals fall, which to them is reminiscent of the samurai's graceful and honourable death suggesting qualities of invisibility but also the ephemeral nature of life.

It was when Vasudeva and Kadambii Barnao met with Hidenori Miura, healer, Qi master and ikebana teacher (flower arranging), that inspiration and timing for the birth of Japanese Essences occurred. Vasudeva feels that every flower in the world has its arena of work, and people's need of certain flowers generally corresponds to the healing properties of the flowers that grow in that area.

There is a distinct speciality to the healing qualities and attributes of the Japanese flowers that the whole of humanity can benefit from; first they highlight the strong sense of community responsibility and work collective; second they assist in balancing individual expression and personal development of relationships between people.

Fuderindou Flower (*Gentiana zellingeri*) **Manifesting the Goal** This essence gives the ability to go forward, manifest one's goals or complete plans no matter the fear, disruption or obstacles one encounters. Enhances the positive qualities of courage, manifesting strength and perseverance. Clears procrastination. For those who are despondent, easily discouraged and lack perseverance. It encourages courage and strength to pursue our convictions, being ready to act on our visions and plans for the future and not be waiting eternally for the 'perfect time'. For the person who is more into planning than doing and is discouraged when plans go wrong, feels anxious and helpless and who, as an insurance against failure, is afraid of commitment.

Hitorisizuka Flower (*Chloranthus japonicus*) **To Have Respect** For respecting the rights of others and the right to enjoy your share of collective resources. It transforms the hearts of tyrants whose desire is to control the hearts, minds and resources of others for their own ends. Encourages integrity, respect for human rights, selflessness dissolving ruthless and controlling behaviour and extreme selfishness. For the insensitive person obsessed with ambition. For selfish 'control freaks'. For those who use people to fulfil their desires and goals. Inspires detachment from desire for fame and power.

Kasumisakura Flower (*Prunus serrulata*) **The Unique Treasure** For being true to one's individuality amidst community life. It helps one to break free from unhealthy social obligations and stimulates a desire to contribute to the collective welfare using your own unique talents. Encourages social balance, individuality, responsibility. Clears rebellious feelings, and the feeling that your true nature is being compromised due to social pressure and subservience. For those who are tired and unmotivated because they are always conforming to the social expectations of others, who are rebellious towards collective or social life and feel a sense of frustration and resentment because it is 'not correct' for them to express their individuality within their community. The flower's qualities help the mind to focus on the true welfare of community life, and heal the resentment and rebelliousness created by such pressure.

Kobushi (Magnolia) Flower (*Magnolia kobus*) **The Higher Responsibility** Relieves the burden of feeling overly responsible and frees one from the subconscious fear of things falling apart for oneself and others. It gives strength, calmness and courage amidst chaos. Encourages responsibility in perspective, freedom and calmness. Chaos and failure are as important to life as order and success and when chaos and failure are accepted as learning opportunities then the birth of new ideas and new understandings manifest. For the person who feels overly responsible for the welfare of others, who feels exhausted and burdened because of the load they carry for others. For the person who feels weighed down because of their own desire for perfection and because they subconsciously fear things going wrong. Frees those with overprotective and overresponsible natures from duties and responsibilities that are not theirs to shoulder. As the healing balance is established, courage, strength and an inner calm and trust in the processes of life is born.

Mitsubatsutsuji Flower (*Rhododendron dilatatum*) **Open to Counsel** Helps to keep an open mind to the advice and ideas of others, and show respect for another's viewpoint, even when possibly faulty. Encourages being open, respectful and tolerant and dissolves obstinate, overly independent, wilful behaviour. For the person who believes that advice from others will be a hindrance rather than a benefit or who is obstinate and self-willed and refuses to listen because they can't trust the advice from others. In bypassing mental blocks due to bad advice in the past, a person is able to view all information on its own merits and can determine its true value.

Mizubasyou Flower (*Lysichiton camtschatcense*) **Wisdom/The Universal Student** This essence is for deepening one's intelligence and expanding one's ability to handle life with spiritual wisdom. Helps parents deal with and understand difficult children so that they may rear them with wisdom and help them so that their deepest goals and wishes are fulfilled. Encourages the positive quality of insightful, wise and inclusive intelligence and the ability to act inclusively for the benefit of all. Clears problems of lack of true wisdom, exclusive intelligence and intellectual arrogance. For those whose life is a mess due to intellectual arrogance and who use their intelligence to manipulate in order to satisfy their own ambitions. Gives the realization of the deeper side to intellect, that of true wisdom. This wisdom is all-encompassing and therefore improves the quality of life for all concerned. This understanding of life fills the person with an inner joy.

Murasakikeman Flower (*Corydalis incisa*) **Love Without End** For letting go of loved ones. Bonds of love are strong, so when separation comes, for example through death, travel or one's child leaving home, a sense of loss, grief and emotional upheaval often ensues. Allows letting go and feelings of inner peace, showing how a beautiful heart does not need to control a person or have them next to them to love them fully. Encourages a selfless love, self-sufficient, inner strength. Aids in recovery from sadness, devastation and loss. For those who feel lost and lonely because of separation from a loved one and who find it hard to re-establish their life after losing that person. Gives an inner peace and a restful heart, helping the person to overcome the trauma of losing a loved one, stimulating the urge to move on with life positively.

Nojisumire Flower (*Viola yedoensis*) **The Gift of Giving** Inspires unconditional benevolence, the desire to be impartial, giving in response to genuine need. This expansion of the consciousness leads to all-round spiritual enhancement. Due to personal desire a person can be partial or selective in their giving, subconsciously giving when there are personal rewards

(emotional or physical). If conscious, inevitably giving is used to manipulate a desired response from another. Encourages integrity, unconditional benevolence, compassion. Dissolves manipulative, selfish and insincere behaviour. For those who control personal relationships through their calculated benevolence, for example the parent who gives to their child on the basis of what they achieve or how good they are and not from the understanding of their genuine needs.

Uguisukazura Flower (*Lonicera gracilipes* Miq.) **Self-Determination** This essence is for finding the strength to break free from unhealthy relationships. Unhealthy dependency that leads to constant pain is destructive to body, mind and soul. Often one stays in these relationships to try to fix them, or to try to make the other person see their point of view. Encourages self-determination, courage, not blaming, and dissolves trauma, hurt and dependency. For the person continually hurt or traumatized by their partner, the child continually traumatized by their 'so-called' friends and the person in a destructive co-dependent relationship who is abused physically or emotionally. This essence evokes courage, independence and forgiveness, freeing the person to go ahead and explore their life.

Wasabi Flower (*Wasabia japonica*) **The Observant Mind** Gives the ability to perceive the function and purpose of the small parts that make up a bigger whole. Understanding life from this vantage point gives respect and appreciation for all life forms. An inability to do this makes it hard to discover the cause of a problem and take steps to solve it, and is often the cause of learning difficulties. For mental sharpness, comprehension of detail, and problem-solving ability. It stimulates wisdom, providing solutions for the more involved problems. For those who find problem-solving hard, who conceive simplistic solutions to involved problems and become frustrated and confused when tackling problem areas in their own lives. Also for those who understand the problem but are unable to dissect and understand agreements, written or verbal, or find the solution. Inspires you to take one step at a time, allowing the mind to observe the detail of how things work in relation to each other.

Yamabuki Flower (*Kerria japonica*) **Sweetness of Service** This essence brings awareness beyond one's self-centred world. It enhances the desire to help, compassion and service. Clears selfish, uncooperative behaviour and indifference to the hardship of others. For the person who likes to pursue their desires and wishes without interruption and who refuses or fails to give a helping hand to others in need, yet seeks help from those very people when they experience difficulties in their own life. For those who are totally insensitive to the hardship of others. Inspires heartfelt warmth to stay in touch with the hardship of others, and help out when possible.

Yukiyanagi Flower (*Spiraea thunbergii*) **The Cosmic Student** Opens the mind and frees it from preconceived ideas and opinions. It inspires focus and understanding of how the universe works. Fosters humility, open-mindedness and wisdom. Dissolves arrogant, know-all attitudes. For the person who feels they have pretty much learned all there is to know on any one subject, the dogmatic opinionated person who sees no point in exploring new sciences or philosophical arenas as they believe their understanding is superior. Gives a true understanding of the limits of the human mind and its ability to understand the universe. This attitude stimulates open-mindedness for all thoughts and opinions, for one understands that no mind has a monopoly on truth or infinitely understands it.

Zazensou Flower (*Symplocarpus foetidus*) **Coming Together** For the carefree joy of sharing oneself with other people. Gives the freedom of uninhibited self-expression while remaining true to yourself, your values and ideals. Encourages sociability and interest in others. Clears reclusive tendencies, isolation and dislike of people. For reclusive personalities who feel uncomfortable in social situations, and who think human relationships are nothing but trouble. Inspires the joy of sharing and communicating with others. It stimulates social interaction and interest in others.

FLOWERS OF THE ORIENT (FO)

Having thought and emphatically said that I would never ever make flower essences (*I have since learnt never to say never!*) I was enticed by spirit to do just that when I won a trip to Thailand and landed in a fabulous spot full of flowers and beauty near Pattaya. Having taken my carendash coloured pencils with me, I thought I would get back into to drawing and started with a beautiful exotic pink Orchid that seemed to dance before my very eyes as I was focusing on it.

The more I drew, the more intense was the energy emanating from the Orchid; the feeling of sexy, sassy, graceful womanly energy surrounded me. Politely waiting till I'd finished, a gently but clearly commanding voice said 'Now it is time to make some essences! Please go get what's needed' and that started the process of making essences especially designed for women.

The Flowers of the Orient have a special energy appropriate for women. So, to create this range I was led to journey throughout the Orient, which included Bali, Phuket and in particular special areas in mainland Thailand, which is a country lush with exquisitely perfumed blooms. In its purest unadulterated form, it is a deeply powerful and sensual land that calls to a woman's inner beauty. The essences were made at a sacred site in beautiful gardens with pagodas dedicated to Quan Yin, the Chinese goddess of grace, beauty, love and femininity.

Flowers of the Orient are 'Essences created especially for women'.

Frangipani (white) (*Plumeria*) Awakens passion and joy. Boosts confidence, inner beauty and feeling complete as a woman. Works on the sacred fire, awakens a passion for life, the joyousness of being a woman, calling to her inner beauty, bringing confidence in her beauty and feminine self. Feeling complete within herself. Frangipani returns her original state of purity and innocence, which is the true 'spirit of woman'.

Hibiscus (*Hibiscus*) Clears nervous stress, calms, cools and relaxes the nervous system. Invaluable for insomnia. Calms a woman's inner core, works in the sphere of the nervous system. It penetrates through all the subtle anatomy, relaxing, refreshing and chilling out the nerve endings. Supports the Qi of the nervous system helping to maintain the integrity of the nervous system's network and strengthens the inner matrix that makes up a woman's delicate structure, this being unique to a woman.

Orchid Queen (*Oncidium altissimum*) Helps a woman to have a clear insight into her own unique nature and tap into the wonder of being a woman. The Quan Yin of essences. Helps to tap into free-flowing dancing, magnetic energy of the goddess within. A sacred essence, giving a clear insight into the nature of womanness, and how it is expressed in her own unique way. It heals the female psyche, inspiring the wonder of being a woman, touching the heart and mind with joy and creating a soft strength.

Pink Orchid Strengthens and stabilizes the inner core, expands the aura's magnetism, tingeing it pink, it softens the edges, dissolving overprotectiveness allowing positive uplifting energies to infuse the auric field and enhancing attractiveness.

Water Lily (Nymphaeaceae) For times of passion, balances sensuality/sexuality and spirituality. Combines night and day, warm balmy nights and hot summer days. For nights of passion. Soft flowing energy gently balances and blends the energy of the chakras especially the heart chakra, allowing a woman to be open to receive, yielding with softness and sensuality. Heightens touching, as well as encouraging the desire to express love through the sensuousness of touching. Guaranteed to send a shiver of delight throughout your partner's entire body right down to his very toes.

Combination essences

Sensuality Blend (Frangipani, Water Lily, Orchid Queen, Hibiscus and Pink Orchid) A combination of exotic and sensual flowers from Thailand created to bring back the passion into one's life. With its silky smooth energy, it acts as a magnet that sets up a powerful vibration within the body and auric field. A subtle and harmonious blend of spirituality with sensuality. For extra effect use in combination with Spirit Lift Spritz.

On my second and third trip to Thailand near the royal city Hua Hin at a wonderful natural orchid farm I made the following essences:

Sacred Banyan Tree A de-coder in order to re-code. Its use clears away the propensity for disease encoded in the DNA, wakens and ignites the cells, holds the pattern for healthy DNA. Fast acting, it actuates and rebuilds. It encourages 'thinking outside the box'. Just because something has been 'so' for generations, doesn't mean it is set in stone. We can change, regenerate, re-invent ourselves, almost on a daily basis.

White Spider Lily Multilevelled protection. For the very sensitive who are just opening up more spiritually. Provides protection from deep within spreading throughout the whole energy system. This essence is a strengthener which strengthens and rebuilds the auric field, so that all the energy originally spent in keeping up defences can be utilized elsewhere. Provides an umbrella-like form of protection, especially whilst the subtle system needs to adjust to a natural form of filtering, which is a more refined and accurate filtering and protective ability. Dissolves overprotectiveness gained through trauma and shock, and readjusts and rebalances energy bodies, offers multilevelled protection.

The Pink Lotus was made near the shore line in Phuket, a year after the tsunami where the land needed much healing from the still visible loss and trauma. After completing the making of this essence, a portion of the essence mother tincture and the Pink Lotus flower itself needed to be offered back to the sea, as an integral part of the process of making this essence.

Pink Lotus 'The flower of the heart', the way of the compassionate spirit. Pink Lotus spiritualizes the heart chakra, so the perception is through the window of the heart. This adds warmth and compassion in interactions with others, enhances feelings of love, allowing the space for true intimacy to develop. Encourages spontaneity, a lightness of spirit which springs from a joyous heart which is a joy to be shared.

Red Torch Ginger A cleanser and multilevelled detoxer, cleansing the mind and emotions, as well as the blood and lymphatic system, it has a beneficial effect on the liver. Emotionally it is a comfort in healing heartbreak and any personal relationship upset or trauma. Creates space for renewal and fresh hope for the future.

Alma Kee Orchid Acts as a catalyst for the spirit of optimism and rejuvenation; through an overall relaxation of the mind it allows the body/mind to recharge and regenerate. Encourages awareness of sense of inner beauty and from that standpoint influences external life in a creative and positive way.

Singapore Orchid Designed for those who find themselves resistant to change, acts as a catalyst, a motivator, enabling a change of direction away from old unhealthy patterns and a positive movement forward towards productive patterns of emotional and physical health.

Red Frangipani/Temple Tree Reconnects a woman to her true inner wisdom, touching into a place of deep joy, encourages a radiant inner smile and maturing sense of sensuality.

Papaya flowers and fruit Nourishes a woman's femininity, balancing the hormonal levels as well as nourishing the reproductive organs. Papaya is an excellent digestive aid; in normalizing blood sugar levels it discourages the desire to crave addictive foods and encourages the body to find its natural balance and optimum weight. Helpful for general water retention but especially for oedema in pregnancy.

Pink Waterlily Instigates passion for life, and a renewed zest and enthusiasm for life, particularly when feeling disinterested and disconnected from all things that make 'the heart sing'. This passionate reconnection will run through all daily interactions with others but partially in relation to our unique direction and purpose in life.

Pink Powder Puff A cleanser for the more subtle levels of the energy system roots out any corners of discordant energy, fine tunes and is like a feather duster in its adjustments whisking away impurities.

Banana A potent male essence that encourages confidence in being a man, enhances vitality and a sense of inner strength, re-empowering the 'inner man'. This has a balancing effect on the hormones and nourishes the reproductive organs.

Positive Change (The Sacred Banyan Tree and Singapore Orchid) The Sacred Banyan Tree embodies the qualities of inner strength, courage, and transformation. The essences can encourage thinking outside the box. Just because a pattern has existed for generations, it doesn't mean it is set in stone. You can change, regenerate, re-invent yourself daily. Designed for those who find themselves resistant to change, acts as a catalyst, a motivator, enabling a change of direction away from old unhealthy patterns and a positive movement forward towards productive patterns of emotional and physical health.

Female (Papaya flowers and fruit, Red Frangipani and Orchid Queen) Nourishes a woman's femininity, balancing the hormonal levels as well as nourishing the reproductive area. Papaya is an excellent digestive aid, in normalizing blood sugar levels it discourages the desire and craving for addictive foods and encourages the body to find its natural balance and optimum weight. Helpful for general water retention but especially for oedema in pregnancy. Helps to reconnect with inner wisdom, encourages a radiant inner smile and a maturing sense of sensuality and feeling good about being a woman! This is one for the males in our lives.

Male Vitality (Banana and Alma Kee Orchid) A potent male essence that encourages confidence in being a man, enhances vitality and a sense of inner strength re-empowering the 'inner man'. This has a balancing effect on the hormones and nourishes the reproductive organs. A relaxation of the mind allows the body/mind to recharge and regenerate, so the spirit of optimism and rejuvenation can influence external life in a highly creative and positive way.

Stress Less (Hibiscus and Alma Kee Orchid) Calms the inner core, encourages the mind to take a rest. Works on relaxing and stabilizing the nervous system, cooling the nerves, recharging and refreshing. Supports the Qi of the nervous system helping to strengthen and maintain its overall integrity especially in times of stress and high demand on reserves. When the mind can relax the body/mind can recharge and regenerate and therefore stress less.

Clear & Detox (Red Torch Ginger and Pink Powder Puff) Red Torch Ginger is a cleanser and multilevelled detoxer, cleansing the mind and emotions, as well as the blood and lymphatic system; it has a beneficial effect on the liver. Emotionally it is a comfort in healing heartbreak and any personal relationship upset or trauma. Pink Powder Puff cleanses the more subtle levels of the energy system clearing discordant energy, whisking away impurities. Creates space for renewal and fresh hope for the future.

Zest & Vitality (Pink Waterlily, Hibiscus and Alma Kee Orchid) Renews energy, zest and enthusiasm and instigates passion for life, particularly when feeling disinterested and disconnected from all things that make 'the heart sing'. So the spirit of optimism and rejuvenation can influence external life in a highly creative and positive way. This passionate reconnection will run through all daily interactions with others but partially in relation to our unique direction and purpose in life.

Shield & Protect (White Spider Lily and Pink Orchid: multilevelled protection) Provides protection from deep within, and an umbrella-like form of protection. Strengthens the inner core and auric field, so that the energy spent in keeping up defences can be utilized elsewhere. The subtle system can then adjust to a natural form of discernment which has a more refined and accurate filtering and protective ability. Softens the edges and dissolves overprotectiveness as result of trauma and shock, and readjusts and soothes energy

THE PRACTITIONER'S ENCYCLOPEDIA OF FLOWER REMEDIES

bodies, magnetizes the aura drawing in positive life-sustaining Qi while providing multilevelled protection.

Spritzes

Spirit Lift Spritzer A blend of exotic oils of Ylang Ylang, Jasmine and May Chang combined with essences of Frangipani (White and Pink), Hibiscus, Orchid Queen and Pink Orchid and White Spider Lily. Designed to uplift a woman's spirit and enhance her sensuality. Spritz the aura with this evocative and delightful aroma whenever you need to feel sexy and sassy!

Pizzazz A heady spicy blend of Cinnamon, Ginger, Bergamot and Cedarwood with the flower essences of Banana, Alma Keen Orchid, Singapore Orchid, Hibiscus, Red Torch Ginger and White Spider Lily. Tailor-made for any man in your life.

A healing skincare range: Spirit of Beauty
To be as nature intended: 'unique'

Another area of exploration for me was the development of my skincare range. Having worked for 20 or so years with mainly women and on seeing how disempowered they felt about themselves as women, I wanted to find a way to reach as many as I could in a different way.

That night I was woken up at 3 am with an overwhelming, powerful yet supremely feminine presence and a vision of what can only be described as the goddess of a woman, the perfect balance of the deva and the diva!

From that encounter, a poem was given to me about the essences of beauty 'The Spirit of Beauty' and what it really means to embody that inner spirit of 'true woman' and that it needed to be embodied and be brought alive in a skincare range through using the flower essences of Orchids and other exotic blooms. As this was the one thing that most women

did on a daily basis, applying moisturizer to their faces, a skincare range seemed to be a natural medium, and is how Spirit of Beauty Skincare came into being.

There were specific requirements, for example, which flower essences to be used to achieve the desired result, etc., and the essences used are a blend of Korte essences with kind and generous permission of Andreas and my Flowers of the Orient.

Also it was my wish to be able to give women a wonderful gift.

So my brief was: to create a skincare tailor-made with a unique formulation that includes flower remedies (Orchid flower essences from the rainforest designed to heal from within) to enhance inner beauty whilst balancing and regenerating the skin, helping a woman to feel truly good about herself, and to be as nature intended, 'totally unique'.

To truly encourage a woman to find her inner beauty, feeling empowered, sensual and sassy, and absolutely fabulous about herself!

My feeling was, like us women, skincare should be able to multitask by doing two or more things at once, and not only naturally heal our skin, nourishing, detoxing and vitalizing, but also create a sense of wellbeing, enhancing our mood by uplifting our spirit bringing a sense of peace and happiness. Synergistically blending flower essences with essential floral oils designed to refresh, revitalize and renew was another key factor, as it was just as important that it was at least 98 per cent natural, with organic ingredients and paraben preservative free!

With a bit of nature's magic, inspired by the rainforest, the energetic healing qualities and revitalizing ingredients of the flower's essence and its oil care for the skin as well as directly affect our perception of life and ourselves.

We all know instinctively that engendering a positive, happy self-image contributes to a stress-free body/mind and has a powerful physiological effect: the less stress, the more opportunity to regenerate, regain balance and vibrancy. Stimulating that inner glow of health and vitality therefore slows down the ageing process.

Spirit of Beauty de-stressing moisturizers Delicate yet powerful creams enriched by the liquid energy from exotic flowers from the Amazonian rainforest, all designed with sensitive skin in mind. Paraben preservative free with a three-year shelf life.

Sun Orchid Skin Replenishing De-stress Moisturizer Designed for those who have a tendency to dry, sensitive, irritated or stressed skin. Floral oil blends of Sweet May Chang to cool and calm the skin, Mandarin to soothe irritation, and Rose which is not only calming, but anti-inflammatory, gently nourishing and rehydrating. With Ho leaf oil with its added anti-inflammatory properties contributing to the skin's replenishing effect. The Sun and Angel Orchid essences bring a light, uplifting sunny disposition and a *joie de vivre*. Spring Gold Rose, the flower of love, helps a woman express her unique inner beauty. Suitable for dry or sensitive skin where skin needs deeply rehydrating; also suitable for eczema, allergic skin and any skin irritations/inflammations.

Dancing Orchid Skin Rebalancing De-stress Moisturizer Designed for those who have a tendency to combination skin/normal. With floral oil blends of Jasmine to refresh, uplift and calm the nerves, Rose which rehydrates, clearing stressed skin, while Geranium balances and clarifies the skin. Lotus Blossom and Paradise Lily Flower essences revitalize and harmonize mind/body and spirit. Wild Rose and Dancing Orchid flower essences boost vitality and nurture a sense of confidence, beauty, grace and positivity. Suitable for combination or sensitive skin; also balances a tendency towards oiliness, helps with hormonal break outs.

Bird of Paradise Skin Renewing De-stress Moisturizer Designed for those with a tendency to oily/maturing and sensitive skin. Floral essential oil blend of Ylang Ylang for nourishing, rejuvenating the skin, Bergamot, and Grapefruit for stimulating circulation, slightly astringent and detoxifying, Lavender for relaxing and de-stressing, strengthening, and Geranium for tonifying, balancing. Carrot seed oil, a natural source of vitamin A benefiting the skin's elasticity, contributing to the skin-renewing effect. Passion Flower and Tibetan Rose Flower essences encourage a passion for life, a sense of sensuality and confidence as a woman. Bird of Paradise helps you to 'love being a woman'. Suitable for maturing or sensitive skin, anti-ageing in effect.

Orchid De-stress Cleansing Gel Orchid and Mandarin facial cleansing gel. A gentle cleansing gel combining glycerin, plant-based cleansers and beeswax. Echinacea flower essence to deep cleanse and Zest of Mandarin to soften and refresh, Lemon flower and Orchid essences to restore energy and promote inner wellbeing. A smooth moisturizing gel that leaves your skin clean, moist and soft to touch. Use morning and evening either warmed in the palms of the hands and worked into the face or using the accompanying facial brush gently working in with a wet brush to exfoliate, splash off with warm water. Ideal for sensitive and all skin types. Also can be used as a face mask: leave on for 10 minutes, rinse off. NB: For those with a tendency for dry skin or sun damage, dry patches may appear as damaged skin brought to the surface, to be healed and cleared; stay persistent as this encourages new baby skin to renew itself.

Floral Toning and Moisturizing Mists The Floral Mist is designed to enhance and complement each of the three moisturizers' effectiveness. Its luxurious base is from the tropical golden palm oil (from sustainable source) which has a toning, nourishing and protective effect allowing the cream to penetrate into deeper levels of the skin structure.

Lightly perfumed with fragrances of the floral oils of Sun Orchid, Dancing Orchid and Bird of Paradise. Highly refreshing and uplifting, which can be used after moisturizing to lock the moisture as well as it being ideal as a perfect overall body spritz which nourishes, softens, moisturizes and energizes the skin, especially when used just after a shower or bath, leaving the skin with a delicate overall fragrance.

A patented product. For flower essences containing medicaments, topical creams, that are particularly useful for alleviating stress. Patent No. GB2409645.

C.

NEW ZEALAND

New Zealand is an unspoilt land which boasts spectacular scenery and vast open spaces. Since c. AD 500 the North Island has been inhabited by the Maori people, who recognize and respect the spirituality of nature.

Despite being a traditional warrior-like people, they show great appreciation for every fish or bird they catch, every seed they pick, every tree they use for building their houses – realizing that these things are provided by the god, Tane. They communicate with the spirit in nature and have no wish to exploit the gifts it has to offer. Their respect and love of nature has contributed to the energy of New Zealand. Many early European settlers were drawn by the philosophy that everything is alive, a philosophy shared by Celtic and Oceanic people as well as the Maori, and brought with them their desire for freedom which has added to the positive feelings of this land. The flowers growing here are imbued with combination of energies.

FIRST LIGHT FLOWER ESSENCES OF NEW ZEALAND (NZ)

Franchelle Ofsoské-Wyber is a New Zealander of Native American and Russian descent. Born with highly developed clairvoyant and healing gifts she comes from an ancient lineage of medicine men and woman. Franchelle began making her New Zealand native flower and plant remedies in the early 1970s. In 2008 she was awarded the New Zealand Health Industry Distinguished Services Award for Research and Development.

This award was in recognition for more than 30 years of research into the nature power of New Zealand and for 'pioneering, developing and establishing New Zealand native flower and plant essences to facilitate holistic healing'. Internationally recognized as a shaman and modern-day medicine woman Franchelle has appeared on a number of international television programmes and documentaries focusing on shamanism and natural healing.

Franchelle has been fully initiated into the Kura Huna, the mystery school of the New Zealand Maori, and is described by highly respected Maori elder, traditional tohuna and ancient wisdom keeper Dr Rangimarie Turuki Arikirangi Pere. Franchelle is also described in Maoridom by traditional guardians of the old wisdom as a genuine *matatuhi*, 'one who can read what is written in the wind' and a *matakite*, 'one who sees with the healing or third eye'.

Franchelle is extensively trained in the protocols and traditional sacred plant lore of Aotearoa. She is highly attuned to the devic and unseen realms and is able to communicate directly with the ancient people and the atua or gods and goddesses of Aotearoa.

She is the author of *The Sacred Plant Medicine of Aotearoa* and *The New Zealand Native Flower Essence Handbook*. She is co-founder of New Zealand's first range of native flower essences – First Light Flower Essences of New Zealand specialist producers, suppliers and training providers for New Zealand native flower and plant essences. Highly respected in her field and described as a world authority on the sacred plant medicine of Aotearoa, Franchelle is a sought-after presenter who transmits the passion and power of working co-operatively with spirit, nature and the ancient healing tool of energy medicine for powerful healing outcomes.

Anthony Wyber has had many years of experience in producing and working with vibrational medicines for holistic health and wellbeing. He experienced a deep affinity with nature from an early age and, to deepen his understanding of devic forces, spent time at the Findhorn Foundation in Scotland. He is well known and respected for his knowledge of and expertise in the field of energy medicine and of the nature power of Aotearoa.

First Light Flower Essences of New Zealand Flower Essences Nos 1–36
Transform your attitude – change your life

- 36 flower essences that address the 36 personality archetypes, expressions and predispositions that can express in a positive or negative manner.

- A complete personality maintenance kit.

- Transforms negative attitudes, emotions, mindsets, moods, responses and states.

Flower Essences Nos 1–36

The 36 First Light Flower Essences focus on the personality, addressing the 36 personality archetypes, expressions and predispositions that can express in a positive or negative manner. They also address the negative attitudes, emotions, mindsets, moods, responses and states we can all experience at a personality level at any time.

No. 1. Pohutukawa
Keyword: Initiative.

Negative condition: Weak willed, can't say no, over-eager to please, easily influenced, submissive, anger.
Positive outcome: Self-awareness, self-assertion, power used with wisdom, personal will and strong sense of self.

No. 2. Native Flax
Keyword: Enthusiasm.
Negative condition: Impatient, tense, frustrated, irritable, flares up quickly, impetuous, abrupt, headstrong, overly enthusiastic, tires easily.
Positive outcome: Eager, forthright, motivated, lively, quick thinking and acting, patient.

No. 3. Cook Strait Groundsel
Keyword: Self-confidence.
Negative condition: Lack of self-confidence, despondency, convinced of failure, doubts abilities so won't try.
Positive outcome: Direct self-focused action, self-motivated, undeterred by challenges.

No. 4. Marlborough Rock Daisy
Keyword: Self-worth.
Negative condition: Low self-worth, nervous, anxiety prone, specific fears of known things.
Positive outcome: Feels good about self, trusts instincts, clear values, quiet courage, positive relationship with life.

No. 5. Native Passionfruit
Keyword: Abundance.
Negative condition: Procrastination, Monday morning blues, temporary mental fatigue, tiredness, doubts ability to cope.
Positive outcome: Inner vitality, strength to cope with difficulties, clear-headed.

No. 6. N.Z. Jasmine
Keyword: Perseverance.
Negative condition: Exhaustion, workaholic, struggles on despite adversity, exaggerated sense of duty, shoulders others' burdens.
Positive outcome: Endurance, resourceful, turns negatives into positives, knows own strength.

No. 7. Mountain Parahebe
Keyword: Communication.

Negative condition: Utter mental despair, has reached limits of endurance but not suicidal, future feels dark.

Positive outcome: Inner release, powerful balanced mental activity, astute, sees new options.

No. 8. Matata

Keyword: Adaptability.

Negative condition: Mental hyperactivity, mind chatter, always worrying, distressing unwanted thoughts, nervous tension.

Positive outcome: Flexibility, versatile, open-minded, optimistic, mentally alert, discernment, tranquillity.

No. 9. Koru

Keyword: Understanding.

Negative condition: Mental blocks, repeats mistakes, poor or slow learner, can't concentrate, feels mentally inferior or misunderstood.

Positive outcome: Concentration, mental discipline and organization, learns from experience.

No. 10. Starry Hibiscus

Keyword: Tenderness.

Negative condition: Over-possessive of others, clingy, needy, demands attention, manipulative, self-pity, interfering, martyr-like.

Positive outcome: Selfless love, cares for self, motherliness, inner emotional security.

No. 11. Chatham Island Geranium

Keyword: Nurturing.

Negative condition: Excessive concern for others, worry or over-attachment to loved ones, fearful for others' wellbeing, over-protective.

Positive outcome: Caring, love of family, emotional independence.

No. 12. Native Harebell

Keyword: Tenacity.

Negative condition: Dwells in the past, nostalgia, homesickness, sad memories, emotionally stuck, difficulty with change.

Positive outcome: Loyalty, emotional resolve, resilience, maturity, stability, lives in the present.

No. 13. Kanuka

Keyword: Spontaneity.

Negative condition: Total exhaustion of body, mind and spirit, no reserves left, feels unable to cope with life.

Positive outcome: Regeneration, restored inner vitality and strength, feels special and loved, spontaneous self-expression.

No. 14. Rengarenga Lily

Keyword: Creativity.

Negative condition: Pre-occupied, indifferent, daydreams, can't focus on reality, absent-minded, disoriented, withdrawn, listless.

Positive outcome: Positive idealism, healthy ego, demonstrative, highly creative.

No. 15. Mingimingi

Keyword: Dignity.

Negative condition: Black depression that comes and goes suddenly with no apparent known cause, feels sad and low.

Positive outcome: Cheerfulness, serenity, self-respect, consistent creativity.

No. 16. Small White Rata

Keyword: Perfection.

Negative condition: Feels unclean, ashamed, not good enough, self-dislike and disgust, obsessive compulsive, perfectionist.

Positive outcome: Purity, order, discernment, composure, energetic integrity, wholeness.

No. 17. Akepiro

Keyword: Synthesis.

Negative condition: Critical, tense, narrow-minded, intolerant of others, focuses on negatives, over-analytical, rigidity of body or mind.

Positive outcome: Tolerant, sympathy, constructive criticism, appreciation of difference, inclusivity.

No. 18. Purple Koromiko

Keyword: Simplicity.

Negative condition: Guilt, blame, regret, self-reproach, self-doubt, victim mentality.

Positive outcome: Sees the obvious, keeps it simple, practical service, desire to assist others in need.

No. 19. Lover's Daisy

Keyword: Love.

Negative condition: Indecision, uncertainty, lacks inner balance, fluctuating moods, power games in relationships.

Positive outcome: Poise, balance, stays true to self, empowered relating, intuitive decision-making.

No. 20. Wineberry

Keyword: Co-operation.

Negative condition: Hides worries or anxieties, mental anguish disguised by cheerfulness, plays down difficulties.

Positive outcome: Diplomacy, social skills, peace loving, generosity, fairness, sees problems in the right light.

No. 21. Hinau

Keyword: Sacred Space.

Negative condition: Self-doubt, uncertainty especially of own ability, easily influenced, needs approval of others, seeks others' opinion.

Positive outcome: Inner certainty, trusts own knowing and intuition, listens to inner voice.

No. 22. Manuka

Keyword: Purification.

Negative condition: Jealousy, hatred, suspicion, intense frustration, rage, temper.

Positive outcome: Self-regeneration, metamorphosis, in touch with own power, depth of inner experience, balanced sexuality/sensuality.

No. 23. Lacebark

Keyword: Fearlessness.

Negative condition: Overwhelming apprehension about breakdown or losing one's mind, coping mechanisms overloaded.

Positive outcome: Openness, composure, expresses deeper feelings easily, sharing and intimacy.

No. 24. Poroporo

Keyword: Willpower.

Negative condition: Resentful, bitter, self-pity, blames others, sulky, 'a wet blanket', victim of fate attitude, smouldering anger.

Positive outcome: Staying power, personal resolve, constructive emotional and mental responses.

No. 25. Kowhai

Keyword: Growth.

Negative condition: Finds change painful or difficult, difficulty adjusting to changes in life circumstances, unhealthy risk-taking.

Positive outcome: Personal development, able to move on or break bonds with the past, the spirit of adventure.

No. 26. Karo

Keyword: Foresight.

Negative condition: Unchannelled talents, uncertainty regarding life meaning, purpose, goals, life path, dissatisfaction, boredom.

Positive outcome: Finds one's life purpose, potential, skill and ambition and open to where this might lead.

No. 27. Karaka

Keyword: Knowledge.

Negative condition: Easily discouraged and depressed, pessimistic, can't see the meaning in anything.

Positive outcome: Knows each day brings opportunity, believes everything will work out. Passes on wisdom and experience.

No. 28. Chatham Island Forget-Me-Not

Keyword: Aspiration.

Negative condition: Dominating, ruthless, over-ambitious, power seeking, inflexible.

Positive outcome: Carries self with authority and conviction, secure in one's place in the world, self-recognition.

No. 29. Mairehau

Keyword: Achievement.

Negative condition: Temporary feelings of inadequacy, overwhelmed by task or responsibilities.

Positive outcome: Detached, neutral, uninvolved, performs at optimal level, strong and capable, leadership abilities.

No. 30. Ngaio

Keyword: Responsibility.

Negative condition: Utter despair, hopelessness, despondency, apathetic, has lost sense of humour.

Positive outcome: Consolidation, commitment, accepting limitations, rekindled optimism.

No. 31. Native Iris

Keyword: Individuality.
Negative condition: Lives on nerves, overbearing, inflexible, fanatical, excessive zeal, inciting unrest.
Positive outcome: A torchbearer, able to inspire and uplift others, the activist creates change.

No. 32. Ice Plant

Keyword: Freedom.
Negative condition: Self-denial, hard on self, rigid strict views and outlook, sanctimonious, intensely dogmatic.
Positive outcome: Adaptability, open-minded idealist, broadminded, high-principled standards.

No. 33. Rewarewa

Keyword: Participation.
Negative condition: Aloof, a loner, appears proud but feels emotionally isolated and lonely, social alienation or withdrawal.
Positive outcome: Tactful reserve, wisdom, approachable, social consciousness and awareness.

No. 34. Heketara

Keyword: Unity.
Negative condition: Anxiety, foreboding, apprehension, fear of unknown things, escapist tendencies result in not managing material responsibilities.
Positive outcome: Compassion, sensitivity, aware of others' pain, grief and suffering.

No. 35. Creeping Pratia

Keyword: Empathy.
Negative condition: Self-centred, seeks attention, saps others' energy, a poor listener, fixated by own troubles.
Positive outcome: The psychic, clairvoyant, interested in others, helpful but able to say no without feeling guilty.

No. 36. Native Linen Flax

Keyword: Service.

Negative condition: Resigned, apathetic, lack of interest, underdog, no effort for self-improvement.
Positive outcome: Devotion, kindness, self-directed, inner motivation, lives one's ideals and dreams.

Fern Essences Nos 37–43

Each of the seven fern essences addresses one of the layers of the aura. There are seven types of fundamental traumas that we can experience and these are held in the aura. The seven native fern essences address these traumas and work to clear the respective layers of the aura.

Moving beyond pain – clearing the aura

- The seven fern essences focus on the layers of the aura, addressing the seven types of fundamental traumas that we can experience.

- A complete aura maintenance kit.

- Clears the layers of the aura to support aura wellbeing.

No. 37. King Fern

Keyword: Security.
Negative condition: Physical/survival trauma, physical abuse, insecurity, de-vitalization, avoidance issues around life or death, accident-prone.
Positive outcome: Self-preservation, feels alive, present and physically safe and secure.

No. 38. Rasp Fern

Keyword: Boundaries.
Negative condition: Emotional/sexual trauma, emotional abuse, insecurity, dependent, needy, volatile, emotional/sexual dysfunction.
Positive outcome: Healthy emotional or sexual boundaries, feels emotionally safe, emotional consistency.

No. 39. Shaking Brake Fern

Keyword: Empowerment.

Negative condition: Disempowerment trauma, feelings of inadequacy, mental insecurity or disconnectedness.

Positive outcome: Self-definition, empowered by life experiences.

No. 40. Silver Fern

Keyword: Trust.

Negative condition: Heartfelt trauma, loss, abuse or betrayal of love or trust, grief, rejection issues, heartbreak, hatred, jealousy, issues around giving or receiving love.

Positive outcome: Self-acceptance, self-trust.

No. 41. Prince of Wales Feathers Fern

Keyword: Respect.

Negative condition: Humiliation trauma, judgement, shame, issues around speaking out or being heard, lacks respect for self or others.

Positive outcome: Self-respect, feels heard, creative expression.

No. 42. Star Fern

Keyword: Self-reflection.

Negative condition: Reality trauma, self-doubt, sense of unreality or disillusionment, life in constant turmoil, invalidation of one's personal reality.

Positive outcome: Knows one's own reality, living authentically.

No. 43. Plumed Maidenhair Fern

Keyword: Direction.

Negative condition: Spiritual trauma, confusion, feels directionless or lost, uncertainty, escapist or self-destructive tendencies.

Positive outcome: Self-knowledge, sense of purpose, clear expression of spirituality, inner direction.

New Zealand Tree Essences Nos 44–50

Each of the seven tree essences is associated with one of the seven major chakras.

Balance, strengthen, protect and clear the chakras

- The seven tree essences focus on clearing and balancing the seven main chakras that can become imbalanced and blocked.

- A complete chakra maintenance kit.

- Balances the chakras to support chakra wellbeing.

No. 44. Kahikatea

Keyword: Structure.

Negative condition: Addiction to security, materialistic, overly strict routines, avoids responsibilities, feels unsupported.

Positive outcome: Base chakra. Stable, self-sufficient, grounded, structured, feels supported, safe and secure.

No. 45. Matai

Keyword: Fluidity.

Negative condition: Reactive emotional responses, obsessive emotional attachments, addiction to pleasure, emotional dependency or manipulation.

Positive outcome: Sacral chakra. Flexibility, ease, emotional balance.

No. 46. Totara

Keyword: Inner Power.

Negative condition: Dominating, power hungry, temper tantrums, weak will, feelings of inferiority, the bully or the victim.

Positive outcome: Solar plexus chakra. Personal power, balanced use of power, strength of will, positive self-image.

No. 47. Kauri

Keyword: Beauty.

Negative condition: Co-dependency, clinging, inability to give of one's self or respond to love.

Positive outcome: Heart chakra. Self-acceptance, loving, empathic, self-loving, healthy intimate relationships.

No. 48. Maire

Keyword: Healing.

Negative condition: Too much talking, poor auditory comprehension, unkind speech, difficulty communicating or expressing oneself.

Positive outcome: Throat chakra. Communication, self-expression, knows when to speak and when to be silent.

No. 49. Miro

Keyword: Intuition.

Negative condition: Overly idealistic, obsessions, delusions, hallucinations, poor memory, blocked intuition, difficulty imagining possibilities or alternatives.

Positive outcome: Third eye chakra. Inner awareness, ability to see limitless possibilities.

No. 50. Rimu

Keyword: Connection.

Negative condition: Overly intellectual, addicted to spiritual beliefs and practices, extreme nervous anxiety, rigid, limited beliefs.

Positive outcome: Crown chakra. Spiritual wisdom, spiritual clarity and focus, open-minded.

New Zealand Seed Essences Nos 51–62
Restoring the master patterns for living

Each of the 12 seed essences focuses on an aspect of the energetic aspect of DNA and the ancestral and past-life patterns that prevent us from reaching full potential. They have the power to release us from powerful hereditary, ancestral or past-life negative core beliefs and the primary fears that sustain those beliefs, beliefs that have blocked or limited us from being who we truly are.

- The 12 seed essences focus on the energetic aspect of DNA and ancestral and past-life patterns that prevent us from reaching full potential.

- A complete DNA energetic maintenance kit.

- Restores the light codes or master patterns for right living.

No. 51. Broadleaf

Keyword: Reverence.

Negative condition: Negative hereditary beliefs, life patterns and fears around life, death, money and material matters.

Positive outcome: Right living. Care for one's physical environment, self and family.

No. 52. Nikau Palm

Keyword: Non-attachment.

Negative condition: Negative hereditary beliefs, life patterns and fears around emotional expression, sex, sensuality, enjoyment, pleasure, nurturing and partnership.

Positive outcome: Right emotional behaviour. Enhance emotional awareness.

No. 53. Wharangi

Keyword: Non-Judgement.

Negative condition: Negative hereditary beliefs, life patterns and fears around inner power, empowerment, expression of power.

Positive outcome: Right use of power. Empowered from within; measured responses.

No. 54. Houpara

Keyword: Compassion.

Negative condition: Negative hereditary beliefs, life patterns and fears around intimate relationships, compassion, trust and beauty.

Positive outcome: Right relationship. Compassion, empathy, deep genuine heartfelt relatedness.

No. 55. Hangehange

Keyword: Truth.

Negative condition: Negative hereditary beliefs, life patterns and fears around creativity, communication and humiliation.

Positive outcome: Right speech. Truthful, sincerity, integrity, high levels of creativity, ease of communication.

No. 56. Inkberry

Keyword: Vision.

Negative condition: Negative hereditary beliefs, life patterns and fears around ideals, dreams, intuition, facing reality.

Positive outcome: Right thought. Being guided by inner wisdom, insight, create a new personal vision, inspired revelations.

No. 57. Cabbage Tree
Keyword: Sovereignty.
Negative condition: Negative hereditary beliefs, life patterns and fears around spirituality, religion, losing control mentally.
Positive outcome: True independence of spirit, able to recognize one's true priorities and path.

No. 58. Ramarama
Keyword: Life Purpose.
Negative condition: Negative hereditary beliefs, life patterns and fears around life purpose and place in the world.
Positive outcome: Purposeful living, releases one's personal will to higher will, instrumental in the restoration and creation of order.

No. 59. Star Lily
Keyword: Unconditional Love.
Negative condition: Negative hereditary beliefs, life patterns and fears around unconditional love and the oneness of life and being spiritually forsaken.
Positive outcome: Universal Love. Divine love and compassion, sees all-encompassing beauty and unity of all life.

No. 60. Dragon Leaf
Keyword: The Will to Good.
Negative condition: Negative hereditary beliefs, life patterns, fears or depression around right creation and participating in the Divine plan.
Positive outcome: Compassionate wisdom, consciously working with Divine mind.

No. 61. Mount Cook Lily
Keyword: Peace.
Negative condition: Negative hereditary beliefs, life patterns, fears around the Divine Feminine as a powerful force in the universe.
Positive outcome: The Divine Feminine. Peace, forgiveness, natural expression of feminine power.

No. 62. Raupo
Keyword: The Will to Be.

Negative condition: Negative hereditary beliefs, life patterns, fears around the Divine Masculine as a powerful force in the universe.
Positive outcome: The Divine Masculine. Benevolence, natural expression of masculine power.

New Zealand Plant Essences Nos 63–84
Each of the 22 plant essences helps enhance life's experiences and to assist the soul to move through the 22 universal archetypal life challenges and situations encountered on the journey of life

Enhance life's experiences – live consciously

- The 22 plant essences focus on enhancing individual soul and soul growth.

- A complete soul support kit to enhance life's experiences.

- The 22 archetypal challenges the soul meets on its journey.

No. 63. Karamu
Keyword: Manifestation.
Negative condition: Unable to cope or to manifest what one needs, overwhelmed by life, scattered energies, unable to tap into one's full potential.
Positive outcome: Focused intent, belief in oneself and abilities, multitasking, the juggler.

No. 64. Koromiko
Keyword: Wisdom.
Negative condition: Feels isolated, misunderstood, empty inhibited, questions validity of one's own 'knowing'.
Positive outcome: Use of intuitive processes, spiritual equilibrium, inner poise and tranquillity.

No. 65. Tree Fuchsia
Keyword: Feminine Power.
Negative condition: Emotional dissatisfaction, suppressed or unsuccessful creativity, always giving, neglects own feelings and needs.

Positive outcome: Abundance, receptivity, inner harmony, secure within one's femininity.

No. 66. Rangiora
Keyword: Masculine Power.
Negative condition: Dominating, stubborn, unemotional, needs to prove oneself to others, intimidated by authority figures.
Positive outcome: Leadership, foresight, organization, personal authority, autonomy.

No. 67. Red Rata
Keyword: Guidance.
Negative condition: Extreme conservatism, superstitious, fearful of what others will think, ignores own inner prompting.
Positive outcome: Spiritual autonomy, receives a flow of guidance, open to signs and messages of everyday life.

No. 68. Puriri
Keyword: Discernment.
Negative condition: Inner conflict, poor choices in love or in life, entering into relationships for the wrong reason.
Positive outcome: Discrimination, appropriate life choices, balance, inner unity and wholeness.

No. 69. Bracken Fern
Keyword: Triumph.
Negative condition: Contradictory thoughts and emotions, feels defeated by obstacles, afraid of opposition or competition.
Positive outcome: Overcoming challenges, bounces back from adversity, willpower, drive for success.

No. 70. Hen and Chicken's Fern
Keyword: Strength.
Negative condition: No passion for life, inner rage at not being centre of attention or getting one's way, infantile.
Positive outcome: Passion for life, inner strength, courage of heart, control over one's animal instincts.

No. 71. Coastal Convolvulus
Keyword: Reflection.

Negative condition: Overly introspective, aloof, melancholy, refuses to take advice or learn from experience.
Positive outcome: Capacity to go within, contemplation, restoration of spirit, self-reliance.

No. 72. Shining Spleenwort
Keyword: Synchronicity.
Negative condition: Missed opportunities, unlucky, trapped in negative cycles of karma, lost inside issues.
Positive outcome: Timely action, going with the flow, attuned to natural cycles, rhythm and timing.

No. 73. Coastal Lobelia
Keyword: Decisiveness.
Negative condition: Lack of objectivity, difficulty making a decision, prejudice, biased attitude, victim mentality.
Positive outcome: Equanimity, mental strength and clarity, cool logic, fairness, neutrality.

No. 74. Golden Corokia
Keyword: Grace.
Negative condition: Resignation, stuck in limbo, midlife crisis, meets situation with lack of grace.
Positive outcome: Inner grace, patience, devotion, sacrifice, letting go, seeing matters from a different perspective.

No. 75. Whau
Keyword: Release.
Negative condition: Fear of death and endings, inertia, burnt out, feels dead or utterly lost inside.
Positive outcome: Rebirth, regeneration, death-type situations, loss, endings, eliminating and shedding the old, ready for change.

No. 76. Native Hawthorn
Keyword: Moderation.
Negative condition: Mood swings, wastes one's energy, over-reactive, intolerant, out of balance, everything feels in a muddle.
Positive outcome: Restraint, forbearance, diplomacy, steadiness of effort, adaptability.

No. 77. Clematis
Keyword: White Light Protection.

Negative condition: Fear, manipulation, gives one's power away, attracts negative energies, addictive repetitive scenarios.
Positive outcome: Humour, able to keep one's spirits up, power used wisely, faces one's fears.

No. 78. Akeake
Keyword: Change.
Negative condition: Hides behind a façade, inner paralysis, state of shock or disbelief, unable to be comforted.
Positive outcome: Initiates and responds positively to change, re-orientation after shock or crisis, faces the truth.

No. 79. Fragrant Fern
Keyword: Hope.
Negative condition: Hopelessness, depression, utter despair, feels lost and abandoned by God or spirit, 'dark night of the soul'.
Positive outcome: Healing, connection to higher spiritual energies, help, protection, inspiration, luck.

No. 80. Raglan Roseberry
Keyword: Clarity.
Negative condition: Total confusion, feelings and emotions run high, feels lost or completely in the dark, feels one is going crazy.
Positive outcome: Listens to one's gut feeling, accesses super-sensory and psychic abilities.

No. 81. Tanekaha
Keyword: Joy.
Negative condition: Despondent, gloomy, jaded outlook on life, doubtful, weary, pessimistic, boredom.
Positive outcome: Happiness and optimism, sunny disposition, ordinary activities give pleasure, freedom at a soul level.

No. 82. Golden Tainui
Keyword: Renewal.
Negative condition: Stuck at the crossroads, delays decisions, closed mind to new possibilities, refuses to respond to inner call.
Positive outcome: Renewal, responds to the soul's call to action, new possibilities, revitalization.

No. 83. Kakabeak
Keyword: Completion.
Negative condition: Instability, life out of balance, lack of composure, has not learned the lessons.
Positive outcome: Fulfilment, successful closure, sense of true self, total transformation, the dancer ready to begin a new dance with life.

No. 84. Kawakawa
Keyword: Faith.
Negative condition: Blind faith, folly, recklessness, foolish, naive attitude to life, careless.
Positive outcome: Moves forward fearlessly, ready to take a leap of faith, enthusiasm, able to be in the moment, ready for next adventure.

New Zealand Healers Essences Nos 85–96

The 12 healers' essences address the area of advanced flower essence therapy. For practitioners, those in the healing and helping professions, shamanic healers, energy workers, counsellors, massage therapists, naturopaths, doctors, homeopaths, nurses, hospice workers, care-givers and all those who are personally walking the healing path or working with those in need of assistance.

Working in harmony with nature

- The 12 healers' teacher plant essences focus on the 12 essential rites of passage of the healer.

- A complete healers' kit for those walking the healing path.

- The 12 essential skills and abilities of the healer.

No. 85. Black Mamaku
Keyword: The Healer.
Opening up to the healing journey; connecting with one's inner healer; stepping onto the path of the healer; moving into timeless healing space; invoking the healer's powers; hearing the call to heal.

No. 86. Ancient Kauri
Keyword: Path of Heart.
Staying in heart; maintaining a heart-centred healing focus; tapping into the wealth of healing knowledge of the ancestors of the land; accessing the wealth of knowledge of the past; healing from the heart.

No. 87. Maire Tawake
Keyword: Staying in Neutral.
Staying in your own power centre; self-reliance; not needing anything from the client; not being swamped by others' processes; learning to prevent negative energy from clinging to you.

No. 88. Wheki
Keyword: Caring for Your Healer Self.

Caring for your healer self; knowledge of and practical application of the principles of holistic healing and living; being alert to your own needs; staying open to expansion; continuing to grow on your path.

No. 89. Black Shield Fern
Keyword: Double Protection.
For maximum energetic protection; to close off energetically; take time out; choosing to be energetically unavailable; recharging your batteries; for high levels of sensitivity to any stimuli.

No. 90. Smooth Shield Fern
Keyword: Healers' Protection.
For those in the counselling, healing, caring or health professions; allows one to stay open and empathetic while maintaining personal objectivity and energetic autonomy.

No. 91. Triangular Fern
Keyword: Triangle of Power.
Activating the triangle of healing power; linking yourself and client with highest spiritual energy, calling on the highest spiritual forces for assistance or information.

No. 92. Lace Fern
Keyword: Energetic Integrity.
Restoring and maintaining the auric pattern and auric energetic integrity; recalibration of one's own perfect auric pattern; honouring one's uniqueness and gifts; fulfilling one's healing destiny.

No. 93. KioKio
Keyword: Metaphysical Sensitivity.
Feeling for the energy; enhances clairsentient abilities; useful for the practitioner wishing to feel, sense, identify and physically register their clients' energies clairsentiently.

No. 94. Five Finger
Keyword: Supersensory Gifts.
Equal development and use of the five subtle senses; activating the five subtle senses – clairsentience, clairvoyance, clairaudience, clairknowing and clairgustus.

No. 95. Toothed Lancewood
Keyword: Psychic Awareness.
The power of thought; awareness; truthfulness; creating your own reality; for understanding thoughts are things; for the after-effects of a challenging client; helps remove psychic barbs or arrows of negative thought from the energy field.

No. 96. Sword Fern Keyword
Keyword: Cutting Ties.
Maintaining objectivity; identifying the main issue; valuing others' viewpoints; relaying information concisely; clarity of communication; not twisting words to suit; severing outworn energetic cords or ties.

New Zealand Shamanic Essences Nos 97–120
The 24 shamanic essences address the deeper areas of advanced flower essence therapy encountered in flower essence practice. A specialist range of native New Zealand teacher plants of a particular potency and high order, these ancient power plants address the age-old question of 'Who heals the shaman-healer?'

Treat the cause – heal the spirit

- The 24 shamanic teacher plant essences focus on the 24 essential rites of passage of the shaman.

- A complete shamanic kit for those walking the healer-shaman path.

- The 24 essential skills and abilities of the shaman.

No. 97. Parataniwha
Keyword: The Shaman.
Accessing the spirit world; walking between the worlds; connecting with one's inner shaman; bridges the gap between ordinary and non-ordinary reality; connecting with one's guide to the spirit world.

No. 98. Native Daphne
Keyword: Reading the Signs.
Being guided daily by the signs in life; interpreting correctly the signs in nature and the spirit world; recognizing omens and true messages and knowing what they mean.

No. 99. Pale Flowered Kumerahou
Keyword: Devic Connections.
Linking in with the spiritual forces of the land/place; sacred offerings; payment for accessing magical pathways; Earth magic; nature power; linking into the fairy folk.

No. 100. Mahoe
Keyword: Inner Fire.
The shaman's drum; arousing the inner fire; entering the shamanic state; moving into an altered state of consciousness; raising the vibration; the excitation of light; accessing the web of oneness.

No. 101. Horopito
Keyword: The Past.
Accessing the lower world or underworld – the place of the past; for wisdom, information and healing connected to past lives or events; connecting with your power animal.

No. 102. Tree Daisy
Keyword: The Present.
Accessing the Middle World – the magical version of our conscious or everyday reality; to gain information or solve everyday problems pertinent to waking life.

No. 103. Native Angelica
Keyword: The Future.

Accessing the Upper World – the place of the future and our spirit guides; to obtain guidance for the future; anchors us safely into the time after 2012 as we evolve into *Homo spiritualis.*

No. 104. Red Matipo
Keyword: Soul Retrieval.
Calling or singing the soul back home after soul loss; causing the spirit to re-enter the being; welcoming the scattered, fragmented, lost or traumatized parts of the self back home.

No. 105. Tawa
Keyword: Self-Integration.
Integrating the experience of healing; identifying and addressing the needs of newly found aspects of self; synthesis; absorption into the existing matrix of a new awareness and reality; uniting into one healed whole.

No. 106. Kawaka
Keyword: The River of Time.
Accessing the eighth chakra; soul scripts; past lives; meeting past keepers; travelling through the river of time; the channel; operating outside the time-space continuum.

No. 107. Tree Nettle
Keyword: Shaman's Death and Rebirth.
The shaman's guardian; dying to the old self; endurance tests; breaking though self-imposed realities; growing in power through facing one's fears; pain or shadow self; support, protection, care for body and spirit while we travel to other realms.

No. 108. Tarata
Keyword: The Hero.
Reconfiguration; telling the story; overcoming the odds; to cleanse, heal and close psychic wounds; suffuses the being with cleansing healing energies after exposure to negative energy; a psychic disinfectant.

No. 109. Marsh Ribbonwood
Keyword: The Spiritual Warrior.
Being in divine ego; discipline; true obedience; the healed feminine and masculine energies in alignment; a spiritual antidote for intrusive energies; curses; difficult energies.

No. 110. Pukatea
Keyword: The See.
Going into the dreamtime; dreaming a new reality; seeing new possibilities; shape shifting; facilitates the expelling of elemental entities associated with alcohol, drug addictions and medication.

No. 111. Giant Flowered Broom
Keyword: The Sage.
Reclaiming or finding your power place; the power of the womb; sweeps clear the karma and energetic debris transmitted from sexual encounters or past relationships.

No. 112. Broken Heart Tree
Keyword: Initiations of Heart.
Retrieval of one's 'heart'; keeping your 'heart' intact when in heartrending situations; recovery from loss or shattered dreams; staying love-full and connected to divine heart.

No. 113. Titoki
Keyword: Initiations of Power.
Retrieval of one's power or will; keeping your power, will or intent intact when in devastating or challenging situations; emerging victorious by staying power-full and connected to divine power.

No. 114. Taraire
Keyword: Initiations of Mind.
Retrieval of one's 'mind'; keeping your 'mind' intact when with a strong-minded other; staying mind-full and connected to divine mind.

No. 115. Bridal Tree
Keyword: The Maiden.
Intent; seeking to dedicate oneself; working together in dedication to the path of service to spirit; sending out a 'call' for the spiritual partner; the intent to unite with the next appropriate life's situation, phase or relationship.

No. 116. Alpine Baby Fern
Keyword: The Mother.
Breath of spirit; times of spiritual gestation or inner growth; giving birth to oneself; to connect with and call in the spirit of a child, creation or enterprise; to assist or make peace with a child in spirit.

No. 117. Clutha River Daisy
Keyword: The Crone.
Spiritual initiations; birth, life; death; assists the spirit of those in transition on the web; releases and clears souls who are lost, stuck or grounded in otherworld realms; clears ancestral lines.

No. 118. Silver Pine
Keyword: Language of the Stones.
Environmental shamanism; ghost busting; lays the spectre, ghosts or grievances of the past to rest; clears or liberates the energies trapped in locations, land or buildings; transformation of the energy of spaces; liberates old stuck unproductive energy.

No. 119. Hutu
Keyword: Council Fire.
Calling on higher forces for divine intervention; divine justice; mediation on behalf of another; the restoration of divine order; invoking universal law; the Knowledge Tree; aligning with the ancient path; a warning in spirit to those cutting across the oneness.

No. 120. Golden Speargrass
Keyword: Standing for the Sacred.
Standing for a better world; master of light; light in extension; awakening the kundalini, a conduit through which the power of the creator can flow; the small still point; the thunderbolt; dispeller of the darkness associated with possession.

Orchid Essences Nos 121–128: alchemical elixirs of transformation
The eight Orchid essences are elixirs of spiritual light that hold the divine eightfold-energies of cosmic consciousness at a chakra level. They are a safe, natural and vital vibrational energetic chakra upgrade for those on the spiritual pathway and offer support for the wave of highly sensitive children and souls often known as indigo, crystal or star children who are now appearing on the planet in ever greater numbers.

The fairy remedies of the Patupaiarehe – children of the stars

- The eight Orchid teacher plant essences focus on the energetic upgrading and attuning of the chakras.

- A complete chakra support kit for *Homo spiritualis* – spiritual humankind.

- Energetically aligns the chakras with the higher vibrational frequencies coming into the planet at this time.

No. 121. Forest Orchid
Keyword: Fairy of the North.
Creates a powerful magical connection with the element of Earth; anchors in spiritual light from the north; energetically prepares, tones and upgrades the base chakra to facilitate a quantum shift to cosmic awareness and attune with the higher energetic frequencies coming into the planet at this time.

No. 122. Fairy Bouquet Orchid
Keyword: Fairy of the West.
Creates a powerful magical connection with the element of water; anchors in spiritual light from the west; energetically prepares, tones, aligns and upgrades the sacral chakra to facilitate a quantum shift to cosmic awareness and attune with the higher energetic frequencies coming into the planet at this time.

No. 123. Spring Orchid
Keyword: Fairy of the East.
Creates a powerful magical connection with the element of air; anchors in spiritual light from the east; energetically prepares, tones, upgrades and aligns the solar plexus chakra to facilitate a quantum shift to cosmic awareness and attune to the higher energetic frequencies coming into the planet at this time.

No. 124. Fairy Sceptre Orchid
Keyword: Fairy of the South.
Creates a powerful magical connection with the element of fire; anchors in spiritual light from the south; energetically prepares, tones, upgrades and aligns the heart chakra to facilitate a quantum shift to cosmic awareness

and attune to the higher energetic frequencies coming into the planet at this time.

No. 125. Elfshood Orchid
Keyword: Fairy of the Rainbow Bridge.
Linking into the magical power of the soul self; anchors in spiritual light from the rainbow bridge; energetically prepares, tones, upgrades and aligns the transpersonal/etheric heart chakra to facilitate a quantum shift to cosmic awareness and attune to the higher energetic frequencies coming into the planet at this time.

No. 126. Tree of Life Orchid
Keyword: Fairy of the Lower Earth.
Linking in with the magical power of lower Earth; anchors in spiritual light from the dragon power at the Earth's core; energetically prepares, tones, upgrades and aligns the throat chakra to facilitate a quantum shift to cosmic awareness and attune to the higher energetic frequencies coming into the planet at this time.

No. 127. Sun Orchid
Keyword: Fairy of the Upper Heavens.
Linking in with the power of the above; anchors in spiritual light from the upper heavens, the 12 far flung heavens; energetically prepares, tones, upgrades and aligns the third eye chakra to facilitate a quantum shift to cosmic awareness and attune to the higher energetic frequencies coming into the planet at this time.

No. 128. Horned Orchid
Keyword: Fairy of the Infinite.
Linking into the power of the infinite; anchors in spiritual light from the source; energetically prepares, tones, upgrades and aligns the crown chakra to facilitate a quantum shift to cosmic awareness and attune to the higher energetic frequencies coming into the planet at this time.

Fern Ally Essences Nos 129–136: alchemical elixirs of spiritual transmutation

The eight fern ally essences are elixirs of spiritual light that hold the divine eightfold-energies of cosmic consciousness at an aura level. They are a safe, natural and vital vibrational energetic aura upgrade for those on the spiritual pathway and offer support for the wave of highly sensitive children and souls often known as indigo, crystal or star children who are now appearing on the planet in ever greater numbers.

The sacred Kaitiaki – guardians and protectors

- The eight fern ally teacher plant essences focus on the energetic upgrading and attuning of the aura.

- A complete aura support kit for *Homo spiritualis* – spiritual humankind.

- Energetically aligns the aura with the higher vibrational frequencies coming into the planet at this time.

No. 129. Owls Foot Clubmoss
Keyword: Guardian of the North.
Energetically prepares, tones, upgrades and aligns the first layer of the energy field with the higher energetic frequencies coming into the planet at this time.

No. 130. Cascading Clubmoss
Keyword: Guardian of the West.
Energetically prepares, tones, upgrades and aligns the second layer of the energy field with the higher energetic frequencies coming into the planet at this time.

No. 131. Upright Clubmoss
Keyword: Guardian of the East.
Energetically prepares, tones, upgrades and aligns the third layer of the energy field with the higher energetic frequencies coming into the planet at this time.

No. 132. Hanging Clubmoss
Keyword: Guardian of the South.
Energetically prepares, tones, upgrades and aligns the fourth layer of the energy field with the higher energetic frequencies coming into the planet at this time.

No. 133. Naked Fern
Keyword: Guardian of the Rainbow Bridge.
Energetically prepares, tones, upgrades and aligns the fifth layer of the energy field with the higher energetic frequencies coming into the planet at this time.

No. 134. Fork Fern
Keyword: Guardian of the Lower Earth.
Energetically prepares, tones, upgrades and aligns the sixth layer of the energy field with the higher energetic frequencies coming into the planet at this time.

No. 135. Adder's Tongue
Keyword: Guardian of the Upper Heavens.
Energetically prepares, tones, upgrades and aligns the seventh layer of the energy field with the higher energetic frequencies coming into the planet at this time.

No. 136. Octopus Flower
Keyword: Guardian of the Infinite.
Energetically prepares, tones, upgrades and aligns the eighth layer of the energy field with the higher energetic frequencies coming into the planet at this time.

Sacred Mountain Grass Essences Nos 137–144

The eight sacred mountain grass essences are elixirs of spiritual light that hold the divine eightfold-energies of cosmic consciousness at DNA level. They are also highly sensitive children and souls often known as indigo, crystal or star children, who are now appearing on the planet in ever greater numbers.

Alchemical elixirs of spiritual transcendence – blessings on the wind

- The eight Sacred Mountain Grass teacher plant essences focus on the energetic upgrading and attuning of DNA.

- A complete DNA support kit for *Homo spiritualis* – spiritual humankind.

- Energetically aligns DNA with the higher vibrational frequencies coming into the planet at this time.

No. 137. Mt. Tititea Blue Grass
Keyword: Blessings of the North.
Energetically prepares, tones, upgrades and aligns the first layer of DNA with the higher energetic frequencies coming into the planet at this time.

No, 138. Mt. Te Aroha Forest Grass
Keyword: Blessings of the West.
Energetically prepares, tones, upgrades and aligns the second layer of DNA with the higher energetic frequencies coming into the planet at this time.

No. 139. Mt. Hikurangi Toe Grass
Keyword: Blessings of the East.
Energetically prepares, tones, upgrades and aligns the third layer of DNA with the higher energetic frequencies coming into the planet at this time.

No. 140. Mt. Maungapohatu Holy Grass
Keyword: Blessings of the South.
Energetically prepares, tones, upgrades and aligns the fourth layer of DNA with the higher energetic frequencies coming into the planet at this time.

No. 141. Mt. Tapuae-o-Uenuku Gossamer Grass
Keyword: Blessings of the Rainbow Bridge.
Energetically prepares, tones, upgrades and aligns the fifth layer of DNA with the higher energetic frequencies coming into the planet at this time.

No. 142. Mt. Rakiroa Wind Grass
Keyword: Blessings of Lower Earth.
Energetically prepares, tones, upgrades and aligns the sixth layer of DNA with the higher energetic frequencies coming into the planet at this time.

No. 143. Mt. Horo Koau Temple Grass
Keyword: Blessings of the Upper Heavens.
Energetically prepares, tones, upgrades and aligns the seventh layer of DNA with the higher energetic frequencies coming into the planet at this time.

No. 144. Mt. Aorangi Snow Grass
Keyword: Blessings of the Infinite.
Energetically prepares, tones, upgrades and aligns the eighth layer of DNA with the higher energetic frequencies coming into the planet at this time.

D.

EUROPE

Throughout Europe there exist ancient traditions of healing with plants and flowers. In many countries such as Britain, France and Switzerland, folk remedies handed down from generation to generation are still alive today. Not surprisingly, many of the most renowned herbalists – from Nicholas Culpeper to Paracelsus – came from this part of the world. Dr Edward Bach himself was a native of Britain and prepared many of his remedies from flowers growing in the fields and hedgerows of Oxfordshire. Throughout Europe many others are following in his footsteps.

BACH FLOWER REMEDIES (B)

In the 1930s Dr Edward Bach rediscovered the art of healing with flowers and created 38 remedies from flowers growing in the British countryside. After his death his close companion Nora Weeks kept his work alive; she in turn entrusted the Bach Centre to Nickie Murray for many years. Since then it has changed hands again; Judy Howard now runs the Bach Centre and is responsible for preparing the Bach Flower Remedies. To meet increasing demands the company Nelsons, makers of homeopathic preparations, are now involved in their production and Robert Wilson makes the mother tincture.

Julian Barnard and his then wife Martine also prepared a range of remedies according to the dictates of Dr Bach at their home on the edge of the largest area of national park in Britain (Hertfordshire). They were invited to work at the Bach Centre by Nickie Murray in 1984 and were involved in establishing the Bach Educational Programme before setting up their own Healing Herbs company in 1990.

Julian, a medical herbalist, feels it is important to follow Dr Bach's instructions to the word, so he adheres scrupulously to his original methods. He goes to some of the wildest and most inaccessible places to seek flowers, and uses only pure, fresh mountain water to make the essences. His is the only company, as far as is known, who make the remedies with full-strength brandy as did Dr Bach himself. The remedies are strongly endorsed by Nickie Murray.

The remedies have earned a reputation for integrity and quality and Julian now runs a flourishing education programme, and lectures throughout the world.

Agrimony (*Agrimonia*) For those who appear cheerful, jovial and uncomplaining, hiding mental torture and anxieties behind this mask – they may be restless and seek excitement to overcome their worry, or may use alcohol/drugs to dull and forget their pain. Helps us acknowledge and transcend such feelings so real peace and humour can be found.

Aspen (*Populus tremula*) For irrational, vague, inexplicable fears of unknown origin; sudden apprehension, fear of unseen power or force, of sleeping and dreams; headaches, sweating, trembling, sudden faintness, sleep walking/talking, fatigue and anxiety.

Brings a sense of security and an ability to trust that we are safe and protected.

Beech (*Fagus sylvatica*) For those who are critical, dissatisfied, intolerant, unsympathetic, irritable, always finding fault, seeing only the negative side of things; for tension affecting the upper-chest area, jaw and hands. Brings compassion and tolerance, relaxing strict attitudes.

Centaury (*Centaurium erythraea*) For timid, quiet, kind, gentle, conventional people who are anxious to please. They may have a tendency to lose their identity and direction, be submissive and be exploited. Physical symptoms affect the shoulders and back. Encourages self-determination and an ability to trust and follow our good judgement, to act decisively.

Cerato (*Ceratostigma willmottiana*) For those who doubt their own abilities, lacking faith in their own intuition and judgement, always asking others' advice, they tend to be mercurial and are easily led astray.

Cherry Plum (*Prunus cerasifera*) For desperation, fear of being unable to control negative thoughts, feelings and impulses of losing control, suicidal feelings, obsessive fear, delusions, nervous breakdown. Enables us to feel strong and safe enough to deal sanely with issues that scare us.

Chestnut Bud (*Aesculus hippocastanum*) For those who do not learn by experience, repeating the same mistakes over again, always looking ahead and failing to see what is happening. They can be careless, clumsy, slow to learn and inattentive. Enables us to observe, remember and make logical connections which help us make sense of life and formulate wise responses and choices.

Chicory (*Cichorium intybus*) For those feeling empty inside who become manipulative and possessive to get the attention they crave, who dislike being alone, needing their loved ones near to control and direct their activity. For 'the mothering type' as well as children who demand attention. Helps those who are self-pitying, fussy, bossy, critical, smothering, tearful and thwarted. Nourishes by instilling feelings of love and security.

Clematis (*Clematis vitalba*) For dreamers who are absent-minded, lacking concentration and vitality; for quiet people preferring dreams and fantasy to reality, who are romantic and imaginative but unrealistic, prone to drowsiness, excessive sleep, sensitivity to noise and faintness. Helps transform ideas and visions into actuality, developing talents and creating a life that is interesting and fulfilling.

Crab Apple (*Malus pumila*) A cleansing remedy for those who feel unclean and polluted, leading to despondency and self-disgust. For those obsessed with and repelled by what is seen as bad in themselves and the environment. Enables us to process impurities and negativity, and create sensible priorities.

Elm (*Ulmus procera*) For capable people who shoulder responsibility and occasionally take on tasks that are unreasonably demanding, making them feel exhausted, overwhelmed and temporarily inadequate. Enables us to let others handle the excess responsibility, so we are free to enjoy what you are doing.

Gentian (*Gentiana amarella*) For those easily discouraged by difficulties, who doubt and lack faith in their ability to succeed. For the negativity that breeds feelings of failure, disappointment, scepticism, gloom and sadness. Encourages perseverance and the realization that we cannot fail when our goal is to learn more about ourselves and the nature of life.

Gorse (*Ulex europaeus*) For times when life seems a misery, bringing hopelessness and despair. For those resigned to feeling nothing can be done to help and that any attempt will be futile. These feelings can result in conditions that apparently cannot be cured, or repeated failure or disappointment. Heals the inner will to see light in the darkness and embrace suffering as a positive aid to self-realization.

Heather (*Calluna vulgaris*) For those who feel needy of and greedy for attention of others. They may be obsessed with their own affairs, constantly chattering, unable to bear being alone, seeking sympathy and living off the energy of others. For those who are self-centred, overconcerned with themselves, lacking interest in others or prone to hypochondria. Enables us to stand alone and find a wider, less self-centred view of life.

Holly (*Ilex aquifolium*) For when we are enveloped in negative and aggressive emotions such as anger, jealousy, bitterness, envy, rage, suspicion, revenge, hatred, bad temper, contempt, selfishness, frustration. Encourages the ability to show good will and love to others, in the awareness that what enhances us enhances all.

Honeysuckle (*Lonicera caprifolium*) For nostalgia, getting stuck in the grief, regrets and memories of the past, longing for happier days gone by, romanticizing the past. Also for homesickness. Helps us to live in the moment, using past experiences as a guide and solid foundation, rekindling interest in life.

Hornbeam (*Carpinus betulus*) For temporary feelings of being overwhelmed, mental/physical weariness, lack of energy, boredom, the feeling that everything seems too much, an inability to get up in the morning and face the day. Also for convalescents. Encourages creation of a balanced lifestyle which is sufficiently stimulating and varied to allow inspiration to flow.

Impatiens (*Impatiens glandulifera*) For impatient, impulsive people who dislike restraint and are driven by urgency and hastiness, who like working at their own speed, act quickly and are critical of others. For those prone to nervous tension, overexertion and accidents, temper outbursts, irritability, sudden pains and cramps, indigestion. Releases pent-up tension and encourages the patience to enjoy being as well as doing. Brings sensitivity to situations and relationships.

Larch (*Larix decidua*) For lack of confidence, feeling trapped in self-doubt, inferiority, expecting failure so not bothering to try, hesitating and procrastinating. Also for the despondency and general depression often associated with impotency. Develops our sense of realism about our talents, builds confidence and self-assurance, and clears old patterns of limitation.

Mimulus (*Mimulus guttatus*) For fear of specific or known origin, often undisclosed due to shyness; fear of illness, death, others and being alone. Symptoms may include stuttering, blushing, shallow breathing and oversensitivity to noise, crowds and confrontations. Allows us to value our sensitive disposition and have the strength, courage and safety to enjoy life.

Mustard (*Sinapis arvensis*) For overwhelming black clouds of depression of unknown origin, causing deep sadness and melancholy that lifts as unexpectedly as it descends. Brings the realization that every day is an opportunity to get more deeply in touch with ourselves, to grieve for what is amiss so healing can occur in preparation for new growth.

Oak (*Quercus robur*) For strong, reliable, responsible and patient people, who shoulder their burdens without complaining, though have a tendency to take on more than they can manage. Their perseverance can lead to exhaustion, though they find ill health frustrating because it imposes limitations.

Olive (*Olea europaea*) For total mental/physical exhaustion. Useful after prolonged illness or during convalescence, for combating the effects of overwork and over-worry, and to help us get through crises such as divorce or conflict.

Pine (*Pinus sylvestris*) For those taking the blame for others' mistakes or situations not of their making. For the guilt and self-reproach that has become part of their lives. Also for those who are self-critical, overconscientious and constantly striving, leading to tiredness and depression. Allows forgiveness of shortcomings, releases responsibility, brings true understanding and acceptance of the human condition.

Red Chestnut (*Aesculus* × *carnea*) For those who are fearful and anxious for the welfare of loved ones, anticipating trouble, imagining the worst, being overconcerned about world problems and projecting their anxiety onto others. Develops trust and calm confidence in the ability of others to look after themselves.

Rock Rose (*Helianthenum nummularium*) For fear, panic, feeling paralyzed by terror, and the hysteria due to emergencies, sudden illness or accidents. Symptoms include coldness, trembling and loss of control; nightmares. Brings calm so we can respond adequately and appropriately to problems.

Rock Water (*Aqua petra*) For rigidity and self-repression, being ruled by logic and hard on oneself and others. Also for fantasists and idealists prone to obsession, punishing self-discipline and spiritual pride. Facilitates open flexibility and a sense of balance in our approach to life.

Scleranthus (*Scleranthus annus*) For indecision, mood swings, lack of concentration and balance, restlessness, changeable outlook, problems making oneself understood. Also for those prone to travel sickness. Helps us to discover inner balance so we can become clear and decisive.

Star of Bethlehem (*Ornithogalum unbellatum*) For all forms of shock: sudden and traumatic, long and slow over a period of time, delayed from the past, the shock of birth. Clears shock from the system bringing a sense of being centred, soothed and comforted. Restores the body's self-healing mechanisms.

Sweet Chestnut (*Castanea sativa*) For anguish and despair, desolation, feeling at the limits of our endurance, that nothing is left but destruction and oblivion – the dark night of the soul. Reveals the light at the end of the tunnel, restoring hope and an awareness that all transforming processes have a purpose. Brings the understanding that we must experience darkness to appreciate the light.

Vervain (*Verbena officinalis*) For those who are overzealous and forceful in their beliefs, enthusiastically trying to convert others by imposing their own will and ideas. For those who are highly strung, argumentative, strong willed and prone to overexertion, thus setting up a stress pattern for physical tension, muscle strain, headaches, migraines, eyestrain and exhaustion. Releases the stress pattern and built-up tension, enabling us to relax and let others lead their own lives.

Vine (*Vitis vinifera*) For self-assured, proud, dominating, bossy people who use authority to gain power; leaders who are of great value in emergencies but who can be ruthless in pursuing their goals; tyrants and dictators; those prone to back problems and high blood-pressure. Brings flexibility, allowing us to put our skills and abilities to the general good while letting others develop their potential.

Walnut (*Juglans regia*) For protection from outside influences and from major life changes (puberty, a new career, etc.) which have unsettled our foundations. Helps us to break with the old and those influences that impose on our free will. Enables us to establish new patterns, to break free and be ourselves.

Water Violet (*Hottonia palustris*) For loners who retreat and isolate themselves, appearing aloof and quiet. They are self-reliant and contained, knowing their own minds, seemingly condescending because they believe they are different and special, never interfering with others and intolerant of interference; prone to physical tension, stiffness and rigidity. Brings the ability to ask for help when needed; allows us to appreciate and enjoy others.

White Chestnut (*Aesculus hippocastanum*) For persistent unwanted thoughts, restless mental chatter, congestion, preoccupation, insomnia, confusion, depression, nervous worry and headaches. Quietens and calms mental processes, allowing the mind to function clearly and efficiently.

Wild Oat (*Bromus ramosus*) For feeling uncertain of one's direction in life; dissatisfied, undefined or unfulfilled ambitions; despondency, frustration and boredom. Gives definite knowledge of and clarity to one's purpose in life.

Wild Rose (*Rose canina*) For resignation and apathy; feeling unable to cultivate interest or make an effort; being fatalistic, lacking vitality; prone to dullness and fatigue. Restores motivation, creativity and energy; rekindles enthusiasm.

Willow (*Salix vitellina*) For resentment and bitterness, blaming others, feeling hard done by, being self-centred and self-pitying, bearing grudges, feeling wronged. Often linked with arthritic problems. Brings the ability to take full responsibility for life in order to make a fresh start. Cultivates optimism and a sunnier disposition.

Special combinations

Five Flower Remedy (The rescue combination) A blend of Cherry Plum for loss of control, Clematis for unconsciousness, Impatiens for stress, Rock Rose for panic/ terror, and Star of Bethlehem for shock.

BAILEY FLOWER ESSENCES (Bal)

These essences have been developed over a period of 40 years by Dr A.R. Bailey at his practice in the north of England. As a child Arthur was drawn to flowers and loved going on long walks in the woods and fells near Grange-over-Sands, England, with his 'Uncle George' (his grandmother's housekeeper's husband) who taught him the names of the local wildflowers.

He first discovered flower essences when he was suffering from post-viral syndrome. He consulted Dr Aubrey Westlake, a homeopathic doctor whose wife assisted in the selection of homeopathic and Bach Flower Remedies by dowsing. Arthur made a speedy recovery and subsequently found he could heal others by laying on of hands and worked with the Bach Flower Remedies. Sometimes none of the remedies seemed suitable although he instinctively knew the flowers could help. He began his own investigation and prepared essences from flowers in his own garden. To his surprise he found them very effective. The range steadily expanded and are mainly prepared from flowers found in the Yorkshire Dales and Ilkley Moor, though many come from all corners of England (and indeed some are from abroad). Some plants such as Firethorn were an exception to the rule and gave better results when their fruits were used.

Arthur discovered the main properties of 'Bailey' essences through meditational insight and realized that they were for attitudes of mind – how people see and relate to the world around them. Indeed, it is our attitudes of mind that give rise to negative emotional states. As the series continued to expand he realized that there was far more to flower essences that he had dreamt possible, and came to realize that we are all multidimensional beings. When we experience difficulties the root of our problems may not be in just the body-mind area; it is necessary to take a much broader view.

The present range of Bailey essences is primarily concerned with personal growth and transformation. This is not to suggest that essences cannot help physical illnesses – far from it. Yet their main emphasis is of helping to integrate mind, body and spirit and break the hold of old conditioning and beliefs which can so deny us our freedom.

The original six essences have steadily expanded since they were first developed. There are now 60 essences in the standard full set, 21 of which are composites made from the essences of several flowers. The composites are: Anger & Frustration, Cellular Memory Childhood, Confusion, Dependency, Depression & Despair, Fears, Grief, Grounding Essence, Insecurity, Liberation, Obsession, Protection & Clearing, Sadness & Loneliness, Self-Esteem, Shock & Trauma, Stuck in a Rut, Tranquillity, Transition, Unification, Yin/Yang Balancer.

Arthur and his wife, Christine, in partnership with their son-in-law Simon Hunter, have also created an acupuncture set of 12 composite essences for use with the five elements. The flowers used to make these composites are not included here, though they can be purchased from Bailey Essences – see Useful Addresses.

In total, there are 101 single essences available, although just the 39 available in the standard set are listed here. All are handmade by members of his family using spring water and vodka as a base.

Algerian Iris Can ease our path in life and make us less susceptible to getting sexually involved in relationships that are inherently flawed.

Almond The supportive inner teacher, the guide. Forms links with our soul and encourages intuition.

Arizona Fir To help us to celebrate life and existence as spiritually based beings.

Bistort To provide loving support at times of major change in our lives.

Black Locust For protection against the negative influences of other people, including psychic attack.

Bladder Senna For escaping from feelings of guilt and being unworthy, brought about by judging ourselves far too harshly. It brings compassionate understanding of our past actions.

Blue Pimpernel Rediscovering our spiritual nature whilst growing up in a superficially material world.

Bog Aspodel For the 'willing slave' – those who help others yet frequently ignore their own needs.

Bracken Aq. For when intuitive sensitivity was blocked in childhood, resulting in a fear of the intuitive side of one's nature.

Buttercup For those who find it difficult to let the 'sunshine' into their lives. Helps one to let go of embittered feelings.

Conifer Mazegill For sudden, irrevocable changes in our life. Continually activates energies of positive change.

Cymbidium Orchid Relates to the hidden side of our nature; brings peace and harmony to the subconscious parts of our mind.

Cyprus Rock Rose For deep terrors and fears that are difficult to expose and resolve. More powerful and deeper-acting than common Rock Rose.

Dwarf Purple Vetch For deep-rooted, hidden patterns usually originating in childhood and often resulting in sexual difficulties.

Early Purple Orchid For unblocking the energy centres in the body and protecting any vulnerable spaces so created.

Flame Azalea Helps us to regain our vital life force and sense of community after major changes in life.

Giant Bellflower The clarion for change. It is the catalyst for action when old habits have been holding us back.

Hairy Sedge For those who worry and find it difficult to keep their minds in the present moment. This inattention can result in poor memory.

Himalayan Blue Poppy The essence of spiritual lineage. To fulfil our potential in this lifetime, we need to build on strengths gained in the past. Furthers insight and psychic skills.

Leopardsbane For those who are at a major change point in their lives. They may feel as if they are living on a knife-edge.

Lilac For those whose personal development has been stunted by dominant influences, usually in childhood or adolescence.

Lily of the Valley For yearning. For those who have become blocked by desiring the unattainable.

Magnolia For unconditional love. This essence helps to bring and awaken within us the energies of love and compassion.

Meadow Rue For discerning what is worth striving for in our life and what is unhealthy. Brings clarity to see where we need to be heading to fulfil our true purpose in life.

Mediterranean Sage For the 'Earth' qualities of warmth, comfort and wisdom. Helps to catalyze insight from a firm earthed base.

Milk Thistle This remedy is for those who do not love themselves. Often they try to make up for this by trying to please others.

Monk's Hood For difficulties of long standing that have their roots in the distant past. Helps to bring one up-to-date.

Oxalis For things that 'have you by the throat' and seem so overpowering that there appears to be no way out.

Red Frangipani The essence of awakening. Reunites us with the true source of our being which lies beyond the spiritual dimension. Brings joy and new levels of perception and confidence.

Sacred Lotus A powerful essence to open the heart to the love of the universe and the divine.

Solomon's Seal For the busy mind. This remedy helps bring quietness and detachment.

Spotted Orchid To help us overcome difficulties and blocks on our path of personal growth.

Spring Squill For freedom after breakthrough. Helps us to soar like a bird, finding our own true path in limitless space.

Thrift For helping to open up to psychic sensitivity but keeping the person firmly grounded at the same time.

Tufted Vetch For sexual difficulties caused by an incorrect sexual self-image – usually due to childhood conditioning.

Welsh Poppy For those who have lost their fire and inspiration and become daydreamers.

White Lotus For bringing peace and unification to body, mind, spirit and soul.

Wood Anemone For use where there are very old difficulties – genetic or karmic.

FINDHORN FLOWER ESSENCES OF SCOTLAND (F)

Scotland conjures up images of mist and magic, with a wild landscape of rugged mountains and magnificent lochs and a Celtic spirit that like its environment is known for courage, honesty and tenaciousness.

The Findhorn Flower Essences are subtle infusions of Scottish wildflowers which, when used for healing, can enhance spiritual awareness and growth by restoring equilibrium throughout the different levels of being. They are made by Marion Leigh, who first joined the Findhorn Foundation in 1976, then temporarily returned to her native Australia to become a qualified homeopath. Through her study of homeopathy and work with the Australian Bush Flower Essences she came to appreciate the extraordinary healing properties of flower essences. On returning to Findhorn she found the whole region carpeted with gorse in full bloom, and was drawn to preparing an essence from this flower. She decided to use water collected from a local ancient secluded well with known healing properties. The magical energy of the flowers from the Findhorn gardens is well known and the strong connection with the nature spirits has produced some wonderful flower essences.

Marion feels the flowers tend to find her when the time is appropriate. One exception was the rare Scottish Primrose, a plant found only in certain areas on the north coast of Scotland and in Orkney. Marion actively went in search for this flower after receiving a message that its essence had remarkable powers for promoting feelings of inner peace and stillness in times of struggle, strife and conflict.

Findhorn Flower Essences

Ancient Yew (*Taxus*) Emergence
Realize your life's purpose. Cast off burdens that hold you back and take spontaneous action that leads to new directions for growth.

When you come to the realization that the time has come to release your attachment to someone or something that is holding you back, like the irrepressible Yew tree you are propelled onwards to change, adapt and make choices, and that will allow you to be free to grow, expand and regenerate. Ancient Yew flower essence can assist in letting go of whatever is standing in the way of achieving your purpose.

Apple (*Malus*) Purpose
Focus on your purpose with enthusiasm and perseverance, and use your will to realize the goal.

Apple essence is an aid to realizing your goals and objectives by cultivating an open attitude and willing body and mind. With willingness, and the power of sustained application, you can pursue a goal without getting side-tracked or procrastinating.

Balsam (*Impatiens glandulifera*) Tenderness
Nurture yourself and others through love and intimacy. Overcome feelings of separateness. Emanate and attract warmth and tenderness.

The Balsam personality 'type' is a self-sacrificing server. They can be out of touch with their own feelings and needs, and often put the needs of others before their own. Balsam flower essence helps in nurturing tenderness and affection without reservation. Love yourself, and your love will radiate out and touch others.

Bell Heather (*Erica cinerea*) Confidence
Have faith and trust in yourself. Release doubt and fear. Stay firmly grounded, flexible and confident.

Bell Heather helps you to let go of anxiety, turmoil and fear of the unknown, and to stand firmly grounded and focus on the positive aspects of a situation whereby you can mobilize your inner forces to overcome any difficulties.

Birch (*Betula pendula*) Vision
Open your mind and broaden your outlook. Banish uncertainty and worry that obscure your vision. Exercise your imagination to see 'the bigger picture'.

Birch flower essence can assist in looking at events with fresh eyes and from different perspectives, to open your mind and free your imagination. It also helps to expand your capacity to visualize and find creative routes to desired goals by releasing your expectations.

Broom (*Cytisus scoparius*) Clarity
Clear your mind and focus your thinking. Dispel emotional turmoil that hinders your powers of concentration.

Broom essence helps to clear the mind so that your thinking becomes more flexible and adaptable, supporting the mental body's capacity in learning, concentration, memory and recall. Clear thinking gives us the confidence and power to apply and express our thoughts through creative, intelligent activity.

Cabbage (*Brassica oleracea*) **Devotion**
Boost dynamism. Convert procrastination into action. Labour with joy.

Cabbage flower essence motivates and encourages you to follow your vision. By trusting 'the flow' of events, the vision can manifest perfectly and in the right timing. Cabbage's dynamism may assist to harness enthusiasm, patience, persistence and perseverance.

Cherry (*Prunus serrulata*) **Compassion**
Be open-hearted and open-minded. Transcend negative, inherited predispositions and consciously conduct yourself with integrity and in the spirit of goodwill.

Cherry blossom symbolizes the philosophy of balance, harmony and co-existence, where seemingly separate or opposing forces are interconnected and interdependent in the natural world. This essence fosters acceptance, without judgement. When you radiate loving kindness with an open and compassionate heart, you expand your ability to love and be loved.

Daisy (*Bellis perennis*) **Protection**
Stay calm and focused. Overcome agitation and anxiety and find your centre of balance.

Daisy flower essence may help you to stay centred, grounded and in command when circumstances which are out of your control threaten to throw you off balance. This essence helps you to centre in yourself, remain calm and composed, collect your thoughts and then move forward with peace of mind.

Elder (*Sambucus nigra*) **Beauty**
Be the light and beautiful being that you truly are. Relax the desire for perfection and stimulate your natural powers of regeneration and renewal. Reveal your youthfulness and vitality.

Elder flower essence stimulates powers of recovery and renewal of the vital life energies that rejuvenate. When body and soul are revitalized, you can be imbued with the sense of wellbeing that boosts vitality and self-esteem. How you appear is a direct reflection of how you see yourself, what you believe about your appearance, and how you feel about your body. 'Energy follows thought.'

Elecampane (*Inula helenium*) **Sensitivity**
Magnetize your abilities to receive and transmit spiritual energies and forces. Be a clear channel through purity of motive, right alignment and attunement.

Elecampane flower essence is of benefit in connecting with the inner dimension of one's spirituality and channelling the higher energies in a balanced way. When the channels and receptors are clear, you are able to correctly register, integrate and transmit the higher vibrations. Purity of motive and the discriminative loving power of the heart need to be engaged.

Elf Cup Lichen (*Cladonia coccifera*) **Liberation**
Release and clear deep-seated negative or destructive emotions. Purify the emotional body and make space for positive change and for growth.

Elf Cup Lichen essence can help you to become clear of your past patterns of reaction. As a reminder that an issue will not just go away if you ignore it, it can help to release and purify negative emotional reactions and detrimental behaviour that cause pain and suffering.

Garden Pea (*Pisum sativum*) **Expression**
Cultivate confident, articulate self-expression. Release negative thought patterns and clear the blocks to heartfelt communication. Speak your truth.

Expressing yourself creatively is an essential aspect of living a life of passion, fulfilment and authenticity. This essence can help you to construct a support system for self-expression and communication by opening pathways for your imagination to follow, and for beauty and inspiration to flow freely and spontaneously.

Ginkgo (*Ginkgo biloba*) **Endurance**

Be enlightened and allow the power of the life force to radiate through you. Rhythmic flow of life force helps harmonize mental and emotional bodies and regulates your responsiveness to light.

Ginkgo flower essence may be helpful in making the connections that allow the proper streaming of the life-giving energies. The power of the light force, penetrating into the mind, brings mental clarity, as equilibrium of the rhythm of life, and cycles, is maintained.

Globethistle (*Echinops sphaerocephalus*) **Strength**

Connect with your powers of patience, persistence and perseverance. Letting go of unnecessary burdens will set you free and ultimately serves the highest good.

Prolonged self-sacrificing service to others can result in your easily becoming overwhelmed, feeling 'put upon' or, in the extreme, the martyr. Globethistle flower essence can help to reconnect with your power, to distance yourself sufficiently to be able to see the whole picture. It also helps in identifying patterns of behaviour that do not serve you or those you serve. Care-giving from the heart brings more life, energy and resources for you to actually do what needs to be done *and* feel a sense of joy and fulfilment.

Golden Iris (*Iris pseudacorus*) **Fidelity**

Realize powers of right perception and discernment. Act from this wisdom and master impulses that impair good judgement.

When you are loyal to the purpose and principles of your true self, and sincere in your aspiration to live your life integrated with and guided by that, you can differentiate between what is real and what is unreal. As you stand in the spiritual authority of the true self with this clear perception, you take the right action recognizing that 'energy follows thought'.

Gorse (*Ulex europaeus*) **Joy**

Bring light into the mind, uplift your heart and activate enthusiasm and dynamism. Overcome resistance to fully engaging by kindling the inner flames of joy and passion.

Gorse flowers are bearers of light and joy. True joy is a sublime state of feeling yourself to be at peace with your true self. Through identification with this self, the life energies flow and radiate through all the being, lighting up and uplifting body and mind, which vibrate with 'joie de vivre'.

Grass of Parnassus (*Parnassia palustris*) **Openness**

Open the heart to healing. Let down your barriers and release your fear. Restore your faith in the healing power of love.

Grass of Parnassus flower essence opens the heart to the healing power of love. When you have the courage to open your heart, to be more open and trusting, you radiate warm love and are sensitive to love in return. Real happiness comes when you give your love, and yourself, openly and freely.

Harebell (*Campanula rotundifolia*) **Alignment**

Believe in yourself. Have trust and confidence in your abilities to be well and prosper.

Harebell flower essence can help you to align thoughts, words and actions that are in harmony with manifesting the success you desire in life. When you are in alignment with your true self that knows no limitations, by thinking and speaking with words that build confidence and keep you motivated towards achieving your goal, you begin to manifest positive results instead of dwelling on potential negative results.

Hazel (*Corylus avellana*) **Freedom**

Be free to 'go with the flow' and travel forward in wonder of your new unfolding potential. Transform expectations into explorations.

When life seems like a struggle and you are creatively stuck, Hazel flower essence aids in releasing the sources of frustration and unhappiness by helping you to let go of expectations and patterns of thinking that cause doubt, fear and discontent. Focusing on the things you can control and releasing the things you can't brings inner peace and calm. Hazel flower essence gives you the freedom to explore new directions and to follow your inspiration.

Holy Thorn (*Crataegus*) Acceptance

Open your heart. Let down the barriers that inhibit love's expression.

Holy Thorn flower essence brings gentleness to people who may have become hardhearted, or who are hard on themselves and others. This creates barriers to being able to express yourself authentically in relationships. When the heart chakra is awakened, the impulses of spiritual inspiration and altruistic love pour in and through you, allowing you to express yourself freely without fear that enables you to reach out to, understand and empathize with others.

Iona Pennywort (*Umbilicus rupestris*) Transparency

Live with integrity in the light of truth. Banish guilt, self-judgement and fear. Let light illuminate the dark corners of your mind.

Iona Pennywort essence helps to penetrate the darkness by shining soul light on a problem that you are hiding, denying or covering up. Light protects from darkness and also lets you see what is real and what is imaginary. This flower essence may help to bring in the light of awareness. The discriminating mind united with the soul's light of wisdom can dispel the fogs that cloud the consciousness.

Lady's Mantle (*Alchemilla vulgaris*) Awareness

Bring to light all your inherent power and intelligence. Dissipate false impressions in awareness and cognition by bridging the mind-body connection.

This flower essence may help to strengthen the mind-body connection. By connecting rational and intuitive elements of the mind, we open doors into mindfulness. Through this unification we can realize deeper levels of awareness for optimal mental and physical performance.

Laurel (*Prunus lusitanica*) Resourcefulness

Hold your vision, get organized and bring your plan into manifestation.

Laurel flower essence helps to organize, direct, plan and structure your thoughts in line with your intention. Inspired with the idea and formulating a clear and concise mental picture and vision of exactly what you want, by your intention, your highest dreams become a reality.

Lime (*Tilia platyphyllos*) Universality

Cultivate harmonious relationships. Transform feelings of separateness. Be at peace with yourself, your neighbours and your world.

Lime cultivates peace and harmony in the heart and mind. It teaches that inner peace exists within you right now and can be accessed when you choose to accept things as they are. Peace in the outer world arrives when we make peace with ourselves. We develop universal love and compassion through harmlessness and selfless service to others, by doing the most loving thing in each situation, letting love determine the way.

Mallow (*Malva sylvestris*) Grace

Unite thinking with feeling by accessing the wisdom of your true self. Think and communicate from the heart.

When you are overly detached from your feelings or preoccupied with your own thoughts, you can get stuck in your thinking pattern and hardened in your feelings. There is no separation between thought and feeling for they ultimately exist in a continuum. Mallow flower essence helps to 'think with your heart'.

Monkey Flower (*Mimulus guttatus*) Personal Power

Stand in confidence to uphold your truth. Access the source of your personal power and transform insecurity and fear.

Monkey Flower helps to transform and transmute fears held in the unconscious mind that limit your personal power in the world. When you are centred within yourself, in the heart, there is no need to cover up your vulnerability or fear. The sense of security that arises when you stand in your power gives you confidence to face any challenge head-on.

Ragged Robin (*Lychnis flo-scuculi*) **Purification**

Purify your body and clear the way for your energies to flow freely and abundantly. Release obstacles to realizing soul energy.

Suppressed emotions, fixed ideas and rigid thinking all contribute to creating obstacles that impede your energy flow. These may become harmful and give rise to weakness in one or more of the subtle bodies, thereby affecting general health and wellbeing. Ragged Robin flower essence may help to remove the obstacles that cloud your perception of what is good for you and what is not, so that you can consciously choose what you eliminate, absorb and transmit in your life with the highest respect for the sanctity of your mind-body's integrity and wholeness.

Reindeer Lichen (*Cladonia mitis*) **Transmutation**

Open the heart to love and let it revitalize you. Open to free circulation and radiation of the life force through the heart centre.

When the heart is afflicted by grief or loss, the heart chakra is affected and the etheric channels that convey the life force can become restricted or blocked. Reindeer Lichen essence revitalizes the etheric heart centre. By opening to the power of love, you can purify, transform and transmute your suffering. You breathe in peace and you breathe out peace when you find your centre of balance in the heart.

Rose Alba (*Rosa alba*) **Power**

Connect with your creative power. Trust and follow your intuition. Speak and act from your inner authority.

Rose Alba flower essence represents the vital, creative principle of power. This is the positive, 'yang' principle that initiates and purposefully calls on and applies the inner driving force or impetus to activate, build and create. The essence stands for the best use of this power. You can channel your creative

powers in the most appropriate ways, acting spontaneously and trusting your intuitive knowledge. When you trust and follow your intuition, right speech and right action follow.

Rose Water Lily (*Nymphaea*) **Presence**

Feel the presence and draw strength from your source deep within. Rise above the emotional pressures and demands of daily life and reconnect with your spiritual roots.

When you get caught up in the commotion and the drama of your life, you can become disconnected from your spiritual self, metaphorically lose your way, your devotion to your purpose, and become dreamy and ungrounded. Rose Water Lily flower essence can help you to cultivate your awareness to stay present in the moment, to rise above the pressures and demands of daily living to a place of inner serenity and peace, and deep, abiding trust.

Rowan (*Sorbus aucuparia*) **Reconciliation**

Be at peace with yourself and others. Take responsibility to heal the past. Surrender, forgive and move on.

Rowan flower essence helps to accept and take responsibility for behaviour and actions that have caused pain or suffering, in order to learn from the experience. Negative emotions that are not resolved can manifest again in other situations and relationships that have nothing to do with the original trauma. In some instances, this may mean reaching back into the past to process events and make amends.

Scots Pine (*Pinus sylvestris*) **Wisdom**

Trust the source of wisdom within you. Overcome the insecurity of uncertainty by tuning in and listening. Be guided by your inner voice.

Scots Pine flower essence helps to access the source of wisdom and knowing from within yourself and supports you in finding the confidence to trust the choices and decisions you make, and the directions you take in life.

Scottish Primrose (*Primula scotica*) **Peace**

Find inner peace and restore natural rhythms. Overcome conflict, fear and anxiety by opening the heart to the source of unconditional, universal love.

The greatest challenge for anyone who is attempting to cultivate a calm mentality is to become free from negative emotions such as anxiety and fear. For this reason, accessing true peace of mind is vital in achieving a disposition that is free from stress and conflict. Scottish Primrose moves us into a state of loving tenderness, enlightened understanding and compassion, and when this inner peace ultimately radiates out into the collective consciousness, true peace can be realized.

Sea Holly (*Eryngium maritimum*) **Brilliance**
Step forth fearlessly to success and fulfilment. Overcome the limitations of inhibition that restrict the potential for achievement. Let your light shine.

With Sea Holly essence we are able to let down barriers of self-protection and foster a calm and concentrated inner peace by overcoming our insecurities and inhibitions. Sea Holly flower essence helps you to step out boldly and to express your thoughts, feelings and ideas with confidence. You feel truly liberated when you open up to realizing your full potential, standing in your power to be the radiant, enterprising and brilliant being that you are.

Sea Pink (*Armeria maritima*) **Harmony**
Balance your inner dualities. Stay well-grounded and maintain your centre of equilibrium.

Sea Pink flower essence addresses the problems of division or polarization of one or more parts of the self that causes fragmentation, disconnection and being ungrounded. The essence may also help to release energetic blocks within the etheric and subtle bodies, helping to achieve a dynamic balance of the energy-distribution system as a whole. Integrated functioning of the mind: the mental body, and the sentient, astral body, with the physical/etheric body, permits free circulation of energies and a more balanced state of being as a whole.

Sea Rocket (*Cakile maritima*) **Regeneration**

Use your resources wisely. Release insecurity and the desire to hold on. Connect to your source, and trust in your powers to adapt and thrive.

Sea Rocket flower essence helps you to recognize that you have an innate capability to adapt to changing circumstances and environments. Instead of being tossed back and forth by the waves of circumstance, Sea Rocket helps you to be aware of and responsive to your own needs, to know that you have within you the resources to meet the need and to make the most of what you have been given. Trusting that all your needs can and will be perfectly met is the natural outcome.

Silverweed (*Potentilla anserina*) **Simplicity**
Live lightly and simply. Transform that which keeps you bound to worldly things. Raise your consciousness through self-awareness.

Silverweed essence supports self-mastery. By non-attachment to your fascinations and your desires, you realize that virtue and beauty is expressed on the 'golden mean' between the extremes, between needs and wants, sufficiency and deficiency. This flower essence promotes vital enjoyment of the beauty of the simple things in life.

Snowdrop (*Galanthus nivalis*) **Surrender**
Surrender, release and let go. Move forward with renewed hope and optimism. Be still and find your inner peace.

Snowdrop flower essence helps us to triumph over fear, grief and pain, particularly in times of change and transition. When we accept our powerlessness over circumstances that cannot be controlled or changed, we reach a turning point. When we surrender our attachments, we find freedom and new hope. Like the light at the end of the tunnel, a clear vision of the future may be revealed in all its beauty and potential.

Spotted Orchid (*Dactylorhiza fuchsii*) **Equanimity**
Be positive. Surrender your limited viewpoint and keep the greater plan in mind.

Spotted Orchid flower essence helps to bring balance through self-regulation.

Harnessing your willpower, and managing inner impulses and drives, allows you to focus on your greater mission or plan, to rise above narrow views or self-interest and to look beyond perceived imperfections. With a more positive attitude, imaginative and creative solutions emerge that bring the sought-after reward of personal acceptance, fulfilment and contentment.

Stonecrop (*Sedum anglicum*) **Transition**

Embrace change and transformation. Transmute restlessness and frustration. Find peace and stillness within.

We resist change because we feel comfortable where we are. The cost of resistance is discontent, restlessness and frustration. Stonecrop flower essence helps you to shift your consciousness to your centre, to the point of stillness and peace within. Even in the quietude you sense subtle, perpetual movement and accept that in times of transition you need to be patient and respect the process.

Sycamore (*Acer pseudoplatanus*) **Revitalization**

Relax, recharge and revive. When persistent stress leads to exhaustion and burnout, be gentle with yourself. Let the smooth flowing of energies lift and lighten body and soul.

The way we think determines our feelings and behaviour and how we respond or react to outer circumstances, whether with calm and ease or hurriedness and stress. Sycamore flower essence can help to relax unrealistic expectations you have of yourself and others. When you feel constrained, this essence helps to ease inner tension, thereby giving strength and the power of perseverance.

Thistle (*Cirsium vulgare*) **Courage**

Find inner strength and courage and let go of the fear. Stay in command and act with confidence and certainty.

Thistle flower essence can help to give you the courage to cope with a crisis. Courage is not the absence of fear but the power to triumph over fear. This essence helps to access

inner strength and willpower, to remain calm and think clearly in any emergency, and to harness the willpower to respond with positive, intelligent action.

Valerian (*Valeriana officinalis*) **Delight**

Be open and responsive in the moment, lighten up and have fun. Make time to enjoy the simple joys in life that bring you true happiness.

Valerian flower essence helps you to focus your attention in the present. One of the main benefits of living in the present moment is an improved ability to concentrate – your mind does not wander, you do not dwell on the past nor worry about the future. Many of life's pleasures have to be enjoyed in the moment. There are opportunities to experience joy every day, if you open your heart to take a moment to find the joy in living. Be aware of the times when you get caught up in the buzz. Slow down, then stop and smell the flowers.

Watercress (*Rorippa nasturtium aquaticum*) **Wellbeing**

Clear stagnant energies and sound a vibrational note of purity. Transform your thoughts and emotions and reveal the true you.

Watercress flower essence facilitates a cleansing process that aids the release of stagnant energies in the subtle bodies so that your energies are free to flow 'like a river'. As you come into harmony with your true self and homeostasis is restored, the emotions are calmed and you can find peace of mind.

Wild Pansy (*Viola tricolor*) **Resonance**

Clear the pathways to the free flow of life energies from the heart.

Love is the energy that fuels your life and if its flow is obstructed it is similar to the lifeblood flowing through the veins being obstructed. All manner of unsettling thoughts, sensations and emotions may then arise such as anxiety, fear, panic and disorientation. Fear blocks love and without love you cannot truly thrive. Wild Pansy flower essence gives the sense of stability, and the feeling of safety from which you can open your heart, and feel your emotions.

Willowherb (*Chamaenerion angustifolium*) Self-Mastery

Harness your fiery, passionate nature through mindfulness and the right use of will and power.

Negative emotional reactions to stressful events are natural and human and, to some degree, inevitable. Willowherb flower essence helps to calm your emotional body through awareness and conscious mindfulness. You may not be able to eliminate adverse emotional reactions but you can change your response to your emotions through knowing you have control of your feelings, much like you have control over other choices you make in your life.

Wintergreen (*Moneses uniflora*) Gladness

Mobilize the spiritual will. Dispel darkness and stand in the light of the self. Open to love and support.

Wintergreen flower essence initiates the awakening or expansion of consciousness that invokes support from the soul. We call in our higher power to persevere, no matter how disinclined we are to do so, and no matter how extreme the inner turmoil. Pain opens the heart to love and understanding. Surrendering to receive love and guidance from the soul opens the heart to love and support from others.

Findhorn combination flower essences

Baby Blues
Supporting emotional change after birth.

Sudden separation following the achievement of a cycle can cause upheaval and the sense of an emotional anti-climax. Baby Blues can help you to tap inner reserves of energy and strength to overcome weariness, uncertainty and anxiety and to be reassured and to stay calm.

Birthing
Open up naturally to conscious birthing.

Anxiety, fear or self-limiting belief patterns can inhibit the spontaneous processes of giving birth. Birthing essence can help you to relax and let go with open-hearted expectancy to the successful culmination of a new birth and a new beginning.

Bon Voyage
To offset the negative effects of travel stress and fatigue.

Travel can disturb natural rhythms. Bon Voyage can help you to find balance to cope with motion and calm to overcome fear, so that you arrive feeling 'ready to go'.

Calm Me Down
Focus dynamic energy into intelligent creative activity.

Foster calmness of mind and body through self-mastery of negative emotions that impede clear thinking, concentration and composure. Calm Me Down helps to integrate the mental and emotional bodies, which aids your ability to pay attention and channel energies into the right action.

Clear Light
For bringing about a peaceful state of mind.

By stilling and focusing the mind, Clear Light can influence mental clarity and brightness and assist in attuning to higher wisdom and inspiration. An excellent aid for meditation and study.

Energy Shield
To cleanse and protect the energy field.

Energy Shield helps you to stand in strength and create the positive energy that you need to feel more confident to handle detrimental vibrations that affect you. Energy Shield helps to purify, transform and release negative energies and influences.

Eros
Nurture love, sensitivity and intimacy.

Without self-acceptance it is difficult to love and nurture yourself or be a loving partner. Eros can help you to relax, enjoy and be in tune with your body.

Femininity

Support for women's issues and cycles.

During times of changing rhythms or mood swings, Femininity can help you to release tension and restore emotional balance and wellbeing.

Fertility
Co-creation of a new heart and soul.

Stress and emotional imbalance can impede the processes of naturally conceiving. Fertility can help open your heart to love, to being impregnated with a new way of being and creativity, and to the emergence of a fresh impetus in life.

First Aid
Calming, soothing relief in any crisis.

In times of stress or trauma, First Aid can help to relieve associated fear and anxiety, and ease pain and tension.

Go with the Flow
Enjoy the freedom of movement.

When limitations that restrict ease of movement hold you back, Go with the Flow can help you to release tension and relax. When your energies flow smoothly, so do you, and with graceful, effortless movement.

Healing the Cause
Strength and support to get well.

Deep-seated or long-standing negative emotions hinder the ability to get well. Healing the Cause can help you to take charge of your own health, surrender obstacles to wholeness and wellbeing, and heal the past and sources of suffering.

Heart Support
To heal the heart when affected by trauma or grief.

For all issues connected with the heart and love, Heart Support can help you to feel supported during major life changes that cause stress and tension.

Holy Grail
To integrate and harmonize the physical, emotional, mental and spiritual bodies.

Holy Grail can help bring balance and harmony into all aspects of your life through alignment and synthesis of body, mind and soul. Embody and express your full creative potential.

Inner Child
Nurturing your inner child.

When you react from childhood emotional wounds and attitudes, your experiences of the past dictate how you respond to life today. Inner Child may help to change your behaviour patterns and to honour the child you were, in order to love the person you are.

Karma Clear
To release the tensions that bring pain, suffering and unhappiness.

Karma Clear can help you heal the past through compassion and forgiveness and by awareness and understanding of the underlying causes of life's predicaments and ailments.

Life Force
To overcome tiredness, low energy or burnout.

Life Force can help to uplift body and soul when you feel weary or drained of energy. Activate the vital life force and stimulate the body's powers of renewal.

Light Being
Be content and enjoy life.

Light Being can help to uplift your spirits when feelings of despair, sadness or hopelessness weigh down on your soul. Identifying with a greater sense of purpose and nurturing an optimistic outlook on life, contentment and happiness can be achieved in the present moment.

Masculinity
Discovering the secret of the masculine soul.

Masculinity may help when you get caught up in cultural and traditional 'masculine' roles and expectation, to get in touch with and free your feeling nature. The willingness to move from power to love reveals a soul strong enough to accept vulnerability and to be authentic.

Prosperity
Manifesting an abundance of wellbeing.

Prosperity can help foster a sense of inner security and faith in yourself, and to align with the source of universal, limitless supply to manifest your dreams and goals.

Psychic Protection
Protecting the emotional body against negative forces.

Feel calm and centred by creating a safe space within you and around you. Psychic Protection can help in detaching from negative thought forms or energies when you feel vulnerable or in overwhelming situations or environments.

Seasonal Affections
Sunshine in the soul when feeling under the weather.

Seasonal Affections can help you to release emotional congestion, discomfort and irritation. Feel protected and supported, no matter what the season or prevailing conditions.

Sexual Integrity
Awaken to loving intimacy.

Sexual Integrity can help you to break old patterns and learn how to channel sexual energy in ways that nurture the body as well as the soul.

Spiritual Marriage
Integrate and harmonize the masculine and feminine qualities.

Spiritual Marriage can help balance your inner pairs of opposites. Dynamic union of intuition and consciousness with intelligence and activity can free your full potential and maximize richness in the joy of right relationship.

Sweet Dreams
Good night, sleep well.

Sweet Dreams can help calm your energies and restore natural rhythms, with the result that you find balance and peace of mind.

Teens
Spontaneity, focus and balance.

Teens can help overcome the limitations that greater self-consciousness creates and help foster self-acceptance, understanding and confidence.

Transformation
Supporting personal growth and transformation.

Transformation can help to harmonize seemingly opposing parts of you, cultivate your inner strength to persevere and stay on course, and help you to willingly make sacrifices that serve your highest good.

Voice Confidence
Express and radiate inner beauty and confidence. Elecampane, Garden Pea, Holy Thorn, Lady's Mantle, Rose Alba, Scots Pine, Sea Holly and Thistle.

Voice Confidence can help you to free your expression and let creativity flow. With trust, and the motivation to succeed, your performance reflects calmness, composure and self-confidence.

Findhorn elemental essences

The elemental essences work essentially to restore the health of the elements in the body and to strengthen the receptivity of life energies, or *prana*, in the related chakra or centre.

Earth Earth elemental essence works at the level of the first or base chakra and embodies the will to be oneself. It represents stability, security, balance and the ability to stand in strength in your power.

The Earth element and therefore the essence strengthens the receptivity of life force in the base centre through concentration, patience, perseverance and discipline and leads to calm, dependable grounding of ideas, practicality and material abundance.

Water Water elemental essence works at the level of the second or sacral chakra and nurtures love of family, friends and one's group. It fosters empathy, sensitivity and tenderness and the power to create harmonious emotional relationships.

The water element and therefore the essence strengthens the receptivity of life force in the sacral centre through receptivity, understanding, adaptability and imagination and assists in relaxing and maintaining a peaceful and magnetic personality.

Fire Fire elemental essence works at the level of the third or solar plexus chakra and stimulates aspiration towards the ideals of the soul through self-confidence, enthusiasm, optimism, passion and the desire to help others.

The fire element and therefore the essence strengthens the receptivity of life force in the solar plexus centre through cognition and alertness of mind that brings self-reliance, courage and leadership skills, increasing vitality in all areas of life and the ability to take forthright action.

Air Air elemental essence works at the level of the fourth or heart chakra, as well as the fifth or throat chakra, and upholds the intuition, and the expression of unconditional love, sympathy, emotional independence and personal refinement.

The air element and therefore the essence strengthens the receptivity of life force in the heart centre through perceptiveness and objectivity, leads to clear comprehension and discernment and helps in developing dexterity and enterprise skills in intuiting practical solutions.

Ether Ether elemental essence works at the level of the fifth or throat chakra, as well as the sixth or ajna chakra and seventh or crown chakra, and exists as quintessential life force. It concerns the expression of the consciousness.

The ether element and therefore the essence strengthens the receptivity of life force in the throat centre, develops the instinctual intuition, mental flexibility, creative intelligence and right speech and manifests as spiritual love and the power of synthesis. Ether element essence is the 'quintessence', the fifth element, the mother and creator of the four elements. All the other elements arise from the fifth or spiritual etheric realm.

Exaltation Exaltation essence works at the level of the sixth ajna or brow chakra. Soul or universal love energies work through the 'third eye', through the ajna, and coordinate all the other centres in unison to bring forth the spiritual will.

It blends the energies of ajna, heart and crown chakras and manifests as the spirit of goodwill expressed through the heart and mind.

Spiritual insight gained through the intuition, pure reason and comprehension of ideas can then be expressed through the formulation of ideals. When illuminated by purity of motive and loving purpose, the energies of love and wisdom work out in true spiritual activity on the physical plane.

Wesak Blessing Wesak Blessing essence works at the level of the seventh or crown chakra and brings consciousness from the subtle and higher planes into definite working awareness. This is achieved by opening to divine inspiration and receiving those higher spiritual qualities of clear-sightedness, understanding and enlightenment into the crown chakra and distributing them through the ajna.

Intention is the invocation, by opening to the processes of spiritual perception through the intuition and by the clear pure light of divine understanding.

Mist and sprays

Clear Light Mist
Birch, Broom, Lady's Mantle, Rose Alba, Scots Pine and Wild Pansy. For bringing about a peaceful state of mind. By stilling and focusing the mind, Clear Light can assist in attuning to higher wisdom and inspiration, and influence mental clarity and brightness. An excellent aid to meditation and study.

Eros Mist
Balsam, Elder, Gorse, Grass of Parnassus, Holy Thorn, Rose Alba, Sea Pink and Sycamore. To nurture love, sensitivity and intimacy.

Without self-acceptance it is difficult to love and nurture ourselves, or be a loving partner. Relax, enjoy and be in tune with your body. Also available in Aloe Vera gel for external application.

Prosperity Mist
Bell Heather, Cabbage, Elder, Harebell, Laurel, Rose Alba and Sea Rocket. Manifesting an abundance of wellbeing. Foster a sense of inner security and faith in yourself. Align with the source of universal, limitless supply and manifest your dreams and goals. Recognize your inherent power and follow the keys to success: work with the spiritual laws of money and abundance; affirm creative abundance; experience and feel gratitude for the abundance in your life; magnetize inner resources needed to implement a plan and attract your heart's desire ('hold the vision'); build towards manifesting your ideas and ideals; and follow your inner guidance and intuition.

Psychic Protection Mist
Ancient Yew, Daisy, Iona Pennywort, Rose Alba, Thistle, Watercress and Wintergreen. For protecting the emotional body against negative forces. To feel centred by creating a safe space in and around yourself. Psychic Protection can help in detaching from negative thought forms or energies when feeling vulnerable, or in overwhelming situations or environments. Also helpful in cutting the ties that bind. Also available as a spray mist for external use.

Sacred Space Mist
Findhorn Elemental Essences of Earth, Water, Fire, Air and Ether and pure essential oils of Rose Alba and Frankincense. Revitalizing and energizing space clearing spray mist, to help clear and transmute negative energies. Use to refresh and energize your personal space, cleanse and purify your aura, promote happiness and harmony around your home, bring forth light, clarity and serenity.

HAREBELL REMEDIES (Hb)

The Harebell Remedies are made from the wild flowers from a remote area of southwest Scotland, on the Southern Upland Way. Galloway is a gentle place of rolling hills, quiet lochs and wooded estates, sheltered from the extremes of the Scottish highlands.

It was established by Ellie Web in 1985. A flower essence maker and practitioner for more than 20 years, Ellie was inspired to make flower essences after having explored various spiritual and healing paths. When her interest in herbs and natural remedies grew, it was natural for Ellie to bring together nature and healing, evolving it into a flower essence therapy for inner wellbeing. Ellie was strongly drawn to making essences from the healing qualities of plants immediately around her. Helped by the strong nature spirit of the place and by her two small daughters, she made mother essences of many flowers in her large garden and surrounding countryside. The Harebell Remedies are named after one of Scotland's favourite wildflowers, and the essences eventually settled into the set of 64 essences described here. They are made from a mixture of familiar wild flowers and garden favourites. All are made in the purest of habitats far from pollution and wherever possible in places where the flowers are naturally established and abundant. In recent years combination essences, mist sprays and roll-on essences have been added to complete the range.

Alkanet (*Anchusa officinalis*) Inner strength. For the ability to centre and strengthen ourselves in preparation for change. Unifies opposing energies. Helps us move through transformative experiences safely.

Bluebell (*Endymion non scriptum*) Cooling. Deeply cooling, calming and grounding. Works well on a hot temper or in times of overexcitement, stress, injury and trauma. A good 'rescue' remedy with a pleasant after-effect.

Borage (*Borago officinalis*) Cheerfulness. Gives emotional strength and courage. A tonic to fortify the heart, renew confidence and promote a cheerful outlook. For the discouraged or downhearted.

Broom (*Cytisus scoparius*) Perseverance. For strength of will and endurance. Supports a calm, mindful response to difficulties. For the ability to start afresh and keep going.

Buttercup (*Ranunculus acris*) Appreciation. Increases capacity for pleasure and fun and helps you to value life in the present moment. Balances negativity, overseriousness, impatience, cynicism and lack.

Chamomile (*Chamaemelum*) Harmony. For emotional stability. Like the herb, the essence calms and soothes, bringing a release of anxiety. Beneficial for deep relaxation and acceptance of a situation.

Comfrey (*Symphytum officinale*) Integration. To make whole. Good for injury, tiredness, memory loss and for balancing natural cycles. Relaxation, repair and renewal. Positive visualization and deep-level healing.

Cornflower (*Centaurea cyanus*) Individuality. Makes us comfortable and happy with our difference. Gives a healthy self-knowledge and worth. Protects sensitivity and special gifts from harmful, ignorant attitudes and institutional conditioning (e.g. from schools, hospitals and prisons).

Cymbidium (*Cymbidium*) Self-possession. Gives confidence and strength and allows us to embrace the tiger within. Gives power and potency to the heart. Helps us to overcome fear of disapproval and show our true colour. For a fast and truthful response.

Daffodil (*Narcissus pseudonarcissus*) Uplifting. Lifts us out of a low, inward-looking mental state. Opening up to lighter, brighter energies, and banishing blues, casting out doubts. Depression, tiredness, low self-esteem and SAD (seasonal affective disorder).

Dandelion (*Teraxacum officinalis*) Relaxing. A deep letting go with profound effect. Release of fear and of being overwhelmed. Gives us a trust in our ability to cope. Turns a 'driven' energy to calm strength and natural vitality.

Elder (*Sambucus nigra*) Assertiveness. Brings self-protection out from a deep place inside. Balances timidity and helplessness. Good for helping us deal with bullies and tyrants. Gives us the strength to say 'no' consistently.

Eyebright (*Euphrasia officinalis*) Perspective. An uplifting essence bringing understanding and gladness. Brings a wider and wiser viewpoint, connecting heart and mind.

Flowering Currant (*Ribes sanguineum*) Flowing. Assists the natural breath. Relaxes tightness and control in the chest and shoulders. Expands and softens the lungs. Warms and opens the heart.

Forget-Me-Not (*Myosotis sylvatica*) Balanced. Emotionally grounded. Helps us remember reality and release fear. Brings us back to Earth from flights of fantasy or paranoia. Good for working with dreams.

Forsythia (*Forsythia suspensa*) Energy. Brings an awareness of how we gain and lose energy. Helps us to make use of it better. Gives a greater appreciation of life force. Helps us choose energizing activities.

Geranium (*G. atlanticum*) Manifesting. Makes things manifest and visible. Helps us to bring cherished ideas to reality and see well-grounded plans through to the end. Aids in making us let go of being 'not ready'.

Harebell (*Campanula rotundifolia*) Wildness. Healing separation from nature. Allows us to stay close and connected to the wild spirit within us. Encourages freedom and a gentle strength of character.

Hawthorn (*Crataegus monognya*) Hope. Defends the spirit, bringing hope and deep compassion to sorrow and despair. Protects the heart through grief to recovery.

Heartsease (*Viola tricolor*) Comforting. Helps a closed heart to open or eases an open heart in pain. Comfort for overwhelming emotions. Encourages compassion and self-forgiveness.

Heather (*Calluna vulgaris*) Courage. Helps us facing loneliness and fears in order to grow and find peace. Accepting silences and solitude, feelings of emptiness or lack of certainty.

Honesty (*Lunaria annua*) Openness. Truthfulness and clarity. Can help us to stay present when the truth is complex and emotionally difficult. For confusion, memory blanks or lapses in consciousness.

Hyssop (*Hyssop officinalis*) Anxiety. A tonic to lessen and release the burdens of guilt and blame. Understanding the true reasons behind some of the thoughts and deeds which trouble us.

Iris (*Iris germanica*) Empowering. For coming into one's own personal power. Being our own authority and withdrawing that invested in others. Releasing blocks to creativity and living to our full potential.

Jacob's Ladder (*Polemoneum caeraleum*) Receiving. Learning how to ask for, recognize and receive assistance. Both practical help and spiritual guidance. For when we feel we must resolve all our problems alone.

Jasmine (*Jasminum officinale*) Processing. For absorbing what we need and eliminating what we don't. Stimulates us to be decisive, practical and less confused. For efficiency and self-esteem.

Lady's Mantle (*Alchemilla vulgaris*) Prayer. Awakening or reaffirming a belief and trust in a divine feminine influence. Invoking protection and inspiration. For prayer and meditation.

Lavender (*Lavandula spica*) Serenity. Soothes and cleanses. Brings peace to the mind and balance to the emotions. Can help us to develop a sense of composure, space and healthy detachment.

Lilac (*Syringa vulgaris*) Flexibility. For a relaxed attitude and ease or grace of movement. Opens and aligns our posture. Helps us to surrender; to bend and not break.

Lungwort (*Pulmonaria officinalis*) Clearing. To create a clean and peaceful space in and around our body (lungs) and mind (psychic space) through meditation and awareness of breathing.

Marjoram (*Origanum vulgare*) Supportive. Enables us to put our trust in creation. Comforts and protects through danger and difficulties. Brings emotional release, especially of fear. Heals lack of security; helps us feel safe.

Marsh Woundwort (*Stachys palustris*) Security. Gaining reassurance and love. For the tendency to worry and fret unnecessarily. For letting go of the distress from unmet needs in the past and being content in the present.

Monkshood (*Aconitum napellus*) Judgement. To help us recognize and banish bad influence from our life. Good judgement in protecting ourselves and our spiritual integrity. To keep us from harm.

Nettle (*Urtica dioica*) Connection. Warmth, expression, communication and sharing. For withheld feelings resulting from past hurt, and the cool and distant personality. For easier relationships.

Oriental Poppy (*Papaver orientale*) Facing. Making the choice to live, to fully be here in the present moment instead of escaping, numbing or pretending. Endurance and joy in being alive.

Pansy (*Viola wittrockiana*) Resistance. Promotes hardy strength and builds up the ability to recover from frequent illness. Use when tired, overwhelmed and vulnerable. Claim the power of the warrior within.

Plantain (*Plantago lanceolata*) Acceptance. For turning resignation or a heavy heart around to grounded strength. For when there is a holding on to negativity preventing good things in the present.

Potato (*Solanum tuberosum*) Calming. For feeling safe, centred and grounded, and calming down from an overstimulated state. For the feeling of coming home and enjoying the ordinary or commonplace. Use before or after intense experiences.

Primrose (*Primula vulgaris*) Opening. For the release of whatever is held. Lightens and cleanses as though a weight is lifted. For the lifting of any heavy, lethargic or 'poisoned' feeling. Helps with eating imbalances.

Purple Foxglove (*Digitalis purpurea*) Growing. For learning through difficulties and accepting responsibility for life's lessons without becoming bitter. For dealing with wounds and betrayals.

Ragwort (*Senecio jacobaea*) Centring. Surrendering to the physical. To build respect for our body's natural wisdom. Calms an emotionally confused and mentally overactive mind. For intuition and trust.

Red Clover (*Trifolium pratense*) Release. Letting go of fear. For shock or fright. Gently calms, soothes and reduces panic or inappropriate reactions. For taking care of our own immediate needs.

Red Rose (*Rosa floribunda*) Passion. For being true to our desires and against shame. For boldness, passion, love and romance. Living with enthusiasm and delight and follow our heart.

Red Rosebud (*Rosa floribunda*) Sensitivity. Openness and tenderness. Feeling safe to be loved and touched. Good for new relationships and also the passage through puberty. Giving and receiving love and bringing eroticism into whatever we do.

Red Tulip (*Tulipa 'darwinii'*) Outgoing. Being lively without losing one's centre. To overcome shyness or mistrust of the spirited side of our nature. Giving birth to the whole self.

Rhubarb (*Rheum nobile*) Boundaries. Brings awareness of others and their boundaries. Compassion for our insecurities; allowing feelings and silences. Balances uncensored behaviour.

Rosebay Willowherb (*E. angustifolium*) Responsive. Lasting release of old fear and conditioning. Brings awareness of the ways we are numb to others and a willingness to change stubborn and defensive patterns. Sensitivity in relationships.

Rosemary (*R. officinalis*) Remembering. Active remembering means putting back together. To strengthen the power of recall; linking heart and mind. Encourages trust and strengthens bonds.

Rowan (*Sorbus aucuparia*) Attachment. For following the path of the heart and deepening attachments to people, places and culture. For positive connection to our ancestors. Drawing on our rich personal heritage.

Sage (*Salvia officinalis*) Enlightenment. For connection with Higher Self. For wisdom and joy. Helps us to find the fool within and not take life too seriously. Practising good judgement whilst retaining a humorous detachment.

Self-Heal (*Prunella vulgaris*) Responsibility. Taking charge of our own wellbeing and nourishment. For inner health, self-love and acceptance. Trusting the body's self-healing process. Heals self-doubt and confusion.

Snapdragon (*Antirrhinum majus*) Expression. Brings bold expression of emotion. Aids in loosening the facial muscles. Helps us move on from frustration and release anger, fear or sadness held tightly in the face or jaw. For voice work and speech problems.

Snowdrop (*Galanthus nivalis*) Regeneration. Deep cleansing and renewal wherever there is felt to be a loss of innocence. For issues of safety and trust, and healing the child or adolescent inside. For self-forgiveness.

Speedwell (*Veronica officinalis*) Change. To look forward to a new direction so that the trauma, discomfort and disorientation of any kind of travel, big change or crisis are reduced.

St John's Wort (*Hyp. perforatum*) Holding. Calm protection when we are vulnerable. An essence to hold and contain us. The effect is to greatly reduce fear. Promotes trust, healing and sleep.

Thistle (*Cirsium vulgaris*) Integrity. To be steadfast in our own truth. Encourages us to have pride and self-respect which empowers both ourselves and others. Balances a compliant nature.

Tormentil (*Potentilla erecta*) Confidence. To bounce back from small setbacks. Cheerfulness and renewal. For countering negative beliefs and turning the other cheek. Not easily defeated.

Violet (*Viola odorata*) Kindness. Allowing the heart to open and bring love into our lives. Letting go of negative critical thoughts. For practising loving kindness towards others. For letting in the love around us.

White Foxglove (*Digitalis purpurea*) Dreamy. To free the mind of thought, making us less aware of time. Encourages us to be more imaginative, dreamy and wild. Use to deepen meditation, explore an altered state or simply loosen up a little.

White Narcissus (*N. actaea*) Spontaneous. To be guided by the heart and the spontaneous child within. For those who think too much. For being aware of our own and others' feelings.

White Rosebud (*Rosa floribunda*) Blessing. To keep us in a state of grace and growth toward fulfilling our potential. For infants and babies in the womb to rest and keep a sense of Heaven on Earth. For blessing and thanksgiving.

Wild Thyme (*Thymus polytrichus*) Purify. To strengthen one's thoughts and intentions. Helps us to reflect on our appropriate motivations and clear the mind of doubts and fears.

Yarrow (*Achillea millefolium*) Protection. Brightens and strengthens our energy field. To allay fears and protect from outside negative influences in situations where we are vulnerable.

Yarrow in Sea Water (*Achillea millefolium*) Cleansing. Protective Yarrow made in cleansing sea water. Take during and after exposure to radioactive, electrical or chemical pollution. Helps us to release harm.

Combination remedies

Acceptance and Peace A well-tried combination useful in many situations as well as promoting general wellbeing. Heather gives the courage to face fears or difficulties; Lungwort promotes a quiet meditative state; and White Rosebud encourages appreciation and thankfulness.

Confidence New but already popular this combines three simple essences: Borage for emotional strength, courage and cheerfulness; Tormentil for the ability to bounce back from small setbacks and for countering negative beliefs; and Red Tulip for overcoming shyness and being bold and outgoing without losing one's centre.

Inspiration A new combination to bring a breath of life into whatever you are doing. Contains Flowering Currant which relaxes tightness and encourages going with the flow; Lady's Mantle to invoke a little divine influence; and White Narcissus for spontaneity and being guided by the heart.

Motivation An aid to 'doing' of any kind. Broom gives purpose, perseverance and determination; Oriental Poppy helps us keep on making that choice to live and to come out of 'stuck' or negative places; Wild Thyme is cleansing and strengthening, focusing the mind on appropriate intention and clearing away any doubts and fears.

Physical Trauma Another well-tried combination. A beneficial aid through rescue and recovery from accident, operation or any harm to the physical body. Useful for all kinds of shock. Use long term as an aid to recovery from serious injury or drug abuse. With cooling Bluebell, calming Chamomile, healing Comfrey and soothing Red Clover.

Purify & Cleanse This is one to turn to when you feel unwell. Jasmine to help with processing things wisely on both a physical and emotional level; Lungwort for awareness of breathing and clearing the space around you; Primrose for cleansing and the release of toxins; and Wild Thyme for purifying thoughts and clearing the mind.

Relaxed & Grounded A useful mix of some favourite essences. Dandelion brings a letting go of tension and renewal of trust; Forget-Me-Not for emotional balance with a firm hold on reality; Lilac encourages grace of the body and flexibility of mind; Potato keeps us calm and down to earth.

Stress Release One of the first Harebell essence 'combinations', it has stood the test of time. Containing Chamomile for emotional stability and release of anxiety; Lavender bringing peace to the mind and a sense of composure or healthy detachment; Red Clover for the release of fear or panic; Sage for connection to the Higher Self who is wise and able to find the humorous side to life; and finally Self-Heal for staying focused on and taking charge of one's own wellbeing.

Travel Has been made for many years and proved useful to promote a calm and positive experience of journeys and life changes of any kind. With Potato for calming down from over stimulation; Speedwell to encourage looking forward to the new direction so disorientation is reduced; and Yarrow to brighten our own energy and protect from any negativity along the way.

Uplift A popular combination as a party essence or general daily tonic. Contains Bluebell which is joyful as well as being cooling and grounding; Daffodil to lift and open up to lightness and brightness; Hyssop helps with releasing any troubled thoughts; Primrose lightens, cleanses and dispels lethargy; and Sage gives wisdom and humour.

Seasonal combination remedies

Twenty-five ml combinations to take over several weeks. Begin when you feel the need, which does not always coincide with 'official' season change.

Autumn Reflection

Heather, Honesty, Hyssop, Rowan and White Foxglove flower essences. To deepen and enrich, a time of completion, of gathering in, of sifting and sorting. Take stock and prepare for turning inwards. Process and release the past, mourn your losses. Protect and hold the seed of the coming year. Take any time from late August onward.

Spring Renewal

Primrose, Lungwort, Snowdrop and Wild Thyme. To lighten, cleanse and renew as winter's dark mantle is shed. Clearing and purifying for both body and mind. Promotes release of negativity and a lightening of thoughts. Take as early as January till about May.

Summer Love

Buttercup, Eyebright, Geranium, Sage and White Rosebud. Time to run with life, let go of negativity, lack and of being overserious. Appreciate and think of others, create a little happiness. Feel your heart, enjoy your life, watch things happen and give thanks. Take from May onwards. Take forever.

Winter Strength

Jasmine, Pansy, Self-Heal, St John's Wort and Yarrow. To give strength through the winter months. Take from November through to about February/March. A time to draw on inner resources. The remedy supports positive action to process things wisely, protect ourselves and build up resistance.

Mist sprays and roll-on remedies

Peace & Harmony Rollette

Essences of Chamomile, Forget-me-not, Heartsease, Heather, Lavender, Lungwort, Marjoram and White Rosebud. With essential oils of Lavender and Chamomile for calmness and peace of mind. A soothing topical flower essence which is convenient to carry around and safe for children to use. An all-round beneficial blend for many of life's fearful, anxious moments. Has proved a useful aid for calm travel or peaceful sleep.

Scottish Wildflower Mist

Essences of Broom, Harebell, Rowan, Thistle and Wild Thyme. Bringing qualities of strength, integrity and freedom. With the sweet and mysterious essential oil of Bog Myrtle. A subtle hint of the Scottish countryside to use as room spray or personal mister.

Space Cleansing Spray

Essences of Jasmine, Lungwort, Primrose and Wild Thyme. With the fresh and uplifting Bergamot essential oil. A purifying blend which helps to dispel stale air and negativity from rooms. Useful for cleansing the home or workspace. Especially beneficial after the use of electrical equipment – computers and televisions, etc.

GREEN MAN TREE ESSENCES (GM)

Our relationship with trees is as old as time itself. For centuries humans have regarded certain trees as having healing qualities, and have revered and cared for them as sacred or even magical beings. Trees are among the most ancient living organisms on this planet. They are protectors and regulators of their surroundings, offering food and shelter to many other forms of life. We now realize that our existence is totally dependent on the great forests and woods that cover the Earth. They not only regulate the atmosphere ensuring a life-sustaining balance of oxygen and carbon dioxide, but also control weather systems and enrich the soil.

Trees flourish and survive by adjusting their form to harmonize with the prevailing conditions, and they succeed in maintaining this balance for hundreds, sometimes thousands of years. This ability to be balanced and flexible, to absorb and let go, is a lesson from which we could all benefit.

Each species of tree shows different characteristics and you can sense their particular energies when walking in ancient woodlands or forests. Integrating this energy into our own system helps us to act more responsibly towards nature. The Green Man Tree Essences were created by Simon Lily and his partner Sue as an aid to meditation and self-healing. In traditional British folklore the Green Man is the perfect blending of human and plant life. He is the spirit of nature, an embodiment of fertility, and is celebrated every May Day.

The Green Man range comprises 74 tree essences. The first essence made was from the flowers of the Hazel tree, whose qualities encourage the growth of new skills and information.

Alder (*Alnus glutinosa*) Release. Reduces nervousness and anxiety. Brings clarity of mind and eases stress. Increases *prana*/Qi.

Apple (*Malus domestica*) Detoxification. Helps the elimination of toxins on all levels and brings in spiritual energies. Transforms negative emotions.

Ash (*Fraxinus excelsior*) Strength. Harmony with your surroundings. Feeling in tune. Brings flexibility and security.

237

Aspen (*Populus tremula*) Delight. Intuition and intellect; balances overanalysis; calms fears and gives a broader perspective. Brings amusement and wise laughter.

Atlas Cedar (*Cedrus atlantica*) Resilience. For the removal of out-of-date patterns and achieving a personal path. Gives resilience to cope with change and adversity.

Bay (*Laurus nobilis*) Energy. For deep-rooted vitality. Releases blocked and suppressed emotions. Spiritualizes physicality.

Beech (*Fagus sylvatica*) Easy-going. Brings confidence and hope in oneself and one's life. For relaxation and release of held-in trauma. Confidence in self-expression and speaking out clearly.

Bird Cherry (*Prunus padus*) Sensuality. For unblocking deep emotional wounds. For those who have become overdefensive of emotional attachments. Helpful where there are sexual difficulties, mental rigidity and being overcritical or uncomfortable with physicality.

Black Poplar (*Populus nigra*) Nurture. Creates a powerful peacefulness; a sense of security and inner clarity. Very comforting. Blends all energies.

Blackthorn (*Prunus spinosa*) Circulation. Helps absorption of energies necessary for life. Stabilizes emotions; brings hope and joy. Stimulating.

Box (*Buxus sempetvirens*) Clarity. Strengthens the mind and will. Clears the head and eases irrationality and confusion. Links you with your Higher Self.

Catalpa (*Catalpa × erubescans*) Joy. Stabilization of emotions, helps find peace of mind. Reduces anxiety, increases self-confidence in what one can achieve.

Cedar of Lebanon (*Cedrus libani*) Turmoil. Physically cleansing, a breath of fresh air. Where there is suffering this essence lessens the resistance to needed change. Brings clearer messages from the deep mind and universe regarding appropriate actions. Increases peaceful flow, reduces turmoil.

Cherry Laurel (*Prunus laurocerasus*) Balance of mind. For all problems with the mind and head. Imagination and inspiration used practically. Helps maintain molecular and genetic integrity of the body. Subtle perceptions accessed. Gives high-level protection and support.

Cherry Plum (*Prunus cerasifera*) Confidence. For wisdom and security of the inner self; helps remove fears. Tension and rigid mental concepts are eased. For opening up on emotional levels. Helps shyness.

Copper Beech (*Fagus sylvatica var. purpurea*) Depression. Brings a deep, enlivening sense of peace and detachment from worries. Energizes emotions in a positive, non-aggressive way.

Crack Willow (*Salix fragilis*) Spiritual sun. For letting go and allowing things to happen. Brings a sense of oneness with the world. Aids communications with the Higher Self, the planet and the energies of the sun.

Douglas Fir (*Pseudotsuga menziesii*) Standing alone. For relatedness and finding one's place. Brings spontaneous energy and freedom to be oneself.

Elder (*Sambucus nigra*) Self-worth. Calms aggression, brings stability, love and forgiveness. Balances self-image. For times of transformation and change. Good for fretful children.

English Elm (*Ulmus procera*) Enthusiasm. Desire to progress, move on. Re-energizes the mind when fatigued and balances the heart when feeling drained or overemotional. Brings clarity for decision-making and study.

Eucalyptus (Cider Gum) (*Eucalyptus gunnii*) Sustenance. For opportunity; restoration of energy; smooth integration of energy; and correct relationship and flow.

Field Maple (*Acer campestre*) Aching heart. Brings balance to those hearts reaching for love. For understanding and contentment when overwhelmed by a sense of responsibility or remorse for mistakes, accidents, etc. Aligns heart chakra to higher love.

Fig Tree (*Ficus carica*) Generator. For expression of needs; soul food; feelings of emptiness resolved; letting go; dancing; and energy to achieve.

Foxglove Tree (*Paulownia tomentosa*) Harmonious flow. For ending of turbulence; strengthens aura and life force; brings happiness, relaxation and smooth waters.

Gean, Wild Cherry (*Prunus avium*) Soothing. Focuses energy in the physical and stimulates self-healing. Calms the heart and mind. Creates a smooth flow of energy. Useful where there is emotional pain.

Giant Redwood (*Sequoiadendron giganteum*) Weight of responsibility. For those who are too hard on themselves or on others. Brings a sense of balanced responsibility, tolerance and relaxation that allows wisdom the space to develop. Releases energy blocked in lower chakras.

Ginkgo (*Ginkgo biloba*) The ancient way. Brings harmonization with the universe; invisibility; flowing with the tides. For a smooth flow of emotions and internal harmonization.

Glastonbury Thorn (*Crataegus monogyna biflora*) Out of the woods. Helps find a clearer direction. What feels right to do and be emerges from indecision and chaos. This brings immediate relaxation and release from tension, increasing subtle information and intuition.

Gorse (*Ulex europaeus*) Integration. Eases restlessness, frustration and jealousy. Brings joy from emotional security and growth.

Helps integrate new forms of energy or knowledge in a useful, personal manner.

Great Sallow (*Salix caprea*) Soul. Allows the mind to expand and link with the soul. Brings an understanding of life purpose. Energizing. Links to Earth energy.

Hawthorn (*Crataegus monogyna*) Love. Stimulates the healing power of love. For trust and forgiveness. Helps to cleanse the heart of negativity.

Hazel (*Corylus avellana*) Skills. For the flowering of skills. For the ability to receive and communicate wisdom. Helps all forms of study; clears away unwanted debris. Brings more stability and focus in order to integrate useful information.

Holly (*Ilex aquifolium*) Power of peace. Agitated states, balance of mind. For people with a loss of control, panic, lack of self-worth, unhappiness, loneliness. Active expression of love. Non-aggressive, peace-loving yet assertive.

Holm Oak (*Quercus ilex*) Negative emotions. Relieves emotions and restlessness related to thwarted expression such as guilt, jealousy, anger, etc. Activates personal creativity and balances emotional and mental energy.

Hornbeam (*Carpinus betulus*) Right action. Deep energizing on many levels clearing blocked or stagnant energies. For clarity of purpose. Standing up for personal experience. Increased security in working with others.

Horse Chestnut (*Aesculus hippocastanum*) Agitation. Harmonizing flows of energy to and from the individual, eases agitation caused by contrast and difference. Brings clarity of mind and a flow of intuition. Peace. Ability to ground and dissipate excess energy.

Italian Alder (*Alnus cordata*) Protected peace. Brings peace, love and protection for delicate energies. Helps with shyness or overaggression. Courage for new starts.

Ivy (*Hedera helix*) Fear. Eases hidden fears and anxieties. Helps to release true feelings and identify needs. Balances the heart chakra and its nadis.

Judas Tree (*Cercis siliquastrum*) Channelling. Brings access to completely new thought patterns and ideas. Openness and acceptance of very subtle levels of energy and the ability to communicate it to others. For the ability to discriminate and discern the validity of given information.

Juniper (*Juniperus communis*) Doorway. For renunciation of the past; generosity; relaxation; releases old stresses; ancestral patterns; and brings inner versatility.

Laburnum (*Laburnum* × *watereri Vossii*) Detoxification. For a balanced release of stress and tension. Increases detoxification processes and the growth of creative potential, optimism, positivity and expression of personal wisdom.

Larch (*Larix decidua*) Will to express. Helps the communication of personal wisdom from new levels of peace and healing. Brings inspiration and creativity. Enhances physical and sexual energy. Balances heart and mind, will and desire.

Lawson Cypress (*Chamaecyparis lawsoniana*) The path. Helps identify correct action and one's true needs. Initiates change in the right direction. Brings increased communication between mind and body, and discipline to attain one's goals and spiritual direction.

Leyland Cypress (*Cupressocyparis leylandii*) Freedom. Helps ease hidden fears and anxieties, increases positive attitudes and sense of humour allowing a sense of freedom in which to grow and feel comfortable. For those who dislike being by themselves.

Lilac (*Syringa vulgaris*) Spine. Eases all energies of the spinal axis. Activates all chakras.

Eases tension. Lilac is closely aligned with many different types of nature spirit.

Lime (*Tilea* × *europaea*) Development. For shifting levels of consciousness without disorientation. Calms anxiety where related to practical use of one's psychic and healing potential. Doubts and fears ease. Past programming is lessened.

Liquidambar (Sweet Gum) (*Liquidambar styraciflua*) Sweet tongue. For self-aware dynamic energy. Brings personal energy integrity; care for self and others; and a calm mind.

Lombardy Poplar (*Populus nigra 'italica'*) Aspiration. Discrimination; acts of unique creativity; understanding deep drives; inspiration to aspire.

Lucombe Oak (*Quercus hispanica 'lucombeana'*) Creative energy. For life-supporting creativity, inspiration, ideas. Increased mental focus. Commitment to act and bring change. Wisdom and compassion.

Magnolia (*Magnolia* × *soulangeana*) Restlessness. Eases restlessness and lack of clarity. Helps to maintain balance when difficult changes have to be made. Increases sense of freedom and relaxation. Learning from past experiences, brings a clearer idea of one's true identity.

Manna Ash (*Fraxinus ornus*) Happy with oneself. Heals the heart and emotions. Brings honesty with oneself about how one feels. Helps with unresolved emotional issues. Increases understanding and access to creative levels of consciousness.

Medlar (*Mespilus germanicus*) Boundless. Brings energy to core personal patterns; motivation, enthusiasm and drive. Boundless energy to achieve goals. Increase in joy and happiness. Total security. Strength, humour, brightness and creative intelligence.

Midland Hawthorn (*Crataegus laevigata*) Expansion. Energizes aspects of the heart chakra and its relationship with personal growth and spiritual awareness. Enthusiasm to enjoy and explore life.

Mimosa (*Acacia dealbata*) Sensitivity. Brings increased awareness of what is going on inside self. Intuition is better understood. Ability to stand up and express oneself. A sense of peace.

Monkey Puzzle Tree (*Araucaria araucana*) Fierce compassion. Calms aggression but allows creative, forceful action. Strongly energizing, earthing, protecting. Perception of cycles of time and space, expanded awareness of continuity and change on this planet.

Monterey Pine (*Pinus radiata*) Connectedness. Helps remove very deep trauma. Artistic blocks eased. Balances emotions, calms anxieties. Brings a deep peace and connectedness to everything. At ease in one's body, physical wellbeing. Past-life information.

Mulberry (*Morus nigra*) Wrath. Powerful emotions released constructively. Freedom from remorse and past pain. For those hurt by the world and who react with anger and cynicism.

Norway Maple (*Acer platanoides*) Healing love. Brings love and acceptance; healing and nurturing energy for emotional shock and trauma. Lightness, happiness, relaxation. Taking back control of life and power for oneself.

Norway Spruce (*Picea abies*) Trust. Helps in understanding change. Brings lightness and openness to experience. seeing clearly; axis; beacon.

Oak (*Quercus robur*) Manifestation. For absorption and integration of very deep, hidden energy underlying this reality. The desire for stability whilst experiencing the polarities of existence. Brings the ability to manifest one's goals. Channelling energy.

Olive (*Olea europaea*) Valour. Warmth; solar energy; truthfulness motivation; passionate clarity.

Osier (*Salix viminalis*) Spiritual void. To contact Higher Self. Energy to adapt, change and grow. Useful when everything seems empty and useless. Brings energy and understanding.

Pear (*Pyrus communis*) Serenity. Helps you be happy to be who you are. Brings clarity, simplicity, confidence. Reduction of stress in the nervous system. Increased enthusiasm, drive and energy. Deep peace.

Persian Ironwood (*Parrotia persica*) Alienation. Brings energy, emotional strength, drive, enthusiasm. Grounds spiritual energy into the physical body. Activates deep-level healing. Connectedness to the highest level of planetary consciousness. Strong sense of connectedness, belonging and joy. For feelings of alienation and weakness.

Pittospora (*Pittosporum tenuifolium*) In two minds. Helps to clarify how one truly feels. Useful when loyalties are divided. Helps find solutions to mental worries and conflicts. Increases perspective and sense of humour.

Plane Tree (*Platanus × acerifolia*) Fine judgement. Brings ability to discriminate subtle levels of the truth. Helps prevent introspection, melancholy and overanalysis. Broadens viewpoints and gives a peaceful space to meditate.

Plum (*Prunus domestica*) Empowerment. Helps the highest spiritual energy enter into the material world. Practical solution to problems. Increased awareness of surroundings and effective use of personal power. Self-worth, self-motivation.

Privet (*Ligustrum vulgare*) Old wounds. Works with subtle bodies to repair physical shock and trauma. Creates harmonious vibration that helps to heal on fine levels. Increases life force to allow letting go of old wounds.

Red Chestnut (*Aesculus × carnea*) Fear for others. A feeling of serenity and protection at a deep level of being, both for oneself and others. This reduces fear and anxieties and brings a peace and detachment from the worries of what may, but probably won't, be. Helps create a clear, positive, unselfish link with others. Fears and phobias ease.

Red Oak (*Quercus rubra*) Practical support. Energizes the body's structural systems. Growing conviction of one's place and purpose in the world. Clearing of self-doubt and false views. Very practical searching for the spirit.

Robinia (Black Locust) (*Robinia pseudoacacia*) Awakening. For a calm mind; dissolves 'glamour' and obsession. Brings optimism; clearing emotional and mental clutter.

Rowan (*Sorbus aucuparia*) Nature. Attunement to the energies of nature, particularly wood and Earth. Enlarges perspectives to a cosmic level, allowing deep understanding of the universe.

Scots Pine (*Pinus sylvestris*) Insight. Helps activate third eye and development of subtle awareness in a balanced way. Brings penetrating insight and increases tenacity and patience. Broadens one's outlook.

Sea Buckthorn (*Hippophae rhamnoides*) Pioneer. Fresh perspectives; uninvolvement; protection from harmful influences; understanding emotions.

Sequoia (*Sequoia sempervirens*) Anchor. Creates space to deal with energy blocks, stabilizing our anchor to the planet and opening to the universe. Eases difficult emotions giving clarity of thought.

Silver Birch (*Betula pendula*) Beauty. Ability to experience beauty and calmness. Tolerance of self and others. For those who find it difficult to express themselves.

Silver Fir (*Abies alba*) Enthroned. Empowering; going with the flow; transformation; open crown; brightness; brings a flow of healing and creativity.

Silver Maple (*Acer saccharinum*) Moods. Helps balance the flow of energy through the body and regulates mood swings. Realigns the meridians, so useful for acupuncture.

Spindle (*Euonymus europaeus*) Self-integration. For understanding one's true nature and needs. Brings increased sense of security, reducing the need to compare oneself to others. For feelings of superiority/inferiority. Energizes soul, accesses energies of the shadow-self in an integrated, positive way.

Stags Horn Sumach (*Rhus typhina*) Meditation. Energizes brow chakra. Eases flow of information. Balances energies for meditation. Stills mental and emotional processes while allowing clear intuition and communication at deep levels.

Strawberry Tree (*Arbutus unedo*) Quietude. Quietens and clears the mind of all unnecessary thought. Brings stillness and silence, which allows change to occur on deep levels. Energizes the crown chakra. Good for healers and meditation.

Sweet Chestnut (*Castanea sativa*) The now. For focusing and centring in the present moment. Helps release guilt, particularly alienation with physical world. Creates detachment and understanding to regain wider perspective. Finding ways out of difficult situations.

Sycamore (*Acer pseudoplatanus*) Lightening up. Energy levels increase, so helps with lethargy. Brings awareness of the sweetness of life, harmony and relaxation. Lifts heavy moods.

Tamarisk (*Tamarix gallica*) Fire of transformation. Helps in finding spiritual direction, freeing up energies for personal expansion and growth. Deeply cleansing and uplifting, cleanses age-old dross for the true self to emerge.

Tree Lichen (*Usnea subfloridana*) Wisdom. Accesses past knowledge and ancient wisdom. Brings a sense of independence and detachment without isolation. Letting go of things no longer needed in order to grow.

Tree of Heaven (*Ailanthus altissima*) Heaven on Earth. Dynamic, energizing, spiritual energies. Maintains integrity of self whilst removing barriers and allowing growth of new levels of awareness. Brings practical spirituality and practical wisdom.

Tulip Tree (*Liriodendron tulipifera*) Spiritual nourishment. Nourishing on spiritual levels, particularly for those feeling restless and dissatisfied or those with addictive tendencies. Helps in finding positive outlets for energy and expression. Artistic. Brings balance for meditation.

Viburnum (*Viburnum tinus*) Reassurance. Support and reassurance. For those who feel unsettled, vulnerable or unhappy. Helps to establish identity and direction, particularly after life-threatening situations.

Walnut (*Juglans regia*) Liberation. For purification and cleansing; sturdiness; helps in the removal of all sorts of intrusions and influences; brings personal power and integrity; security.

Wayfaring Tree (*Viburnum lantana*) Far memory. Recognition of similarities of circumstance and patterns in the present relating to the past. Re-establishing personal boundaries and independence to create a protective space.

Weeping Willow (*Salix* × *chrysocoma*) Ego. For proper use of personal power and energy. Useful for those who get annoyed by others' views and attitudes. Tolerance of others and acceptance of one's own short-comings. Energizing and motivating in a wise, balanced way.

Western Hemlock (*Tsuga heterophylla*) Open grace. For cleansing, clearing, quietening and focusing. Brings serenity; acceptance. For new beginnings.

Western Red Cedar (*Thuja plicata*) Constancy. Brings underlying peace; play of emotions; and belief in oneself. Helps screen harmful influences. For subtle tides of consciousness; steadiness.

White Poplar (*Populus alba*) Starting again. Increases wisdom, joy and contentment. Heals mind and emotions. Gives energy and courage to recover from emotional setbacks.

White Willow (*Salix alba*) True self. The perception of the self is put in the context of its universal existence. This clarity brings a truer balance within oneself. Ego is cleansed and filled with a sense of bliss and love welling up. Spiritual cleansing.

Whitebeam (*Sorbus aria*) Otherworld. Stimulates finer levels of perception. Understanding of the animal and plant kingdoms. Opens heart and mind to finer levels of creation.

Wild Service Tree (*Sorbus torminalis*) Unfoldment. Brings expansion of awareness and an understanding of motives. Also for past-life healing; self-definition; hidden currents.

Willow Leaved Pear (*Pyrus salicifolia*) Dance of life. Brings security within the self; dance of joy; healing; personal power and vitality; creative living; enjoyment.

Wych Elm (*Ulmus glabra*) Attainment. The mind is brought to clarity. There is a more positive, life-affirming outlook. Brings confidence in personal strengths and abilities and peaceful awareness, no matter what state. Meditation touches many subtle realms.

Yellow Buckeye (*Aesculus flava*) Devas. A way to link to devas, elementals and nature spirits in all environments. Modifies personal energy patterns in order to understand different sorts of communication.

Yew (*Taxus baccata*) Protection. Protects from harm by activating the highest spiritual values of survival and protection. Aids the memory and discrimination, helps the immune system and increases energy.

SUN ESSENCES (Sun)

Sun Essences have a policy of hand-prepared flower essences where living flowers are held in the bowl, in addition to the picked flowers. As the remedy is potentizing, it remains connected to the ongoing stream of life force, which strengthens the healing potential of these English flower essences.

Sun Essences were created by Vivien Williamson, whose passion for flower essences evolved from a decade-long love affair with the Bach Flower Remedies and the unforgettable experience of making her first flower essence – White Chestnut in 1989. She started her company, Sun Essences, in the early 1990s and lives near Cromer, a much loved haunt of Doctor Edward Bach.

Right from the beginning Vivien had an intuitive sense that essence combinations would be a significant part of the future of flower essences and with the help of Jane Stevenson (of Sun Essences for Animals), she began developing ranges of blends for people and animals.

Vivien believes that, as in ancient traditions, the rainbow is a bridge between Heaven and Earth. It is also thought to be the colours of the human soul. As we strive to build a bridge between the needs of our inner self and the demands of this busy world, a good colour balance can enhance our natural life force. With this in mind, Sun Essences has taken care to blend the colours of the flowers chosen, to create a rainbow in each bottle.

These flower essences support an inner radiance, so the soul colours can shine through and we can function more effectively in our daily lives.

An active member of the flower essence community in the UK, Vivien was Chairman of the British Flower and Vibrational Essence Association (BFVEA), and was editor of its *Essence Journal*. Her book *Bach Flower Remedies and Other Flower Essences* was published in 2000, and during that year Sun Essences was asked by Bioforce to supply the essences for the Jan De Vries range of flower essences. Living Essences and Be Blends are some of her ranges.

The English Collection

Living flower essences (all individual essences made by Vivien Williamson and Jane Stevenson).

Alkanet (*Pentaglottis sempervirens*) Calm in a storm. Alkanet can help you to keep your own inner sacred space centred and contained. It becomes easier to focus and communicate clearly, thus finding a way through challenging situations.

Autumn Leaves (All colours) Transition. Some people today find themselves living many lifetimes within their single lifespan, seemingly dying and being reborn to new circumstances, not unlike the cycles of nature. This can be a very challenging process. This essence eases the way through periods of profound personal change and may clarify anything that might be blocking the way.

Bluebells (Mixed colours) (*Endymion nonscriptum*) Uplifting stillness. Bluebell is nature's panacea. Use whenever life seems full on and you are feeling overwhelmed, vulnerable and finding it difficult to cope with the pressure. Consider also when there is trauma, anxiety or grief, or when feeling crowded, isolated and depressed by circumstances. Bluebell brings a balanced connection with the Higher Self, stillness and tranquillity.

Chalice Well Renewal This essence is made with water from the Chalice Well, a red iron spring in Glastonbury. This ancient and deep source of water helps to dissolve imprints from the past. These old patterns can be quite aggressive, draining energy and taking a real hold. This essence brings renewal, unblocking channels of energy and bringing in new light. It is ideal when there is a need to rejuvenate in a natural way.

Copper Beech (*Fagus sylvatica*) Rooted and present. Copper Beech is indicated when you are feeling disorientated, panicky, scattered and unable to focus. There may also be times when you forget where you are or what you've done. These symptoms can drain confidence, as you feel anxious and out of control of your life. Such withdrawal of consciousness from reality can be a habitual response to unpleasant life circumstances. Copper Beech helps you feel secure and rooted in yourself so nothing can throw you off centre. You will notice that it is pleasurable to be on life's journey, despite the challenges.

Dark Mullein (*Verbascum nigrum*) Supporting mental clarity. This essence is an ideal choice when a clear mind is desirable and there is taxing mental work to be done. It helps the body stay straighter and feel supported, which enhances consciousness and promotes high energy levels. Prevents heavy energies from the surrounding environment from draining or zapping energy, so an aid to vulnerable and sensitive types who need to keep functioning in intrusive situations, for example, busy offices, trains, planes, etc.

Double Daffodil (*Golden Dukat*) Abundance. Double Daffodil can help those who have a rigid and constricted attitude and find it difficult to be expressive. It opens the heart to the rich abundance of life and allows in feelings of joy and happiness.

Elderflower (*Sambucus nigra*) Integration of the shadow side. Elderflower can help us come to terms with the dark side that is within us all. It gives a sense of protection as we face this fearful challenge and promotes a deeper understanding and acceptance of the self.

Eyebright (*Euphrasia nemorosa*) Clear sight. Eyebright is indicated when there is a need to live life through someone else, as it is easy to lose your sense of identity and way in life. This essence can bring a wider viewpoint and helps you to embrace new and independent opportunities in life.

Feverfew (*Tanacetum parthenium*) Flexibility. In quick-moving, challenging situations, this essence can help you to 'think on your feet', encouraging the quality of adaptable and flexible thinking. It is an ideal choice when travelling or moving house as it brings out strength and tenacity.

Jack by the Hedge (Hedge Garlic) (*Allaria petiolata*) Fragility. For sensitive, fragile and delicate individuals, easily run down. This essence is ideal when emotional pain, for example, grief, has weakened the constitution, leaving you feeling low. Jack can strengthen the heart, which can bring valuable support to the system's defences. Partners well with Ramsons.

Lady's Mantle (*Alchemilla vulgaris*) Honours the female side. This essence can help protect your sensitive, female side. Ideal for men struggling to be comfortable with their vulnerabilities and holding back emotions through fear. Whatever your sexuality, Lady's Mantle helps give more understanding and acceptance of the feminine aspect.

Lungwort (*Pulmonaria officinalis*) Energizes auric field. Lungwort opens the breath, and connects you more fully with the universal life force which can mend and revitalize

245

your energetic body. This process is gentle and ideal for those of a delicate constitution who need strengthening.

Meadowsweet (*Filipendula ulmaris*) False persona. Meadowsweet is for those who tend to present a false, superficial front. They are usually popular, but their flattering ways are often a guise for control and an insurance that others will continue to like them. This essence helps them feel safe enough with who they are inside to be more genuine with others.

Mixed Poppy (*Papaver*) (various species) Restriction. This essence is indicated when you are restricted by life. Perhaps you are trapped in your head with many pressured thoughts, or you may be hemmed in by physical circumstances you can't change, for example, elderly people in a home, so escape is not an option. With Poppy essence, pent-up pressure is dissipated and some sense of inner control within the self is regained, despite the situation. Also suggested for animals in kennels and people immobilized by various domestic or work-related circumstances.

Orange Hawkweed (*Pilosella aurantiacum*) Realization and rejuvenation. Orange Hawkweed throws off anything that is not 'of the self'. It stops things settling into the system, so can be used as a protection against psychic pollution, or the effects of trauma. It very effectively clears and recharges the system, so is an ideal choice when you are really 'stuck' with life or feeling very low or run down. It creates more inner space and brings an expansion of consciousness, filling the system with renewed energy and light, so is an aid to meditation. You begin to understand the true self and get a more objective view on life.

Primrose (*Primula vulgaris*) Lightness to one's inner child. This essence is indicated when there is unexplained melancholy or deep sadness, which is often the sign of a repressed inner child. Primrose can gently nurture this crushed spirit bringing comfort, hope and release. It is as if you can start anew, pure, unblemished and refreshed to life.

Ramsons (Wild Garlic) (*Allium ursinum*) Cleansing and cooling. Ramsons can invigorate the body with an explosion of cleansing white light. If you feel congested, it can 'burn' off the dross and take strength where it is needed. It is helpful in reducing the effects of heat, as it can balance the four elements thus bringing harmony to the system. Ideal for people who become quickly dehydrated, or easily feel overheated.

Snowdrop (*Galanthus nivalis*) Purity. For frozen, numbed or locked-down emotions, perhaps due to past abuse, sometimes sexual. Snowdrop will help to cleanse and purify emotions and move you to a place where you can start again. It brings new light on situations and initiates forgiveness and trust. You can learn to be more open or creative, and connect to loving situations in a new way.

Trine Tree (*Carpinus betulus quercifolia*) Synthesis. A rare form of Hornbeam bearing 'leaves like the Oak' hence its Latin name. This tree can bring strength and endurance when struggling to harmonize opposing aspects of life. It helps you see how it is possible to give equal importance to the diverging needs of the body, mind and spirit, so is helpful during times of personal growth or crisis.

Viper's Bugloss (*Echium vulgare*) Balances loving forces. Viper's Bugloss helps to realign how love flows in the system. When this is out of balance, people may become the perpetrator or victim of manipulative patterns in an effort to get their needs met. This flower can help dissolve these stubborn and distorted patterns, thus helping the loving forces to flow more freely.

Wild Daffodil (*Narcissus pseudonarcissus*) Appreciation of talents. Wild Daffodil is indicated when your talents seem insignificant or do not appear to fit into society. This essence can help the recognition of their worth. Once they are used with this positive attitude, they can blossom and grow with abundance.

White Violet (*Viola odorata*) Acceptance of the spiritual self. This essence is indicated when there is a strong awareness of the spiritual side of life but through a fear of rejection, you deny this aspect of the self. White Violet brings feelings of self-acceptance, truth and trust, so it becomes safer to be open with others.

Yellow Archangel (*Lamiastrum galeobdolon*) Happy on your path. This essence is for when you lose spiritual direction, maybe through rushing to get somewhere or even arrogance. There can be an urge to keep up with everyone else, so maybe you pretend to be other than who you really are. This essence helps you to learn your lessons, and pay more attention to your Higher Self. You become content to move at your own pace, at peace with the self and happy to be where you are on your life journey.

Be Blends Sun Flower Essences

Hand-prepared, the Be Blends are easy to choose and simple to use and are nature's gentle way of soothing our minds and emotions from the various challenges of everyday living.

Be Balanced For when the system needs some tender loving care. This gentle blend eases anxiety, tension and frustration, thereby restoring balance during the natural cycles of life. Also brings essential vitality during times of change and is therefore an ideal choice for women.

Be Calm The crisis blend. This blend of flowers is designed to bring ease during those times when much is demanded and there is extreme anxiety or pressure, for example, shows, interviews, tests or exams. It helps the mind and body relax, thus enabling the individual to feel focused, productive and in control. Use also for mishaps, unsettling news, the acute stages of bereavement, etc. Take 7 drops on the tongue or sip in water as often as required, the effect being cumulative.

Be Comforted This blend of flowers is designed specifically to comfort and ease the enduring pain of losing a treasured friend or family member. It gives support when moving through the wide range of emotions that are a natural part of the grieving process, such as anger, guilt, blame, sadness or despair. It enables you to come to terms with the loss in your own way, and in time brings hope of a new beginning.

Be Confident This blend of flowers is for those who lack confidence in their ability to achieve goals or perform as well as others. Also suggested for individuals who may have had disappointments or setbacks in life. This essence brings determination and self-belief while staying focused on the task in hand. If needed for a specific occasion, start at least two weeks prior to the event.

Be Courageous If you suffer from everyday anxieties or apprehensions, this blend of flowers helps reduce them to a manageable level, by enhancing feelings of courage and inner safety. They help you to forget the original cause of the problem, which is what often triggers the attack. For particularly difficult conditions these essences may be used to complement and support other treatments, as they stimulate inner strengths.

Be Decisive Ideal for those who worry about making the wrong choice and need to feel more decisive. This blend offers support during times of personal change, as it facilitates a letting go of the past and provides a stable inner centre from which to choose a way forward. If there are issues present that inhibit this progress, for example, extreme fear, these will come to light and can be dealt with appropriately.

Be Focused Lack concentration? Exams? Computer weary? Then this is the one for you. This blend of flowers helps to clear the head, improve motivation, stimulate creativity and restore interest in daily tasks. If working under pressure, then this essence may be taken more frequently.

Be Free This blend is ideal for letting go of the things that control your life. Depending how serious these habits are, this blend of flowers may either be used on its own or in conjunction with other modalities. This blend supports a positive self-image and is particularly helpful when there has been a setback. It can also boost motivation and the drive to make progress each day.

Be Loving Ideal for dealing with everyday situations that call for greater love, forgiveness and acceptance, for example, relationships, children, at the work place. Particularly helpful when strong feelings emerge and there is a need to diffuse them and gain greater insight. Its effectiveness can be boosted if taken by partners/family members at the same time.

Be Positive Whatever the reason is for feeling down, hopeless, negative or discouraged, this blend of flowers will help you to lighten up and become more positive. Releases the need to focus on personal problems and helps create a new optimistic frame of mind. Life can become more enjoyable, bright and promising.

Be Relaxed A key blend for hectic modern living, so is ideal for those leading demanding lifestyles or with high-pressure jobs. This blend enables you to relax, unwind and feel more refreshed on all levels. It is then easier to enjoy increased focus and productivity in daily life.

Be Resistant This blend of flowers is designed to support the system at times when you might be feeling at a low ebb. Ideal for when you go down with everything that's around and it is hard to shake things off. Gives you a much-needed lift and, if taken regularly, strengthens the system.

Be Restful Being unable to settle at night can be a frustrating downward cycle. This blend of flowers helps to overcome restlessness and supports the return of natural patterns, with improved quality of rest. Ideal for people who cannot switch off, and suggested for children who feel unsettled at night.

Be Vitalized Exhausted, no get-up-and-go? Lack staying power? This blend of flowers is particularly useful when feeling drained after a period of overwork. When taken as part of a positive move towards a more holistic lifestyle, this essence will gradually recharge your batteries.

WILDFLOWER ESSENCES OF ENGLAND (WF)

Paul Strode is also someone who I've had the great pleasure in guiding and nurturing through the birth and development of his wildflower essences. As he jokingly says, he was 'under my wing' and now he is in full flight!

Deeply woven into England's ancient landscape is a concentration of healing energy found in nature. The mountains, coastlines, old Oak forests and the countryside of this isle hold great beauty and also the key to this abundant healing energy. Our ancestors knew of this wisdom and built great stone circles not only to understand the cosmos but also to focus Earth's healing energy. The wildflowers of England are steeped in the healing wisdom of this land, from which we can now benefit.

The growth of farming over the past four decades has contributed to a steep decline in wildflowers throughout the UK. The use of pesticides and fertilizers, as well as the wide-scale clearing of hedgerows, hay meadows and wildflower pastures, has created a huge imbalance to the natural environment in which wildflowers used to flourish. In turn this has had a devastating impact on our insect friends such as bees and butterflies which are essential for wildflowers to thrive, and on the birds that feed from the insects.

Paul Strode started making wildflower essences in 1999 in response to the urgent need to preserve our English wildflower heritage and with the aim of bringing plant energy medicine to a wider audience. To play a small part in correcting the imbalance, Wildflower also invests in beehives to encourage pollination, as well as in the flowers themselves, and does not use the hives for commercial purposes but leaves them alone to thrive naturally. Paul's passion for the health-giving properties of the wildflowers has developed into a deeply intuitive connection with nature and he encourages the growth and spread of wildflowers by cultivating seeds from mature plants and distributing them at other wild sites to return a greater diversity of natural flora into the environment.

Paul's range of English wildflower essences was created to aid and nurture a natural way of helping and maintaining emotional wellbeing, and he continues to explore and research natural healing methods to ensure that wildflower essences offer the best possible accompaniment to our healing journey.

Paul is a craniosacral therapist with more than 14 years of clinical experience specializing in the treatment of children and horses. He brings warmth and enthusiasm to his work and enjoys helping others find their path to wellness.

The essences are handmade from natural ingredients, using only spring water and organic brandy as a preservative. There are many different ways to produce essences. Wildflower produces 'living flower essences' from plants where the flower has not been picked or cut. The essences are drawn from flowers which are still attached to the plant and its roots – drawing on the energy from the whole plant and the environment in which it resides. Great care is taken to find the right location of each wildflower so the healing properties of the Earth can be gained too.

Traditionally glass bowls are used in producing flower essences. At Wildflower they use crystal geodes, which can help amplify the energetic signature of the wild flower, and infuse the mineral's essence into every tincture. The combination of wildflower and mineral essences can offer a deeper healing than when used singly.

The crystal geodes used are Bluelace Agate, Clear Quartz, Celestite and Rose Quartz.

Mineral essences

Bluelace Agate
Benefits: Highly inspirational when working with our inner wisdom.
Offers: Peace and calm.
Chakras: Fifth and seventh.

Celestite
Benefits: Communication with the higher spiritual realms.
Offers: Peace from anxiety and worry.
Chakras: Fifth, seventh and ninth.

Clear Quartz
Benefits: Energetic cleansing and fortification of our energy body.
Offers: Clarity of thought.
Chakras: First, second, third, fourth, fifth, sixth and seventh.

Rose Quartz
Benefits: Supports unconditional love in our energy body.
Offers: Emotional stability.
Chakras: Fourth and eighth.

The Wildflower Essences

1. Bluebell
Benefits: Encourages us to look inwards to find our true feelings and communicate with others. Bluebell urges us to be 'in nature' and to listen to our hearts. The natural world can

help us find the inner space and stillness to listen to our feelings. Finding the words to truly express our inner feelings can help create clear and healthy boundaries in our lives.
Chakras: Fifth and seventh.
Mineral: Celestite.

2. Bramble

Benefits: Offers us the protection we need while we face feelings of vulnerability and fear. As we try to come to terms with grief and loss in our lives, frustration can express itself through anger. Just as the rabbit will hide deep within a bramble thicket for protection from a fox so Bramble can help us feel safe to explore the dark side of grief and heal deep-seated emotions.
Chakras: First and sixth.
Minerals: Bluelace Agate and Clear Quartz.

3. Cow Parsley

Benefits: To rest our overactive nervous systems and bring stability to our lives. An overactive mind can create a spiral of negative thoughts and feelings. During sleep, which should be a time of healing for our physical selves, our mental confusion can get the better of us. Peace of mind is imperative for its calming influence on our bodies. Cow Parsley reminds us of the innocence of summer and of being in sweet meadows of wild flowers.
Chakras: Second, fourth and seventh.
Minerals: Bluelace Agate and Clear Quartz.

4. Dandelion

Benefits: To help us remember to be gentle on ourselves and take it easy. Stress is woven into the very fabric of life and a certain amount is healthy. However, anxiety and worry can manifest physically in many ways such as tightness in the neck and shoulders or disruption of our digestive system. As stress builds up so our energetic body reacts negatively. Dandelion can remind us to breathe deeply and remember not to take life so seriously.
Chakras: Second and third.
Minerals: Bluelace Agate and Clear Quartz.

5. Great Willow Herb

Benefits: To help us embrace our fractured soul and reconnect to our heart's energy so we can feel safe to love again. To know one's self is more than a simple matter of intellectual understanding; it is the compassionate embrace of our fractured soul. Emotional wounds can create such fractures in our energy body that we disconnect from our own hearts. Great Willow Herb can help to heal these past traumas.
Chakras: First, second, third and fourth.
Mineral: Clear Quartz and Rose Quartz.

6. Herb Robert

Benefits: To help clear the body and aura of vibrational toxicity and prepare us to shift our focus to the inner planes of knowledge and wisdom. Stagnant energy or low Qi in our bodies can make it difficult for us to focus when we want to listen to our intuition. Herb Robert can weave our mind and heart together as one to find stillness and wisdom within.
Chakras: Second and fifth.
Minerals: Bluelace Agate and Clear Quartz.

7. Honeysuckle

Benefits: To help us feel safe without being vulnerable, allowing us to let intimacy back into our lives. Relationships in our past may have closed down our hearts as a form of protection. Sometimes these experiences can be so shocking to us that we never want to feel as vulnerable again. We can create a metaphoric wall around our heart to keep further pain out. But this can close our hearts to any new and loving experiences as well. Honeysuckle can help us to let love back in, so we can heal the past and move forward again with our lives.
Chakras: First, fourth and sixth.
Minerals: Clear Quartz.

8. Lesser Celandine

Benefits: To boost our confidence by finding the strength and courage to overcome life's challenges. To evolve as a spiritual being we must face the fears which hold us back. Scattered thoughts can overwhelm us and make it confusing to know how to proceed with

confidence. Lesser Celandine can help us focus our minds to see the path ahead and have the courage not to give up but to persevere.
Chakras: First, fourth and sixth.
Mineral: Celestite.

9. Pink Purslane

Benefits: Balances our heart centre helping us to reconnect to life by showing a greater perspective into our thinking. When we are trying to be creative or working with new ideas we can feel we are chasing our thoughts and are unable to see the bigger picture. Our bodies may have a certain level of restriction within the connective tissues which may lead to restrictions of our thoughts and ideas. Pink Purslane can help to free these restrictions by expanding in our energy body and bringing clarity of vision.
Chakras: First, fourth and seventh.
Minerals: Bluelace Agate and Clear Quartz.

10. Moon Daisy

Benefits: To help get our feet back on the ground and bring a more balanced approach to our spiritual seeking and self-development. In our eagerness to grow spiritually and to find truth in our lives we can sometimes become ungrounded in a swirling mass of information and personal insight. This can put excessive strain on our energy body and we can lose focus on what life is actually all about. Moon Daisy can help us see that there is no rush and to take our time as each step we take on our life path reveals truth.
Chakras: First, seventh and ninth.
Minerals: Bluelace Agate and Clear Quartz.

11. Nettle

Benefits: To help purify and fortify our aura and, if we feel especially sensitive to hostile environments, provide psychic protection. The human energy body or aura is an extension of ourselves and a mirror of our physical health. The aura allows us to receive and interpret information from our environment at a subtle energetic level. Nettle can help if we have low energy or Qi, which makes our aura sensitive to electropollution or negative thoughts and feelings from others.

Chakras: First, third and sixth.
Mineral: Clear Quartz.

12. Pink Campion

Benefits: Helps us in weaving our emotional and spiritual self together by connecting with inner wisdom. Our life is a journey and, to connect our hearts and minds, we must move into our spirit. As the Buddha said, 'the only wisdom is compassion' and to find truth in our lives we must move into the world of true wisdom. Pink Campion actively supports our spiritual growth and shows us that compassion and a gentle heart is a true spiritual path.
Chakras: First, fourth and seventh.
Minerals: Bluelace Agate and Clear Quartz.

13. Primrose

Benefits: To help us feel that we are safe, nurtured and secure in the world we live in. Modern life can make us feel disconnected from the natural world. Emotions such as confusion, worry and anxiety can bring disruption to physical and emotional health and relationships. Feeling disconnected from the Earth can create feelings of instability and exclusion. Primrose can help you see that we are a part of a bigger picture in that as all creation is made with love, so we are made with love too.
Chakras: First and third.
Mineral: Celestite.

14. Purple and White Clover

Benefits: To help clear and balance our energy bodies. We all understand the importance of maintaining a balanced approach to the many aspects of our lives. With the challenges that life can offer us our energy body can fluctuate greatly. So that our energy body does not feel overloaded or compromised, it is important to recharge and bring it back into harmony. Purple and White Clover can help us function at our optimum energy level so we are ready to deal with life's challenges.
Chakras: Third, fourth, fifth, sixth, seventh and ninth.
Minerals: Bluelace Agate and Clear Quartz.

15. Purple Foxglove

Benefits: Allows us to distance ourselves from emotional turmoil and reveal with remarkable clarity truth behind our feelings. When we hold on to emotional turmoil or painful experiences so tightly, it is sometimes difficult to understand them; we become confused and unable to move on in our lives. Purple Foxglove allows us to see with the inner eye which becomes activated and the veil of illusion is lifted.

Chakras: First and sixth.

Minerals: Bluelace Agate and Clear Quartz.

16. Purple Spotted Orchid

Benefits: To help us change deep-seated patterns in our behaviour and to recognize how best to make changes and to support healing. We can bring to this life experiences from our ancestors which can express themselves as memories or past-life experiences. We may sometimes find that we keep repeating the same old patterns over and over again. Purple Spotted Orchid can help heal ties from the past freeing you to experience present life into the full.

Chakras: Third, fourth, sixth, seventh and eighth.

Mineral: Clear Quartz.

17. Ramsons (Wild Garlic)

Benefits: To help us feel protected while we discover what it is that fear is trying to shield us from. Fear is so misunderstood in our lives. It can literally freeze us into inaction and can create less fluid movement within our energy body. Fear can make us feel vulnerable, unprotected or weak. But fear can save our lives. Ramson fortifies and clears our energy body and can help create a bridge of understanding so we can work more closely with and understand fear.

Chakras: Fourth, seventh and ninth.

Mineral: Celestite.

18. Red Archangel

Benefits: To help us understand that anger is nothing to be afraid of. Anger can be so misunderstood when actually it is a necessary part of life. It is a natural emotion which is a part of our fight or flight mechanism, but it can be held so deeply within us that only the subconscious remembers its true origins. Red Archangel can help us feel protected as we experience this troubling emotion and can help us understand what it is that we have chosen to protect so deeply within ourselves.

Chakras: First, sixth and seventh.

Mineral: Celestite.

19. St John's Wort

Benefits: Offers us peace of mind and positivism, which in turn will help us to laugh with ourselves again and not take life so seriously. Life can sometimes become so serious, that we become overburdened with our perceived failings, weighed down, ungrounded and unable to laugh. This can make it challenging for us to sustain positive thoughts or feelings. St John's Wort can show us how to lighten up and feel grounded within ourselves.

Chakras: First, second, third, fourth and seventh.

Mineral: Celestite.

20. Snowdrop

Benefits: To help us see the opportunity in darker moments and to rekindle our personal connection with spirit. Grieving can bring a great darkness that can envelop our lives. We can lose hope, feel lost and disconnected and even abandoned by spirit. Snowdrop offers us hope, a light at the end of the tunnel. It reminds us of the promise of spring, of renewal and allows us to experience joy in our lives again. It will show us how to embrace the grieving process and not be afraid.

Chakras: Second and ninth.

Mineral: Celestite.

21. Tutsan

Benefits: To help us expand beyond our self-limiting thoughts and feelings, to a more creative space, free from our perceived constraints. At times in our lives we can feel caught in a rut or feel boxed in by our emotions. We can feel frustrated with not finding a clear path ahead and seeing a new perspective. Tutsan encourages us to lighten up, laugh more and not take it all so seriously. The joy is in the journey.

Chakras: First, second and sixth.

Minerals: Bluelace Agate and Clear Quartz.

22. White Archangel

Benefits: To help balance out emotions between ourselves and others. Our journey into healing can sometimes raise difficult memories, feelings and emotions. It may bring to the surface past traumas generating anger towards others and ourselves. White Archangel reminds us of our lightness of being and our connection to spirit. It can help remind us that we are all spiritual beings in human form and encourage forgiveness.

Chakras: First, fourth and ninth.

Mineral: Celestite.

23. Wound Wort

Benefits: To help realign our whole energetic body matrix and remind us that we are all connected and loved. Emotional trauma may be so deep-rooted that we do not know where it stems from. We may find relationships hard to commit to or even sustain. If not healed, over time this can create disruption in our energy body, eventually disconnecting us from life and making it hard for us to feel with our emotional heart. Wound Wort can be seen as a 'heal all' flower essence which reboots our whole energy system and brings our heart back on line.

Chakras: First, second, third, fourth, fifth, sixth, seventh, eighth and ninth.

Minerals: Bluelace Agate and Clear Quartz.

24. Wild Marjoram

Benefits: To help us out of a negative rut; to reprogramme our thoughts and feelings so we can connect with our emotional heart again. By expressing the same negative thoughts or beliefs about ourselves or a situation, we can create entrenched patterns in our lives. We can feel numb to our emotions, trapped inside our heads and disconnected from our bodies. Wild Marjoram can help us align ourselves to love and positivity and to trust that all will be well in our lives.

Chakras: Fifth, sixth and seventh.

Mineral: Clear Quartz.

25. Wild Rose

Benefits: It can remind us that we are all good at something. Life can feel like a treadmill and we can easily lose heart to what in life is really important. We can lose our way and become unsure where to go next. Wild Rose can help us feel real worth in what we are doing and give us honour on the path we have chosen. It is important to feel joy in our hearts and to lighten up and enjoy life, whatever it is we chose to do.

Chakras: First and fourth.

Mineral: Bluelace Agate and Clear Quartz.

26. White Foxglove

Benefits: Helps us distance ourselves from our over-loaded thoughts. When we are unable to switch off an overactive mind, the body responds by restricting the flow of energy to our bodies. As our body tries to cope with excessive mental activity we may feel ungrounded and our thoughts can feel as though they are spiralling out of control. White Foxglove encourages us to be in the here and now and trust that through our hearts we will find the stillness within.

Chakras: Second, fourth, sixth and seventh.

Mineral: Clear Quartz.

27. Wild Basil

Benefits: Offers us a chance to take a metaphoric breath and find the space we need to ground our overactive minds. In our quest to evolve as spiritual beings we can grab at life for meaning and understanding. We can reach out so far that we can overload our energy body becoming lost in the fog of overactivity and lacking focus. Losing the present moment we disconnect from our emotional heart. Wild Basil brings us back to the present and reminds us to have faith and trust in life.

Chakras: Fourth, sixth and seventh.

Minerals: Celestite and Clear Quartz.

28. Yellow Archangel

Benefits: To help us to reinvigorate ourselves and bring vitality to our digestive process. Digestion is a metabolic action but it can also be understood as the way we process life's lessons. If this process gets sluggish we can start to feel heavy and blocked with unprocessed emotions which can bring frustration to our lives. Yellow Archangel encourages us to release locked-up feelings and resentments and be unafraid of showing our emotions, in order to digest life's lessons, however painful they may be, and offer movement and growth to our lives.

Chakras: First, third and seventh.
Mineral: Celestite.

HABUNDIA SHAMANIC FLOWER ESSENCES (HUB)

Shamans of many different spiritual traditions have been communicating with the spirits of flowers and plants in order to learn and understand their healing qualities for many generations.

Peter Aziz has been involved in shamanism for 37 years. He has trained in Pueblo Indian, Kahuna and Hungarian shamanism, is a trained ayahuascero and has been in retreats in the jungle in which he learned to communicate with the plant spirits. These retreats usually involve eating only one plant, until the spirit of that plant comes to teach its secrets. He is also a qualified homeopath. He has been preparing flower essences since 1987. His inspiration originally came on one of his wilderness retreats, when the flower spirits told him how they wanted to be prepared. He only uses flowers that ask him to use them. They are taken and prepared in a sacred way, using songs taught by the plant spirits, and are thereby imbued with a great deal of power. Peter works as a healer, and has been teaching these shamanic skills for 18 years.

General remedies

Alfalfa (*Medicago sativa*) Strengthens the root. Self-worth. For honouring and communicating your needs. Earthing.

Aloe Vera (*A. barbadensis*) Soothes emotional pain, shock and emotional traumas, new or old.

Apple (*Malus sylvestris*) Develops the heart. Giving and receiving. Generosity, trust, magnetism.

Artichoke (*Cynara scolymus*) For feelings of weakness, helplessness, impotence and emotional exhaustion, after devastating experiences or long, drawn-out emotionally painful situations.

Bramble (*Rubus*) Teaches us to approach love with respect.

Butterfly Orchid (*Oncidium papilio*) For speaking one's own truth, rather than impressions picked up from others. Clears the psychic gate. Strengthens the tongue and spine.

Chickweed (*Stellaria media*) Being happy with yourself, so you don't need to seek approval from others, and do not attract 'draining' relationships.

Comfrey (*Symphytum officinale*) For letting go of the past, and flowing with new impulses.

Cowslip (*Primula veris*) Strengthens the solar plexus and comforts and uplifts the emotions. For when you are feeling vulnerable.

Cyclamen (*Cyclamen persicum*) For healing childhood deprivation.

Dandelion (*Taraxacum officinale*) Centring. Understanding one's emotions and the cause of one's reactions. Helps release hatred and resentment.

Date (*Phoenix dactylifera*) Strength of character and vital energy to complete goals.

Dock (*Arctium minus*) Quiets and calms. Lessens the ego and fears around one's vulnerability.

Figwort (*Scrophularia nodosa*) For overcoming judgement towards matter. For those who love material existence and see it as a vehicle for spirit.

Fleabane (*Inula dysenterica*) Provides the quiet vitality that allows one to build health. Gives immunity against parasites on many levels.

Ground Ivy (*Glechoma hederacea*) For rebuilding when you have given out too much.

Harebell (*Campanula rotundifolia*) Faith in oneself and one's own judgement. Guards against giving away power and authority to others.

Hedge Woundwort (*Stachys sylvatica*) For healing deep hurts and tapping a source of inner strength.

Honesty (*Lunaria annua*) Maintains peace and beauty amongst stressful surroundings.

Ivy (*Hedera helix*) Patience, strength, stability, rooting. Links one to the Earth Mother.

Jasmine (*Jasminum*) For finding peace, rest and recharging in the darkness. Overcomes fear of darkness, and judgement towards that which is dark in ourselves.

Lily of the Valley (*Convallaria majalis*) Safety, by enshrouding the negative tendencies of the subconscious mind that could draw in trouble.

Madonna Lily (*Lilium candidum*) Opens one to joy, and releases all shame and judgement towards one's sexuality.

Marigold (*Tagetes*) Vitality. A great catalyst in healing. For any difficult conditions which are taking much energy to heal.

Navelwort (*Umbilicus rupestris*) Security, safety, self-esteem. Heals the shock of the umbilical cord being cut too soon.

Papaya (*Carica papaya*) For those involved in therapy and self-discovery. Papaya helps assimilate experiences faster, and brings out memories and deep feelings.

Rosemary (*Rosmarinus officinalis*) Brings clarity when there is great emotional stress, loss of trust or confusion.

St John's Wort (*Hypericum perforatum*) Uplifts the emotional body, eases fears and nervousness and aids calm, peaceful sleep. Good for nightmares.

Snowdrop (*Galanthus nivalis*) New hope. Helps one deal with rejection by finding nourishment within.

Solomon's Seal (*Polygonatum biflorum*) For disappointment. Restores courage, hope and the will to live.

Stonecrop (*Sedum*) Becoming really still inside, so that you grow more easily.

Sunflower (*Helianthus annuus*) True enthusiasm and balanced masculinity. For those who are disconnected from the feelings, stress and deprivation of others.

Sycamore (*Acer pseudoplatanus*) Increased flow of life force. Fertility on all levels.

Tansy (*Tanacetum vulgare*) Causes you to look at yourself and examine your motives, while providing some protection against outside influences.

Trefoil (*Trifolium*) Gives courage to shy, sensitive and nervous people. Also offers protection on the astral level when breaking through into new dimensions.

Wayfaring Tree (*Viburnum lantana*) Cleansing and healing the sexual chakras.

Wild Rose (*Rosa* × *pruhoniciana*) Bringing out the beauty of your wildness. Overcoming limited conditioning and beliefs. Love and appreciation of all life, including self.

Yarrow (*Achillea millefolium*) Strengthens the aura. Protection. Overidentification with other people's energy.

Yellow Iris (*Iris pseudacorus*) Understanding commitment in its true sense, that is, keeping one's vision, and working towards it with constancy.

Yellow Poppy (*Eschscholzia californica*) Calms emotions and brings clarity of mind. Helps to memorize, synthesize and adapt.

Spiritual remedies

Arrowhead (*Sagittaria sagittifolia*) Provides the urge to all spirituality, and realigns our dark urges.

Blackthorn (*Prunus spinosa*) Balancing beauty with power. Gives security in showing your inner beauty.

Bluebell (*Endymion non scriptum*) Trust in the source of all abundance. Joy, spontaneity, connection to Pan.

Cherry (*Prunus serrulata*) Overcomes fear of death. Trust in what is beyond material life.

Daffodil (*Narcissus pseudonarcissus*) Good for meditation. Enlivens the spirit, aids connection to one's Higher Self and allows faster spiritual growth.

Edelweiss (*Leontopodium alpinum*) Opens the crown chakra and attunes us to the highest vibration we can reach. Brings trust in spirit, and helps us know our destiny and true will.

Elder (*Sambucus nigra*) Wisdom to rise above apparent opposites and encompass dualities. Overcomes judgement. Recognizing the importance of all things, each in its own place.

Laurel (*Prunus lusitanica*) Aspiration. Helps break through into higher dimensions.

Oxtongue (*Helminthia echioides*) Builds power and vitality within, while overcoming the urge to give it out too soon.

Pyramidal Orchid (*Anacamptis pyramidalis*) Develops a warrior spirit and urges us to follow our true will.

Scarlet Pimpernel (*Anagallis arvensis*) Strengthens and nourishes the navel chakra and etheric body. Brings out resentments. Replenishes creative and sexual energy.

Spearmint (*Mentha spicata*) Opens one to take joy in receiving.

Spinach (*Spinacia oleracea*) Develops a higher octave of the heart chakra, to universal love. For growing out of repeated patterns.

Stinking Hellebore (*Helleborus foetidus*) For breaking out of conditioning and outer pressures to conform, while maintaining a strong, loving heart. Freedom and individuality.

Stinking Iris (*Iris foetidissima*) Withdrawing for spiritual transformation and vision. Makes you unreachable to those who drain you.

Thistle (*Cirsium vulgare*) Spiritual value. Trust in spirit. For maintaining one's spiritual integrity in spite of undermining company.

Tree Mallow (*Lavatera maritima*) Develops the spiritual heart chakra. Allows rapid growth through adversity.

Water Lily (*Nymphaeaceae*) Provides a sense of space. For detachment, stability and safety, while providing inner nourishment.

Wild Garlic (*Allium ursinum*) Enhances one's projections of power in such a way that they are able to put a stop to any negative energies in their environment.

Wild Pansy (*Viola tricolor*) Develops a strong, loving warm heart. Heals traumas of love, and overcomes feelings of being undeserving.

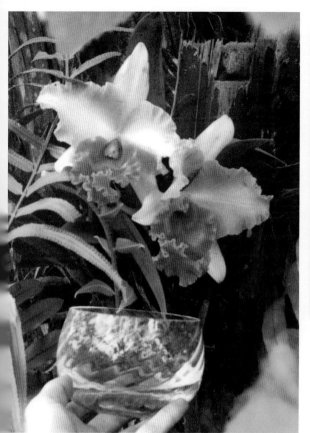

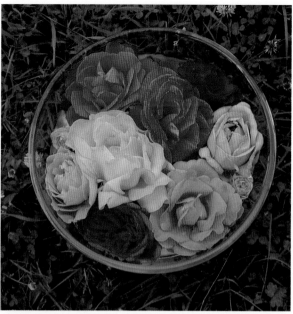

Roses: Mother Essence in the process of creation
(courtesy of Jane Thrift; IFVM – Flower Essence School)

Dancing Orchid Queen: Crystal method,
process of connection with the aura of the
flower to make Mother tincture in Thailand

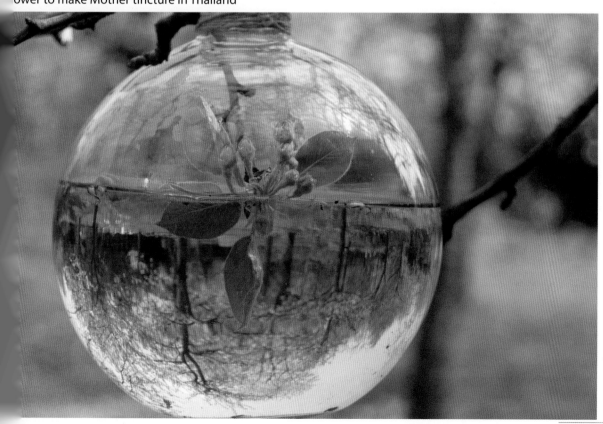

...thod of making mother tincture in the Netherlands (courtesy of Bram and Miep Zaalbergis)

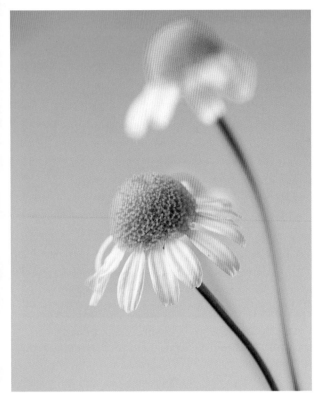

Chamomile (FES, AK, Dv) (source: Dreamstime)

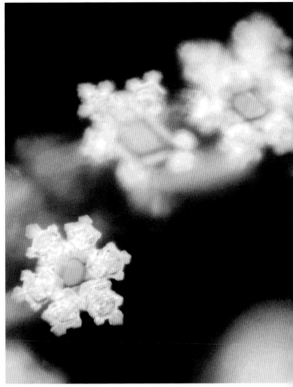

Water crystals of chamomile essence (courtesy of Dr Masaru Emoto, *Messages from Water*)

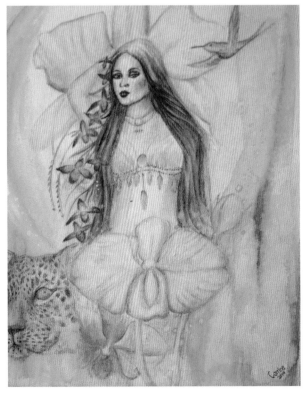

Artist's impression of Orchid Deva (by Corrine Cyster)

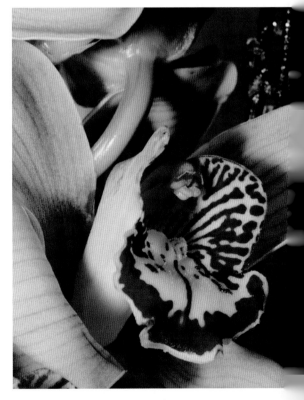

Pink Orchid (FO) (courtesy of Savio Joanes)

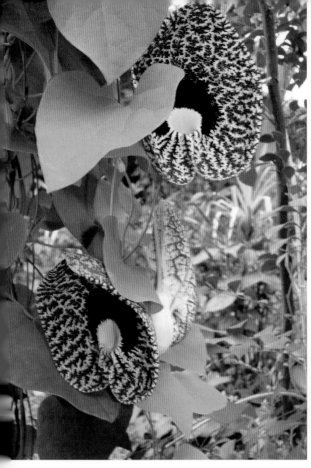

Dutchman's Pipe (SME) (courtesy of Sheila Hicks Balgobin)

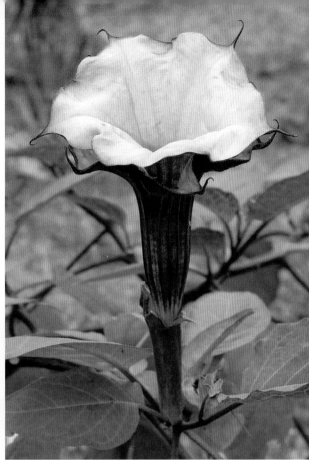

Devil's Trumpet (SME) (courtesy of Sheila Hicks Balgobin)

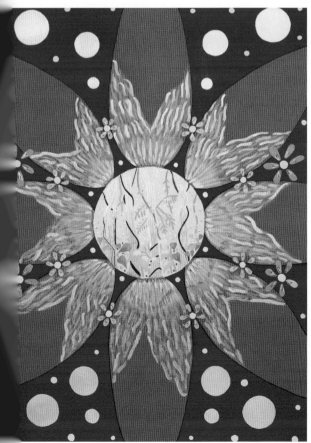

Chuhuasi (AmT) (by Mimi Buttacavoli)

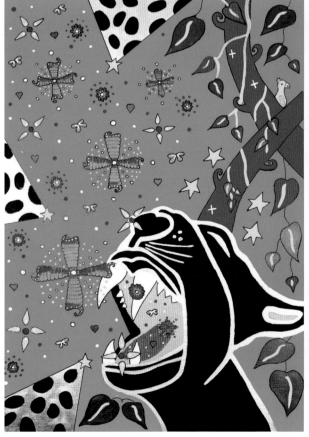

Una De Gato (AmT) (by Mimi Buttacavoli)

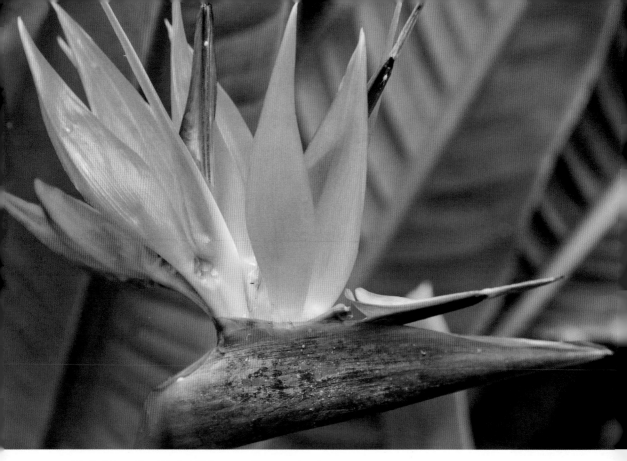

Bird of Paradise (Haii, AK) (source: Dreamstime)

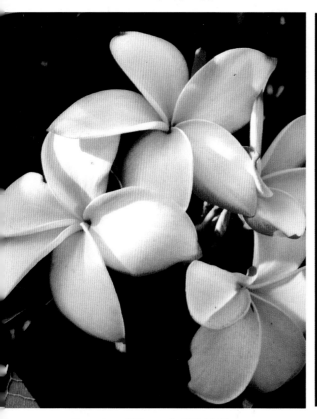

Frangipani/*Plumeria* (FO, Haii)
(courtesy of Cathie Welchman)

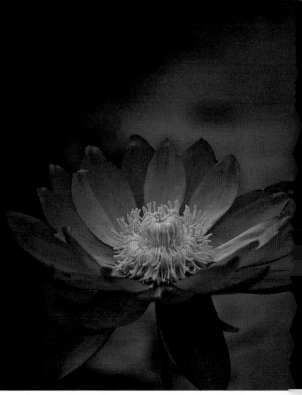

Blue Lotus (courtesy of Savio Joanes)

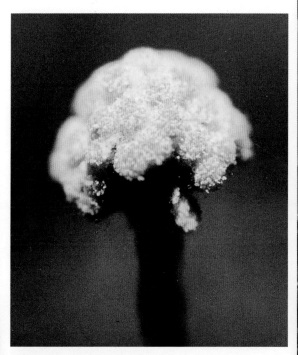

Above: Antiseptic Bush (Aus L)
(courtesy of Vasudeva Barnao)

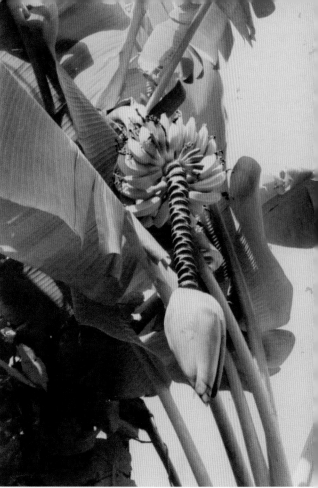

Right: Banana (AK, FO)

Below: Fringed Mantis Orchid (Aus L)
(courtesy of Vasudeva Barnao)

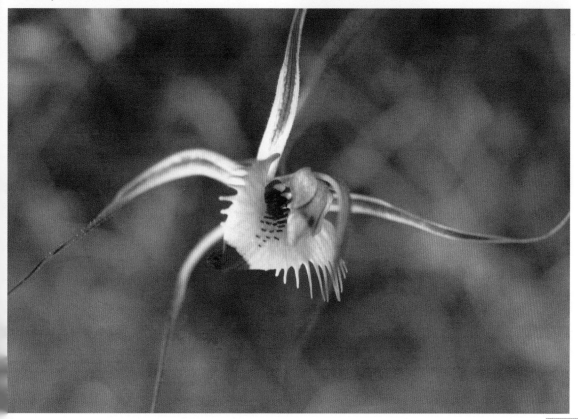

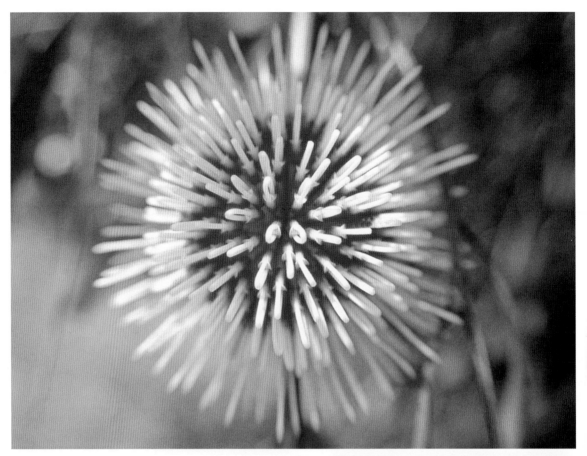

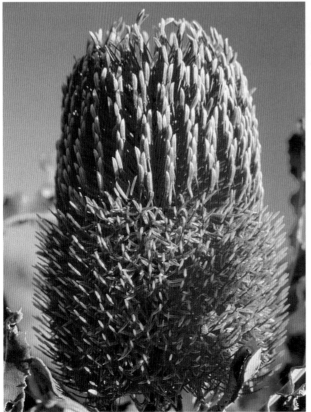

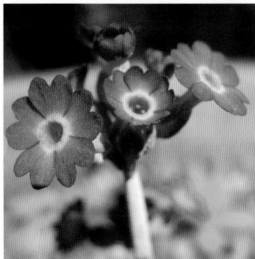

Top: Pincushion Hakea (Aus L)
(courtesy of Vasudeva Barnao)

Above: Scottish Primrose (F)
(courtesy of Marion Leigh)

Left: Menzies Banksia (Aus L)
(courtesy of Vasudeva Barnao)

Right: Princess Gum (FE Aus)

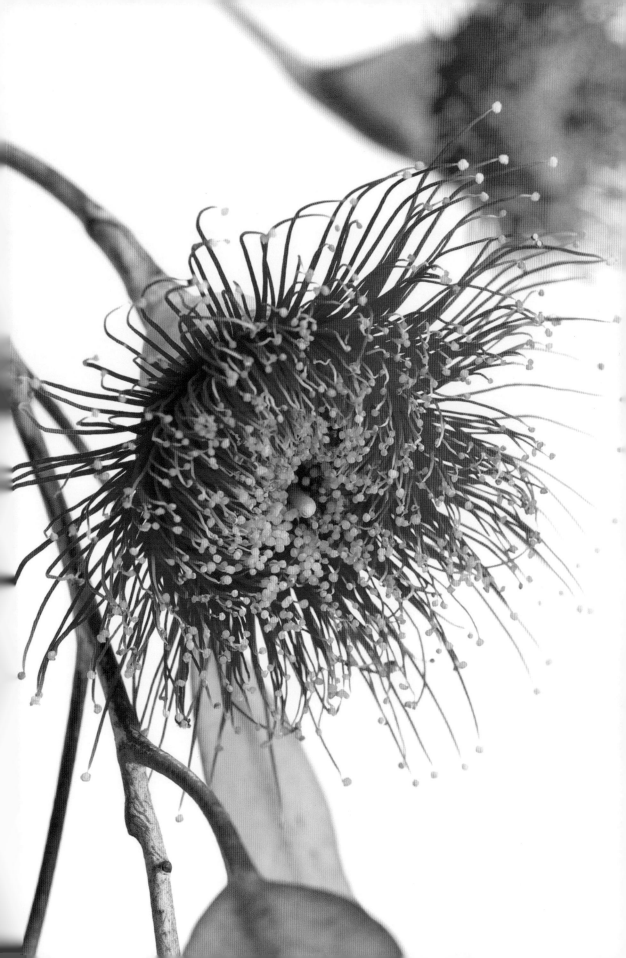

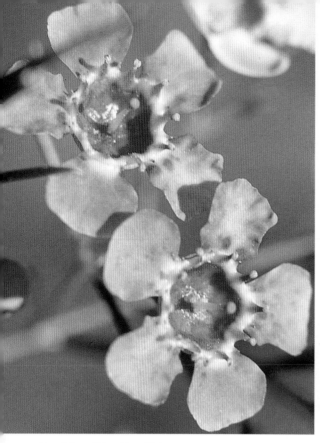

Geraldton Wax (Aus L) (courtesy
of Vasudeva Barnao)

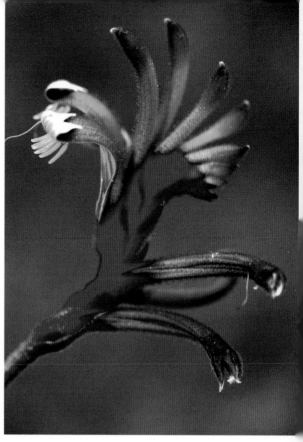

Kangaroo Paw (FE Aus)

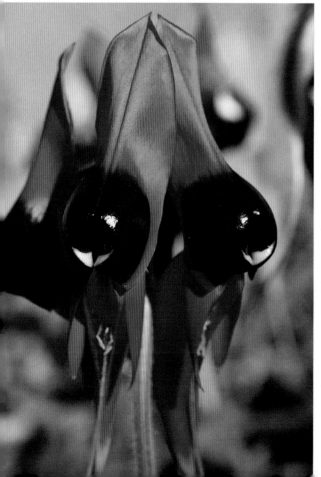

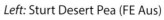

Above: Wild Garlic (AK) (courtesy
of Regina Hornberger)

Left: Sturt Desert Pea (FE Aus)

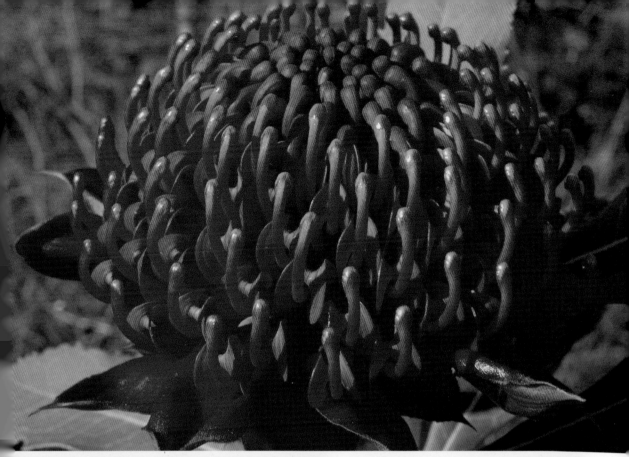

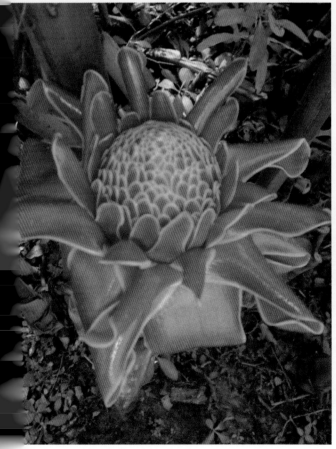

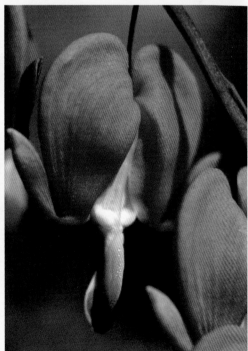

Top: Waratah (FE Aus)
(courtesy of Erik Pelham)

Above: Bleeding Heart (AK) (courtesy
of Regina Hornberger)

Left: Red Torch Ginger (FO)

9

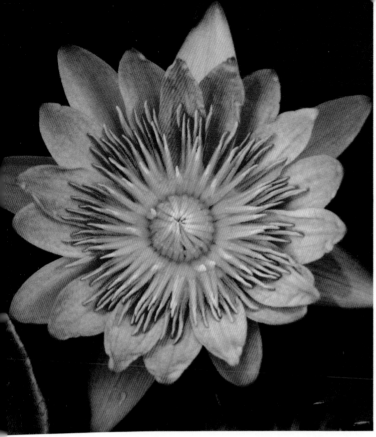

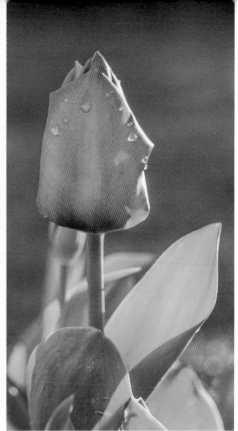

Pink Water-Lily (FO) (courtesy of Cathie Welchman)

Dew on Tulip (courtesy of Amida Harvey)

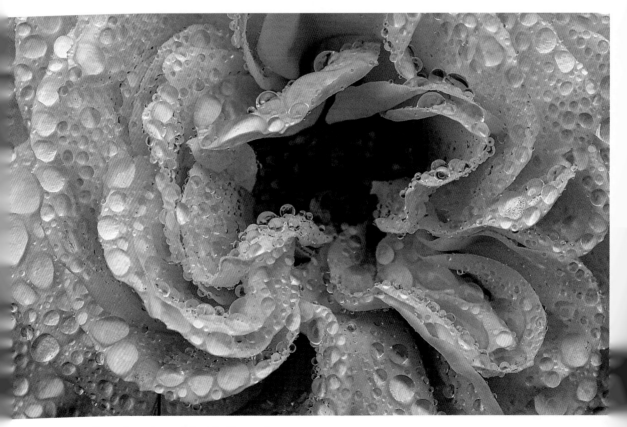

Dew on Roses (courtesy of Amida Harvey)

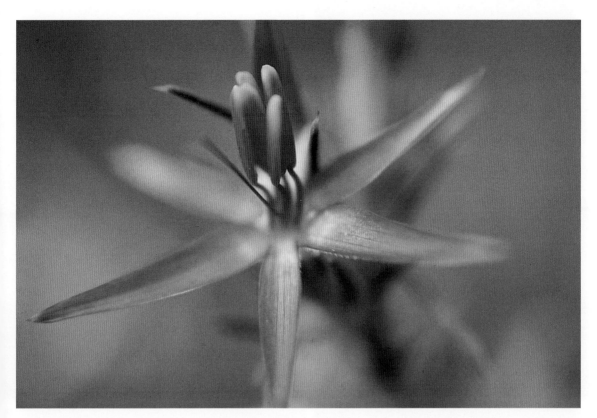

Star of Bethlehem (Aus L) (courtesy of Vasudeva Barnao)

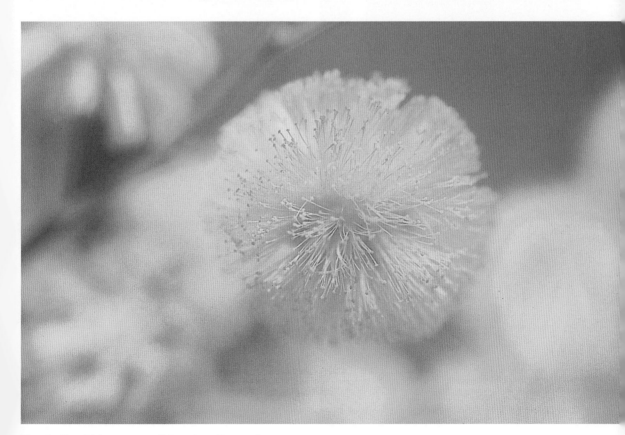

Illyarie (Aus L) (courtesy of Vasudeva Barnao)

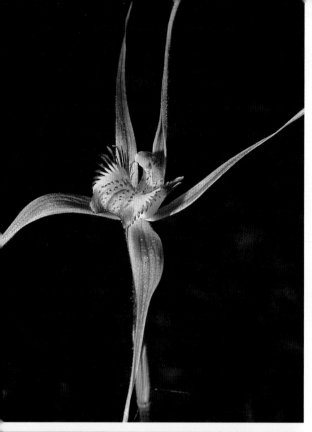

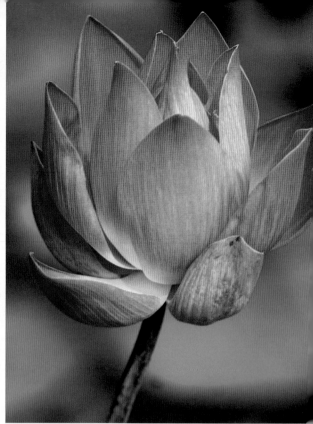

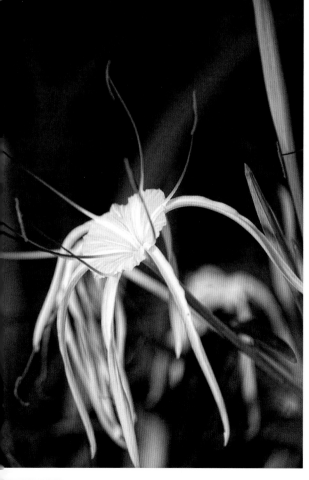

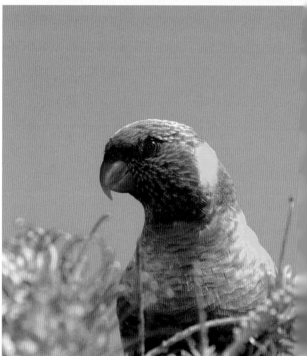

Top left: Spider Orchid (Aus L)
(courtesy of Vasudeva Barnao)

Top right: Pink Lotus (FO)

Above: Rainbow Parakette (source: Dreamstime)

Left: White Spider Lily (courtesy of Savio Joanes)

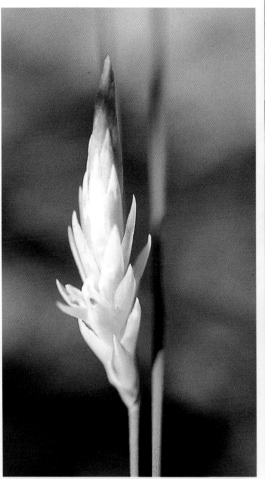

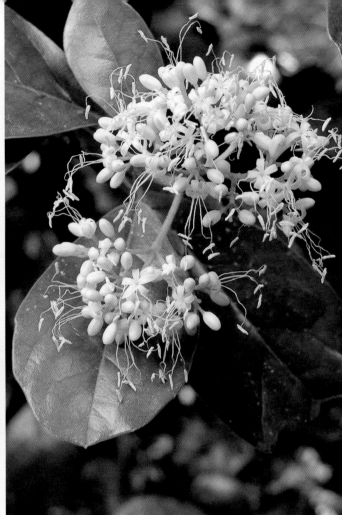

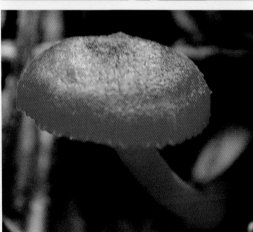

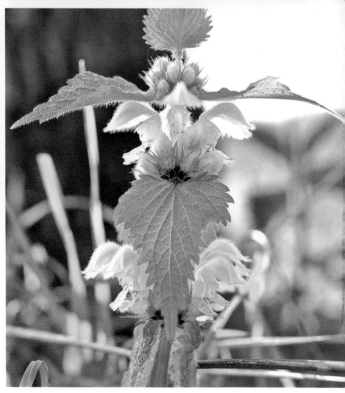

Top left: Candle of Life (Aus L)
(courtesy of Vasudeva Barnao)

Top right: Bridal Tree (NZ) (courtesy
of Franchelle Ofsoské-Wybe)

Above: Red Kali Mushroom (Tasmanian
Wilderness Mushrooms) (courtesy of Tanmaya)

Right: White Archangel (WF)
(courtesy of Paul Strode)

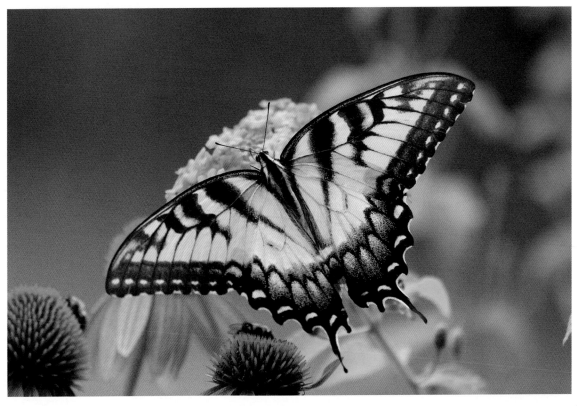

Tiger Swallowtail (Butterfly Essences) (courtesy of Erik Pelham)

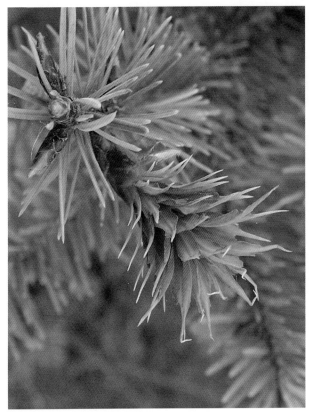

Douglas Fir (GM) (courtesy of Simon and Sue Lilly)

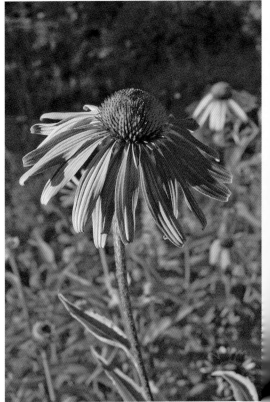

Echinacea (PF, FES) (courtesy of Richard Katz and
Patricia Kaminski © Flower Essence Society, used
by permission, permission is required for re-use

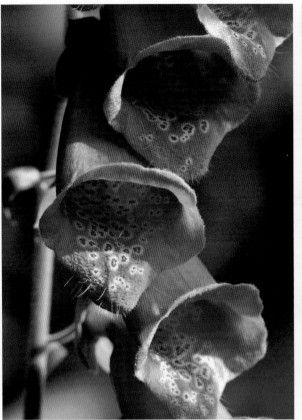
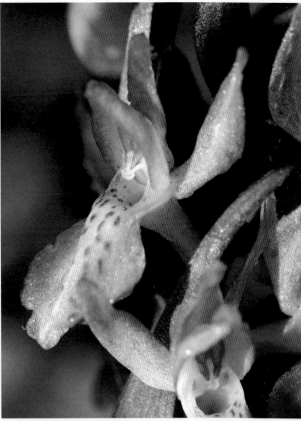
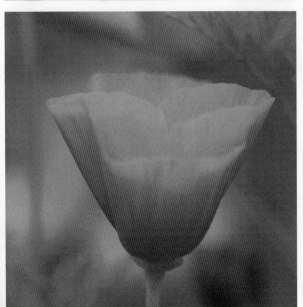
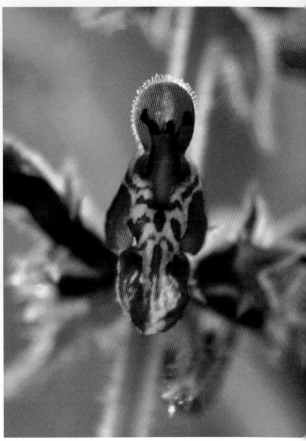

Top left: Purple Foxglove (BL) (courtesy
of Christine and Arthur Bailey)

Top right: Purple Spotted Orchid (WF)
(courtesy of Paul Strode)

Right: Sturt Woundwort (WF) (courtesy of Paul Strode)

Above: Red Poppy (BL) (courtesy of
Bram and Miep Zaalbergis)

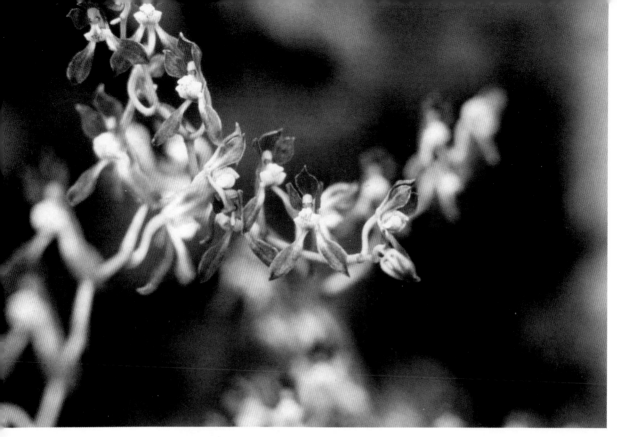

Faith and Courage (Peru) (courtesy of Star Riparetti)

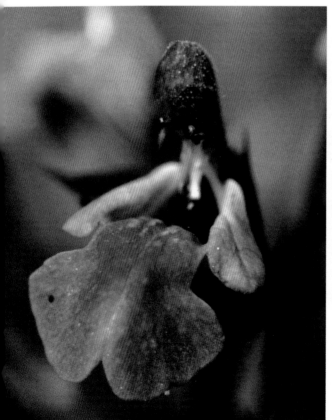

Self-heal (AK) (courtesy of Regina Hornberger)

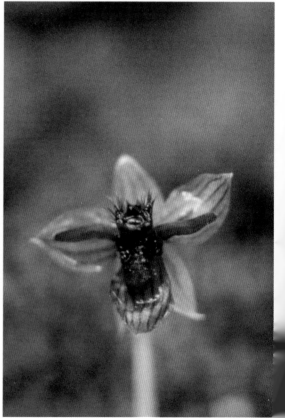

Nature Communion (Peru)
(courtesy of Star Riparetti)

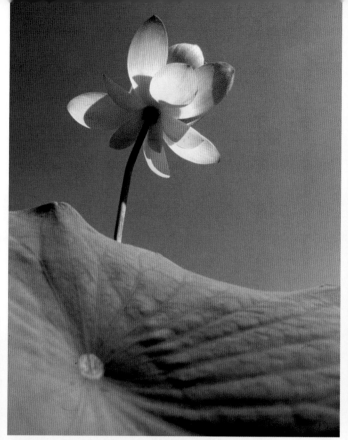

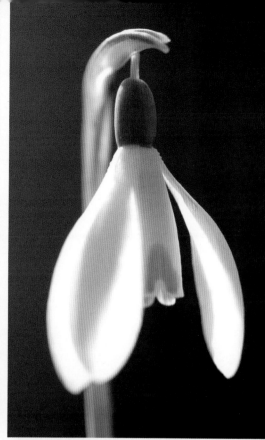

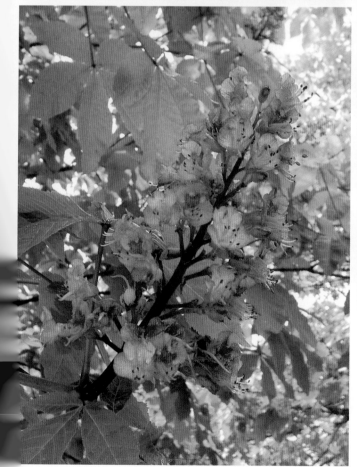

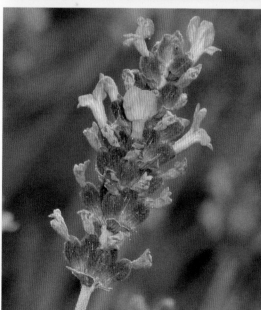

Top left: Lotus (FO, AK) (courtesy
of Helmut Maier)

Top right: Snowdrop (BL) (courtesy
of Christine and Arthur Bailey)

Above: Lavender (FES, AK, PF, Hb)
(courtesy of Deborah Vear)

Left: Red Chestnut (GM) (courtesy
of Julian Barnard)

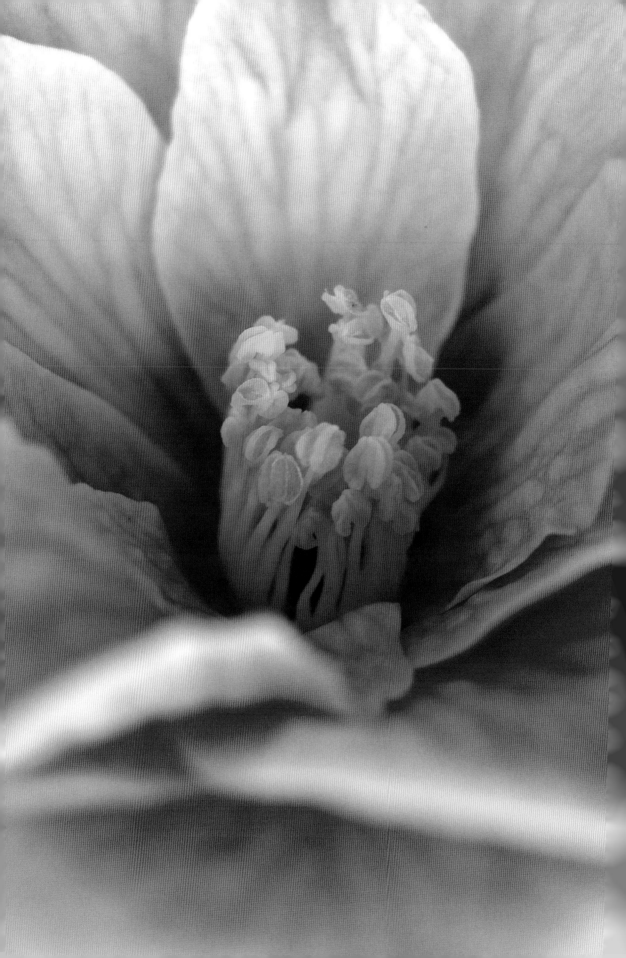

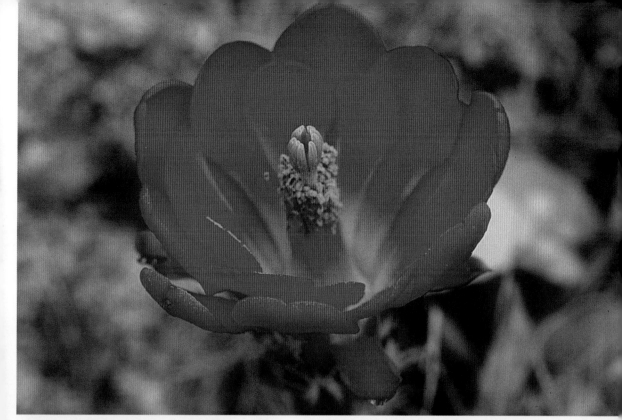

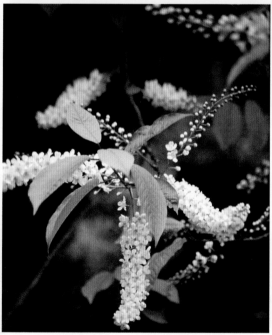

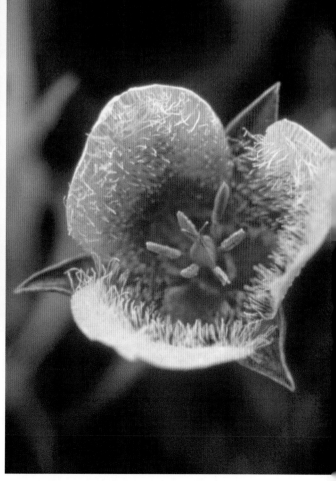

Left: Camellia (PaC) (courtesy of Amida Harvey)

Top: Claret Cup, Hedgehog Cactus (DAl, GH)
(courtesy of Cynthia Athina Kemp Scherer)

Above: Bird Cherry (GM) (courtesy
of Simon and Sue Lilly)

Right: Star Tulip (FES) (courtesy of Richard
Katz and Patricia Kaminski © Flower
Essence Society, used by permission,
permission is required for re-use)

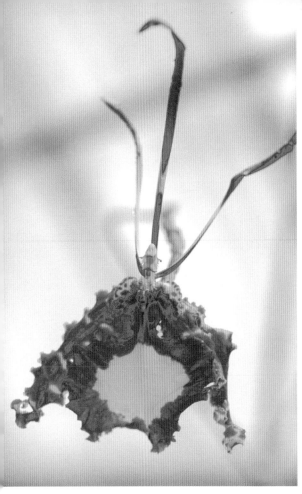

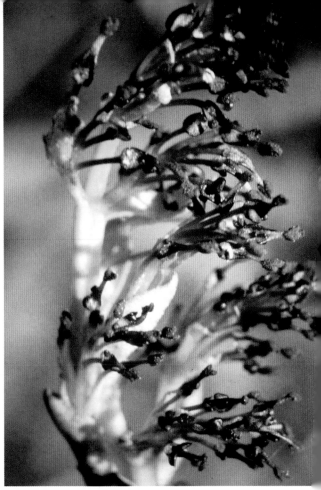

Heart Wings (DL) (courtesy of
Shabd-Sangeet Khalsa)

Ash Male (GM) (courtesy of Simon and Sue Lilly)

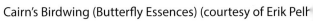

Cairn's Birdwing (Butterfly Essences) (courtesy of Erik Pelh

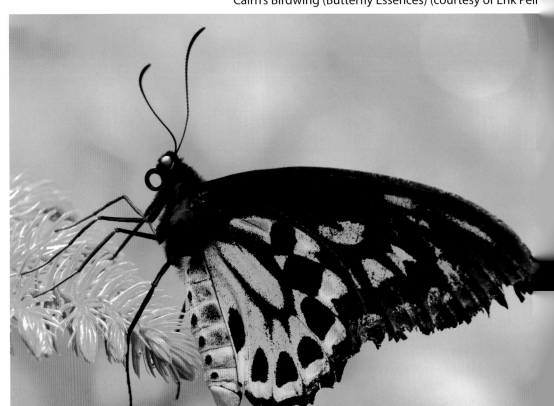

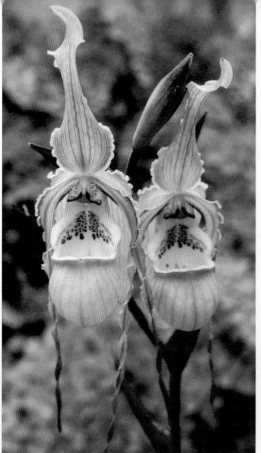

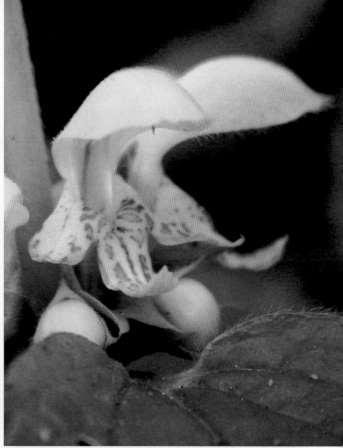

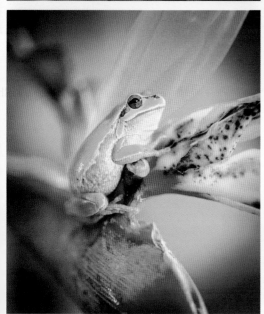

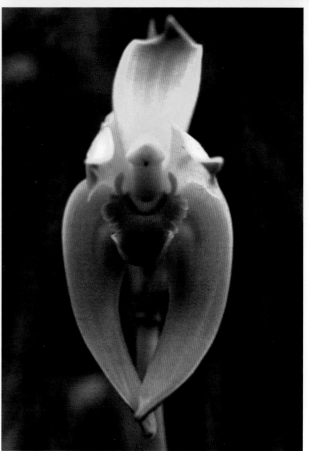

Top left: My Song Calls Me Home (DL)
(courtesy of Shabd-Sangeet Khalsa)

Top right: Yellow Archangel (WF)
(courtesy of Erik Pelham)

Right: Ancient Wisdom (Peru)
(courtesy of Star Riparetti)

Above: Bird of Paradise with
Frog (source: Dreamstime)

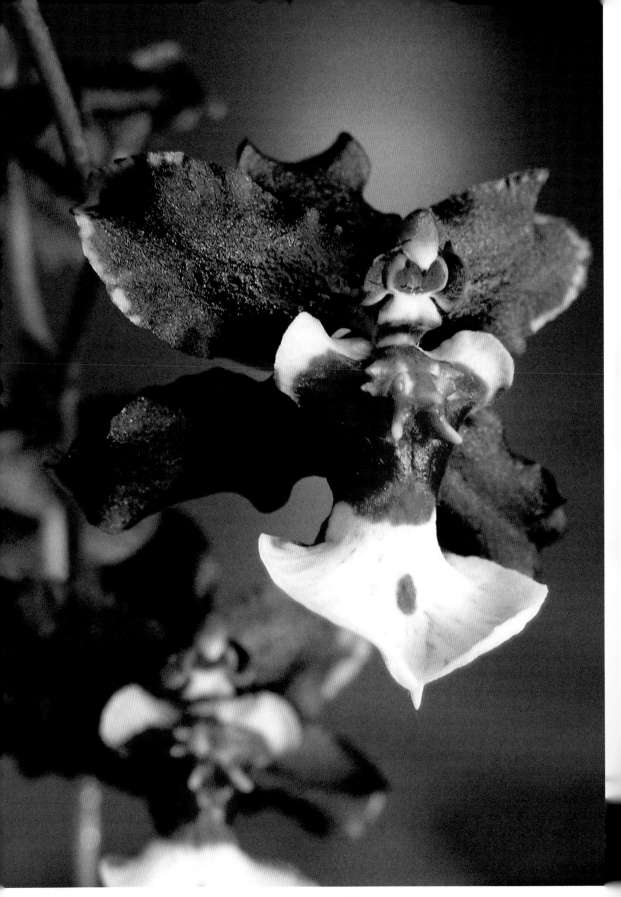

Harmony of the Heart (DL) (courtesy of Shabd-Sangeet Khalsa)

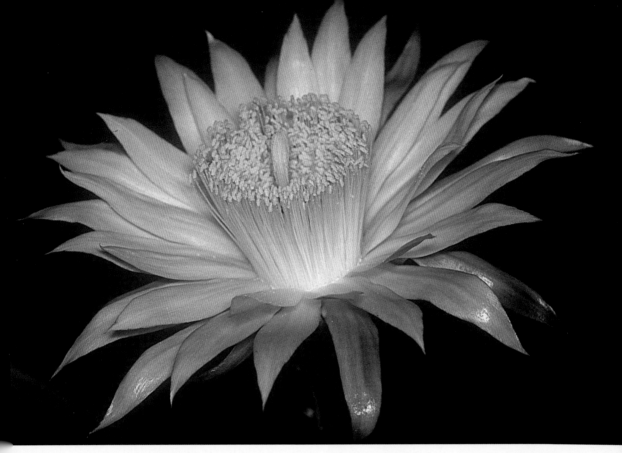

Queen of the Night (AK, Dal) (courtesy of Cynthia Athina Kemp Scherer)

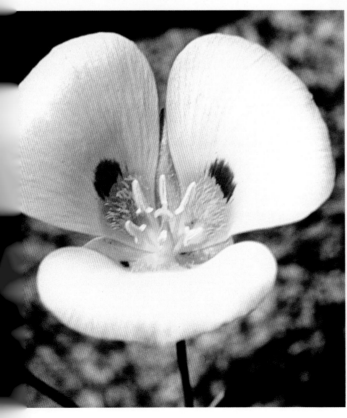

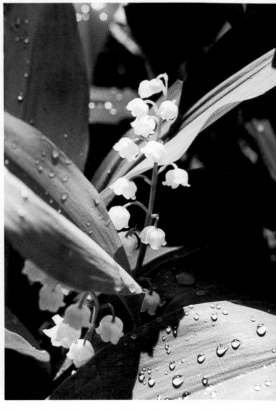

Mariposa Lily (FES, DAI) (courtesy of Richard Katz and Patricia Kaminski © Flower Essence Society, used by permission, permission is required for re-use)

Lily of the Valley (PaC) (courtesy of Sabina Pettitt)

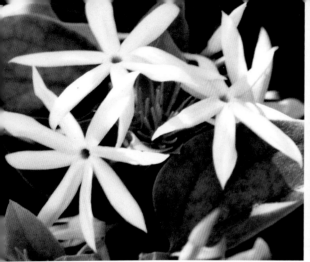

Star Jasmine (Haii) (courtesy
of Cathie Welchman)

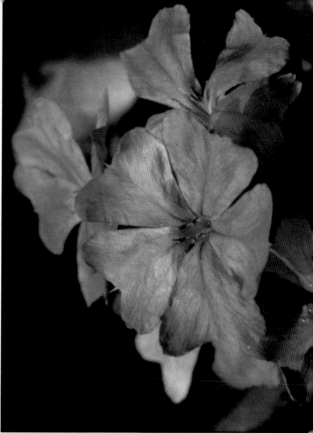

Cerato (B) (courtesy of Julian Barnard)

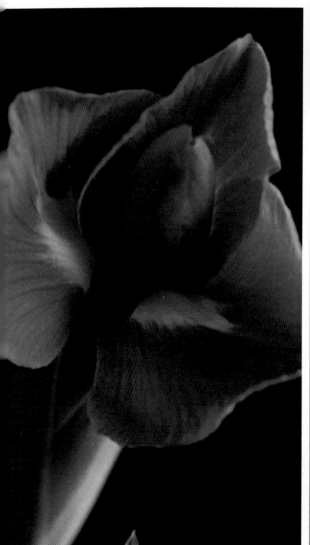

Blue Iris (courtesy of Savio Joanes)

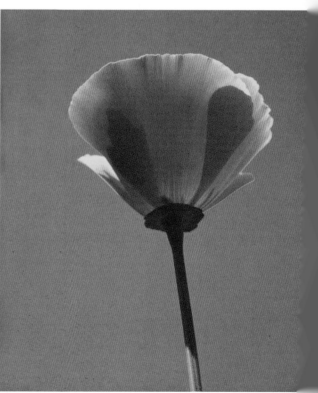

California Poppy (FES) (courtesy of Richard Katz and
Patricia Kaminski © Flower Essence Society, used
by permission, permission is required for re-use)

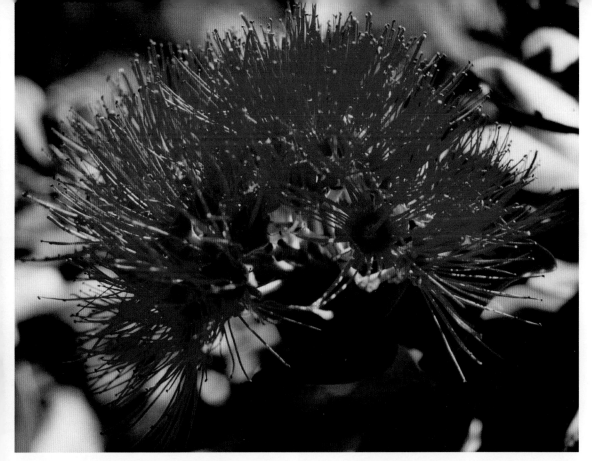

Ohia Lehua (Haii) (courtesy of Cathie Welchman)

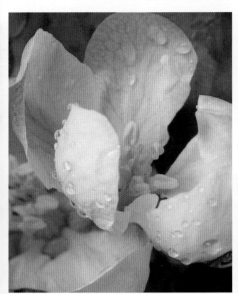

Apple Blossom (courtesy of Deborah Vear)

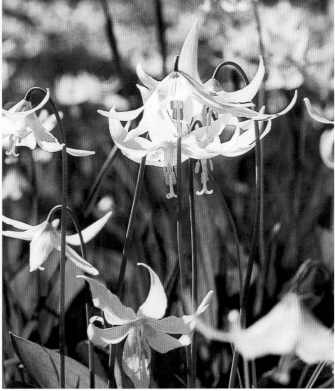

Easter Lily (PaC) (courtesy of Sabina Pettitt)

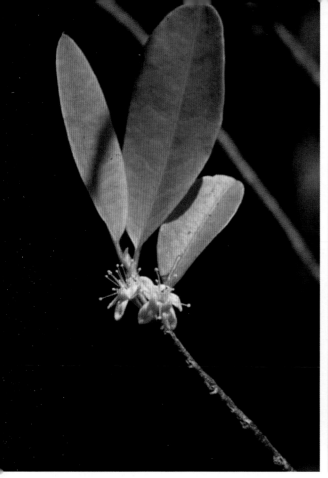

Inocencia Coca (Peru) (courtesy of Star Riparetti)

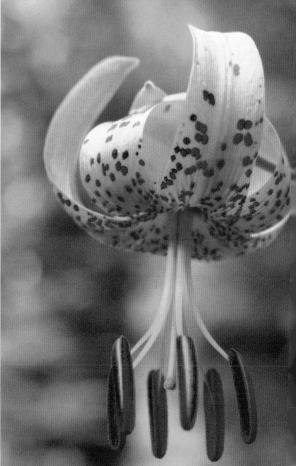

Tiger Lily (FES) (courtesy of Richard Katz and Patricia Kaminski © Flower Essence Society, used by permission, permission is required for re-use)

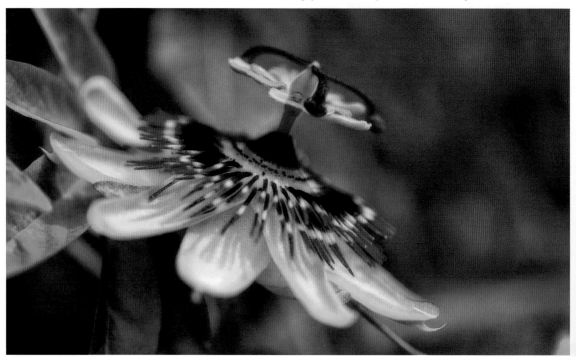

Passion Flower (Haii) (courtesy of Savio Joanes)

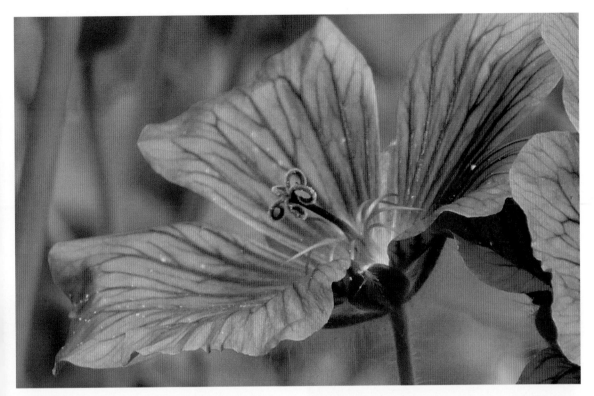

Geranium (Ask, PF) (courtesy of Deborah Vear)

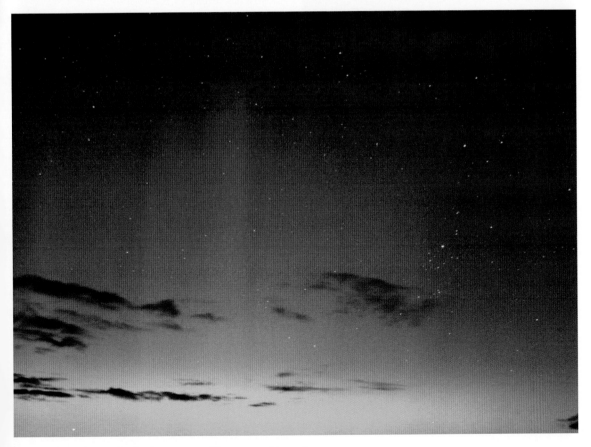

Aurora Borealis in Alaska (courtesy of Lawrence Henry)

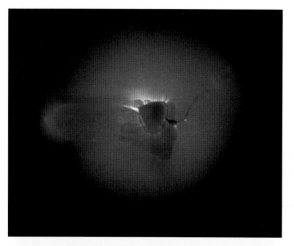

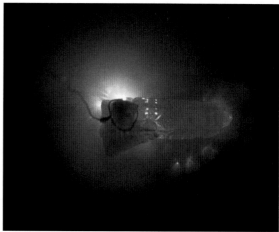

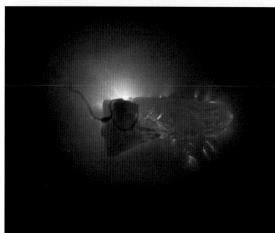

Kirlian Photography

Photographs showing the energetic effects of Cherry Plum essences dropped onto a crystal, starting with a control without any essence, progressing to a few minutes later when the drops have been administered to the crystal (courtesy of Erik Pelham).

Above left: Control
Above: Immediate
Left: After two minutes
Below: After four minutes

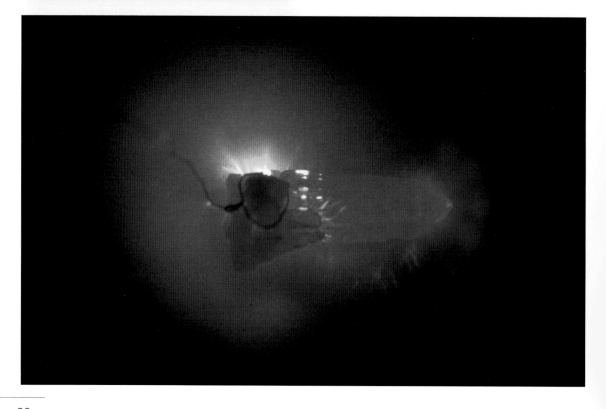

Effect of essences on the subtle anatomy

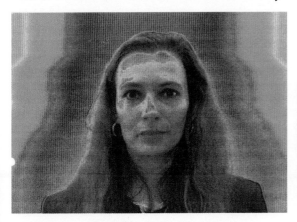

My aura and subtle bodies after a long day at a trade show in Switzerland; the grey and dull areas indicated exhaustion due to contact with so many people; the pink around the eye and nose indicates an open and activated third eye.

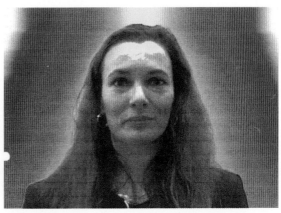

The effect after taking vibrational essences (Star Traveller from Soundwave Essences). The whole aura and subtle bodies are brighter, clearer and refreshed. The column of bright yellow light is the effect just after taking the essences when spiritual energy was drawn down into the crown and third eye chakra.

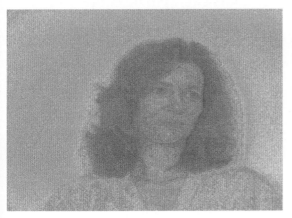

Harry Oldfield's electro-scanning machine 'photographs' the aura and imbalances in the body's energy field. The red/pink areas in the neck and right shoulder regions indicate congestion in the throat chakra and a buildup of muscular tension. I had a slight sore throat and a long motorway journey. The turquoise with yellow indicate a person who heals through changing consciousness.

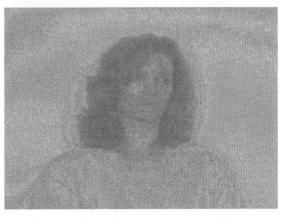

This shows the colour change in the energy field when I held pansy flower essence – an antiviral remedy. The red/pink areas are lessening, clearing the throat and discharging negative energy out through the right side. This also shows pansy's ability to bring violet-coloured energy into the auric field from above, to heal imbalance. (Images courtesy of Harry Oldfield)

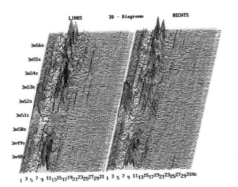
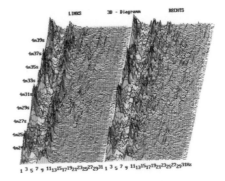

EEG of the effect of dolphin essences (courtesy of Andreas Korte).

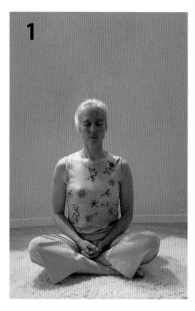
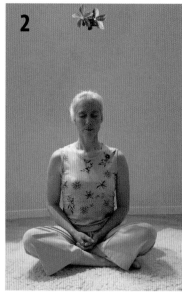
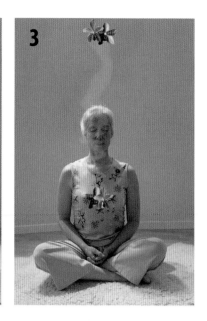

A representation of the process of connecting with the energy of essences

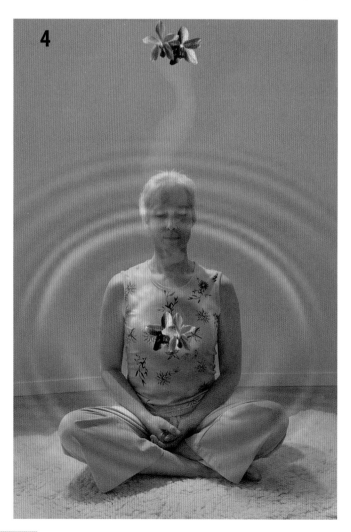

Photo 1:
SSK before taking Acceptance – drops placed on the crown, tongue and heart

Photo 2:
Subtle bodies of the orchids appeared at the 13th chakra as an entry point into the aura. Two orchids were present in combination to make the essence blend into one unified subtle body

Photo 3:
The orchid essence Acceptance was released through the 13th chakra by the orchid essence subtle body as light which softly flowed down through the chakras into the heart chakra.

Photo 4:
At the heart chakra the essence of Acceptance pooled, and then moved outward as ripples on a pool of water. Sit in this softly reverberating pool of watery light allowing yourself to be infused with perceptions of Acceptance wisdom. (courtesy of Shabd-Sangeet Khalsa)

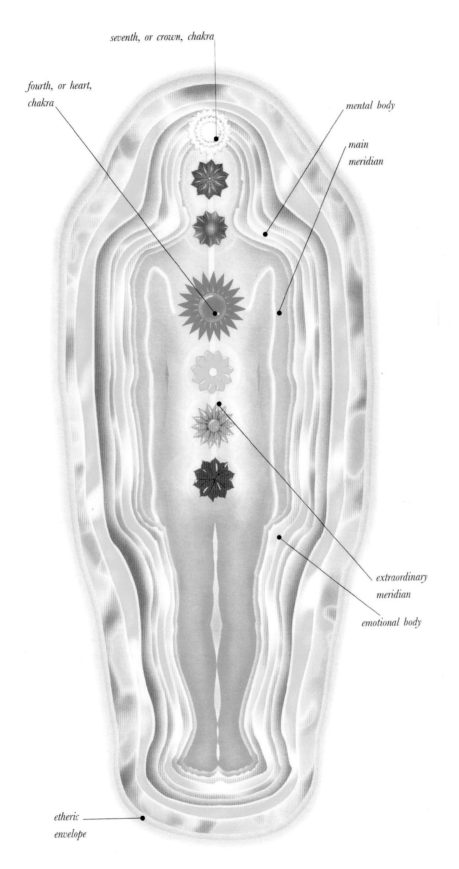

seventh, or crown, chakra

fourth, or heart, chakra

mental body

main meridian

extraordinary meridian

emotional body

etheric envelope

The visual for Clare's explanation of the Subtle Anatomy on pages 40–43.

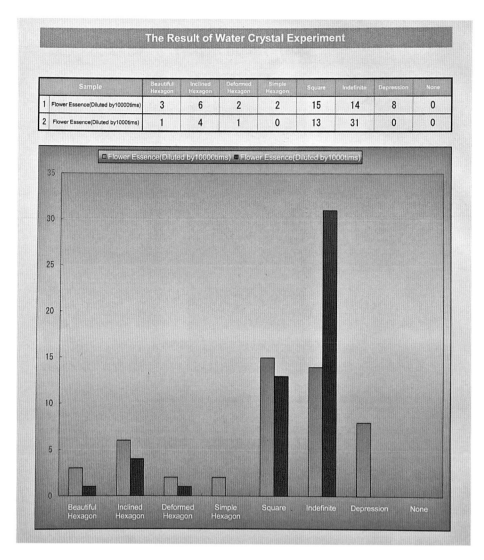

The Result of Water Crystal Experiment

	Sample	Beautiful Hexagon	Inclined Hexagon	Deformed Hexagon	Simple Hexagon	Square	Indefinite	Depression	None
1	Flower Essence(Diluted by10000tims)	3	6	2	2	15	14	8	0
2	Flower Essence(Diluted by1000tims)	1	4	1	0	13	31	0	0

Image courtesy of Dr Emoto and Paul Strode.

This bar chart may offer us an insight into why 'less is more'.

The chart shows the results of 2 different dilutions of Wildflower's White Archangel flower essence.

There are seven different categories of crystal formation that this chart shows. Each category may not necessarily be an absolute representation of the substance tested, but the results of this chart do present a stark difference in the indefinite crystal formations that is worth contemplating.

The indefinite crystal category is when the hexagonal shape that can be seen in the pictures is not fully formed. This may represent a lack of coherence or strength within the substance being tested.

In understanding 'less is more', we dilute a flower essence many times to increase its strength or energetic potency. To understand this, imagine that the packets of energy or life force found within an essence is highly concentrated. When we dilute this concentration, it can increase its availability by making it easier for our energy body to digest (energetic digestion).

We diluted White Archangel flower essence in distilled water by 10,000 times, which the blue bar represents, and 1,000 times, which the red bar represents.

The overall results show a consistent increase in the blue bar, except when we get to the category of indefinite crystal formations, because of the lack of potency. The greater dilution (blue) is constantly showing us better results in all the hexagonal shapes found in the crystal formations.

Magical remedies

Black Tulip (*Tulipa negrita*) Clears the third eye. Brings clarity, perception, vision and originality.

Black Hellebore (*Helleborus niger*) Re-establishes the barriers of the mind, and clears out invading energies from the mind.

Cuckoo Pint (*Arum maculatum*) Protects the spirit from invading entities, and quickly rebuilds vital energy when it has been lost. A great ally in soul retrieval.

Deadly Nightshade (*Atropa belladonna*) Powerful third-eye stimulant and psychic purge. Clears one from psychic interference. To be used as a single dose when required.

Dittany of Crete (*Origanum dictamnus*) Attunes one to positive astral forces, and opens one to help from the spirit world.

Early Purple Orchid (*Orchis mascula*) Makes one fully aware of one's desires, and one's ability to manifest those desires. Strengthens desire.

Enchanter's Nightshade (*Circaea lutetiana*) Acts on the unconscious, so that you draw towards yourself that which you need, particularly spiritual needs.

Four-Leafed Clover (*Trifolium*) The essence of magic. Expands awareness into new dimensions. Aids connection to nature spirits.

Five-Leafed Clover (*Trifolium*) The essence of the magical dynamic of fire. Will, direction, inner strength, purification. (Caution: this essence responds to your thoughts. Always take it with a clear intention in mind.)

Foxglove (*Digitalis purpurea*) Helps one let go of the material plane, of anxiety about one's material situation, or what is to come. Aids transition into other planes. Good for trance work, inner journeying and astral projection.

Henbane (*Hyoscyamus niger*) For understanding death and exploring its realms. Prepares one for death initiations. Connecting with spirits of the dead.

Houndstongue (*Cynoglossum officinale*) Brings out hidden powers from the unconscious, releasing inhibitions and restricting dogma.

Ivy-Leafed Toadflax (*Cymbalaria muralis*) Breaks down inertia on the astral level that builds up through desire for power.

Larkspur (*Delphinium consolida*) Strengthens and clears the aura, particularly the psychic gate. A good protection remedy, it produces a vibration that casts out psychic parasites and external forces.

Lemon (*Citrus limon*) Cleansing and renewal. Removes old, unwanted energies from the person.

Mandrake (*Atropa mandragora*) Connects one with that which is eternal and indestructible within them, and therefore builds confidence by overcoming the illusion of powerlessness.

Marjoram (*Oreganum majorana*) Restores power, will and the knowledge of who you truly are.

Mugwort (*Artemisia vulgaris*) Gives control of the astral plane, and trust in the unseen. Helps creative visualization and the positive use of dreams.

Periwinkle (*Vinca minor*) Prevents energy leakage and recentres one after astral experiences. Focuses energy and prevents dissipation.

Penny Royal (*Mentha pulegium*) A powerful purifier. Activates the crown chakra, earths spiritual energies and unconditional love, and overcomes judgement.

Thornapple (*Datura stramonium*) A very initiating essence that should be taken with clear motivation. Helps movement between different planes of consciousness. Breaks limitations in the mind. Seeing beyond life and death.

Wolfsbane (*Aconitum napellus*) Control of power, and of one's mind. Strengthens visualization and will. Helps awaken latent psychic powers.

Yellow Archangel (*Lamium galeobdolon*) For understanding and accepting the balance of light and dark. Puts one in touch with hidden realms, and helps accept all that one may find in these planes.

Viper's Bugloss (*Echium vulgare*) Understanding primordial powers, and helping them evolve. Helps with the stresses that are due to the emergence of unconscious forces.

Wild Thyme (*Thymus serpyllum*) The essence of feminine power. Creativity, intuition, clairvoyance and psychic power.

CHANNEL ISLAND FLOWER ESSENCES (CHI)

Known for their resplendent wildflowers that can be blooming at any time of the year the Channel Islands are located between the south coast of the UK and France, consisting of the Bailiwick of Guernsey and Jersey. The terrain of the Islands' habitat ranges from fertile soil to barren rocks which ensures a wide and abundant variety of species of flowers. The sea yields its own special flowers: surrounding the shores of the tiny Lihou Island are 130 species of seaweeds.

In the hedgerows and covering the rugged coastline, British as well as Mediterranean flowers grow rampant in a riot of colours, from a swath of Red Sea Campions to a blaze of Yellow Gorse and White Ox-Eyed Daisies. The bright pink flowers of the Fleshy Leaved Mesembryanthemum can be seen colonizing whole cliffs and is truly a sight to be seen.

Created by Susie Morvan, Channel Island Flower Essences originated at the turn of the millennium when Susie felt an inspired connection with the beautiful natural world within the Bailiwick of Guernsey, and made mother tincture from the energetic imprint of flowers she was drawn to in the Islands.

Suzi, a healer and flower essence therapist with a teaching and nursing background, felt that essences' healing qualities were appropriate and effective as dynamic tools for self-healing, emotional balance and harmony, evoking feelings of confidence and motivation, unlocking one's full potential in a natural way.

Combination essences

Borage Carries the vibrational energy of knowing, and resonates with the throat chakra. It aids acceptance of known self; the ability to speak your own truth and feel confident to do so. It promotes a way to see through situations and find coping mechanisms.

Chill Lovingly offers to give a sense of resting the spirit. May be useful for meditation.

Clarity Collection Contains the essence of Borage, Giant Echium and Freesia Rainbow to help you see the way through situations and finding coping mechanisms, to aid personal growth and development, useful with setting and achieving goals.

Connection Collection Contains the essence of Guernsey Lily, Lesser Celandine and Field Violet to enable you to harmonize with the natural rhythm and cycle of life. Promotes a sense of belonging; individually, and on a family global level.

Crisis Collection Contains the essence of Nasturtium, Pink Horse Chestnut/Briza Maxima and Sea Campion to help balance positive and negative emotions, allows healing particularly when in despair.

Directors Cut Designed for those who like to create combinations from this single essence collection: Guernsey Lily, Nasturtium, Lesser Celandine, Pink Horse Chestnut and Briza Maxima, Borage, Giant Echium, Field Violet.

Field Violet Carries the vibrational energy of connection and resonates with the heart and crown chakras. Promotes a sense of belonging; on a family and global humankind level; a gathering together of mutual respect, interest and common goals.

Focus Lovingly offers you a sense of confidence and a belief in your own decision-making abilities.

Freesia Rainbow Carries the vibrational energy of unity, and resonates with the crown chakra. It aids clarity of mood and wisdom. Helps with goal setting and achievement.

Giant Echium Carries the vibrational energy of the visionary and resonates with the brow chakra. It helps to see the bigger picture. Aids personal growth and development, and claiming the right to your own sacred space, and being valued. Enhances relaxation leading to a successful calm repose but also with acute awareness and response to stimuli.

Guernsey Lily Carries the vibrational energy of abundance, and resonates with the root and sacral chakras. It connects with the natural rhythm and harmony of life.

Help Lovingly offers to guard and protect you through times of crisis.

Joy Lovingly offers to help you focus on the joy of this life's purpose.

Lesser Celandine Carries the vibrational energy of individuality, and resonates with the solar plexus chakra. It empowers personal decision-making and connects and harmonizes activity between spiritual and material growth aiding dual direction and stability.

Lesser Toadflax Carries the vibrational energy of confidence and resonates with the solar plexus chakra and the brow chakra forming a linked connection. It helps develop confidence in yourself and belief in your ability to make sound decisions.

Love Lovingly offers to connect you to the natural rhythm and cycle of Life.

Mimosa Carries the vibrational energy of empowerment. It supports a feeling of personal power and belief in one's own abilities. It promotes warmth of persona.

Nasturtium Carries the vibrational energy of balance. Resonates with the sacral and heart chakras. Promotes balance between the positive and negative states of emotion and focuses on the joyful power of this life's purpose.

Pink Horse Chestnut and Briza Maxima Carries the vibrational energy of purification, and resonates with the heart and throat chakras. Gives you the courage to clarify thoughts and feelings towards others. It promotes joyful abandonment and freedom of spirit.

Power Lovingly offers to support a feeling of personal power with warmth of the persona.

Relate Lovingly offers to help you speak your own truth and to feel safe and confident to do so.

Sea Campion Carries the vibrational energy of hope, and resonates with all chakras. It is the choice in crisis, when you are caught up in a whirlpool of despair and need to see through a difficult issue and salvage/awaken hope. It will guard and protect you during this time.

Travel Mate Contains the essence of Guernsey Lily, Sea Campion and Field Violet for feelings of confidence, harmony and relaxation when travelling.

Wisteria Carries the vibrational energy of purpose, and promotes a sense of spiritual grounding and may be useful for meditation.

This unique organically certified range of flower, grass and tree essences encompasses single, combination, multiple gift packs and personal space-enhancing mists.

DEVA FLOWER ELIXIRS (Dv)

In France there exists a very strong tradition of healing with flowers and plants. The doctrine of signatures and principles of homeopathy are widely accepted due largely to the influence of healers such as Goethe and Paracelsus.

Deva Flower Elixirs were started by Philippe Deroide and Dominique Guillet after they had discovered the Flower Essence Society essences (see page 31). The Deva essences are made from the blossoms of flowers growing in the Alps and Mediterranean as well as Deva's own biodynamic gardens. Only the healthiest flowering plants growing in unpolluted environments are chosen; the garden essences are prepared in creative gardens tended according to organic principles.

At the Gaia Institute (the Deva laboratories) homeopaths research the ways in which flower essences exert their benefits. Around 1000 therapists contribute to this work where scientific methodology blends with the intuitive approach to glean information about the healing properties of flower essences.

Almond (*Prunus amygdalus*) For those who fear growing old. Strengthens and regenerates the physical body, joy of living, vitality. Helps us to accept the ageing processes and perceive the beauty beyond superficial physical appearances.

Angelica (*Angelica archangelica*) For emergency situations and each time we feel that our lives are at stake. Offers spiritual protection. Strengthens trust and reinforces resistance in difficult moments. Helps us to face the unknown.

Arnica (*Arnica montana*) To be taken after any physical, mental or emotional trauma. Regenerates and consoles. Repairs damages due to shocks or deep traumas. Re-establishes or maintains our contact with the Higher Self.

Basil (*Ocimum basilicum*) For those who fear and conceal their sexuality – especially when sexuality and spirituality are perceived as opposing forces. Brings sexual integration, helping us to harmonize our emotional and sexual desires with our spiritual worth. Eliminates conflicts of sexual or emotional origins within a relationship by helping us to understand their roots.

Blackberry (*Rubus fruticosus*) For those who cannot materialize their projects, who have difficulties putting their ideas into practice. Also for those hampered by inertia, lethargy and mental confusion. Helps us to overcome confused mental states and develop our hidden talents. Recommended to those who meditate, who practise creative visualization and who work on dreams.

Black-Eyed Susan (*Rudbeckier hirta*) For those who fear looking deeply within themselves and who resist all transformation processes. Aids understanding of hidden emotions and repressed aspects of the self, particularly when the mind censors or disassociates itself from certain aspects of the personality.

Bleeding Heart (*Dicentra spectabilis*) For those who go through a painful experience of separation: loss of a loved one, break-up of a relationship. Fosters the emergence of intense emotions which lie heavy on the heart. Brings harmony and detachment.

Borage (*Borago officinalis*) For depressive temperaments. Fosters courage and self-confidence. Helps us to overcome sorrow, sadness and discouragement when facing trials and danger.

Box (*Buxus sempervirens*) For those who lack will, who are shy, perhaps weak and let themselves become dominated by their nearest and dearest. Helps us develop individuality, detaching ourselves from the domination of others by bringing strength, courage and tenacity.

Buttercup (*Ranunculus acris*) For those who are shy and reserved and have doubts about themselves, who don't know how to appreciate their true worth and underestimate themselves. Brings open-mindedness and trust, and promotes self-esteem.

Calendula (*Calendula officinalis*) For those who listen only superficially and who are often hurtful in what they say. Brings receptivity and understanding beyond words, the real meaning of others' messages. Confers warmth, sensitivity and mellowness in all communications.

California Poppy (*Eschscholzia californica*) Particularly for those who focus on outer means of spiritual development rather than harmonizing with the inner source of spiritual experience. Encourages awakening and recognition of one's qualities and personal abilities. Helps us in our spiritual search by developing attention and inner listening. Safeguards against overfascination with spirituality.

Cayenne (*Capiscum annuum*) A powerful catalyst for overcoming inertia, indecision and immobilization. Develops willpower, brings motivation and enthusiasm. Triggers dynamic transformation when 'stuck' in situations so we can move forward.

Chamomile (*Matricaria recutita*) For nervousness, emotional instability and insomnia. Releases emotional tensions felt mainly in the stomach area. Good for hyperactive children prone to mood changes and to extreme emotional reactions.

Corn (*Zea mays*) For those who live in an artificial environment and need to re-establish contact with the earth (city dwellers). Also for those who tend to shut themselves away when feeling hostile or alienated. Develops the harmonious and balanced relationship between one's social and natural environment.

Comfrey (*Symphytum officinale*) Strengthens and tones up the nervous system. Releases nervous tensions and improves memory. Develops conscious control of physiological processes and improves reflexes. Good for athletes.

Cosmos (*Cosmos bipinnatus*) Allows shy, introverted or hesitant people to express their ideas more clearly and easily, so they can express themselves with calmness and composure when facing the public. Helpful for public speakers, actors and writers.

Daisy (*Bellis perennis*) Helps the mind to synthesize information coming from different sources and integrate them into a global perspective. Useful for those who must plan a project or organize an activity.

Dandelion (*Taraxacum officinale*) For those who do too much and need to learn to release their tensions. Frees muscular, mental and emotional tension. Fosters spiritual openness by relaxing the physical body. Advised for athletes and those doing body work such as masseuses.

Dill (*Anethum graveolens*) For those who feel overwhelmed by the pace of life. Helps us to face up to stress caused by excessive stimulation. Brings liveliness and clear thoughts. Promotes assimilation and understanding of complicated or unusual situations.

Eyebright (*Euphrasia officinale*) Helps healers develop perception of a patient's condition, and increases their sensitivity and intuition.

Fig Tree (*Ficus carica*) For coping with the complexity of modern life in a calm, assured manner. Encourages self-control. Develops mental clarity, confidence and memory. Frees hidden fears and helps in resolving relationship conflicts.

Fireweed (*Epilobium angustifolium*) Liberates tensions and worries caused by traumatizing events. A transformation catalyst which leads one towards a new progressive phase. Promotes regeneration and purification.

Forget-Me-Not (*Myosotis sylvatica*) Releases repressed tensions; stimulates memory, quick wit and insight. Develops our connection with the extrasensory spiritual world. Strengthens the mother–child bond during pregnancy.

Fuchsia (*Fuchsia* hybrid) For freeing deep feelings of anger and sorrow, or feelings linked to sexuality which lead to tension, psychosomatic problems or false emotionalism. An emotional catalyst that encourages the emergence, understanding and elimination of repressed emotions, which often stem from childhood.

Hawthorn May (*Crataegus oxyacantha*) Frees one from outer influences, especially those induced by emotional attachments. Relieves emotional stresses linked to relationship problems. Eases the pain and sorrow of separation. Brings inner freedom.

Hibiscus (*Hibiscus sabdariffa*) For women who have lost all contact with their sexuality. Allows the soul's warmth and feelings to permeate one's sexuality. Frees psychological blocks of sexual origin.

Iris (*Iros germanica*) For eliminating the frustration caused by a lack of inspiration or feelings of imperfection. Brings creative and artistic inspiration.

Lavender (*Lavandula officinalis*) For those whose nervous problems arise from having difficulties integrating spiritual steps to their daily life. A harmonizing essence for those subject to nervous tensions caused by excess stimulation. Brings purification, emotional equilibrium.

Lemon (*Citrus limonum*) Stimulates and lightens the intellect by pushing aside emotional interference and coordinating thoughts. Fosters analytical reasoning.

Lilac (*Syringa vulgaris*) For balancing the flow of energy in the back. Good for those who are fed up. Regenerates the spinal column, corrects posture and brings flexibility.

Linden (*Tilia platyphyllos*) Develops receptivity to love and imbues all communication and exchanges with respect and cordiality. Brings out qualities of protection, nourishing warmth, softness and calmness. Strengthens the relationship between mother and child.

Lotus (*Nelumbo nucifera*) A universal essence for all aspects of the human being. For blossoming and spiritual harmony. Dynamizes and amplifies other remedies. Encourages reception and spiritual openness. Harmonizes the soul forces and purifies the emotions.

Mallow (*Malva sylvestris*) For accepting the transformation processes that occur in life. For overcoming insecurity and introvertedness. Good for those who feel ill at ease socially. Eliminates tension and stress that arise from a fear of ageing. Develops trust and heartiness in shy people.

Martagon Lily (*Lilium martagon*) Recommended for women with fears linked to sexuality, as well as warlike, aggressive, dominating and authoritative individuals. Develops co-operation, solidarity and the ability to listen to others. Helps group work and the search for a joint success.

Morning Glory (*Ipomea purpurea*) For liberating oneself from harmful habits such as dependence on alcohol, coffee, tobacco. Balances vital strength and tones the nervous system. Regularizes the rhythms of daily life.

Mullein (*Verbascum thapsus*) For those in doubt about which moral values to follow.

Encourages awareness of the 'inner voice'. Facilitates and promotes group work by creating unity and developing harmony.

Nasturtium (*Tropaeolum majus*) To be used during 'funny spells', such as when overloaded by work or in a pre-influenza state. Also for those who tend to overindulge the intellect to the detriment of their physical wellbeing. Stimulates vitality.

Nettles (*Urtica dioica*) For resolving psychological problems encountered in perturbed homes. Relieves emotional stress and brings calmness and courage after a family split or break-up. Strengthens family unity.

Onion (*Allium cepa*) For women who have suffered domestic violence or sexual abuse. Eases the process of introspection and the emergence of repressed emotions in psychotherapy. For emotional liberation and 'letting go'.

Passion Flower (*Passiflora incarnata*) Frees physical tensions, allowing us to consider life's events calmly and serenely. Brings stability and eliminates emotional confusion. Opens us up to higher levels of consciousness. For spiritual balance.

Pennyroyal (*Mentha pulegium*) For those disturbed by others' negative thoughts. Reduces the mental confusion provoked by the ill will of others. For protection.

Peppermint (*Mentha piperita*) For those who tend to be dull-minded due to excess mental activity. Helps us to overcome mental laziness and psychic lethargy. Develops mental clarity and a quick wit; encourages active and awakened thought processes. Good for students and intellectuals.

Pink Yarrow (*Achillea millefolium*) For those who are too emotional or who identify with the emotions of others. Protects against emotional tension emitted from the surrounding environment. Reinforces the emotional structure of those who are oversensitive and easily influenced.

Pomegranate (*Punica granatum*) For emphasizing all the feminine qualities. Helps women to resolve conflicts whose origin is an imbalance between career and family life. Balances feminine creativity.

Quince (*Cydonia oblonga*) For women confronted with power conflicts who have difficulty integrating their outer ambitions such as professional ambitions – with maternal love. Balances the feminine aspect of the personality.

Red Clover (*Trifolium pratense*) For keeping one's psychic equilibrium. Recommended in emergency situations such as disasters, conflicts. Allows us to remain calm and centred while facing fear, panic or the collective hysteria generated by certain groups or certain collective states of mind.

Rhododendron (*Rhododendron ferrugineum*) For those inclined to sadness, melancholy and discouragement when confronted with a difficult and harsh environment. Brings warmth, consolation and a sense of joy; encourages emotional liberation in the thoracic area (linked to breathing).

Rosemary (*Rosmarinus officinalis*) For those who are disorientated, prone to forgetfulness and drowsiness, find it difficult to be present in their body. Develops clarity of mind and sensitivity. Helpful for introverted and sullen temperaments. For inner peace.

Sage (*Salvia officinalis*) Promotes reflection on the meaning of life's events. Brings understanding, inner peace and consciousness of our spiritual dimension. Allows us to look more objectively at life's experiences.

Scarlet Monkeyflower (*Mimulus cardinalis*) For those who repress powerful emotions linked to anger and aggressiveness, fearing a loss of self-control or the disapproval of others. Liberates these emotions, helping to resolve power struggles and angry situations in relationships. Frees the vitality that may be concealed by repressed negativity and resentment.

Scotch Broom (*Cystisus scoparius*) For pessimism, discouragement and despair. Helps us to consider life's hardships as opportunities for growth and evolution. Brings tenacity and perseverance to those who are continually confronted by obstacles.

Self-Heal (*Prunella vulgaris*) A catalyst for inner healing and transformation, enabling us to develop our inner power of healing. Supports us when we are fasting or convalescing. Helps the body assimilate most nutritional substances. Good for those who try many therapies unsuccessfully.

Snapdragon (*Antirrhinum majus*) For those who find it difficult to express their feelings. Encourages us to give voice to our repressed emotions. Encourages verbal 'letting go' and the expression of truth.

Spruce (*Picea abies*) For those suffering from tenseness, austerity and coldness, who lack flexibility and refuse to make compromises or concessions. Brings grace and harmony.

Sticky Monkeyflower (*Mimulus aurantiacus*) For integrating love and sexuality, discovering the sacred meaning of all life's aspects. Frees fears and resolves conflict or confusion linked to sexuality and intimacy. Balances out sexual energies.

St John's Wort (*Hypericum perforatum*) For children prone to restless dreams. Offers freedom from nightmares, nocturnal fears, night terrors, feelings of obscurity and the fear of death. For courage, protection and freedom.

Sunflower (*Helianthus annuus*) For resolving conflicts linked to parents or parental images. Balances the ego when it is excessive (vanity) or lacking (low self-esteem). Develops the harmonious expression of our spiritual nature, helping us to work in a creative manner. Encourages our individuality.

Sweet Corn (*Zea mays*) Balance. Balances out and energizes the individual in his or her relationship with the Earth (vertical) and with other human beings (horizontal). Develops harmonious relationships with one's social and natural environment by bringing about love and understanding. This essence is advised for those living in an urban environment, especially those confronted by overpopulated environments. For those who tend to shut themselves up when feeling hostile and alienated. For those who live in an artificial environment and who need to re-establish a contact with the Earth.

Valerian (*Valeriana officinalis*) To overcome insomnia, stress and nervous irritation. Brings tranquillity and peace.

Watermelon (*Citrullus vulgaris*) For birth: the development of a harmonious and correct attitude before, during and after conception in couples wishing to have a child. Eliminates emotional stress during pregnancy.

White Yarrow (*Achillea millefolium*) For those who feel too vulnerable and those who, through their professions, are confronted with the problems of others. Reinforces the energy structure of the individual and protects against disturbing environmental influences (radioactivity, electromagnetism and the electronic radiation of computers).

Wild Garlic (*Allium sativum*) For eliminating fear, anxiety, insecurity and nervousness. Releases tension around the solar plexus. Strengthens any part of us that is prone to repeated infections and to general weakness.

Zinnia (*Zinnia elegans*) Cheerfulness and joy. For those who are depressed, restless or hypersensitive and need to laugh. Helps us to accept that laughter is a very effective therapy. Releases tensions. Helps adults who have communication problems with their children to rediscover the child within them.

Zucchini (*Cucurbita pepo*) For a harmonious pregnancy. Helps pregnant women balance out their emotions and eliminate physical tensions. Generally stimulates and increases feminine creativity, especially when it has been smothered and repressed due to difficult social and cultural environments.

24 complementary essences

Alpine Lady's Mantle (*Alchemilla alpina*) Unconditional love, confidence, protection. For those suffering from, or who have suffered from, the lack of a bond with the mother, who are incapable of expressing tenderness towards their parents, family and those close to them, and who are in permanent need of love. Favours the letting go of repressed emotions. Helpful in rediscovering the capacity to love.

Amaranthus (*Amaranthus caudatus*) Going beyond one's limits. For situations of deep distress. Permits you to overcome feelings of devastation, hostility, solitude and rejection. Helps in confronting and coping with extreme suffering, the most total sense of desolation, hopeless situations in which there is no way out. Reinforces the organism when feeling under attack, weakened or off balance.

Apricot (*Prunus armeniaca*) Joy, plenitude. For intellectual temperaments, with multiple responsibilities, who are subject to rapid mood swings, who are not at ease in their bodies and who display a tendency to hyperglycaemia. Helpful in overcoming mental and emotional tension. Facilitates the resolution of inner conflict.

Birch (*Betulus pendula*) Vitality and regeneration. Greater dynamism, revitalization. For overcoming sclerotic tendencies, related to ageing. Helpful for understanding the meaning of one's existence by going beyond rigid attitudes and behaviour.

Bistort (*Polygonum bistorta*) Openness, self-control. For remaining faithful to one's own aspirations while recognizing and respecting those of others. Helps in overcoming feelings of disorientation, dispersion and lack of presence. For returning to one's centre. Strengthens those who do not have, or no longer have, their feet on the ground, particularly in times of great change.

Echinacea (*Echinacea purpurea*) Integrity and wholeness. Recommended when the dignity and moral integrity of the being are shattered by violent acts and situations. Helps in recovering one's profound identity through self-respect and self-esteem.

Elder (*Sambucus nigra*) Regeneration, purification, vitality. Helps in overcoming feelings of shame, of dirtiness or of imperfection. For dull temperaments, the withdrawn, submissive person lacking in vitality. For those who reject their body or hide behind false appearances. Recommended when one feels abandoned or filled with uncertainty. For moments when one feels at a loss, when one lacks self-esteem following a shock or a difficult event in one's life.

Eucalyptus (*Eucalyptus globulus*) Enthusiasm, faith in life. For overcoming melancholy, sadness and chagrin provoked by conflict in relationships or by unresolved emotional traumas that remain blocked in the respiratory sphere. Gives help in getting over past traumas and moving on.

Golden Yarrow (*Achillea filipendulina*) Openness, protection. For hypersensitive and vulnerable temperaments, who have a tendency to cut themselves off from the outside world to protect themselves. Favours the growth and development of the personality within an active social-life setting, while preserving individuality and sensitivity.

Greater Celandine (*Chelidonium majus*) Self-expression, exchange, openness. Facilitates communication, exchange and receptivity.

For obtuse, obstinate temperaments that are closed in on themselves and have difficulty in communicating.

Hyssop (*Hyssopus officinalis*) Repentance, pardon. For getting over feelings of guilt when one is convinced of having done wrong. Allows one to understand and to go beyond the attitudes and behaviour patterns that are at the root of this guilt.

Jasmine (*Jasmine officinalis*) Purification, self-acceptance. For those who put themselves down, who have a negative image of themselves or who lack self-esteem. For feeling at ease with oneself and at home in the body. Favours the opening of the heart and the rediscovery of one's true spiritual identity. Eliminates toxins, real or imagined.

Lady's Mantle (*Alchemilla vulgaris*) Maternal consciousness, accomplished femininity. For women who reject their femininity in its maternal and nourishing aspects. Attenuates the effects of any shock concerning the genitals. Helps in overcoming feelings of loss, of need or emptiness associated with troubles in the area of reproduction. On another level, strengthens the connection with nature and the Earth.

Lily of the Valley (*Convallaria majalis*) Innocence, spontaneity, freedom of action. For those whose lives are dictated by duties, obligations and social conventions. For those who seek the approval of others and are prisoners of external conditioning. For rebellious temperaments, ever on the defensive, who refuse conformity but find themselves dependent on outside conditions which do not correspond to their true nature. Recommended for adolescents who have left the world of childhood too abruptly and cannot find their place in the adult world.

Maple Tree (*Acer campestre*) Vitality, dynamism, fluidity. Favours the balancing out and circulation of energies. For those who feel immobilized, in periods of stagnation.

Tones up and revitalizes the organism when energy is not flowing. Recommended in acupuncture.

Mimosa (*Acacia dealbata*) Openness, empathy. For timid temperaments, introverts, independent people who turn in on themselves and cut themselves off from others. Facilitates opening up to others and the world. A flower essence recommended in periods of discouragement and depression, in moments of solitude, when one feels abandoned.

Orange Tree (*Citrus sinensis*) Emotional release. A powerful catalyst used to favour emotional catharsis. Liberates emotional tensions and helps in coping with conflicts related to them. Appeases frazzled emotions.

Pansy (*Viola tricolor*) Interior strength, resistance. For those who feel vulnerable, who lack strength and are subject to repeated infections. Strengthens and protects the organism.

Peach (*Prunus persica*) Altruism, letting go. A healing catalyst that facilitates the liberation of tensions. For those who are over-concerned with their problems and are unable to open up to others and the world. Recommended for external application.

Pear Tree (*Pyrus communis*) Balance, bodily ease. Helps to recentre after all situations of imbalance. Brings balance to the spinal column and favours the alignment of the body in its vertical axis.

Petunia (*Petunia* hybrid) Mental clarity, enthusiasm. For those who lack enthusiasm or are, on the contrary, too exuberant and dispersed in what they are doing to reach a determined goal. Helps for examining priorities, eliminating the superfluous, looking at the essential and getting straight to the point.

Pimpernel (*Anagallis arvensis*) Self-affirmation. For problems related to authority and the father image. For those who have difficulty in taking part, getting involved in the action and lack willpower.

Tabacum (*Nicotiana tabacum*) Opening of the heart. For nervous temperaments, dry and tense people who have lost all heart connection with their environment. For loss of sensitivity, emotional coldness. For overcoming the mechanistic tendencies of the modern world.

Tansy (*Tanacetum vulgare*) Decisiveness, action. For undecided, slow and apathetic temperaments, who refuse to take action, refusing to get on with things, always putting things off until later, afraid of constraints, of getting involved, and wanting to be left in peace.

Wild Carrot (*Daucus carota*) Perspicacity, sensitivity. Favours the awakening of clairvoyance and parapsychic qualities. For those who are overmental or overemotional and do not allow the other psychic faculties to develop.

Wild Cherry (*Prunus avium*) Gaiety, good humour. For pessimistic and gloomy temperaments who see only the negative side of things. For developing a serene and optimistic view of life.

Wood Betony (*Stachys officinalis*) Harmonious sexuality. Helps to resolve inner conflict related to sexuality. Brings balance to sexual expression when it is perturbed (excessive sexual activity, degrading sexual practices). For overcoming compulsive needs provoked by sexual fantasies and desire.

Wood Violet (*Viola sororia*) Healthy sensitivity. For timid, vulnerable and self-effacing temperaments who like solitude. Cold and reserved in appearance, they are afraid of being exposed and have difficulty in opening up to others. Helps them to communicate and overcome excess.

Combination essences

Also available as 10 and 30ml sprays. Note: all combination essence bottles and sprays (except 'Assistance') are only available upon request.

Assistance (also available as a cream)
Contains the five essences that comprise Bach's 'Rescue Remedy' plus Lotus.
Positive outcome: Assistance, balance, stability, regeneration.
Patterns of imbalance: Emergencies, crisis situations, shock. A basic combination for use in all crisis situations, in moments of great tension and for getting over hardships of all sorts. Used for remaining calm and collected and for keeping a cool head when confronted with difficulties, it can also be used in a preventive way when some sort of stressful event is expected, to deal with apprehension, fear of losing control or feeling lost and confused, (exams, unusual situations, etc.). (This combination formula is not intended to be used over a long period.)

Physical Ease
Positive outcome: Vigour, suppleness, litheness and ease, gracefulness, psycho-physical harmony.
Patterns of imbalance: Physical and emotional tension. This combination formula is recommended for sportsmen and people who do strenuous physical activity. Taken before and after physical exertions it keeps the body supple and lithe, and the muscles relaxed. It improves coordination between the mind and body helping to prepare for action, and favours recovery after strenuous activity. This formula is also recommended for hyperactive people, who tend to do too much, stretching their physical capacities to the limit.

Protection
Positive outcome: Protection, well-adjusted openness to others and balanced sensitivity.
Patterns of imbalance: Vulnerability, fragility, negative influence. This combination formula is recommended for those who feel vulnerable to others and their surroundings.

It provides protection from disturbing influences present in the environment. These can be psychic (negative thoughts and intentions) or physical (radioactivity, electric and electromagnetic pollution, computers). For sensitive people, the easily influenced, those with emotive temperaments who tend to identify too easily with their surroundings. For the extremely sensitive person who tends to withdraw and turn in on him or herself, it provides protection from negativity in the environment and assistance in overcoming feelings of insecurity.

Balanced Sexuality

Positive outcome: Brings balance to emotional life and the heart, healthy and harmonious sexuality.

Patterns of imbalance: Sexual troubles. Brings the emotional life and sexuality into harmony. Makes it easier to express deep feelings and develop an honest appraisal of one's love life. This formula is recommended when there is difficulty in expressing sexuality in a harmonious way, when it becomes predominant to the detriment of other values or is the cause of conflict in a relationship. Brings about a harmonious blending of loving feelings with physical passion, and gives warmth and vitality to sexual expression.

Self-Balance

Positive outcome: Spiritual resource, inner peace, groundedness.

Patterns of imbalance: Overwhelmed, stress of city life, disorientation. This formula is recommended for those who live in a difficult environment and suffer because of it. It is for those who have the feeling of being strangers on this Earth, for getting back in touch with one's roots and finding inner stability. By helping the soul to express its spiritual nature it makes us aware we can overcome the limitations of the physical world. Used for the stress of city life (sensorial overload caused by too many stimuli, noises, sights; the impression of being imprisoned in crowded places).

Peaceful Sleep

Positive outcome: Calm, relaxation, restful sleep.

Patterns of imbalance: Insomnia, nervousness, mental agitation. This combination formula is recommended for calming children and adults alike when they are unable to relax, have difficulty in getting to sleep or have restless nights (nightmares, disturbed sleep, etc.). Children who tend to have mood swings and extreme emotional reactions become peaceful and relaxed with this combination formula. It is also recommended for people with hyperactive temperaments who find it hard to wind down at the end of the day, as well as for those whose minds are full of repetitive thoughts or constant worry.

Studies and Tests

Positive outcome: Attention, concentration, creativity, ability to synthesize.

Patterns of imbalance: Difficulties in expression and concentration. To optimize the intellectual abilities and facilitate verbal expression. Develop intellectual sharpness and the ability to synthesize by favouring global understanding and avoiding focus on details. Helps overcome mental lethargy and express thoughts clearly and with coherence. To arouse creative potential and integrate the learning processes. For research, studies, exam periods, teaching and writing. Recommended for students, researchers, speakers.

Family Unit

Positive outcome: Listening, understanding, fellowship.

Patterns of imbalance: Rejection, lack of understanding, stress and conflict. Strengthens the family unit. Develops emotional bonds. Favours communication, understanding and the expression of deep feelings within a group or family. Helps overcome emotional disorders related to transgenerational conflicts, as well as the resulting suffering and confusion. Favours the understanding and resolution of negative family conditioning that parasitizes community life. Recommended when everyday situations tend to create barriers between family or group members.

Pregnancy

Positive outcome: Emotional balance, confidence, vitality, receptivity.

Patterns of imbalance: Hypersensibility, vulnerability, uneasiness. Helps the pregnant woman both physically and emotionally by balancing the emotions and eliminating physical stress. Reduces nausea and soothes gastric disorders. Helps overcome nervous stress and hypersensitivity. Reinforces the bonds with the baby before it is born. Facilitates the arousal of maternal qualities and develops confidence in the ability to be a mother.

Evolution

Positive outcome: Courage, clarity, commitment, determination, letting go.

Patterns of imbalance: Inertia, being prisoner of the past, inability to move forward. A complex for periods of change, transformation and self-questioning, when it is necessary to give up old habits in life and behaviour that is not adapted to the present situation and that does not have any reason to continue. Recommended in all phases of minor or major transition: moving, change of social environment, change in career, break-ups. To free oneself from past emotional bonds that prevent moving forward. Help remain centred in periods of major change and look towards the future with courage and confidence. Stirs up the will for change and to not remain bogged down in inertia and inaction. To follow one's road outside of all external influence. Recommended when one wants to become free of a self-image that is false and conveyed by others.

Maturity

Positive outcome: Vitality, joy of living, perspective.

Patterns of imbalance: Fear of ageing, loss of interest, stagnation, lack of satisfaction. Helps get some distance from life's experiences and develop new meaning. For those who feel that life is behind them and who are feeling bitter, harsh, weary and discouraged. Revitalizes and helps overcome the sclerotic tendencies of age. To overcome the fear of ageing or seeing oneself age. Helps break habits that prevent evolution. Facilitates the passage of menopause and helps women go through this period like a healthy and positive transition.

Adolescence

Positive outcome: Will, enthusiasm, affirmation and self-acceptance.

Patterns of imbalance: Self-withdrawal, rejection of others, feeling of isolation and lack of understanding, lack of satisfaction, apathy, immaturity. This complex helps overcome adolescent identity crisis. For those who don't feel comfortable with themselves. To harmoniously integrate sexual identity. To positively affirm one's individuality and defend one's ideas when confronted with family, social and cultural pressures. To avoid letting the adolescent withdraw into illusory experiences that weaken the will (drugs, abuse of passive situations). For those who are confused as to their future and who still have not found a direction in their life. Frees the creative potential of the individual.

Early Childhood

Positive outcome: Openness, self-esteem, social enthusiasm, creativity.

Patterns of imbalance: Feeling of abandonment, self-withdrawal, lack of self-confidence, timidity or aggressiveness. A complex to facilitate the learning of social skills and encourage the child to open up to the world. To develop harmonious relations with the environment, whether within or outside the family unit. Balances the mother–child relationship. Stimulates the affective warmth and favours tenderness between the child and those around him or her. Develops the spirit of companionship and helps overcome the fear of others. Favours balanced self-esteem. Preserves and encourages spontaneous artistic creativity in the child, especially when the social or environmental context tends to stifle creativity. Recommended in situations of ill-treatment and abandon.

MEDITERRANEAN ESSENCES (Med)

The azure-blue, crystalline waters of the beautiful Alboran, Ligurian, Adriatic and Aegean seas, and the sea of Crete are all waters of the Mediterranean. The large islands of Cyprus, Crete, Sicily, Corsica, Sardinia and Majorca, coupled with Greece (which alone counts more than 2000 large and smaller islands, of which only 100 are inhabited), are all within the Mediterranean's umbrella.

The Mediterranean has been a melting-pot, a crucible that generated agriculture and alphabets, empires and democracy, mythologies and major world religions, and was perhaps once the most significant source of civilization in the world. With all its diversity it is evident the Mediterranean area is broad minded, open to exchange, philosophy and other people. Everywhere you turn there is the influence of thousands of years of human exploration, expanding horizons, spiritual searching, creativity and a fountain of innovation. There is the fascinating meeting of diverse peoples with strong temperaments, cultures and languages.

It has been said that 'the Mediterranean blends thousands of substances at a time'.

Mediterranean folks live in the open as much as they do indoors. Climatic conditions allow outdoor living most of the time and they seek sun, light and air. For centuries, this way of life, often following Roman ways, contributed to developing relations and access to the more remote regions to be found in mountainous areas. This nomad way of life indicates a whole different concept of time, space and freedom and the joy they experienced with the beauty and brightness of the wonderful flora and fauna, land and seascapes.

Launched in 2013, the Mediterranean Essences have been co-created by Angie Jackson and Adam Rubinstein. Their passion for both the Mediterranean and the world of essences came together in 2002 to create this project. Since then they have been making flower, mineral and environmental essences at varied locations and sacred sites all over the diverse

and historic Mediterranean region. The Mediterranean Essences encapsulate the energy and spirit of this rich and magical arena. They connect us with support, inspiration and wisdom, empowering us to move forward on our journey with both insight and grounding.

Angie, the initiator of Mediterranean Essences, has been supporting people's personal development using essences and homeopathy for some 30 years. A gifted practitioner, she is now a sought-after teacher of both essences and homeopathy all over the UK. Adam is passionate about gardening and the sacred experience one can find through nature. He became much more attuned to the energies that surround us through many years of Qi Kung practice and his training as a craniosacral therapist in the 1990s.

They established Healthlines in 1999.

Agave (*Agave americana*) Invites us to stand tall and shine our light, to radiate from our hearts and to reach for the forgiveness in our hearts. Be the beacon of light you would like to see in the world.

Autumn Crocus (*Colchicum autumnalis*) Wraps safe and loving arms around us, invites us to be held and supported. This essence encourages us to let go of the pain, to be willing to open our hearts and receive love again.

Autumn Squill (*Scilla autumnalis*) Helps you to connect with your team upstairs and access the unseen, spiritual support for the challenges of life. You can thereby realign and redefine yourself to fulfil your destiny in the world.

Blue (Environmental essence) For when you are struggling and it feels like you are pushing upstream. Taking Blue you can step into the slipstream, align yourself with the flow of energy and be carried along by it, riding the wave. It is effortless.

Carob (*Ceratonia siliqua*) Promotes harmony and reconciliation to heal rifts or feuds within the family or between tribes. May relate to inheritance issues, including those to do with money. Helps to honour the sacred space between us.

Cyclamen (*Cyclamen hederifolium*) Encourages in us a lightness of being and joyful sharing. I feel totally deserving and worthy to receive. I open my arms wide for balanced giving and receiving from a deep sense of abundance and wholeness.

Cistus (*Cistus monspeliensis*) For confidence and courage when we are exploring relationships, including intimate relationships, and feel shy, inexperienced or inadequate. Cistus promotes a sense of self, and helps us ask 'Who am I? What do I want?'

The Desert (Environmental essence) Indicated for when someone feels lost in their life, empty, alone and unsupported. It helps them to reach inside to realize that they have resources deep within which are available whenever they want or need them.

El Ghriba (Environmental essence) Indicated for people who repeat a story that may not be their own. It invites you to be willing to let go of cultural or inherited beliefs, so that your own story can emerge and serve your soul's purpose. It supports you on your journey of finding your own way and your own truth.

Etna (Environmental essence) For people who are carrying conflict within, smouldering away, waiting to erupt. It encourages letting our fire energy flow in a healthy way. This essence also helps us reconnect with our passion, with inspiration, spontaneity, having fun and with our inner wild selves.

Field Scabious (*Knautia arvensis*) For you if you are sensitive, find expression difficult and tend to keep silent. It helps you to express yourself without fear of being judged, to feel that you are heard and what you have to say matters.

Gateway (Environmental essence) For stepping through a gateway into a new chapter in your life. For letting go of your old life and for embracing uncharted territory. Feeling free, being willing to take risks. Rites of passage.

Ggantija (Environmental Essence) A great earth essence. It is for accessing the limitless abundance, nurturing and warm embrace of Mother Earth. Fertility, fecundity, abundance, nourishment, grounding.

Iron (Mineral essence) For warrior energy, not to be messed with. It is helpful when you feel scared and mouse-like, when you need courage to face your tyrant. It is also an essence for project building with resolve, and steely determination.

Olive (*Olea europaea*) For deep, long-standing exhaustion. It brings energy to those who have felt weary and burdened for a long time. It also brings us connection with the ancestors – with their inspiration and understanding.

Olympos Laurel (*Laurus nobilis*) For all aspects of success and failure, achievement and self-worth. This essence is for people who have fear around success and failure, self-limiting beliefs and anxiety about how others may judge them.

Pomegranate (*Punica granatum*) A very feminine essence. It helps us to embrace and celebrate all aspects and phases of being a woman – virgin, mother, enchantress, crone. It also supports us in healing any hurt or trauma in our relationships with women.

Sea Holly (*Eryngium maritimum*) Helps us to think and act with detachment and logic when we risk being overwhelmed by emotion or too much detail. It supports us in both grasping the overview of a situation and managing the parts, so we can work more efficiently.

Sea Squill (*Urginea maritima*) Enables you to connect with the energy of a supportive group. With this support you can find your unique individuality and strength. It is your time now to step up and into your power!

Solar Eclipse (Environmental essence) Supports us when we feel we have lost touch with the source and the purpose of our life. This essence helps us know that the source of life is constant, so that we can now surrender to the divine plan, and once again feel connected to the energy of life's higher purpose for us.

Wild Carrot (*Daucus carota*) Useful for those who have been displaced or feel they don't fit in. Anyone who feels they stand out like a sore thumb, isolated and victimized, shunned and alienated. This essence nurtures a sense of self-respect, which invites respect from others.

BLOESEM FLOWER ESSENCES OF THE NETHERLANDS (Blos)

Water forms a large part of the Netherlands because much as the land has been reclaimed from the sea, so the landmass is laced with waterways. Apart from the cleansing aspect, water has a profound connection with the emotions. The Bloesem essences are made from wild and organic plants, which address issues that living in this water-based environment creates.

Bram and Miep Zaalbergís founded these remedies in 1986 and now produce some 47 essences, a selection of which are included in the repertoire offering some of the first mushroom essences.

Alternanthera (*Alternanthera dentata*) Centred feelings, without fear of expression. Staying centred, undisturbed by people or their issues. Keeping your own counsel. To do the work you believe in and bring your higher truth into reality and expand it. Give full expression to what is. For those

times when you feel like you come from another planet. To find your direction and life purpose. Self-confidence.

Angelica (*Angelica archangelica*) Protection and strengthens help from the spiritual worlds for development and grounding the loving spiritual forces in your life. Gives spiritual protection during pregnancy, birth and dying. Stimulates trust in the Higher Self, personal wisdom and reaching beyond your boundaries.

Borage (*Borago officinalis*) Strengthens the heart in difficult circumstances, bringing gladness and joy. Helps with difficulties or discouragement and when you lose faith, it brings strength to the heart. Helps you with spiritual contact so you can receive support. Helpful when you cannot get pregnant, because you cannot meet the unborn spirit.

Clematis (*Clematis vitalba*) Not only for awakening but gives a clearer picture of one's actions. Clarifying thought processes, improving our capacity for thought enabling a more conscious insight into the handling of daily affairs. Gives a clearer overview of the process of cause and effect and motivation of the unconscious. For working in and for the light and manifesting this light in the world around one.

Coprinus Auricomus (*Coprinus auricomus*) For handling life from the strong source of one's original being; returning to one's own structure. Persevering and endurance despite blockages. Opening the heart and moving towards one's future. Strengthening your feminine qualities. Moving on, being open to your future. Gives strength and space to the physical body. Makes room for the new and transformation.

Evening Primrose (*Oenothera lamarckiana*) This night-blooming flower strengthens the creative forces of the moon. Helps you to rediscover, connect with and reinforce the source of your self-confidence, beauty and the inner feminine (in both sexes). Gives insight in the old, unknown areas of darkness, such as incest, abuse and problems with sexuality. Helps to solve these problems and brings them into the open.

Field Scabious (*Knautia arvensis*) Grounds and supports, especially when there is the feeling of not belonging. Quiets thinking, clears unnecessary thoughts through the Earth. Positive thinking, aids better handling of life, and more perception and openness to others and the environment. Connects us to the higher, serene spheres enabling us to reflect them back out and into the surroundings so the support and warmth of others can be received. Purifies the aura; 2 drops of the remedy in the palm whilst holding them within the aura dispels even the most ancient and tenacious memories.

Foxglove (*Digitalis purpurea*) Eases the mental processes, helps contact the heart. Releases mental structures and behaviour patterns, especially from past lives. To open to and return to the Higher Self as the centre and source of love in your life. Opens up to other sources of information, for example, in dreams. Brings playfulness, joy and pleasure in sexuality. Balances the polarities of the Higher Self and the Earth.

Giant Stropharia (*Stropharia rugosoannulata*) Brings new insight; instead of focusing on the difficulties in life, directs your attention to pleasure and fun. Aids direct action, especially having been thinking rather than doing. All action can then come from the heart, doing for the fun of it rather than feeling one must, or that it's expected. Connects one to the Earth, releasing energy and tension felt behind the eyes.

Goldenrod (*Solidago officinalis*) For individuality especially in a group, feeling inhibited and closed and unable to let go of personal ego, or direct one's attention to the higher qualities. Focused on personal achievements and feeling overdependent on others' opinions. Encourages self-trust and confidence, allowing an openness, enthusiasm, a sense of abundance and co-operation towards others and the environment.

Greater Celandine (*Chelidonium majus*) For men and women alike, balances the right and left hemispheres of the brain, the masculine and feminine; excessive emotionality is purified and grounded. Improves relationships, especially when a wall has gone up between people. Help to purify one's emotional life, so that purity becomes the basis of one's existence. Eliminates emotional toxins and removing feelings of inferiority giving acceptance of one's innermost self.

Ground Elder *(Aegopodium podagraria)* When development seems stuck Ground Elder helps manifest your growth by making better connection with one's true self. Or, when overoccupied with self-development, helps to let go and open to the higher qualities of being. Helpful with difficulty in assimilating experiences. With no need to fight with the environment it provides integration and co-operation through the expression of the heart, coming from the Higher Self.

Ground Ivy (*Glechoma hederacea*) Clears away old emotions, makes you aware of behaviour patterns. For abundance, strength and expansion and a good connection with the Earth. Use for personal development, brings out the finer qualities of your being. Gives self-trust and self-confidence. Useful in healing work to hook out or pull out the toxic emotion out of the physical body.

Impatiens (*Impatiens glandulifera*) Patience and calm; understanding; development of one's deepest true timing and knowing that all life continues in its own unique time. Heightens awareness of disturbances caused by others; helping to express oneself clearly towards others. Aids adaptability towards others without expressing irritation, annoyance; wanting to grow too fast or being drawn too easily out of your own life's timing by the influence of others. Impatiens is also helpful in cases of skin problems and used directly from the stock bottle.

Little Inky Cap *(Coprinus xanthotrix)* Brings emotional strength when feeling vulnerable and gives universal trust. Helps rise above emotions and promotes letting go of old anger and emotions quickly and easily. When others try to bully or to get the better of you it helps one to remain strong giving the ability to stand up, without hesitating, for your own viewpoints and feelings.

Money Plant *(Lunaria annua)* For those who find material, earthly business more important than unity with their own being, the universe and nature. Lack of balance with spiritual development striving after worldly possessions and power. Therefore unable to make contact with his or her own source – retarding spiritual development and creating, as a result, a state of emptiness in the subconscious. An emptiness that is never satiated despite being filled up by activities, feeling compelled 'to do' to keep active. Brings faith in the abundance of the universe. Also good for jealous children.

Motherwort *(Leonurus cardiaca)* The Motherwort flower essence works on and resolves family patterns. Helps those who don't feel at home in their family and on the Earth. For lack of warmth, love and support in the family, resulting in becoming hardened, overorganized, rigid and feeling like a stranger on the Earth. Motherwort essence brings its softness and helps you to stay open to the love and support of family and friends in the here and now.

Mycena *(Mycena polygramma)* A mushroom remedy. For a strong and well-grounded connection with the Earth. To go forward despite difficult situations, especially when everything around you seems to be in chaos. Mushrooms are good cleansers and help your body to eliminate forgotten emotions, especially everything that is hard to digest and Pluto-related problems. Purifying action on and restorative action on the aura.

Peppermint *(Mentha piperita)* For difficult and challenging times. Helps you to digest the problems in your life, and the deep emotions and problems you see in the world around you. Strengthens you and prepares you for many eventualities and difficulties. Gives insight into behaviour patterns and structures held since birth. Makes you awake and alert. Particularly helpful for emotions and energies which have been accumulated in the area of the stomach and the digestive system.

Purple Flower *(Centratherum punctatum)* Brings light into the energy around the head, allows the mind to relax. Heightens awareness in healing; gives you trust in your work as a healer and brings this out into the world. Reflects the light of your being into the different kingdoms (animal, mineral, plant and human); opens for the power of nature, and for the insight and awareness of your environment.

Red Helleborine Orchid *(Cephalanthera rubra)* Strength in all circumstances. Helps you to find and follow your own path. Opens you to 'higher' energies and healing, when you are unsure about the path of becoming a healer. Connects healers with their Higher Selves when they feel depleted and aids being a bearer of light.

Red Henbit *(Lamium purpureum)* Strong earthly bonds and joy in physical activity. Gives clarity in chaotic activities; stimulates organizing with joy: moving, bookkeeping, studying. When you are stuck in chaos, disease, habits or too much work. Strengthens your energy. Apply topically for blockages in the wrists and joints.

Promotes self-expression, activity and is a positive catalyst.

Red Poppy (*Papaver rhoeas*) Strengthens the inner woman and the Earth connection. A warming and empowering essence when you feel vulnerable as a woman. Increases the inner quality of warmth and love. Supports disturbances such as moving, abuse, calamities and disaster. Calms extreme sexuality (in men and women). Good results for all female problems (from menstruation until menopause), as well as insomnia.

Rue (*Ruta graveolens*) Spiritual protection in the psychic realms. Helpful for psychic attack or energy stealing. Especially helpful when this is being done in the area of the crown chakra and the line of connection with the Higher Self. Brings insight in old, deep-hidden and unknown fears. Gives more strength to act from your intuition. Cleanses old physical problems stored in the body.

Sensitive Weed (*Mimosa pudica*) Choosing one's path with certainty, not letting oneself be drawn off course. When others come too close you can feel you can't breathe. For being oversensitive, especially when others get too close. Aids pursuing self-development in all circumstances, feeling protected and supported by the environment and able to accept support and love. Good results with clients with high or low blood pressure.

Smooth Hawksbeard (*Crepis capillaris*) Balance between action and rest. Brings new energy and vitality, softens rigid structures. For feeling at ease with others. Clears childhood emotions. Helps recharge energy and store it in the bones.

Sneezewort (*Achillea ptarmica*) Gives protection on the spiritual path. To follow your direction, physical and spiritual with certainty and without the need to ask others. To strive for your own highest standards and values and to express these. For taking your own decisions and still being open for the help and advice of others, without getting distracted.

Snowdrop (*Galanthus nivalis*) Releases deep pain and trauma, especially when it originates from not being true to yourself. Can bring some tears. To renew the beauty and importance of the self. Brings a strong sense of trust, and joyful and refreshing new energy after a long dark (emotional) winter.

Star of Bethlehem (*Ornithogalum umbellatum*) Helps to remain undisturbed by external influences reconnecting one with universal being. Clears away assimilated blockages not essential for one's being that are hindering one's own unique flowering and the connection with your Higher Self. Anything that's been allowed in, not a part of one's original being, but accumulated throughout life. A truly universal flower essence which helps one believe in one's own beauty.

Sunflower (*Helianthus tuberosus*) This perennial Sunflower works on the father principle, both in men and women. The essence helps you stand up for yourself, restores the connection with the father and helps to release long-standing father problems. Strengthens and empowers the solar plexus renewing the connection with the light or sun as centre of your life. Helps with the manifestation of your dreams. Gives strength, vitality and energy. Allows you to do what you always wanted to do with joy and encourages you to stand up for yourself. Dispels limitations imposed by others.

Tansy (*Tanacetum vulgare*) Use for doubt and the inability to make decisions; brings the insight that indecision will result in stagnation. Tansy brings trust and helps to connect you with your Higher Self. Strengthens the heart and gives insight into the deepest core of doubts on all levels of being.

Trumpet Vine (*Campsis radicans*) Gently breaks through the communication barriers when communication problems need resolving, helping expression of deeper emotions, without being in conflict with oneself. When a thick wall has been set up, it helps to break this down in a gentle way, as it first helps to break down one's own inner wall. Enables courage to do what one really likes, instead of being conditioned to do what one ought or should do. Good results with those who stutter.

Yellow Star Tulip (*Calochortus monophyllus*) For sensitive people who are not sure about their feelings. Connects you with the truth of your heart. For starting projects that you have been aware of for some time, but not initiated. Brings insight into your feelings and connects you with the inner goddess. Gives trust in all changes and stimulates you to act from your Highest Self.

Special combinations of flower essences

4 Elements *Burdock, Impatiens, Stinging Nettle and Tansy.* Allows openness and warmth towards others, while still being yourself. The contact with your soul and the purpose of your soul becomes clearer. Releases hindrances to your evolution, and helps you stay in your own power and accept others as they are. Gives a feeling of freedom, joy and openness.

Cell Phone Combination *Mycena, Terra and Impatiens.* To protect against the radiation emitted from cell (mobile) phones. Hold the essence near the phone when you are using it, also drop the essence on the side of your head in the area you hold the phone. If you already have a pain in your head because of overuse of the phone, put a drop on the painful spot several times a day. Also good for those sensitive to electricity and those who work with computers a lot. One drop of the Cell Phone Combination on a clear quartz will protect you from disturbing electrical and negative frequencies.

Emergency Combination *Angelica, Clematis, Mycena, Red Helleborine and Yellow Star Tulip.* A first-aid remedy for all complaints. First it clears blockages then helps with recovery. Brings peace and calmness in tense situations. Opens the solar plexus. Gives strength in difficult times. Helps with exams, fears, accidents, shock, trauma, moodswings. Recommended use: 2–5 drops straight from the stock bottle under the tongue and/or hold the bottle during prolonged periods of tension. Can be applied locally on the specific area.

Integration Combination *Consists of two mushrooms: Stropharia and Psathyrella candolleana, Angel's Trumpet, Hollyhocks, Impatiens and Pumpkin.* A remedy for integration, protection and the resolution of old emotions which have not been integrated. It helps you to let go of the old and gives insight into how the problem originated. This can be related to past relationships or past misfortunes and abuse. For all situations in which you have been hurt or offended and have lost control over your life. Re-establishes the link to the Higher Self, integrating the various recovery processes and giving protection and confidence.

Living Star Light The Living Star Light is neither a combination nor a flower essence, but a cosmic essence. This essence connects you to the stars. It is an essence from a five-pointed star, with three points directed horizontally, one point directed down and one point directed up. The essence gives relaxation and releases everything that is not part of your being. It helps you to find wholeness on Earth and then deepens the connection of your being with the Earth and with the cosmic energies.

Love *Borage, Foxglove, Greater Celandine, Red Poppy, Red Henbit, Snowdrop and Yellow Star*

Tulip. Awakens love for oneself, others and the earth. Strengthens connection with the earth, opens your heart for the care and love of self-being. As a result pre-conditioned to give this love to others, without denying one's own needs. Giving love with pleasure from the source of one's own self. A powerful catalyst which connects to the Angel of Love.

Protection *Sneezewort, Greater Celandine, Rue and Sensitive Weed.* Gives spiritual and emotional protection. Brings calmness to the centre of your being when there is tension, stress and uncertainty. Protects against all attacks on all levels. Surrounds and protects with a mantle of light.

Purity *Protection, Poppy, Borage, Impatiens, Giant Strophoria and Star of Bethlehem.* A combination remedy for headaches. It purifies the soul and body connecting one to the Earth. Aids a better fit into one's body, and connecting to the original purity of one's soul and origin. Clears unnecessary emotions and strengthens self-confidence.

Rainbow *Borage, Impatiens, Money Plant, Red Henbit and Poppy.* The bridge between Heaven and Earth; a combination essence for personal development. Stimulates creativity, development and new activities. To start the new directly and forget the old. Opens and helps to overcome barriers that block your development; brings awareness to the process of growth.

The Spiritual Path *Borage, California Poppy and Trumpet Vine.* Helps to find your spiritual direction, particularly when choices were not made from a spiritual point of view and when the material world and material things have become the most important aspects of your life. This combination starts to change the choices you have made in the past and gives you the insight that there is no material world without a spiritual world.

Terra Extra (Emergency Combination) *Angelica, Clematis, Coprinus auricomus mushroom,*

Red Helleborine and Yellow Star Tulip. A combination that deals with severe problems for all situations. For those who cannot release their emotions; for those who worry constantly. For excessive stress, Terra Extra helps you to breathe again and makes it possible to move forward in life.

Essences of the new times

Pear (*Pyrus communis* hybrid) Gives balance and strengthens inner power and security. Provides trust in one's inner world and therefore you can release the things in the external world that one has put too much trust in. This gives insight into one's perception of persons and situations. Taken during pregnancy, when out of balance because of all the physical changes. Provides connection with the Earth when the frequency of the universe rises, keeping one's balance between below and above, matter and spirit, Heaven and Earth. Feeds and strengthens the love for oneself. Opens one to the new, and gives the insight into how to manifest oneself.

Cell-Energy Reconnects the cells again with their original structure. Returning to the original frequency of the cell brings the inner cell of humans/animals into harmony again with their original task on Earth, without having to clear all the old emotions. Rather like a spiritual bypass, when blockages are resolved, brings one into power and one can start finding one's own way.

Earth-Protection A new essence made from Smoky Quartz, Himalaya Quartz, Emerald, Tourmaline, Labradorite, Malachite, Garnet and the flower essence of Motherwort. Protects against physical, emotional, mental and spiritual attack, particularly the low energy draining kind. Useful for protection from spiritual and higher consciousness attacks, around the crown and higher chakra area. Strengthens and provides protection from the green energy of the Earth, and when under attack one is assimilated in the protective energy of the Earth.

Bolderik – Corncockle (*Agrostemma githago*) Brings clarity and encourages one to follow the direction of one's heart. Helps assimilate unknown chaotic emotions allowing a vision quest to your centre, bypassing all disturbing influences. Supports one in standing up for oneself and not to give in. Provides insight that in order to move on, growth and development of consciousness is necessary. Releases feelings of revenge opening to the higher consciousness of forgiving and love. Brings the knowledge that one is a child of God (the universe) and when having lost faith in life, the world and humanity, Corncockle brings back a state of purity.

Earth Creation Peace and faith to be, without struggle, to stand in one's power without pain and provide deep roots to complete one's incarnation on Earth. Affords a new level of understanding and initiates cycle of healing of the human race that begins with a true expression of love, opening of the heart and the search for real healing in oneself. Releases what is not important for the fulfilling of the unique role of man in the universe and allows connection to the level of the angels, to be healed after a long search for our original source.

Wintergroen – Round Leafed Wintergreen (*Pyrola rotundifolia*) Helps with digestion of nutrients from the Earth and sustains one. Gives self-confidence and awareness that one often has more qualities inside than is shown. One stands in one's own power enabling the release of old, unprocessed emotions. One can move on, expand and have faith in oneself, so to bring out the qualities hidden deep inside.

Engel en Lemurische Poort – Angel – and Lemurian Portal (with the Orchid *Cephalanthera rubra*) Access the origins of who one is, beyond the limiting codes that keeps one held in old structures. Transformation takes place as one is opened up to the source of higher knowledge. When one is exhausted, running round in circles, it opens connection with the angelic world and aligns one with the wisdom and knowledge of Lemuria. Transforms old grief that blocks the steps to the new and strengthens the connection with your angel/guidance/Higher Self, so one's path can be followed clearly.

Earth Vortex with White Angel An essence for this time, for manifestation, connection with the Earth and strength. Made from a sacred power place with a Black Tourmaline, a Lemurian Quartz and a Super Seven mineral. The sacred power place is a vortex that goes into the Earth and makes a deep connection with a core of light. From this light comes the white angel with a golden globe in her hands.

It not only has a downward spiral, by which the cosmic energy and the star children can incarnate, but also an upward spiral by which the knowledge from old times as Lemuria can be set free. In the centre they come together bringing a strong power of manifestation of the cosmic man. Brings one's focus into reality, into the now of this incarnation, and a strong hold to one's roots in the Earth.

Not only does it make a deep connection with the Earth, but also aids the processing of clearing the shadow side from past lives, as if not properly resolved they can cause problems in this life. The unresolved shadow side can block one's manifestation and growth. Through this deeper connection with the Earth higher qualities of the soul can manifest and strengthen and extend the aura.

Enhances the connection with Lemuria (the heart), with Atlantis (the mind) and connects with Akasha (the golden city of knowledge). Through these connections the power to enhance and manifest who one is can allow change to take place.

A stronger connection with Lemuria is held because the original connection is strengthened. A follow-up of the Angel and Lemurian Portal essence which helps when one cannot enter the portal, and makes the knowledge from Lemuria become available.

It strengthens the inner light and strength to remove the oldest problems that are still present at soul level. When a manifestation of the soul is not finished off, the old problems can get left behind in the consciousness and have a life of their own. Roaming in one's consciousness for ages they can finally manifest as a crisis (for example, a psychosis, a divorce, a conflict or a serious disease).

This crisis mostly takes place at the end of a period of transformations; the problem forces major change, there is no room for delay. Gives you the awareness that you don't have to fight, but release it and that this is the moment to stand in one's power.

Holds a clear relationship with an archetypical pattern: the image of the archangel Lucifer who brings light to humankind, but also the insight that good cannot exist without evil and that everything originates out of a universal source, the trinity. This essence is made on 24 December, the moment of birth of the sun and each year the birth of inner power.

Black Tourmaline works on grounding and cleansing, not only electric fields, but also negativity and evil. It works positively on negative atmospheres and unwanted influences and neutralizes tensions.

The Lemurian Quartz brings light into consciousness, strengthening growth and the divine trust in oneself. The crystal radiates very much love, unity and connects with Lemuria and with who one really is.

The Super Seven or Melody stone opens all chakras, brings transformation and connects with the higher energy, with past lives and is an antenna for receiving knowledge and spiritual guidance.

'I renew, change and manifest the deepest level of my soul, I let go of old unintegrated emotions and give form to my new direction.'

RUSSIAN ESSENCES BY AUSTRALIAN LIVING (AUS L RUS)

With the political and social turmoil in Russia, these remedies reflect the problems that beset the Russian people, and are relevant to all those facing suppression, oppression and the subsequent reactions to these forces.

Made by Vasudeva Barnao, who was invited to the then Soviet Union in 1989 to begin research on essences collected from flowers in the Bush about 125 miles (200km) from Moscow. Their contribution to the essence repertoire is unique and invaluable.

Blue-Topped Cow Weed For the escapist or joker who avoids life's deeper issues – the superficial good-timer who avoids responsibility, lacking empathy, depth of character. Brings a more responsible attitude. Engenders the strength to deal with problems rather than avoid them.

Russian Kolokoltchik For conquering adversity after a long history of struggle when the will to fight has faded. Restores the desire to fight on and not succumb.

Russian Centaurea For brave people who stand up and oppose injustice, regardless of the consequences; for risk-takers who feel opposed or trapped. Teaches that there are times when you cannot act because of negative forces stronger than yourself, when you must keep your flame hidden so as not to attract undue attention from those seeking to destroy you.

Russian Forget-Me-Not For the follower, looking to others for leadership, underestimating his or her own abilities and strengths. Helps you to find hidden strength.

E.

INDIA

India has a very rich floral heritage. The country boasts wide variations in climate, from the icy north to the tropical south, which support the growth of a great variety of flowering plants. In India, flowers are traditionally associated with various deities and with ceremonies, *pujas*, prayers and other occasions. There are also mythological stories regarding various flowers, clearly indicating the effect of flowers on day-to-day life. Flowers still have a role to play in Ayurvedic medicine, a tradition of healing, the principles of which date back at least 2000 years. Regarded throughout the world as one of the most spiritual of flowers, the Lotus is India's national flower.

The Himalayan Mountains in particular exhibit a spectacular floral show every year. Here the land is still relatively unpolluted and uncorrupted by human activity. It pulses with a vibrancy and life force that is fast fading elsewhere on this planet. Each year the peaks grow a few centimetres, a tell-tale sign of the tremendous upward thrust generated from deep within the earth. Pilgrims have traditionally journeyed to the Himalayas to meditate and seek enlightenment. Many sages of old lived in the Himalayas, while others (including the famous Chinese philosopher Lao Tzu) travelled there to end their days having reached a higher state of consciousness, knowing that their final impressions or images of Earth were these eternally snowy peaks. Reaching through the clouds towards the heavens, the Himalayas symbolize the peak of consciousness and the flowers that grow here reflect the extraordinary energies of this land.

HIMALAYAN ADITI FLOWER ESSENCES (Him A)

Aditi is the Sanskrit word for 'Earth'. It is also the spiritual name given to the white Lotus flower, representing divine consciousness. For this reason Drs Atul and Rupa Shah chose Aditi as the name for their collection of flower essences. This husband and wife team are both allopathic doctors who became increasingly interested in complementary medicine. They researched various different therapies before they came across the Bach Flower Remedies. Impressed by the results they achieved with the Bach Remedies, they were prompted to prepare remedies from flowers growing wild on the slopes of the Himalayas and from other particularly verdant spots in this colourful country.

The Shahs have invented a method of preparing essences in situ, so that they can avoid cutting the flowers' stems. This technique involves placing a glass bulb around a flower and pouring water through it. With the intervention of sunlight they have their 'mother tincture'. They try to determine the most auspicious time to do their work and always pray first for permission to collect the essences. The essences are preserved in Ganges water (from the source) as well as brandy. Aware that some people are unable to tolerate alcohol, they are currently looking into making essences with honey.

At their two health centres, where both orthodox and complementary methods work in synergy, the Shahs carry out in-depth research into the properties of their essences. Medical techniques such as X-rays, cardiograms and blood tests are employed to assess the benefits flower essences are bringing to their patients. The Shahs claim to have had much success in treating a broad spectrum of health problems related to stress and tension including infertility, hypertension, breast cancer and arthritis using their own essences as well as others from around the world.

Ashoka Tree (*Saraca indica*) For those who have gone through great trauma such as a bereavement, disease or failure and are suffering from deep-seated sorrow, sadness, grief, isolation and disharmony. Brings a profound inner state of joy, harmony and wellbeing. Especially good for elderly people.

Bougainvillea (*Bougainvillea glabra*) For evoking meditation when we need to re-affirm our connection with our higher spiritual destiny when anxiety, fear or mediocrity swamp us. Rekindles enthusiasm, interest and emotional wellbeing, promoting our sense of the sacred in life.

Butterfly Lily (*Hedychium coronarium*) For those who exercise great power over people in an evil or negative way. For seeing clearly what has been done, wishing to be forgiven and making amends. Brings true remorse for wrong-doing, and inner peace.

Cannonball Tree (*Couroupita guianensis*) For overcoming frigidity in women caused by deep fears in the mind concerning sexual expression. To use in sexual therapy for women when a strong desire to conceive is blocked by inexplicable frigidity.

Christ's Thorn (*Ziziphus spina-christi*) For those in a constant state of internal turmoil for no obvious reasons. Relieves the state of negativity in the psyche and resolves conflicts from the consciousness. A redemptive essence.

Curry Leaf (*Murraya koenigii*) For healing ulcers and hyperacidity caused by mental tension and an imbalanced diet (which may include a lot of meat and alcohol). Produces greater relaxation as well as a balanced awareness and concern about diet and lifestyle.

Day-Blooming Jessamine (*Cestrum diurnum*) For those going through great suffering from painful, debilitating diseases. Brings acceptance and transformation of suffering into positive love, kindness and sensitivity to others. Relieves the burden of fear, nightmares and pain.

Drum Stick (*Moringa oleifera*) For dispelling bitterness, resentment and other pains by building up positive feelings. Also for reducing the desire to smoke and resolving difficult emotions. Good for bronchitis.

Goldenrod (*Solidago virgaurea*) For those who feel insecure and seek negative attention from others in social situations by being naughty, bad or repulsive. Brings real humility, love and mental realism about others and our relationship with them. Eases internal emotional disharmony.

Gulmohar (*Delonix regia*) Spiritual healing for those who have committed acts of sexually related violence in past lives. Restores deep peace and harmony, letting the sexual energy flow so lovemaking becomes fulfilling once more.

Indian Coral (*Erythrina indica*) For bureaucrats and those holding positions of power over society who are self-interested, power-seeking, generally arrogant and insensitive. Brings a transformation of consciousness for those wielding political power and gives them wisdom, enlightenment, understanding and peace. Dissolves the blockages of selfishness and impure intentions.

Indian Mulberry (*Morinda citrifolia*) For groups of people in conflict who are antagonistic and hate one another. Alleviates long-held prejudices, hatred and deep disharmony. Good for dealing with the legacy of negative patriotism and social conflict. Brings reconciliation.

Ixora (*Ixora coccinea*) Relationship enhancer for couples lacking direction or suffering a loss of interest and vitality in their sexual energy. Revitalizes and enhances sexual energy and activity. Enhances and brings responsibility, wisdom, calmness and balance into sexual expression.

Karvi (*Strobilanthes callosus*) For changing distorted attitudes towards sex and the expression of sexuality. For problems of sexual performance, or seeing sex as purely for financial gain. Guides us away from pornography and selfish sexual gratification towards more loving, sensitive and equal sexual relationships and practices. Helps with the problems of frigidity or impotence.

Lotus (*Nelumbo nucifera*) A spiritual elixir and aid to meditation. Calms the mind and improves concentration. Gently releases negative emotions, correcting imbalances. Hastens recovery from illness. Aligns and balances the chakras by releasing, adding and directing energies to them. Clears the entire system of toxins. Balances, cleanses and strengthens the aura. Harmonizes interpersonal relationships. Amplifies the effect of other flower essences when used in combination with them.

Malabar Nut Flower (*Adhatoda vasica*) For those who feel superior to others because of nationality or class. Deals with prejudice, deep-seated pride and snobbery. Enhances love and tolerance and understanding of others.

Meenalih For religious or self-righteous people who repress their sexuality, feeling it is wrong or sinful. For impotence caused by guilt about one's body and the pleasure that sexual urges bring. Transforms old fearful attitudes of guilt. Teaches us that true virtue lies in real love, which embraces everything, and that we have the right to a pleasurable and enjoyable sex life.

Morning Glory (*Ipomoea violacea*) For addiction to opiates and nicotine, benefiting those trying to give up drugs at any stage of treatment. Eases nervous discomfort and physical withdrawal symptoms.

Neem (*Azadirachta indica*) Essence of the heart. For bringing overly cerebral people into their hearts, making them more loving, intuitive, understanding and giving, and less judgemental.

Night Jasmine (Newara) (*Jasminum arborescens*) For those who find it difficult to make love successfully. Can be used to foster long-term synchronization between two people or as an instant tonic prior to lovemaking. A sexual enhancer for attuning and integrating lovers' sexual energies. Produces the state of real pleasure, fulfilment and ecstasy in lovemaking. Revitalizes sexual relationships when taken by both partners.

Nilgiri Longy/St John's Lily/Cape Lily (*Crinum latifolium*) Specifically for teachers and professionals who are too strict and rigid with students. Helps teachers to make learning more creative and fun.

Office Flower (*Portulaca grandiflora*) For those who work in modern, high-tech offices sitting in front of video display screens the whole day, resulting in mental and nervous stress, frustration and associated skin problems.

Old Maid (Pink) (*Vinca alba*) For women who are too promiscuous as a result of mistaken attitudes towards sex, seeing men as playthings for their own sexual gratification and ego, neglecting love and responsibility in sex. For women who have become brutal and insensitive towards men after being used or abused. Brings a loving, caring attitude towards sex and lovemaking.

Old Maid (White) (*Vinca alba*) For men who are too promiscuous through mistaken attitudes towards sex. Helps men change egotistical, self-centred, insensitive attitudes which make them emphasize their own pleasure above all else. Promotes love, caring and greater control over sexual urges. Stimulates deep concern about a partner's experience of the quality of the shared relationship.

Pagoda Tree (*Plumeria alba*) For those who treat sexual partners as mere objects to satisfy their desire and fantasies, putting their own power and satisfaction above love. Dissolves illusions about sex, corrects channelling of sexual energy and cultivates a loving, caring attitude in lovemaking.

Parrot (Flame of the Forest) (*Butea monosperma*) For public speakers who wish to improve the timing of their elocution and coordination between thought and speech. Synchronizes thought, will and speech to improve pronunciation and enunciation. Helps the mind to gain control over the delivery of speech, so enhancing confidence and vocal expression.

Parval (*Trichosanthes dioica*) For hard-hearted people. Opens up the emotions, harmonizing and rekindling compassion and sensitivity towards others. Makes us more spontaneous and joyful.

Peacock Flower (*Poinciana pulcherrima*) For overcoming the effects of long debilitating illnesses or of physical and mental torture. Valuable for any rehabilitation process, such as overcoming drug addiction. Restores the nervous energy flow.

Pill-Bearing Spurge (*Euphorbia plentissima*) For those who are accident-prone, going through a bad patch or feeling powerless to control their own lives. Alleviates the effects of cyclical misfortune and the consequent bitterness.

Prickly Poppy (*Argemone mexicana*) For men who mistreat women sexually, seeing them merely as objects. Brings a caring responsibility and love back to sex without diminishing physical arousal or pleasure. Steers a man towards seeking a fulfilling and caring relationship by teaching that sex can be more fun when responsibly and lovingly undertaken.

Radish (*Raphanus sativas*) For anyone suffering from bereavement and from a sense of being unable to cope. Specifically strengthens and reorders the mind, affording mental objectivity, wellbeing and comfort following the death of someone very close. Integrates the mind after shock and trauma or bereavement.

Rangoon Creeper (Madhumalti) (*Quisqualis indica*) Frees those who are captured in soul and will by very powerful gurus or cult leaders.

Red Hibiscus (*Hibiscus*) For enhancing compatibility between people in one-to-one relationships, thus evoking warmth and responsiveness. Restores mental harmony and emotional wellbeing, and indirectly improves sexual interaction.

Red-Hot Cattail (*Acalypha hispida*) For those who have been abused and wronged in past lives. Opens the heart centre, bringing a warm and loving transformation. Dissolves deep-seated blocks of hard-heartedness and unforgivingness in the psyche. Restores faith in a universal spirit.

Red Silk Cotton Tree (*Salmalia malabarica*) For those drawn to spiritual paths. Cleanses and transforms the inner intention of such people. Liberates them from spiritual glamour and power-seeking by bringing a purity of spiritual intention, humility, love and appreciation for all people.

Rippy Hillox For those who are negative and fearful about sex because they have had difficult or traumatic sexual experiences in the past; for victims of rape or sexual perversion who find the thought of sex too painful to bear.

Sithihea For those who are self-centred in business and their dealings with others. For anyone whose vanity and insensitivity creates a mental block in his or her awareness of others. Evokes qualities of patience, reasonableness, compassion and integrity. Enhances, sensitizes and balances external, financial and material relationships.

Slow Match (*Careya arborea*) For those who feel badly treated in one-to-one relationships such as a marriage or parent/child relationship, resulting in bitterness and resentment towards the other person. Brings real love, openness, trust and understanding of the other person and a will to keep the relationship good.

Spotted Gliciridia (Rikry Rorshia Flower) (*Gliciridia maculata*) For oppressive political leaders. Reforms those who imprison others for their political beliefs, bringing a change of heart as well as enlightenment and wisdom.

Swallow Wort (*Calotropis gigantea*) For those in a state of torment, disharmony and fear in their subconscious minds giving rise to disturbed sleep, nightmares, panic attacks and general restlessness. Alleviates deep disharmony so that peace, wellbeing and courage return.

Tassel Flower (*Calliandra surinamensis*) For deep emotional wounds and disharmony with members of one's own family, particularly for parent/child but also for distant relationships. Fosters forgiveness and aids the reconciliation process. **Teak Wood Flower** (*Tectona grandis*) For vagueness, irrational and confused thinking, mental tiredness. For anyone over 60, especially those with senile dementia. Revitalizes and refreshes the mind, enhancing concentration and keeping the mind alert and interested.

Temple (*Plumeria rubra*) For deepening and strengthening the experience of worship; helpful to anyone who has totally rejected religion. Restores true awareness of the universal spirit.

Torroyia Rorshi Plant (*Fiori viola*) For those living in urban and industrial cultures. Encourages environmental sensitivity and awareness.

Tulip (*Spathodea campanulata*) For those who are aloof and uninterested in their day-to-day lives and in those around them. For anyone unable to wake early due to the intensity of his or her dreams. Brings a willingness to work and an ability to open up to and interact with others joyfully. Promotes early rising and applying oneself more completely to work and daily tasks. Reduces dreaming and astral travelling, helping one to be earthed and to accept physical life fully.

Ukshi (*Calycopteris floribunda*) For elderly women who used to be glamorous or beautiful but who feel rejected, depressed and resentful in their old age. Helps dissolve resentment, bitterness and isolation. Rekindles self-esteem and a sense of *joie de vivre*.

Vilayati Amli (*Fiori bianchi*) For mild envy of those close to us, making us unable to open up to or share/communicate with family and friends because they seem better than us or due to our own inferiority complex. Brings real pleasure in others' success, encouraging us to love and help others with warmth and caring. Improves relationships, particularly those within the family or among close friends.

Water Lily (*Nymphaea alba*) The Kama Sutra among flower essences. A powerful tonic for those with psychological inhibitions about intimacy and sex. Enhances enjoyment of lovemaking by heightening sensuality.

White Coral Tree (*Erythrina variegata orientalis*) For narrow-minded religious people who tend to be dogmatic, critical and simplistic in their assessments of others, seeing the world in black and white. Liberates us from a state of ignorance, broadening understanding and making us more flexible, loving and real in our religious faith.

White Hibiscus (*Hibiscus*) For anyone who feels blocked, tense and out of tune with his or her spiritual nature. Increases responsiveness to the spiritual world and our own spirituality. Increases our psychic and sensory ability to respond to the higher planes of being – the first step towards self-discovery.

Yellow Silk Cotton Tree (*Bombax ceiba*) For those who long to be free of a subconscious craving for spiritual power. Brings a pure, clear will to do spiritual work selflessly, humbly and without the desire for spiritual power over others.

Combination essences

The Shahs have formulated combinations to target specific problems; here is a selection below.

Formula 1 First Aid For moments of intense stress, trauma or emotional shock; helps one to deal calmly under difficult circumstances without panic.

Formula 2 Stress and Tension A soothing remedy that brings relief from stress-related disorders such as tense muscles, headaches and anxiety.

Formula 7 Urban Stress Assists with dealing with urban stress.

Formula 14 Environmental Stress For protection against harmful effects of environmental stress caused by radiation from appliances such as TVs, mobile phones and computers.

Formula 17 Sleep Brings relief to insomniacs and those experiencing disturbed sleep by helping the body to rebuild its natural sleep rhythm.

Formula 18 Travel Aid For those constantly on the move who are exposed to different foods, climates, etc. Boosts personal immunity and keeps good health.

Formula 19 Cleansing Aid A multipurpose combination for multilevelled cleansing.

Formula 20 Acne Effective remedy for treating acne which purifies the system.

Formula 23 Menopause Helps women pass through a turbulent phase of menopause smoothly. Diminishes the physical and emotional discomfort caused by menopause.

Formula 24 Anti-Addiction Aid For those who earnestly wish to give up their addictions. Works on the mind to help to achieve a complete release from destructive habits and patterns.

Formula 38 Immunity Booster Enables one to maintain a good state of health by building the body's immunity against disease.

Formula 43 Sinus/Cold Offers relief from the common cold and sinusitis.

Gels

The Shahs have formulated some successful gels that address arthritic conditions and other painful symptoms.

Arthritis Aloe Vera Gel Fast-acting, cooling gel that uses remedies from Himalayan flowers to ease the swelling and discomfort of painful joints.

Floral Relief Gel This gel is made with Indian flower energy essences. Aloe vera juice is added to a gel base. Use to give relief to bites and itchy eczema as well as minor discomforts such as the following:

Backache Apply over the centre of the spine and on either side of spine. It is desirable to apply over the abdominal muscles.

Burns Relieves mild burns. *Do not* apply to open wounds or exposed burnt skin.

Calf pain Apply over the painful area including back of knee and ankle and also apply to the front of the leg.

Headaches For frontal headaches, apply over forehead and on either side of head. For deeper headaches, apply over painful area through hair, back of neck muscles and in the centre of upper part of abdomen.

Heel pain Apply over the heel and the back of the ankle and to front of heel under the arch.

Injury On any painful area due to injury or sprain. (Not to be applied to open wounds.)

Knee pain Apply over the painful area of knee joint in the front and back. Also apply to front and back of thigh completely. This is important as it will help you to recover fast.

Neck pain Directly apply over the painful area and over the muscles starting from back of neck to the base of neck.

Premenstrual pain or painful menses Apply over lower abdomen and around the navel.

Shoulder pain Apply over the painful area and also on the neck muscles.

Sneezing Apply on the nose and cheek and also on the forehead. Avoid putting it in the nose or in the eyes.

Toothache Apply externally over the painful side of cheek. Do not apply in the mouth.

HIMALAYAN FLOWER ENHANCERS (Him E)

These essences are made from flowers that grow 3000m (10,000ft) above sea level in the Parvati Valley of the Himachal Pradesh region of the Indian Himalayas. Their creator is a man called Tanmaya, a former landscape gardener who left his native Australia to spend the next 20 years as a nomad and spiritual seeker in India. He has always been passionate about flowers, and discovering these flower essences marked a turning point in his life for they brought him out of his reclusive lifestyle.

Tanmaya calls his essences 'enhancers' because of their ability to empower each of the body's main chakras or energy centres. The enhancers shine their light into these centres, dispelling any blockages or stored negativity. The first enhancer he created was for the crown chakra; he named it 'Flight'. Unlike many other prepared essences, the names of Tanmaya's enhancers derive not from the plants themselves but from their therapeutic qualities, such as 'Let Go' or 'Ecstasy'. He makes his 'enhancers' by placing the blossoms directly into pure, locally-produced alcohol – made from wild White Roses, mountain spring water, wheat and sugar. The same White Rose is the source of his 'Happiness' essence. Tanmaya believes we can learn a great deal from the flowers growing in the Himalayas: 'They push up through the Earth and rocks with such determination and courage… [they] are a celebration and a gift from the earth which share their beauty, individuality and uniqueness willingly with us.'

A further development to Tanmaya's collection is the Astro Essences range which addresses the particular vibrational energies of the sun and moon in each of the 12 signs of the zodiac.

Flowers of the world

Endurance Date Palm (*Phoenix dactylifera*), Indian olive (*Olea cuspidata*) (Sinai Desert/Himalayas). Eases inappropriate attitudes and belief systems around ageing. Supports youthful vigour, vitality and endurance.

Goddess Purple Orchid Tree (*Bauhinia purpurea*), Web Rose (*Rosa webbiana*), Rain Tree (*Albizia saman*) (India/China). Enhances the goddess, the wise woman. Provokes beauty, grace, receptivity, feminine strength. Connected to the energy of the moon and Venus.

Isan Neem (*Melia azadirach*) (India). Made from the flowers of an old Neem tree beside the ancient Tantric temples of Khajuraho. Helps integrate body, mind and spirit, creating wisdom referred to by the Zen Master Isan. Good to take after meditation sessions. Strengthens the ability to live one's truth.

Lotus (*Nymphaeaceae*) (India). The philosopher's stone of flowers, a symbol of enlightenment. General tonic and cleanser for the entire system. Activates the crown chakra and enhances all forms of healing; acts as a booster for other flower enhancers, herbs and gem elixirs. Excellent to use in conjunction with meditation. Made under the Taurus full moon.

Morning Glory (*Ipomoea nil* or *Ipomoea purpurea*) (India). Helps you get up and greet the morning with enthusiasm. Enhances vitality and tones the entire nervous system, thus reducing nervous behaviour. Helps break addictive habits such as smoking. Good for restlessness at night.

Rapa-Nui Mira-Tahiti (Easter Island). Evoking ancient Earth energy, healing past-life wounds, merging into the wisdom of Gaia. Made with seawater at the oldest sacred site on Easter Island, under the dark of the moon, with obsidian from the island's largest volcano, and the flower of Mira-Tahiti – the last native shrub remaining on the island.

Renaissance Air Plant (*Tillandsia stricta*) (Brazil). Rebirth. Assists in letting go of all that is not real and dissolving into that which has always been. Helps in letting go of emotional attachment to the past. A support for seekers during difficult times, giving understanding that flowering can happen in any moment regardless of external circumstances and conditions. (This essence was made under a full Pisces moon, with Sandra Epstein, co-creator of the Brazilian Rain Forest Essences.)

Veil of Dreams Cactus (*Acanthocereus Horridus*) (India). Enhances ability to dream consciously and step through the veil of dreams so that you can understand the mysteries behind dreams. Excellent to take before going to sleep. Brings awareness of dream patterns in the waking state, allowing them to dissolve into the here and now. Use in conjunction with 'Clarity' and 'Blue Dragon' (see below) for psychic work.

Warrior Tamarind (*Tamarindus indica*), Grass Tree or Blackboy (*Xanthorrhoea australis*), Plantain (*Musa paradisiaca*) (Australia/India/China). Enhances masculine strength, grounding, courage, male sexuality, strength of purpose. Best taken in conjunction with the flower enhancer 'Ecstasy' (see below). For women it helps re-establish the flowing of energy which is stuck in feelings of intimidation and overcriticism, allowing the energy to move in a more creative way. Connected to the energy of the sun and Mars.

The seven chakras

There are seven Himalayan flower enhancers for the seven major energy centres or chakras of the human body. These chakras each have their own particular quality and resonance, and have a corresponding relationship to one of the various glands in the body's endocrine system. Their exact position varies with the individual. They can be viewed as booster stations, or transformers, for the journey of the energy from the base of the spine to the top of the head, the crown.

First/Base: Down to Earth Himalayan Honeysuckle (*Leycesteria formosa*), Hardy Calanthe Orchid (*Calanthe tricarinata*) Enhances life force energy, connection with the Earth, helps with ungroundedness, sluggishness, anxiety around material existence, subtle or hidden fears, psychological wounds around sexuality, low libido, stress and lack of drive. Enhances sexual energy. Balances hyper-excitement, excess energy in the head, for example, dizziness, mental fatigue.

Second/Hara: Wellbeing Wallflower (*Erysimum melicentae*) Enhances connection with one's power, centring, stimulating creativity and integrating emotions. This chakra is the storehouse of energy and the centre for transforming base energy. Helps diffuse internalized anger, birth traumas, fear of death, imbalances of emotions.

Third/Solar Plexus: Strength Spearwort (*Ranunculas lingua*), Marsh Marigold (Badmia) (*Caltha palustris var. himalensis*) Enhances one's individuality, personal creativity, honesty and self-worth, self-identity, and the power to manifest in the material world. Helps overcome lack of self-esteem, self-doubt and inability to express one's innate creativity. Dispels feelings of insecurity, lack of personal power, lack of direction and motivation in life, sense of hopelessness, depression and oppression. Helps release early childhood conditioned patterns.

Fourth/Heart: Ecstasy (*Rosa webbiana*) Enhances love, compassion, sincerity, truthfulness, depth of feeling, empathy with all living things and transpersonal love. Helps with bitterness, jealousy, feelings of contraction, feeling unloved, undernourished, overcritical of others, disillusioned and lack of truth. Enhances feelings of expansion and universal love.

Fifth/Throat: Authenticity (*Delphinium incanum*) Enhances expression, verbal communication, appreciation of beauty, creativity, refined experience, questioning, seeking, singing, sharing ideas, stimulating dreams, imagination, embracing humanity. Enhancing conviction and self-authority. Helps in cases of timidity, shyness, fear of speaking one's truth, difficulty in communicating, stress, tension, apprehension, claustrophobia, lack of conviction, stage fright and unwillingness to change.

Sixth/Third Eye: Clarity Columbine (*Aquilegia pubiflora*), Blue Oxalis (*Parochetus communis*), Wild Thyme (*Thymus serpyllum*) Enhances clarity, awareness, sharpness of intellect, perception, intuition, sense of spirituality, understanding, ability to see into the heart of things, bliss. Sense of universal self. Meditation, insight and clairvoyance. Aids poor concentration, unawareness, lack of clarity and direction. Helps with headaches, balances excess sexual energy. Dispels isolation, alienation and feelings of meaninglessness.

Seventh/Crown: Flight Jasmine (*Jasminum officinale*) Enhances oneness, meditation, prayer, Higher Self, union of mind, body and spirit, sense of formlessness and the ability to experience nothingness. Helps with feelings of separateness, isolation, lack of meaning, feelings of insignificance. Enhances universal love, brotherhood, universal sharing, wonder, awe. Catalyst for all essences. Helps with egocentric, selfish and judgemental attitudes. Gives receptivity and acceptance of the beauty of oneself and others.

Himalayan flower enhancers

Astral Orchid (*Dactylorhiza hatagirea*) A higher octave of the third eye. For connection with one's Higher Self and channelling.

Aura Cleaning Himalayan Indigo (*Indigofera heterantha*), Baby's Breath (*Gypsophila cerastioides*) Cleans and refreshes the aura, adding a lightness and sparkle to the energy field. Excellent for use in the bath or spraying over the body or around the house.

Blue Dragon (*Corydalis cashmeriana*) Gentian (*Gentiana ornata*), Prickly Blue Poppy (*Meconopsis horridula*) Enhances focus, concentration and single-pointedness. Excellent for meditation. Pierces straight to the heart of the matter, dissolving the illusion of separation revealing only one sky.

Cedar (*Cedrus deodara*) Gives grounding and courage, stability, strength and vitality. Encourages deep roots in the earth so one's branches can reach to the sky.

Champagne Kashmir False Spirea (*Sorbaria tomentosa*) For celebration – particularly good at night. Take with the floral enhancer 'Ecstasy' for a night of celebration, 'Clarity' for a more mysterious night, or 'Down to Earth' and 'Ecstasy' for a night of passionate lovemaking.

Children's Flower (*Androsace primuloides*) Primula (*Primula gracilipes*), Strawberry (*Frugaria nubicola*) Protective essence for children. Helps the child to maintain their original connection with the natural world. Invokes delight, playfulness, innocence, resilience, a sense of wonder and awe in the mysteries of life. Connects adults with their inner child.

Chiron (*Thermopsis barbata*) Gives insight into the wound which has disconnected us from our essence; the key points that keep us from living our truth/being our true selves. Opens the senses to refined experiences. For healers evokes shamanistic energies and clarifies the point of disconnection in the client. Good for channelling. Can clarify Chiron transits.

Expansion Common Chicory (*Cicorium intybus*) Specifically for the chest area, opening and releasing tension – bringing expansiveness to the heart chakra and the experience of letting go. Dissolving the perceived boundaries of the heart and merging into the heart of all things.

Gateway Indian Horsechestnut (*Aesculus indica*) Assists in times of transition, rites of passage, dark night of the soul. Gives strength and resilience in times of inner turmoil. Helps you turn within when times are difficult. Can help to appreciate the process, the bigger picture.

Golden Dawn Impatiens (*Impatiens scabrida*) Particularly good for women. Releases old wounds around sexual, psychic and physical abuse from male domination. Centres one in the place of stillness where no wounds exist, and so allows disidentification and gentle healing to happen by itself. For example, can bring awareness to the internal restrictions women place on their feminine side due to mental conditioning from growing up in male-oriented societies.

Gratefulness Jasmine (*Jasminum officinale*) Enhances universal brotherhood and sharing, wonder, awe. Catalyst for all essences. Helps counter egocentric and selfish attitudes.

Happiness Himalayan Musk Rose (*Rosa brunonii*) Provokes a radiance from within that sends a smile, a soothing glow throughout the whole body, relaxing the mind. Gives a deep sense of joy in life. Very supportive for laughing meditations.

Healing Indian Poke (*Phytolacca acinosa*), Musk Orchid (*Herminium monorchis*), King Solomon Seal (*Polygonatum cirrhifolium*) For healers. Gives the effect of walking through a pine forest, clearing the channels for the healer, centring and bringing them back to their natural relationship with existence. Helps them to be in touch with the basic life forces in nature; especially helpful to healers working in cities or heavy urban environments. Encourages an instinctive relationship between healer and client, particularly if taken in conjunction with the Heart Essence and the essence most suitable to the client. Of great help where the life force is weak. Apply directly onto the hara or wherever there is a marked absence of energy.

Heart of Tantra Impatiens (*Impatiens glandulifera*) Creates a circle of light between the sex chakra and around the heart chakra. For men particularly, this bridges the solar plexus with the heart, thus moving sex from being about power to being about love.

Hidden Splendour (*Iris kemaonensis*) Brings forth the splendour within. For reclaiming your birth right; your inner glory. Helps combat feelings of worthlessness, constriction, insignificance, smallness.

Let Go (*Hackelia uncinata*) A Pisces flower – dissolving into the moment, relaxation, surrender, 'throwing away the oars and letting the boat take you where it will'. Letting go of past hurts, fears and attachments – moving into the present with empty hands. Good for hypnosis and guided fantasy work.

Nirjara Drumstick Primula (*Primula denticulata*) A deconditioning essence, excellent for all work of deprogramming. When there is conscious intent to change conditioned attitudes and patterns, this essence helps to erase outmoded imprints from the cells. Supports transformation. A powerful healing essence.

Nirjara 2 (*Primula macrophylla*) Aids in peeling back the layers of conditioning around our perception of reality – allowing the true face to reveal itself.

Opium Poppy (*Papaver somniferum*) Helping to break free of addictive emotional patterns and compulsive behaviour that keeps us in the past.

Pink Primula (*Primula rosea*) Opening the heart to pure delight and the joy of being alive.

Pluto (*Arisaema propinquum*) Diffuses anger and frustration and old patterns of behaviour whilst helping one to identify with the enormous power of change/evolution, rather than clinging to the old patterns that are being broken away. Brings consciousness to the shadow part of the mind. A powerful essence for embracing the disowned, 'darker' side of one's self. In the act of conscious acceptance, these negative

aspects lose their grip on the unconscious, and no longer have power in our life. In some people this essence can be initially cathartic. Brings strength and clarity to the aspect where Pluto is placed in the birth chart. Eases Pluto transits.

Purple Orchid (*Roscoea alpina*) A doorway in. Accessing great depths within. Good for those who find it difficult to turn their focus inward, this essence draws the attention away from external distractions, towards profound inner spaces.

Rock Primula (*Primula saxatilis*) Quiet acceptance or connection with one's inner beauty/peace – regardless of what may be going on around you.

Roots and Wings Cedar (*Cedrus deodara*), White Orchid (*Cephalanthera longifolia*) Roots and Wings nurtures and reminds us that we are not separate, but one with existence itself. It gives us the courage to live our lives from this place of knowing and understanding. To tread lightly on the earth and interface with all beings through love.

The White Orchid opens wings in our heart, enabling the feeling and recognition of the vast open sky of love that is our nature. Gives courage to live from this heart-space, and meet the world through the eyes of love and openness, rather than through fear and rigidity. The Cedar anchors us to the Earth and so supports us to live our truth, knowing that we are one with our Mother Earth. Our bodies are from the Earth; we are not separate from the Earth. Our spirits are love and we are not separate from love.

Sat-Chit-Ananda A combination of Nirjara, Nirjara 2, Pink Primula, Rock Primula and White Orchid. Meditation essence. An exquisite support for melting into the heart of existence.

Sober Up Himalayan Honeysuckle (*Leycesteria formosa*) For grounding, balances excess energy in the head, gives stability, solidity and stamina. Has been reported to help give balance and stability to people with a tendency to drug and alcohol abuse and related problems.

Trust Anemone Clematis (*Clematis montana*) A bridge between the vertical and the horizontal dimensions (see the structure of the flower itself); the horizontal being the space/time dimension, the vertical being the transcendental/spiritual. Bringing one to a place of trust in the big picture – that one is exactly where one needs to be in this moment. A state of surrender. Also heals wounds between lovers allowing a higher level of union.

Vital Spark Indian Horsechestnut (*Aesculus indica*), *Hackelia uncinata*, Himalayan Musk Rose (*Rosa brunonii*), Himalayan Indigo (*Indigofea heterantha*) Enhances vitality and life force, especially in situations of shock, fear and extreme emotions. Centring. Helps one calm down, relax, let go and surrender to the moment, thereby providing space for healing to take place. Can be given to distressed animals, plants shocked due to replanting, etc.

White Orchid (*Cephalanthera longifolia*) A higher octave of the heart chakra. Accessing the angelic realms of the heart, compassion and bliss.

Himalayan astro enhancer essences

These 24 astro essences offer a doorway into the particular vibrational energies of the sun and moon in each of the 12 signs of the zodiac. Many people may be familiar with their sun sign, most commonly referred to as your zodiac sign, but if you have never had a birth chart done, and do not know your moon sign, you can still use these essences.

Take the essence of your own sun and moon sign if you wish to increase your conscious recognition of these energies, and/or to reveal that of which you have previously been unaware. Take your sun sign essence to help clarify your direction and add vitality; take your moon sign essence to help clarify your emotions and revitalize flagging feelings.

It can be beneficial to take essence of other sun and moon signs, if your current situation would benefit from a particular energy, or to reveal the energy of that sign. This revelation may be especially pertinent if you have another planet or point (such as the ascendant) in your birth chart in that sign. Briefly experiencing the energy of a sun or moon sign that is not your own may also help your understanding of how these energies are experienced by others.

Taking these essences may increase your awareness of the difficulties for each sign. Although possibly uncomfortable, revealing these difficult energies can add insight and assist healing.

Aries Sun essence Lost contact with your inner warrior? Need courage, enthusiasm, a fighting spirit? Starting a new venture? Start your motor, get moving with this essence.

Aries Moon essence Been feeling blue lately? A little down in the dumps? Need a pick-me-up tonic? This essence may provide the fuel to light your fire.

Taurus Sun essence Haven't seen your Earth goddess lately? Need stability, or help to push through? Assistance could be at hand with this essence.

Taurus Moon essence Feeling wobbly and need to feel grounded with indulgence, pampering and sensuality on the menu? The rich pastures you need could be in this essence.

Gemini Sun essence Need to communicate? Feeling mentally off the boil? The running shoes in this essence could get you off to a good start.

Gemini Moon essence Need to adapt to changes and movement on your inner life?

Feeling stuck for words? Get the words bubbling with this Gemini fizz.

Cancer Sun essence Need to connect with family, put down roots, make a home? Let the mothering influence in this essence help you.

Cancer Moon essence Aching for Mother to nurture and protect you? Feeling numb, closed off, fragile or vulnerable? Pick up the emotional grit in the crab shell of this essence.

Leo Sun essence Is the king in you dead? Stuck with your creative projects, need to be fired up? Get motivated and let this essence put the crown back on your head.

Leo Moon essence Lacking warmth, life feels serious? Take heart, contact your courage and playfulness with this sparkler of an essence.

Virgo Sun essence Can't see the wood for the trees? Muddling along in disorder and lacking routine? This essence may be the tool to perfect, tune and polish your life.

Virgo Moon essence Feel like you've lost your grip on things, everything feels chaotic? The servant in this essence may sort it all out for you.

Libra Sun essence Looking for compromise? Co-operation with others and team effort not working? The harmony you seek may be in this essence.

Libra Moon essence Feeling off balance and finding relationships with loved ones difficult? Add a dose of peace and beauty with this essence.

Scorpio Sun essence Need to shed some skin and to clear out some debris? Do a spot of research and get to the bottom of it all with this detective essence.

Scorpio Moon essence Wish to add some extra spice or bite to your feelings and emotions? Having difficulty connecting with your gut instincts? Put your feelings under the microscope with this essence.

Sagittarius Sun essence Run out of goals and need a new direction? Got itchy feet and yearn for adventure? Cut loose and seek new horizons with this essence.

Sagittarius Moon essence Feel like you've reached a dead end? Feeling restless and restricted? Feel your body and mind expand with this essence.

Capricorn Sun essence Lack discipline and needing to assume responsibilities? Nothing to work on and not achieving? This essence may provide the 'rope and tackle' to scale your next mountain.

Capricorn Moon essence Life feels out of control and feel unable to go the distance? Ache for a dose of stability and practicality? This essence may provide the 'mountain climbing boots' to get you back on track.

Aquarius Sun essence Searching for a new way and different methods? Do you have unusual ideas and want to change your world? Start the revolution by plugging in to this essence.

Aquarius Moon essence Feeling bored with the old you and fed up with being one of a crowd? Feel like a party? This essence could be the 'lightning bolt' you need.

Pisces Sun essence Struggling with trust in your life and forgotten your source of spiritual nourishment and 'the dreamer' inside you? Dive into your ocean with this essence.

Pisces Moon essence Need a dose of sensitivity and intuition and a rest from worldly affairs? Need to switch off and recharge your flat battery? Jump aboard this essence and float away.

Tasmanian wilderness mushrooms: fungi from the far south Tasmanian wilderness

These fungi mostly grow in the wilderness areas of the far south of Tasmania in ancient myrtle forests – only the tip of South America is further south on our planet. These beech-myrtle trees are hundreds of years old and as a species date back more than 780,000 years to Gondwanaland.

The mushrooms, as energies or essences, act across dimensions, independent of time and space, integrating personal, collective and cosmic dynamics. The essences are so powerful that often a single drop on the crown chakra is enough to ignite us into alignment within the greater whole and initiate a personal process.

As individuals, these essences take us down our unique pathways through our own personal psychology, physiology and history. The very personalized world of mental associations, images, memories, meanings and symbols dances in synchronicity with the mushroom energies causing realignment towards wholeness. While the specifics of the inner reorganization of representation and energetics are completely individual and not transferable in meaning or authority to any other, the process of specifically highlighted awareness and energetic re-patterning is identifiable and repeatable.

At the same time as the process of coming-into-personal-wholeness, there is a clear sense of the mushrooms acting simultaneously at the collective level of human consciousness, integrating and harmonizing dissonant energies. From this platform, awareness can expand to the cosmos and opens to an experiential bridge to oneness.

As we engage and work with these Tasmanian wilderness fungi, more and more they seem like old friends, as if they are conscious entities with personalities and domains of activity – they relate and respond in intimate synchronicity as if orchestrated within a huge and intimately interconnected cosmos. Taken once can be enough and act for weeks, maybe longer, a lifetime. They work on the whole being, the expanded energy/spirit through time, space and lifetimes.

Tanmaya has continued his research into essences and produced the following new essences.

Tasmanian Wilderness Mushrooms are taken as 1 drop on the crown and not internally. This is due to the lack of knowledge about potential toxicity of the fungi. Most Australian fungi are not classified or named.

Sorrow This mushroom helps when one is unable to connect deeply with a personal grief or loss, even if unconscious, but shaping one's current life, actions or decisions. Experientially, the process is very deep – one needs to give it time to unfold.

I am Earth pain and churning grief held, supported and integrated within a matrix of stillness.

Assimilation This mushroom offers deep physical, emotional and family healing by clearing old tensions held in the second and third chakras. It is an amazing healer, bringing deep peace, harmony and ease.

I digest life and align with purpose.

Singularity (*Ganoderma applanatum*) Singularity facilitates letting go to cosmogenic forces; it is like White Tara, the Divine Living Mother. Experientially it is a shower of white light vibrating the energy body to a higher frequency.

I balance left and right brain moving consciousness into a spacious domain while aligning with Earth.

Bleeding Heart Bleeding Heart is a wonderful gift. Awareness of the pain of the world is held in equilibrium and stillness, in a balance which is rock solid. The mushroom elicits great compassion like Christ's bleeding heart. This mushroom enables a deep cleansing of the collective heart in these painful times. Experientially, energy imprints courage, power and strength in vulnerability – supporting strength to stand there in my truth in the midst of chaos.

I stand alone, resilient from the blood of the ages.

Green Earth (*Dermocybe austroveneta*) This mushroom gives abiding peace and nurture. Embracing the natural world releases tension in the body which the musculature is holding. The fecundity of this mushroom is the energy of the forest. Experientially, under this energy of the forest, social grief, turmoil and chaotic influences move to settled calm, integration.

I am the human–Earth connection, the untamed Earth. I address the fear of wild nature.

Red Kali (*Hygrocybe miniata*) Red Kali resonates female sexuality and wild love. She initiates a restless spirit journey to the core of being, urging passionate expression. The energy is like a female planet Mars, the yang female, the active female, the wild female – Red Kali, Red Tara.

I am wise old woman, solid with the Earth. I know life and its pathways, rivers and ridges, cut into the contours of time and place.

Orange Trickster (*Clavulinopsis miniata*) Trickster's message and action is to 'Let go' – of thoughts, beliefs, tensions – to switch and snap out of 'states', particularly those where love is blocked. Trickster shakes up the fixed structures to enable free fall into love. Experientially, it is lively and enlivened, daring, reckless, cheeky and light.

I am all for Life, jumping empty handed into the void.

Coming Home (*Cortinarius sanguineus*) It releases, relaxes and restores so you are more fully, authentically, who you are – unshaped by external expectations and compliance. It is like pruning away unwanted but strong, habituated energy pathways which have shaped one's life – to encourage self-supporting growth. Experientially

there is a speeding of energy largely in the chest. A vibrant energy then expands, creating deep vibrant peace felt in the upper half of body, a sense of wellbeing.

The message of this mushroom is 'getting things off your chest'.

Ancient Myrtle (*Northofagua cunninghamii*) Giants in the wilderness forest, the Ancient Myrtles radiate a tangible, powerful presence invoking cosmic connection and awareness. The Ancient Myrtle energy alerts human consciousness to its capacity as a universal opening, a portal.

I am the ancient one breathing the cosmos into the impregnated Earth.

Pagoda People (*Podoserpula Pusio*) Pagoda People are a mushroom community of small yellow to orange mushrooms centred around one Pagoda mushroom. In the forest Pagoda People seem like children. The sense echoes interconnectedness of community which is playful and happy, celebrating the joy in being alive. The community spoke of trust in life and innocence.

I am filled with wellbeing, fully secure and connected.

Past Lives (*Naemataloma fascicularc*) This mushroom addresses deep trauma related to abuse, sex and death which are held in the first chakra. The healing is on both the personal and collective level. Formative wounds shape patterns which cascade through lives, events, relationships. These can be repatterned at their source, namely where energy shapes behaviours. Experientially, from my wound a survival pattern arising from the base chakra is shaken into visibility and re-experienced – the mushroom gives deep insight into the pattern and its effects drawing forth conscious integration.

I loosen and release energy blocks allowing whole-being integration.

Simplicity Simplicity offers deep relaxation and self-acceptance – no action, no doing, no fixing, simply being aware of being.

I am simple, deep, still and ordinary.

Red Ganesh This mushroom facilitates a visceral re-experiencing of obstacles which opens into a horizontal expansion of light and spacious awareness. Experientially, obstacles are felt in all their discomfort then dissolve as light expands and their weight lifts off.

I dissolve obstacles and create clarity.

Get Down This mushroom strengthens vitality in the first chakra. Ordinariness of sexuality and physicality becomes grounded with heightened sensory awareness.

I bring Earth support with a strong, stable, secure foundation.

Stairway to Heaven The white coral fungus grew on the base of the Ancient Myrtle. It offers a stepped and possible pathway to ascending layers of consciousness. It enables greater awareness at times of change, aligning one to be one step ahead. Experientially, waves of awareness rise through the body, clearing the dross in a container which is solid.

I reveal and create readiness for cumulative states of consciousness.

Liver Lover This mushroom cleanses the liver channel, and brings relaxation and release to the area around the third chakra. Experientially, there is an appreciation and gratitude for all the organs in the body – thanking them for their work and apologizing for past uncaring behaviour that burdened them.

I quietly purge tensions and hurts, physically and emotionally, facilitating flexibility.

Radiant Light From the ground of ordinary life, this mushroom expands consciousness. It brings deep relaxation, effortless presence, joyful contentment and delight in being.

I shine joyous golden light into areas of the body that need illuminating – expelling darkness.

Huge Eucalypt And I have been here as Earth from the beginning of time. I am the forest and the mountains. The ocean and all creatures. There is nothing embodied that I am not. I am still and patient, unwavering and undisturbed. This mushroom grounds the soul in its physical incarnation – simple, unwavering and steadfast bringing pleasure in form. I am finely connected and can choose where to attend, anywhere.

My body is the Earth.

Delight in Being This mushroom evokes a sense of being very comfortable in this physical existence – relaxed, undisturbed, contained, quietly being. Experientially, there is a kind of bubbly attunement with the little people of the mushroom world and forest, with a sense of wholeness.

I am delight, joy and a celebration of fecundity.

Buddha's Ears There is acute awareness of sounds and the world around and penetrating into other realms – dissolving the idea of separation into oneness. Experientially, energy extends out resolving 'knots' (blocks in my interconnecting field) – knots in relationships, knots created by ego, obstacles to flow that I created – bringing resolution.

I am right listening.

Fierce Love I cause internal and external shake-up, clearing space and expanding our human capacity for love on a common scale of experience. Love reverberates with this mushroom actively waking new states – wholeness manifests as present and embodied. Experientially, it is rooting out all mind concerns and debris bringing me back to here – it is sifting through the grunge, cleaning, bringing me back to expansion, lightness.

Kelp of the Great Southern Ocean Flexibility, fluidity and acceptance are the gifts of this kelp – flowing with all that comes I am firmly anchored. Experientially, tensions and resistances to life are shed through being immersed in oceanic connectedness.

I am at one with the movements of life.

The Gulaga Essences

Gulaga is a mountain on the South Eastern seaboard of Australia sacred to the Yuin people who regard her as the mother, the source of creation. She is the dominant feature on the coastal landscape, and her presence is felt by all (indigenous and non-indigenous) who live in or visit the area. She inspires, heals, confronts and nurtures, embodying the sacred wisdom and beauty of the Earth.

Yuin Elder: "Our Creation Story on the south coast of Tunku and Naadi coming down from the stars – they came from the stars to this beautiful land. They became this earth, they became part of the stones, the rocks, the clay. They became part of the trees and the mountains themselves...and the oceans. And they developed from the earth, and all our energies and everything else that we are is in those rocks at Gulaga and every other teaching place. And so we became part of the earth. We never profess to own the land, but the land owns us."

Gulaga Red Mushroom (Australia). A powerful essence for transformation. Ruthlessly exposing and clearing away all that is no longer appropriate or serving us our journey. Realigning us with our life's purpose. Made during a solar eclipse from a red mushroom at the sacred ceremonial site on Gulaga Mountain, on the far south coast of Australia's eastern seaboard.

Gulaga Crystal Quartz Crystal (Australia). Made from a crystal shard from a quartz vein connecting Gulaga (the mother) with Natchanuka (her son). Imparts grounding vision reconnecting with source. Aligns the mind, crystallizes intention, grounds new vision, strengthens resolve. Brings lightness, clarity and joy.

Gulaga Orchid King Orchid (*Dendrobium speciosum*) (Australia). Opens the heart to forgiveness of self and others.

Peace (*Magnolia grandiflora*) Opens channels to receive *prana* (life force). Relaxes one deeply into the moment, and accepting life as it is.

Protection Combination of *Black Tourmaline*, *Isan*, *Pink Yarrow*, *Aura Cleaning*, and *Let Go*. Protection from unwanted psychic, emotional energies. Space clearing.

Repatterning Fungus (Australia). Helps open one to new information and ground it in the body. Reboots energy pathways to keep pace with one's growing awareness.

Sludge Buster (*Melaleuca lateritia*) A good spring cleaner of all those murky corners.

Spider Fungus Exposes primal wounds/ dysfunctions in the first chakra, particularly around sexuality. Promotes clear and authentic speaking.

Synergy Fungus Enhances inter-connectedness, a sense of community and co-operation. Helpful for bringing people together at the beginning of workshops.

Tracking (*Ochna serrulata*) Brings clarity to point of disturbance or imbalance in oneself or client, where it may be appropriate to bring healing awareness.

Womb With A View Fungus (Australia). Brings recognition and release from energetics one received *in utero* that are not one's own and do not serve one's higher purpose.

F.

USA, SOUTH AMERICA AND CANADA

For hundreds of years before the arrival of European settlers, the vast and colourful North American continent was inhabited by peoples who knew it as Turtle Island. These Native Americans regarded themselves as caretakers or keepers of the land who were responsible for safeguarding its fertility. They saw themselves as belonging to the natural world and also saw it as their duty not to disturb the balance that exists in nature. The idea of splitting up and owning various bits of land was alien to them. The whole of Turtle Island was their home and they regarded it as sacred. Native North as well as South American legends talk of Gentle Giants who once walked upon the Earth in times when all was peace and harmony. These 'Giants' were reputedly a highly spiritual people, such was their awareness of the Great Spirit – Gitchi Manitou – in all living things and their deep connection with nature. They are said to have possessed the gift of talking with the energies of animals, flowers, the wind, water and thunder. They also had the ability to utilize these energies for healing purposes. Native American traditions live on and are an inspiration to many of those who seek to explore the healing powers of nature.

ALASKAN FLOWER AND ENVIRONMENTAL ESSENCES (Ask)

The Alaskan Flower Essence Project was founded by Steve Johnson in 1984 to coordinate the collection of new flower essences from the extensive ecological regions of Alaska.

Johnson was born and raised in the mountains of Idaho where he developed a deep connection with the natural environment. He spent his childhood playing in the gardens and orchards, walking in the forests and swimming in the nearby lakes and rivers. After graduating from high school he began his career working as a fire-fighter. He was stationed near the largest wilderness area in the United States where he learned the names and uses of all the local plants. He then transferred to Alaska, a land of vast, unspoiled forests and tundra regions which are home to many unusual species of plants.

Johnson's interest in flower essences was kindled in 1980 when he was given two Bach Flower Remedies and experienced a notable change in his health and emotional being. As a result of this experience he decided to find out as much as he could about flower essences and their mode of healing. During the next three years he trained in auric energy balancing, polarity, reflexology and massage before specializing in using vibrational energies for emotional, mental and spiritual healing.

He began making Alaskan flower essences in the summer of 1983, preparing them from the native plants of Alaska which have adapted and flourished over many aeons in a vibrant ecosystem, an environment of extremes from frigid cold to sweltering heat, from long dark winters to summers of perpetual light. These flowering plants reflect the special strength, power and vitality of this land.

Because they have evolved freely, without human intrusion, this community of plants embodies a unique range of vibrational energies and healing qualities that are especially relevant to the growth and evolution of human consciousness.

While the Alaskan Kits 1 and 2 are composed primarily of the essences of flowering trees and plants, and aim to balance the core or fundamental life-energy patterns, Kit 3 features essences from unique and rare plants which work on the subtle or spiritual levels of our being. The majority of essences in these kits come from wild flowers growing in healthy thriving plant communities at the peak of their blossoming stage, while the garden remedies come from blossoms growing in a co-creative garden (nature and the nature spirits co-creating together).

Encapsulating the special energies of Alaska, these flower essences provide significant levels of support for the process of conscious change and transformation and work on issues related to unfolding one's future, opening to higher levels of perception and understanding, and living life in alignment with divine purpose. They are also unique in their orientation towards healing the heart and therefore healing our relationship with each other and all forms of nature.

Johnson further developed combination essences, and Alaskan feng shui sprays to address the toxic build-up in one's surroundings. The environmental essences are an interesting exploration into the concept that we are directly affected and influenced by the forces of nature (see Section J of the Encyclopedia on environmental and sound essences).

Kit 1

Alder (*Alnus crispa*) For clarity of perception on all levels, allowing our seeing to become knowing, recognizing truth in personal experience. Empowers us to move beyond limited mental programming and respond to higher learning.

Balsam Poplar (*Populus balsamifera*) Releases the pain and emotional tension associated with sexual issues (which block the circulation of energy in the body); resulting from shock and trauma or a lack of grounding, associated with sexual trauma; synchronizes sexual energy with planetary cycles and rhythms.

Black Spruce (*Populus balsamifera*)Allows integration of the eternal into awareness and experience in the present; opens us up to information contained within the archetypes of nature. Helps us to learn the wisdom of the ages.

Blue Elf Viola (*Viola* sp.) Helps us to understand the seeds of our anger and frustrations; enables us to express anger in a clear and non-violent way; releases and dissipates the protective energy surrounding unresolved conflicts, bringing the whole process to completion so they can be expressed in a clear and heart-centred way.

Chiming Bells (*Mertensia paniculata*) Peace through understanding one's true nature; joy in physical existence; awakens a spiritual awareness of nature. Good for feeling depressed; despondent; disheartened; no joy in one's day-to-day existence; feeling a lack of support and stability at a basic level. For regeneration, renewal and stability at the physical level of our beings; opens us to the loving energy of the Divine Mother.

Cotton Grass (*Eriophorum* sp.) For letting go of pain held in the body; shock and trauma resulting from an accident or injury of any kind; fixating on one's discomfort rather than on the healing process; unable to heal an old injury completely because of a lack of awareness of what led to its creation. Helps a person come to an understanding of the core issues that led to an accident or injury so that they can release the physical, emotional and mental trauma associated with it. Restores equilibrium after injury or trauma; shifts our focus from pain to healing. Can be applied topically.

Dandelion (*Taraxacum officinale*) Brings awareness and release of emotional tension and stress held in muscle tissue; and the deeper mental attitudes that lead to chronic muscular tension; increases one's level of body–mind communication to be better able to identify the underlying issues and attitudes. Difficulty releasing emotional energy stored in the body. For use both internally and externally.

Fireweed (*Epilobium angustifolium*) Helps us ground and cleanse old stagnant energy patterns from the body so that new life may enter; good when feeling burned out or have a weak connection to the Earth. Strengthens and restores a nurturing flow of energy after a traumatic or transforming experience. Brings new cycles of renewal and revitalization. Useful in emergency situations especially for releasing physical pain, trauma and shock.

Forget-Me-Not (*Myosotis alpestris*) Opens our hearts for the release of pain held deep in the subconscious; facilitates the release of fear, guilt, feeling separate; difficulty connecting to the spiritual dimension; helps us to remember our original innocence. To regain true respect and compassion for ourselves, others and the Earth.

Foxglove (*Digitalis purpurea*) Releases fear and emotional tension centred around the heart; fear of the unknown; lack of perspective on how to deal with a challenging situation; allows us to see through perceptual constrictions to the 'heart' of the matter. During conflict or difficulty enables our perceptions to expand to connect with the truth of the situation.

Green Bells of Ireland (*Moluccella laevis*) For opening our perceptual awareness

to the various levels of energy and intelligence that exist in nature; feeling ungrounded; helps us to reconnect with the energy of the natural world and to feel at home on the Earth. Helps the newly born greet the Earth; strengthens the energetic connection between the physical body and the Earth.

Golden Corydalis (*Corydalis aurea*) Creates the ability to get all of one's talents and skills to work together in a focused way; and make sense of how one's life fits together. For positive growth of the personality. Restores full communication between the soul and the personality; reintegrates our identity according to the needs of the soul after an experience of deep transformation.

Icelandic Poppy (*Papaver icelandica*) For reflecting one's inner radiance to all aspects of life. When survival, sexual and spiritual aspects of life are not integrated. Supports the gentle unfolding of spiritual receptivity; strengthens our capacity to integrate and radiate spiritual energy into all aspects of our lives. Opens us up to and helps us maintain a spiritual focus in life.

Jacob's Ladder (*Polemonium pulcherrimum*) Helps to bring awareness of our attempts to control the events of our lives and be open to receiving the creative impulses of the soul; allows mental control to evolve into a disciplined acceptance of spirit. Resolves unclarity about intention or motivation. When lacking trust in the spiritual world and trying to 'figure things out' brings you to a place of opening to receive the wisdom that is available in each moment.

Labrador Tea (*Ledum palustre*) For addictions, and when attempting to balance one extreme with another. For imbalance in any area of life. When you have difficulty coming back to centre after a traumatic or unsettling experience. Centres energy in the body and calms extreme imbalances of physical, emotional and mental energy; relieves the stress associated with extremes and helps continually learn a new perspective of balance. Useful in times of emotional catharsis or after traumatic experiences.

Lady's Slipper (*Cypripedium guttatum*) Helps us to gain awareness of subtler energy flows in and around the body. Personality. Alleviates resistance to receiving healing energy from others. Fosters the collection, focus and release of energy for healing and regulates circulation in all of the major energy pathways. Works on the chakras and central nervous system and spine – gentle catalyst.

Monkshood (*Aconitum delphinifolium*) Gives fearlessness. For those who feel vulnerable through lack of well-defined boundaries and who have difficulty allowing contact with others. A powerful and precise essence which increases our ability to interact with others through a stronger identification with our divine nature; strengthens and defines our energy fields so we can create and maintain our physical, emotional and mental boundaries to help us function in accordance with our higher purpose.

Paper Birch (*Betula papyrifera*) Helps us gain a clear perspective of our true purpose; reveals the underlying true and essential self present within. Confusion or disorientation about the direction life should take; unable to connect with deeper levels of insight regarding life purpose. Useful when facing important life decisions, or when lost or uncertain how to proceed, helps us gain a clearer perspective of our life purpose and how to live it.

Prickly Wild Rose (*Rosa acicularis*) For openness, courage and renewed interest in life in the face of adverse circumstances. For lacking trust and faith; feeling hopeless; apathetic and uninterested in life; unable to keep the heart open when involved in adverse circumstances. Allows the heart to open in response to conflict and struggle.

Brings courageous interest in life and our hopes to fruition.

Spiraea (*Spiraea beauverdiana*) To overcome resistance to conscious growth and expansion. For feeling unsupported by life; attachment to the way things are, even if they are not to our liking. Brings unconditional acceptance of support, regardless of the form it comes in. To learn to nurture and be nurtured by living things.

Twinflower (*Linnaea borealis*) For those who are defensive or reactive and have difficulty expressing themselves or listening to/understanding others. Improves communication skills, helping us to listen and speak to others from a place of quiet, inner calm and focused neutrality.

Wild Iris (*Iris setosa*) For lack of belief in one's own capacity to create; blocking and disconnected from creative expression because of an unwillingness to share it with others; brings a focused release of creativity, encouraging sharing one's inner beauty and creative energy freely and enables recognition of the beautiful expression of divine creativity.

Willow (*Salix bebbiana*) Brings mental receptivity, flexibility and resilience. Dissolves resistance to taking responsibility for one's actions or for the life one has created; brings awareness of how thoughts create reality. Helps us remove our resistance to consciously creating our lives and a positive reality from the quality of one's thoughts.

Yarrow (*Achillea borealis*) For strengthening the overall integrity of the energy field; knowing and being the source of one's own protection. For those oversensitive to the environment when the integrity of the aura has been compromised by injury or trauma in this or another lifetime. Use to seal energy breaks in the aura and strengthen the aura and the overall integrity of the energy field and build a protective shield against environmental hazards, such as electromagnetic radiation from computers and fluorescent lights. Helps us know and be the source of our own protection.

Kit 2

Alpine Azalea (*Loiseleuria procumbens*) Releases old patterns of self-doubt. Opens your heart to the spirit of love. For living in total unconditional acceptance of yourself; teaches us compassion through understanding. Clears self-doubt and stops us withholding love from ourselves or being unable to have compassion for ourselves.

Bog Blueberry (*Vaccinium uliginosum*) Clears conditional acceptance of abundance; attachment to the form in which anything manifests in one's life. Neutralizes the beliefs that limit the experience of abundance on all levels; encourages us to open to the abundance that is offered with acceptance and gratitude.

Bog Rosemary (*Andromeda polifolia*) Nurtures through the process of trust. For deep cleansing and healing of the experience of life, strengthens trust in divine healing and support. Promotes the release of fear and resistance held deep in the heart; helps one let go of any resistance to being healed. Strengthens one's connection with the infinite life force.

Bunchberry (*Cornus canadensis*) For focusing and directing the power of the will; for mental steadfastness and emotional clarity in demanding situations, especially when easily distracted by or caught up in the emotional turmoil of others. For when we feel we do not have enough time to complete tasks. Strengthens the boundary between the emotional and mental body and promotes coherent thinking.

Cassandra (*Chamaedaphne calyculata*) Quietens and calms the mind; clears anxiousness and increases the depth of perception so that we can sense the currents of life. Acts as a catalyst to improve the quality of our relationship with nature. An aid to relax into deeper levels of meditation in order to receive inner guidance.

Columbine (*Aquilegia formosa*) For self-appreciation, cherishing our unique and distinctive personal beauty regardless of how it differs from others'. For projecting a strong sense of self and the ability to project ourselves out in the world for others to see.

Cow Parsnip (*Heracleum lanatum*) For those who feel powerless to direct their lives. Feeling ungrounded and cut off from one's roots; unsure of one's inner direction; or when having difficulty connecting with or adapting to new surroundings after a move. Promotes inner strength; assists with the process of adapting to a new environment. Helps us to thrive wherever we are. Brings contentment with present circumstances and peace of mind during times of intense transition and change.

Grass of Parnassus (*Parnassia palustris*) Brings a high and pure quality of light into the aura for cleansing, purification and protection; attracts nourishment from nature, re-energizing. Helpful for those who have difficulty maintaining energy levels in toxic environments, or who are living and working in crowded, polluted surroundings. Helps us bring past experiences to completion on all levels.

Grove Sandwort (*Moehringia lateriflora*) For feeling a lack of physical and emotional nurturing; weak bonding connections between mother and child; feeling unsupported by the Earth. Strengthens the physical and emotional bonds of communication and comfort between mother and child; opens us up to support a nurturing relationship between Earth Mother and all living beings, and encourages sharing this support with others.

Horsetail (*Equisetum arvense*) For distorted communication with other levels of one's consciousness; difficulty communicating with the Higher Selves of others, including animals. Helps feeling connected; enhances communication with our different levels of consciousness. Through this we are better able to make true contact with others. Improves inter-species communication.

Lace Flower (*Tiarella trifoliata*) For appreciation of all nature and of ourselves; strengthens self-acceptance and our sense of self-worth; realizing the importance of how a unique contribution enriches the contribution to the whole, however humble. Dissolves lack of awareness, acceptance or appreciation of our own natural beauty and intrinsic value; feeling insignificant; unsure of how our personal or professional contributions fit into the whole.

Mountain Wormwood (*Artemisia tilesii*) For healing old wounds; helps us by releasing unforgiven areas in our relationships with others and with ourselves. Dissolves unresolved anger and resentment; forgiving past actions regardless of the intent behind them. Helps to bring all our relationships into balance.

Opium Poppy (*Papaver somniferum*) For when unable to find balance between activity and rest. For finding a balance between doing and being; helps us integrate previous experiments in order to live fully in the present. Balances extremes of activity and rest, being and doing. Clears deep exhaustion; unawareness of past accomplishments; and difficulties in understanding and integrating lessons and experiences so we may live more fully in the present.

Pineapple Weed (*Matricaria matricarioides*) Encourages freedom from injury and risk through harmony with our physical environment. For those unaware of the support and nurturing that is available from nature and also for weak nurturing bond between mother and child; helps to build affinity between mothers and children. For active young children, mothers and mothers-to-be. Promotes sense of wellbeing during pregnancy.

River Beauty (*Epilobium latifolium*) An essence of emotional recovery, reorientation and regeneration. To help you start over after a devastating experience overwhelmed by grief, sadness or a sense of loss; shock and trauma from emotional or sexual abuse and to see adverse circumstances as a potential for cleansing and growth. Helps us start over.

Single Delight (*Moneses uniflora*) For those suffering feelings of isolation and loneliness during a dark or depressing time; cloudy inner vision. Links us energetically with other members of our soul family. Opens the heart and reminds us of the support we have always had.

Sticky Geranium (*Geranium erianthum*) For getting out of a rut, or 'unstuck'; frees the many aspects of our potential; helps us to go beyond previous stages of growth. For feeling unfocused, lethargic or indecisive; resistance to moving on to the next level or stage of an experience; lacking energy to reach our goals; attached to our current level of consciousness and identity. Encourages us to move from procrastination and lethargy to decisive and focused action.

Sunflower (*Helianthus annuus*) For an unbalanced expression of masculine energy in men or women; weak or dysfunctional relationship to the father, or to one's own identity as a father. Strengthens our radiant expression; harmonizes the active, masculine aspect of energy in both men and women. Promotes a functional relationship and teaches us to accept the authority of the Higher Self, without imposing our will on others.

Sweetgale (*Myrica gale*) For emotional energies blocked in lower chakras. For when emotional communication with others is defensive, lacking clarity, and is characterized by conflict, blame and the assignment of guilt. Aids deep integration and release of emotional pain and tension that undermines the quality of our communication and interactions with others, especially in male/female relationships. Heals the core of our emotional interactions with others. Aids completion of unfinished emotional experiences, enabling us to respond to the present with strength and clarity.

Tamarack (*Larix laricina*) Builds self-confidence through a deeper understanding of one's unique skills and abilities. For a weak sense of self-identity; or those who lack awareness of what they are capable of. Helps us remain centred in the knowledge and self-confidence that our abilities will carry us through challenging times. Encourages the conscious development of individuality.

Tundra Rose (*Potentilla fruticosa*) For hopelessness; lack of inspiration and motivation. For those overwhelmed by the responsibilities they have taken on. Restores hope, courage, inspiration and a love of life. Allows the power of life to be communicated through our living of it; for combating fears of living and dying. Releases deep resistance that has blocked the dynamic expression of spirit in our lives. Encourages a robust expression of joy and enthusiasm to the fulfilment of one's responsibilities.

White Spruce (*Picea glauca*) Unification. For information overload; feeling disintegrated; unable to apply knowledge to life's challenges; difficulty integrating how one feels with how one thinks. Balances intuition, thought and emotion together and unifies them in the present moment. Native Alaskans considered this to be 'the gentle grandfather healer' – a touchstone to our higher knowledge. Brings us to a place of balance and stability. Grounds spiritual wisdom into the body and opens us up to that internal wisdom that will illuminate our current situation.

White Violet (*Viola renifolia*) For highly sensitive people who find contained environments intolerable. For those uncomfortable in closed spaces and constrained environments and those who are fearful of losing their identity in a group or unable to embody their sensitivity in a comfortable way. Supports creation of new energetic boundaries, allowing trust and relaxation to develop regardless of the dynamics of the environment. Opens our hearts to the essence of purity; connects us with the highest in ourselves and in others.

Yellow Dryas (*Dryas drummondii*) Support for those who explore the edge of the unknown; for the expansion and clarification and maintaining awareness of self and family throughout dynamic cycles of growth and change. For feeling estranged from one's soul family; unable to sense the connective thread that links one's experiences into a coherent and understandable whole. For the pioneer in us.

Kit 3

Bladderwort (*Utricularia vulgaris*) Brings awareness of truth and shattering illusion through clear internal knowing so that we see only truth. Promotes discernment when faced with dishonesty in others; strengthens our ability to perceive the truth regardless of the confusion that surrounds it. Enables one to make decisions that support one's highest good. Good for those often deceived or taken advantage of or with a lack of discernment.

Blueberry Pollen (*Vaccinium uliginosum*) For abundance. Releases deep patterns of limitation from the mind so we can attract and be open to receive all we need to live life to the fullest. For those with a lack of belief in the concept of abundance; low prosperity consciousness; difficulty receiving from others and from the Earth. Helps us expand on all levels to accommodate abundance; facilitates the release of mental and emotional attachments that limit our ability to manifest higher purpose in physical form.

Cattail Pollen (*Typha latifolia*) For standing tall in one's personal truth; helps you to find the courage and inner strength to act in alignment with this truth even during pain and trauma; to follow your chosen path even when feeling unsupported by others and weakened by connections and involvements which no longer serve one's highest good.

Comandra (*Geocaulon lividum*) For clearing disharmonious energies from the heart that limit one's ability to be open to and aware of subtle energies in nature. For those whose visionary abilities are undeveloped or ungrounded and of no practical use, and whose focus of their perceptions is limited to the material aspects of the physical world. Supports maintaining the necessary vision to move through the current dimensional shift; opens the heart to be a bridge between the third and fourth dimensions; helps us develop our potential to see the physical world from a higher perspective.

Green Bog Orchid (*Platanthera obtusata*) Gently releases blocked pain and fear held deep in the heart due to lack of trust in one's deeper motivations. For difficulty communicating from the heart. For coming into true balance with the natural kingdom so that we can fulfil our divine co-creative potential. Expands our awareness, sensitivity and ability to perceive life from a place of openness and neutrality and encourages the development of a heart connection with others.

Green Fairy Orchid (*Hammarbya paludosa*) For accepting oneness through total internal balance. For when there is a core imbalance between the masculine and feminine aspects of the self, resulting in difficulty resolving conflicts within the heart. Creates a level of honesty in the heart where nothing is hidden; expands the heart, balancing the inner male/female at the deepest level of the body and being. Releases duality.

Hairy Butterwort (*Pinguicula villosa*) Ascension. Aids acknowledgement or trust in higher guidance and support, especially when confronted with a challenging situation or life lesson; clears lack of awareness of the core issues that need to be addressed in order to resolve a situation. Helps consciously access the support and guidance needed in order to move through threshold points of conflict and transition with grace, ease and deep understanding without creating crisis or illness.

Harebell (*Campanula lasiocarpa*) Removes self-imposed mental and emotional limitations, when feeling unloved and cut off from the source; looking for love outside of oneself. Allows you to open up your life to receive universal love and the presence of the divine and give unconditional love.

Ladies' Tresses (*Spiranthes romanzoffiana*) For lack of awareness of the connection between our life lessons and our life purpose; difficulty reconnecting with the body after a serious injury or traumatic experience. Brings deep internal alignment for releasing deeply held traumas held at the cellular level, helps us reconnect energetically with parts of the body that have been injured or traumatized. Realigns you with your soul purpose in this lifetime.

Lamb's Quarters (*Chenopodium album*) Heals separation when there is a lack of balance and harmony between the mind and heart, the rational and the intuitive. Helps to assimilate information through the heart before interpreting it through the mind. For those who tend to be highly intellectual.

Brings the power of the mind into balance with the joy of the heart.

Moschatel (*Adoxa moschatellina*) For those with an overly intellectual focus on life; believing that everything must come through struggle; creating without joy. Teaches us how to accomplish more by grounding our mental focus into the Earth. Opens our intuitive connection with the plant kingdom and helps us learn how to co-create with nature through celebration and play.

Northern Lady's Slipper (*Cypripedium passerinum*) Reconnects body and spirit. For a weak body/soul connection; traumatic birth experience; pain and trauma held very deeply in the body. Allows one's being to be touched and healed by infinite gentleness. A positive nurturing energy and a catalyst for adults who need to heal the core traumas of their inner child and the wounds that are being held very deeply in the body. Good for children and babies with birth traumas.

Northern Twayblade (*Listera borealis*) Clears resistance to opening of the subtle aspects of our own consciousness. For when we are unable to integrate our spiritual wisdom and divine nature with our most basic needs. Helps us ground our sensitivity to the subtle realms more fully into our physical body and life experience; helps us enlighten our most basic needs, instincts and mundane realities with the finest aspects of our spiritual wisdom.

One-Sided Wintergreen (*Pyrola secunda*) Helps sensitive people become aware of how they impact on and are impacted by others. Teaches us how to work in close proximity with others without losing our centre; helps create functional energy boundaries based on awareness of our own sensitivities. Dissolves dysfunctional energy boundaries when strongly influenced by other people's energy. For creating and maintaining functional boundaries that are in alignment with one's highest truth and

life purpose, especially when unaware of how one's energy and actions affect others.

Round-Leaved Sundew (*Drosera rotundifolia*) For merging with the source of life; relinquishing identification with your ego, blending ego and divine will. Letting go of resistance to change and attachment to the known, fear of the unknown; when struggle rather than change is preferred. Overidentification with the ego; lack of communication between the Lower and Higher Self. Brings the ego into alignment with divine will.

Shooting Star (*Dodecatheon frigidum*) For developing our connection to inner spiritual guidance for understanding cosmic origins and earthly purpose. When a sense of not belonging on the Earth or homesickness for a place that cannot be identified creates an inability to understand consciously why one is here. Strengthens one's connection to inner spiritual guidance; brings a deeper understanding of cosmic origins and earthly purpose.

Sitka Burnet (*Sanguisorba stipulata*) For healing the past on all levels and feelings of internal discord from unknown origins. When unable to locate the source of our problems in life or having difficulty understanding the lessons contained within our learning experiences. Initiates healing completion on all levels – a facilitation essence which helps you identify issues that are contributing to internal conflict, bringing forth the potential in any healing process.

Sitka Spruce Pollen (*Picea sitchensis*) A 'grandfather' essence which acts as a catalyst by supporting the right action for the present moment, fostering a positive relationship with one's power. Dissolves lack of humility in one's relationship to the Earth. Clears and expands our energy channels so that we can accept a strong flow of energy in the body. Connects us with ancient archetypes of mastery, male and female power perfectly joined together, clears imbalance between the masculine and feminine expressions of power within an individual. For reluctance to express or exercise one's power for fear of hurting someone. Balances power and gentleness in men and women supporting the balanced partnership with nature.

Soapberry (*Sheperdia canadensis*) Release of constrictions around the heart associated with a fear of the power of nature, fear of one's own power, or fear of using one's power in irresponsible, inappropriate or unbalanced ways. For understanding and integrating intense experiences in nature and helps us move through fear with an open heart. Supports us in channelling the expression of power through our hearts. Harmonizes both personal and planetary power.

Sphagnum Moss (*Sphagnum* sp.) For those who are overly critical and judgemental of the healing journey and obsessing about the day-to-day details of the healing process. For those who are unable to see the positive side of transformational experiences. Helps us release the need for harsh judgement or criticism of our healing journey; enables us to create a space of unconditional acceptance in the heart so that core issues can be brought there for healing, and helps us learn to see with unconditional love.

Sweetgrass (*Hierochloe odorata*) For the cleansing and rejuvenating of the energy blockages in the etheric and physical body and low energy flow during the day. For difficulties in bringing a healing process to final completion. Good for removing negative energies from the home or work environment. Helps to bring one's lessons and experiences to completion on all levels and removes disharmonious energies from our home or work environment.

Tundra Twayblade (*Listera cordata*) Supports the release of deep pain, anguish and past trauma held at the deepest level of one's being. Opens the heart to allow unconditional love complete access to areas of the body that need healing – supports the clearing of trauma held at the cellular level of the body, especially dysfunctional patterns held within the collective consciousness (abuse being the most prevalent form of these patterns today).

White Fireweed (*Epilobium angustifolium*) For deep emotional healing of shock and trauma from profound alienation from the body after an experience of sexual or emotional abuse. Calms the emotional body after shocking experience, releasing the energetic imprint of the past emotionally painful experiences from our cellular memory so rejuvenation can begin.

Wild Rhubarb (*Polygonum alaskanum*) Promotes mental flexibility, clearing blocked or undeveloped mental faculties and expanding the channel of communication between the heart and mind. Brings the mind into alignment with divine will through the heart; encourages a relaxation of inappropriate mental control; balances the rational and the intuitive. As a result, new thoughts, plans for action and solutions to problems come about.

New essences

Angelica (*Angelica genuflexa*) Promotes effortless acceptance of spiritual support in all situations; letting the light into your life, experiencing the protection that comes from within.

Cloudberry (*Rubus chamaemorus*) Opening to the true source of your being and reflecting this outwardly for others to see; for replacing low self-esteem with an awareness of inner value; helps you see the light of purity deep within yourself; recognizing the 'angelic' level of your being.

Comfrey (*Symphytum officinale*) Supports healing on all levels; heals the etheric body when there has been an injury in this or another lifetime; promotes the embodiment of higher spiritual energies and the expression of our divine potential.

Dwarf Fireweed (*Epilobium adenocaulon*) Helps transform unresolved issues that are held at the core of your being; allows you to be open to and experience transformation with gentleness, pacing and ease; releases pain and trauma from the past so you can reconnect with the original joy of living, helps to fine-tune how we move through a healing process so we do not create more difficulties or pain. Encourages the feeling of 'I have my whole life to live'.

Lapland Rosebay (*Rhododendron lapponicum*) Penetrating insight into the self and all of nature; seeing without distortion; brings a person back to their senses when they have been looking outside of themselves for answers; reminds you to look within for wisdom, knowledge, perspective and direction.

Lilac (*Syringa vulgaris*) Aligns the chakras so that they can more fully receive and embody light; helps you gracefully raise the frequency of your energy fields. For raising energetic vibration in the body; aligning the chakras to receive and embody light energy fully.

Pale Corydalis (*Corydalis sempervirens*) Balances addictive and conditional patterns of loving; helps you see relationships as catalysts for spiritual growth and enlightenment; helps you follow the divine plan in relationships.

Pink-Purple Poppy (*Papaver somniferum*) Purity in form; helps you embody and project universal love through your heart. Helps you maintain balance during rapid phases of evolution, when your entire vibrational makeup is undergoing transformation; enables you to experience deep levels of integration and rest while allowing the transformative process to continue; helps you open to and embody new information from the Higher Self that enhances life in the physical dimension.

Potato (*Solanum tuberosum*) Physical release: helps you 'thaw out' incomplete cycles of experience that are being held in the body; allowing love to penetrate into every cell of the body and into all manifestations of your being.

Purple Mountain Saxifrage (*Saxifraga oppositifolia*) Grounding wisdom from the Higher Self; helps you tune in to higher frequencies of information.

Purple Poppy (*Papaver somniferum*) Balance during rapid phases of evolution, when our entire vibrational makeup is undergoing transformation; enables us to experience deep levels of integration and rest while allowing the transformative process to continue; helps us be open to and embody new information from the Higher Self that enhances life in the physical dimension.

Red Elder (*Sambucus racemosa*) Grandmother wisdom (Native American for wisdom of the ages) helps one view life from the centre rather than from the periphery; and open up to your future potential. Also helps one contract overexpanded states, that is, feeling frazzled and overwhelmed.

Red-Purple Poppy (*Papaver somniferum*) For balancing extremes between physical and etheric levels; blending the survival and spiritual aspects of life together in a balanced way, supports us in making full use of our physical capacities to embody spirit.

Self-Heal (*Prunella vulgaris*) For raising self-esteem, self-acceptance and an expansion of love and compassion for yourself. Helps strengthen your belief in the body's ability to heal itself. Relaxing and calming, slows one down in order to gain perspective on priorities, especially under pressure to do and decide.

Valerian (*Valeriana officinalis*) Helps you slow down in order to gain perspective on your priorities, especially when feeling pressured to do or decide; promotes harmony in relationships finding a peaceful common ground.

Wild Sweet Pea (*Hedysarum mackenzii*) Increases your sense of your own inner strength and stability; helps bring these qualities to the surface to be offered in balance to others; promotes confidence and ease in your interactions with others.

Yellow Paintbrush (*Castilleja unalaschensis*) Facilitates the release of emotional frustrations and feelings of self-limitation that block our creative expression; helps you open and cleanse the heart so that it may act as a focal point for the sharing of your creative energies.

Combination essences

Calling All Angels *Angelica, Chalice Well, Chiming Bells, Kunzite.* Calling All Angels is a combination formula that helps you contact the love, guidance and protection of the angelic realm. It brings a very soft, loving and serene energy into your heart, physical body and environment. Use it to:

- strengthen the knowledge that you are guided, supported and protected by the angels;

- bring more joy and peace in to your life;

- make a stronger connection with the divine feminine;

- create a sacred and protected space for sleeping and dreaming, especially for children;

- come into a stronger awareness of your own angelic nature; experience the love of the angelic kingdom in your physical body.

Fireweed Combo *Fireweed, River Beauty, White Fireweed, Dwarf Fireweed.* Fireweed Combo encourages and supports deep processes of transformation and renewal. Helpful to prepare for a transformational experience, especially useful when in the middle of an intense healing process and needing extra support to get through it. Enables you to access the support you need to face fears, let go of resistance and allow the process to move forward through each stage to its completion. Helps to:

- strengthen your grounding connection to the Earth so your energy system will be more stable and better able to cope with change;

- shift the whole transformative process to a deeper level by releasing layers of deep pain and emotional trauma that are being held at the cellular level of the body;

- stay engaged with the transformative process until you have resolved all of the issues that are connected to it;

- reconnect with the desired levels of joy and happiness that are your birth right.

Add to a bath whenever you need additional support to make it through a period of intense transformation and change.

Guardian *Covellite, Devil's Club, Round-Leaf Orchid, Stone Circle, White Violet Yarrow.* Guardian creates a powerful force field of protection in your aura. It invokes positive, harmonious energies that help you claim your energetic space, maintain your grounding and feel the protection of strong, healthy boundaries. Especially effective for those who:

- are overly reactive to influences in their environment;

- are ambivalent about being present in their body and on the Earth, because they don't feel safe or protected;

- work around computers and other electromagnetic equipment or in a toxic environment;

- have a tendency to take on or absorb the thoughts and emotions of others;

- are unable to embody their sensitivity in a practical and easy way because of a lack of functional boundaries;

- are doing healing work that requires them to be in the working, living or personal energy space of their clients;

- have just moved into a new home or neighbourhood and are having difficulty grounding into their new situation;

- feel tired or run-down and need to rest and nurture themselves, but can't seem to create the space to do it.

Lighten Up *Carnelian, Grass of Parnassus, Orange Calcite, Solstice Sun.* A combination formula that increases your ability to embody light. Its overall effect is to uplift, energize, inspire and nourish. Designed specifically for people who suffer from light deprivation, either due to living in extreme northern or southern latitudes, the limitations of their living environment (in a dark house or apartment) or because of the quality of their energy system (energy pathways blocked or undeveloped). It is also helpful for those who are depressed, caught in negative patterns or situations, or feel cut off in any way from their inner sources of light. It works on three main levels:

- It opens and cleanses the chakras so you can draw more life force energy through appropriate channels already present in your energy system.

- It cleanses and expands the energy pathways in your physical body, and amplifies your ability to assimilate light at the cellular level.

- It strengthens your ability to integrate experience, thereby increasing the amount of energy that can flow through your body and life.

Use when you are fatigued or feel a chronic lack of energy on the physical level. When you want to enhance the qualities of light in your living and working environments. For seasonal affective disorder. With animals that must be kept inside for long periods, especially during the winter months. In the classroom, when you are losing your ability to concentrate. On plants to give them extra light and energy during short winter days.

Pregnancy Support *Balsam Poplar, Bog, Devil's Club, Diopside, Emerald, Grove Sandwort, Lady's Mantle, Northern Lady's Slipper.* This formula was inspired by the work and research of Cynthia Abu-Asseff, a flower essence therapist and mother living in Sao Paulo, Brazil. Cynthia started using the Alaskan essences with mothers and babies at a centre called Projeto Renascer in January of 1999. This centre was started in 1991 by a service-oriented spiritual group led by Cynthia's parents. In the years since its formation, it has helped more than 1000 pregnant women.

Pregnancy Support is designed to strengthen, stabilize and balance a woman and the baby growing within her during the entire pregnancy. Its primary action is to help the mother to meet the physical, emotional and mental challenges that can arise during this life-changing event. Use to help a woman create and nurture a sacred space in her life and body to support the growth and development of her baby. To assist both the mother and the indwelling soul in clearing any ambivalence they have about being on the Earth. Helps mothers strengthen their connection with the Earth so they can provide nurturing energy for themselves and their families. Enables women who themselves suffered from a traumatic birth to heal this trauma so they can offer a stronger body/soul connection to their babies. Develops and strengthens the energetic triad between the mother, father and baby.

Purification *Black Tourmaline, Fireweed, Portage Glacier, Sweetgrass.* Purification is designed to cleanse and purify your home and work environments as well as your personal energy field. Used to break up and cleanse stagnant patterns of energy on any level. Use to:

- release toxic energy from the mind, emotions and physical body;

- revitalize, balance and stimulate the renewal of energy on all levels of your energy system;

- break up unhealthy patterns of energy in an environment where there has been addiction, depression or abuse;

- purify and recharge the environment where there is stagnant energy;

- release old ingrained habits that are no longer useful, necessary or contributing to your wellbeing.

Soul Support *Cattail Pollen, Chalice Well, Cotton Grass, Fireweed, Labrador Tea, Malachite, River Beauty, Ruby, White Fireweed.* Soul Support is our emergency care formula. Provides soul support for the whole family in acute stress, for children and for animals. Maintains strength, balance and stability during any kind of stressful activity or traumatic situation, including:

- accidents involving injury, shock and/or trauma;

- emotional catharsis and violent outbursts;

- fear of flying and motion sickness;

- before, during and after visits to the dentist;

- after a fight, argument or disagreement;

- after receiving bad news;

- for post-traumatic stress;

- before and immediately after surgery and during recovery;

- for abrupt and/or major changes in plans;

- in an animal shelter and for wild animal rescue and rehabilitation work;

- for any transition, challenge, or initiation.

Travel Ease *White Violet, Yarrow, Covellite, Black Tourmaline, Smoky Quartz.* The Travel Ease combination is specifically designed to ease the negative effects of air travel, including jet lag. For those who are environmentally sensitive and have difficulty being confined in small, constricted spaces for long periods of time, supports the establishment and maintenance of functional energy boundaries, enabling us to feel as though we have all the personal space, even on a crowded flight.

The accumulation of 'airborne' pollutants in the auric field during long flights is one of the main contributors to jet lag. This essence maintains the overall integrity of our energy fields, challenged by electromagnetic radiation generated by the plane's avionics and wiring, and by the noise and vibration generated from the plane. Releases any toxic or unwanted energies absorbed during flight.

Addresses the disorientation when travelling to new places and from moving through multiple time-zones, maintains grounding during flight and keeps our body energies synchronized and aligned by constantly updating our energetic system with the Earth's energy as we move from one location to another. So we arrive at the final destination, truly there, energetically as well as physically. For maximum effectiveness, begin taking the Travel Ease combination several days before your flight, at least three times during the flight and for a few days after you reach your destination. For extended travel, the formula should be taken every hour you are airborne. It will also be helpful if you drink lots of water during the flight, stretch whenever possible, and get plenty of exercise before and after your trip.

Sacred Space Sprays

The Sacred Space Sprays, co-created by Jane Bell and Steve Johnson, were designed primarily for space clearing, an ancient practice brought to life by Denise Linn in her book *Sacred Space*, for helping people to create healthy living and working environments. These sprays are further developed from the Alaskan combination formulas: Calling All Angels, Guardian and Purification. Added to these are complementary blends of the highest quality essential oils and absolutes, chosen on the basis of their therapeutic qualities, and their ability to ground and enhance the function of each essence combination.

The Sacred Space Sprays were formulated to address the increasing challenge of maintaining our health in this crowded and fast-paced world. Stagnant and toxic energies accumulate in our living and working environments from computers and other electrical equipment, pollution, emotional upsets, illness, clutter and even from previous occupants. Over time these disharmonious energies can have a detrimental effect on our physical vitality, relationships, productivity, creativity, prosperity and general wellbeing. You can cleanse yourself and your surroundings of these unwanted toxins and bring in the fresh, elementally infused energies of nature by using Sacred Space Sprays along with the simple and straightforward techniques of space clearing.

These sprays were designed to help evolve from a position of being at the mercy of surroundings to having a positive effect on them. The apartments, flats, houses and buildings in which we live and work can become beacons of light that radiate out and positively transform our neighbourhoods, cities, countries and the world.

Calling All Angels Spray *Angelica, Chalice Well, Chiming Bells and Kunzite essences with essential oils of Bulgarian Red Rose Otto, Carnation, Alpine Lavender and Pink Grapefruit.* This spray helps you to contact the love, guidance and protection of the angelic realm and bring a soft, loving, serene energy into your heart, physical body and environment. The joyful and calming oils promote the release of tension, and open our hearts to the love and peace of the angels. This spray came out of Jane's work with children who were having difficulty sleeping, and as a result were keeping their parents up as well. Instead of calling out for Mum or Dad after waking up, they would use this spray, say, 'Calling all angels' and fall back into a peaceful slumber.

- Invokes the love, guidance and protection of the angelic realm into a room after it has been space cleared.

- Creates a sacred, protected space for sleeping and dreaming – works for pets too!

- Strengthens the awareness that all family members are supported and protected by the angels.

- Brings the essence of joy and peace into your life. Makes a stronger connection to the divine feminine.

Guardian Spray *Covellite, Devil's Club, Round-Leaf Orchid, Stone Circle, White Violet and Yarrow; also contains the essential oils of Hyacinth, Litsea Cubaba, Tangerine, Lime and Melissa.* Guardian helps you create a powerful force field of protection in your aura and environment, enabling you to claim your energetic space, maintain your grounding and feel the protection of strong, healthy boundaries. The oils enhance the protective and grounding qualities of the essences and add uplifting notes of joy and playfulness. Especially useful for the highly sensitive: often feeling sensitivity is a curse instead of a blessing, because we don't know how to keep the energies in our environment from penetrating and depleting us. Guardian reminds us that we are the source of our own protection. Connects us with our inner light, helps radiate this powerful energy outward into our surroundings. This helps us stay open and sensitive, while feeling sealed and protected. For those people who:

- need to strengthen their boundaries before entering into another person's living, working or personal space;

- want to invoke an energy of protection into a room that has just been space cleared;

- want to set a more relaxed and grounded energy into the environment;

- want to preserve the energy that they have just invoked into a space;

- would like to decrease the detrimental effects that computers and other electromagnetic equipment are having on them or their employees.

Purification Spray *Black Tourmaline, Fireweed, Portage Glacier and Sweetgrass enhanced by the essential oils of Peppermint, Lavender Mailette, Black Spruce and Frankincense.* Purification cleanses and purifies your home, work environments and personal energy field. Utilized to break up and clear stagnant patterns of energy on any level and contains the four most powerful cleansing and releasing Alaskan essences. The oils enhance the purifying function and add clarifying, sanctifying and refreshing qualities to the spray. The Purification Spray evokes a feeling of cool winds blowing off glaciers. It carries an invigorating blast of ionic energy that washes away tiredness and brings a sense of vital aliveness. This spray transports the purity of the wilderness into our complex man-made environments, awakening our senses and reminding us of our true natures. Spray to release any kind of stagnant energy that

has collected in a room or building – the first step in the space-clearing process.

- Breaks up unhealthy patterns of energy in a space where there has been illness, addiction, depression or abuse.

- Releases toxic energy from the mind, emotions and physical body.

- Purifies the energy in your rental car when you pick it up and in your hotel room when you arrive.

- Revitalizes, balances and stimulates the renewal of energy on all levels of your home, office or aura.

Soul Support Spray *Cattail Pollen, Chalice Well, Cotton Grass, Fireweed, Labrador Tea, Malachite, River Beauty, Ruby, White Fireweed and essential oil of Lavender.* Utilizes the soothing and clarifying properties of an organic Lavender oil from Kashmir. Use it to calm, ground and centre your environment as well as your energy field. It can be used in all of the situations listed above, especially when oral application is impossible or inconvenient.

Travel Ease Spray *White Violet, Yarrow, Covellite, Black Tourmaline, Smoky Quartz and essential oils of Black Spruce, Lavender and Pink Grapefruit.* The essential oils in the Travel Ease Spray support the cleansing, grounding and uplifting qualities of the formula. Using the Travel Ease Spray is a refreshing way to keep your energy field strong, clear and grounded during long flights, train or bus journeys, and when transiting through airports, train and bus stations.

Alaskan Flower Essences: making the environmental essences

Shabd-Sangeet Khalsa (SSK) has kindly provided some of the original notes she made when making the environmental essences. From these one can gain further fascinating insights into these unique essences and the process of attunement and deep connection producers have with the nature kingdom.

As a child SSK would listen to the sound of silence, lie on the ground next to a waterfall and go into the silence beyond her thoughts, hear the music played by trees, and receive profound wisdom while she was 'just being'. Often she would talk to fairies and fell in love with flowers in the garden; she particularly loved the Pansies with their happy little flower faces. Compelled to pick the Roses and breathe in their fragrance throughout the day, she would often sip raindrops from the flower petals – it rained frequently where she lived. SSK felt the natural world deeply. Her desire to commune with the oneness of nature was an ache deep at the core of her being.

She moved to Alaska in 1976 where she studied botany at the University of Alaska and received an undergraduate grant to conduct a taxonomic survey of the wild plants in the arboretum. She marvelled at the wild Green Orchids in the bogs, and the carnivorous plants in the mosses, tussocks and ponds. SSK lived and breathed flowers; it was her Heaven on Earth.

In the 1980s she was drawn to the California Flower Essence Society essences (FES) and was amazed by their subtle magic. She felt compelled to begin making her own.

As she listened to the nature spirits in her garden and in the woods and heard the messages from the flowers on how they wanted to be used for healing, she began to make essences with Pansies, Johnny-Jump-Ups, Fuchsias and so on.

In 1983 she was introduced to Steve Johnson, and as their friendship grew, they started making the Alaskan Flower Essences together. In 1984, they co-founded the Alaskan Flower Essence Project in order to accurately identify each of the wildflowers that were used as essences, as common names can often apply to multiple species and even different genera.

A further development was initiated when in the Arctic winter SSK made the Northern Lights environmental essence, and in the summer she made the Rainbow Glacier, and Glacier River. Together they made the Solstice Sun Essence on the longest day of the year at about midnight with the sun shining brightly between two mountain peaks. They were standing along the banks of the Koyukuk River just south of the Arctic Circle. This was the start of a new concept in making essences and became the range of environmental essences.

According to SSK it is important to keep information about the essences as pure as possible without filtering it through the mind and ego, which changes the information. When opening herself to receive the essence's message she opens her heart, experiencing the flower's essence, allowing it to be expressed in words to convey her experience. She says it is a challenge to bring words to describe such gossamer journeys – words can only give a sense of the essence. Each person who uses an essence can follow the energy of the essence to experience it themselves. It is a delicate line to walk between bringing the energy and information through so that it is not too etheric, but is understandable, and giving free rein to the mind to manipulate the information to fit a personal agenda.

An essence producer has a major responsibility to be aware of when the mistakes of the mind and ego are made as this creates a product of the ego, which is not what a flower essence is about.

Alder 9-9-87 A crown of light to dwell within. Open, move beyond your resistance. Let this crown of light work within you.

Blue Elf Viola – my garden 9-7-84 Dissipates anger through its calming vibration; it cools the nervous system.

Blue Elf Viola – my garden 9-6-87 Draw upon this source of calm in the midst of intensity.

Butterwort 6-18-88 (SSK made this near Bettles, just south of the Brooks Range.) This essence brings harmony to the inner, subtle levels of your humanity. It connects

313

all aspects of the human self to the Higher Self, more vibrant levels of light. Imagine this as threads you can follow to adjust your state of mind, emotions or general awareness. It feels like the freshness of rain. It feels like you slept all night in a wonderful cleansing rain and you awoke very clear and refreshed. It functions as a vehicle to take you deep inside yourself to leave past deprivations behind, to ascend within yourself as you dive deep into your own heart and consciousness to the experience of, 'I want to be you, I know I am you when I look into your eyes and feel the openness of my heart. I want to envelop you, to merge with you, to flow as the identical light we become in this recognition.'

Cattail Pollen 8-10-87 Courage during emergence. To come forth in growth to be as you truly are. Stand tall in your courage, sway if you must but do not yield to forces outside of yourself. Let your spirit soar while you keep your feet planted on the Earth. Stand solid in your truth. This is the essence of standing tall on your truth.

Chiming Bells 6-15-84 Helps you develop the gift of spiritual song. It helps you to open to more life force energy, puts more life into your eyes, opens the heart to the subtle consciousness of the natural world. It helps to shield you from the effects of loud noises.

Combination Poppy – my garden 7-18-89 Joy, willingness to touch into the deep layers of your being to see and share the inner light. To see yourself as separate, compartmentalized is not true. See what is whole, that you are whole and you are a part of the whole.

Crowberry 5-8-91 Feel your own sense of knowing from within your body, your vehicle with which you experience this life. If you resist living in your body this essence will help you sense how much you are in and how much you are out. This essence is

a guide for those who are lingering on the outside of their bodies. The essence will guide you into your body.

Crystal Saxifrage – Rainbow Mt. 6-4-88 (SSK gave it this common name as it had none.) This essence works indirectly with solar energy by bringing it into an etheric crystalline form within the flower. It can assist you in working interdimensionally. The purpose is to expand your awareness and to tap into this tiny source of power which acts as a catalyst for intense creative thought; as a preparation for creative breakthrough this crystalline energy helps you access additional energy, especially when you have reached a point where you need to move through a 'tight squeeze' or meet with inertia.

Focus your thoughts at the heart centre, place the essence on the heart centre and bring the energy to the heart. Let the crystalline energy develop in you; bring your thoughts into the centre of the crystals. Allow for the transformation to take place within you, for the creative flow, the opening, expanding intuitive knowing.

Double Shirley Poppy – my garden Abundance. It begins with where you grow, flourish and blossom. You share your nectar, fruits and seeds. Each stage takes place in its own time. While there is growth there are no fruits or seeds to share, but they are developing out of sight while the plant grows them in fertile ground where the Earth shares her abundance through the roots; the sky shares its abundance through the sun and rain. The sharing of abundance requires patience. Some flowers bloom while others have gone to seed. In abundance there is variety. The Earth is generous and abundant.

Look within; what variety of abundance do you have within and in what stage of development? What are you able to share abundantly with yourself and with others?

Forget-Me-Not 9-4-84 This essence penetrates to your depths to help you bring forth the golden heart within you so you can share this in your life.

Foxglove 9-4-84 This essence assists you when you must navigate through darkness, through tunnel vision. It will help you to be able to see where you are headed because you will be able to follow your inner guidance; your goal will be very clear and precise. Go beyond the forms of darkness; once beyond it you are infinity, you can create what you wish.

Fuchsia – my garden 6-17-84 Abounding joy in having physical form for expression of life. See your inner light, your glow, the rainbows moving all around you. See your own beauty in this creation; you are but another flower in the garden of life. For clarity of mind, breaks the chains of habitual thinking and emotions.

Glacier River 7-18-90 The glacial river embodies the process of release from form. The river carries suspended particles of ground-up mountains. The water in this river comes from melting glaciers and snow. The glaciers glide over the mountains and grind the rocks into tiny particles. The mountains are gradually released from their forms. While the mountains were growing the glaciers were forming. During their creation they were also being destroyed. The mountain pieces are so tiny they remain suspended in the torrential waters flowing rapidly downhill. If you feel rigid, non-fluid, resistant to change, clinging to the form you assume is 'real' this essence will help you release.

Nothing is set in stone, even if it looks like it is. The river is always flowing even in the deep of winter when the world feels so cold in the far north. The waters still flow, the glaciers still slide over the rocks and the grinding goes on. Be like the river, always flowing, always releasing form into formlessness and movement. You can embody disembodiment during the times you find it difficult to let go. You will find this essence in some of the wild divine flower essence combinations.

Green Bells of Ireland – my garden These flowers create illusions to fool the mind to bring you to a place of inner openness. The essence expands a silvery light inside you to create neutral space from which to explore the inner worlds. This essence is a beginning step of travelling into the green light energies of nature, which is the expansive self.

Green Fairy Orchid 7-8-87 (SSK gave it this common name as it has none in the taxonomic key for Alaska.) Accepting oneness. Seeing Helpers. You can look at this Orchid and not see it. It is tiny and elusive. Once you feel it with your heart you will see it. The green light beckons you onward past the sight of your eyes. This tiny bog Orchid helps you to focus in and inward. It is the tiny things in life that help you to see differently. Through this inner focus you are invited into a realm beyond the ego, into the mystical green energies of nature to find the inner light, to let it be focused to a pin point to go through it into the heart beyond the mind. This helps to set you free, to experience your boundlessness. This essence helps you to see when it is time to see what you have not yet focused on. See the light you are, it grows, and you cannot be separate from the divine except in your mind.

Grove Sandwort 6-21-84 It can assist with regaining balance when experiencing a whirlwind of emotions. It helps settle the emotions of the unborn child when the mother is disturbed; happiness returns. This essence can facilitate developing the bonds and communication between mother and child. It will help you to strengthen your own tie with Earth Mother and to be open to being nurtured by her. As you are nurtured so you can nurture.

Harebell – Rainbow Mt. tundra 8-12-87 Connecting open hearts. Connects the hearts of those who love one another. To connect despite barriers. This essence is like an invisible string that keeps the hearts touching, feeling the connection. The connection can be lost if it cannot be felt even when it exists. The heart feels; the head does not. Heartfelt connections need to be felt to be kept alive.

Icelandic Poppy 9-4-84 This bright splash of light in the flower's colours helps to reflect your inner radiance. The flower is a solar collector; it collects light and reflects light. It will help you become bold in your life if that is what you need.

Labrador Tea 6-21-84 Clears shadows away from the mind to help one see what is true and to make new choices.

Lambsquarters 7-17-87 Accessing information through the heart before interpreting it in the mind. Expand into and beyond the vastness of time and space. Be connected, be the flow, let your vision, your wisdom and awareness expand beyond the mind. This essence will help you develop a lighter life. Between the mind and its might follow this green light on the path to the heart.

Lilac – my garden 7-3-90 Garden Lilac calls out, 'Reunite yourself, be one with all things.' (The lilac brings in the purple rays, angels slide to Earth from the heavens on these beams.) The lilac ray, the Christ ray of light. Strength and joy. This lilac essence brings in the purple ray energies. Within this ray is a full spectrum of the purple and violet hues. It relates to ascension. Not the ascension of leaving the body as in the example of the Christ, but in aligning the chakras, opening the energy pathways to receive light, to embody light and to share light.

Monkshood 7-11-87 This essence helps you to remove your earthly burden, to help you disrobe from the heaviness you carry in your mind, emotions and body. It can teach you to walk in the nudity of truth so you can be clothed in light. The entire plant is toxic; truth is toxic to the ego. When you resist truth it can make you sick. Monkshood shares the calmness of the sanctuarial confines where the focus is on the divine without distractions. You can be cloaked in this calm vibration with this essence which makes it easier to touch the divine in yourself and therefore in others.

Northern Twayblade – Rainbow Mt. 7-6-91 Opening to the infinite. Attuning your perceptions to a very subtle level of manifestation. An energy so soft that you cannot develop any resistance to its healing.

Onesided Wintergreen One side of one thing is the other side of another. There is no separation. This essence is to bring you into the awareness that all that you do is affected by others and all that you do affects others. Will you think and behave differently if you are actually cognisant of this, if you can actually feel your connectedness with all?

Opium Poppy Devic Essence 7-6-91 This preparation embodies not only the floral archetype, but also the living presence of the devic energies, consciousness. This essence becomes a living entity, a living potential as an essence. Archetypes are usually well formed unless there is a need for them to be altered.

Pansy – my garden 9-7-84 These flower vibrations spread cheer. They vibrate fearlessness.

Pink Lady's Slipper 6-22-84 Each flower has the ability to stimulate energy in the body, open meridians for the Qi to flow powerfully. It helps to give clear vibrations to the voice.

Pink-Purple Opium Poppy – my garden 10-4-90 This essence is to help you drink in the elixir of love. Not the emotions, but the Big Love, the essence of creation, the purity of form and the love of life, the gift of life, the gift of consciousness. This essence is to help you to drink in the nectar of life, of living freely, not bound by form, but allowing form to become your freedom.

The balance grows finer as you become more developed. The universal love can flow into you, through you. Your heart can keep this pure. This will help you to keep your heart pure so the flow through you will be unimpeded. Let it flow, be the flow and then overflow the elixir of life in your life.

Prickly Wild Rose 6-19-84 Fortitude, expansive clarity of spirit.

Purple Saxifrage – Rainbow Mt. 5-29-91 This essence is a beacon of light, a receptor for stellar light, channelling it into the planetary grid of light. It pulses blue light upward to bring in the needed frequencies. It will help you to clear your own energies so that you can be aligned with the incoming frequencies to assist you with multidimensional living. Do you want to be a clear receiver? It can help open the crown chakra. It will help you make energetic adjustments so you can more readily receive the celestial songs that mingle with the Earth elements. It will help you to shift from living solely in rapport with the limited intellect to living in relationship with your limitless spirit, open heart and ability to manifest beauty on this Earth.

Purple Opium Poppy – my garden 7-9-89 This essence is for when you need a break and there is no break. It is for when you go through very challenging and profound growth that brings you closer to spirit. It is for when your entire vibrational blueprint is being rearranged. When you feel so uncomfortable you don't want to be in your body. This vibration is like a vibrational oasis, rest during evolution. Sometimes the internal changes are almost too intense to bear; that is when this essence is really needed.

Rainbow Glacier 8-11-87 Essence of the elements. Time and space frozen in ice. Then and now moving as one in ancient ice. Power and tranquillity. Elements seemingly in opposition come together as one in glacial ice. Ice as mass of moving, melting, flexing, pushing, grinding frozen water. A river of ice moving, imperceptible. Renewal, cleansing. Earth is scraped bare. This essence of the elements contains the energies that create the beginnings of life.

Grain by grain, mountains are ground into tiny flecks of ground-up rocks, glacial silt. This is how you move a mountain. If you find there are seemingly insurmountable obstacles in your life this is the essence to use.

Red-Purple Opium Poppy – my garden 10-4-90 This essence helps to balance the extremes between Earth and ether, physical and spirit. When the earthly focus takes too much attention then the balance is lost. When the physical is ignored the balance is also lost. These are meant to function together. Not one to negate the other or to be held in more favour than the other. They are part of the one and together they create a balance for dwelling with spirit embodied, with body respected. Life is a yoga, the coming together of the perceived opposites to find out how they synergize to expand your awareness and help you to evolve as a whole being.

Rhododendron – Rainbow Mt. 6-4-88 Pink crystalline energy envelops these flowers, it is more cloudlike, less formed; or more gaseous, etheric and moving than static or structural. This essence will help to reveal small things in all forms. It will help to intensify your awareness of life at this small scale, shift your perception of smallness to equal vastness and then have nothing to do with size at all. It will play with your mind to help you shift and expand and come to perceive this life with freshness, with the not-knowing wisdom of an unconditioned mind. The soft pink light of these flowers and this essence will be like guides for your eyes, for your inner vision.

Single Delight (Toads' Reading Lamp) (*Moneses uniflora*) This flower channels light along the surface of the Earth where it grows. It focuses additional light to the earth's grid, which is a natural aspect of nature. This essence will help you to feel connected to those who also walk upon this earth.

Sitka Burnet – Rainbow Mt. Healing the past so the constrictions around the heart do not return. This essence will assist you in dealing with internal strife, the kind that results from inner conflicts, lack of inner congruency or lack of time given to oneself. This essence will help soothe you, like an internal massage or a sense of the smoothing of your feathers.

Snapdragon 9-4-84 Helps with healing jaw injuries. This essence contrasts 'good and bad' side, positive and negative, yin and yang, to help you be aware of the direction each polarity will take you.

Spireae 6-17-84 Brings the vibrations of the forest's peace and the sensitivity of the heart. Opens one to the love and beauty of flowers, and deep inner strength.

Sweetgrass – Bettles 6-21-88 This essence will make you feel very clean, like you have showered in the cleanest rain and every single facet of your being is very, very clean.

Tundra Twayblade – Rainbow Mt. tundra 7-6-91 (SSK gave this its common name.) Seek the green places in the heart; they will lead you inward. Listen inwardly. This essence has green light rays as sharp as points to help sharpen your vision. Follow the green light within to expand your heart light. The journey is inward; follow the light inward. The green points of light

become crystalline and can be focused in the body to assist with healing. Life begins in the ethers, with thought and energy, your imagination is your tool, like your hands in the subtle playground of the not yet physical form. This essence is an expression of the divine creation in its delicate beauty, and intricate creation. It will show you the power of your heart because as closely as you look at this flower so must you look at yourself.

Twinflower 6-21-84 Helps magnify sound, will help intensify the spoken quiet voice and shows you the power of small thoughts.

Verbena – from my garden Celebration of light, colour, raindrops, sunlight, life and scent. Joy embodied in beauty. Fairy trumpets. Dancing fairies. Attune your ears to the joy; let the joyful dance touch you. Lighten yourself in celebration, in cosmic dance. Light becomes the perfume of flowers. Drink in the colours and cosmic laughter.

White Spruce Cosmic antennae. Call on the infinite wisdom through the spruce. Feel the support of creation. Access your wisdom. When you have trouble doing so, the white spruce will assist you again and again.

Wild Iris 6-27-84 Opens you to your inner health, balance and strength after a difficult confrontation. It helps to bring solar energy inward for strength so you have energy to develop to your full capacity in your life.

Wild Rhubarb 8-5-87 Clearing the channel between the mind and the heart. Flexibility of the mind is like flexibility of the spine; it keeps new life coming in. It is necessary to learn how to bend. The green light of the flowers helps to cleanse the mind. The more you allow it in the clearer you can become. The mind can stand in the way of living from the heart. This green energy is the energy of the heart; it helps to soften the grip of the mind. If the mind becomes rigid, it will affect your flexibility. Use this essence to keep or increase your flexibility on all levels.

Willow 9-9-87 For a strong energy field that cannot be broken. This is the power of regeneration in great abundance. Bring this strength into yourself.

Wormwood This essence is an etheric map into the heart to heal the human soul so that the evolution is not hindered, but that you may experience the hidden treasures of nature that are in your own nature; there is no separation. It is a journey into the self through healing, or releasing the constrictions around the heart so that your own light may expand and you know your truth. There is no separation. There is limitlessness. There is ultimately the light and bliss, of which we are all expressions.

Zinnia – my garden 9-7-84 This bright red orange flower vibrates powerfully. It can help you to penetrate dense vibration so that you can move through them as though they were not there.

DANCING LIGHT ORCHID ESSENCES (DL)

Inspired by the indefinable spiritual nature of orchids, after her work with the Alaskan Essences SSK went on to develop her delightful range of Dancing Light Orchid Essences.

Orchids have an exceptionally high vibrational quality and are said to be 'the queen of the plant kingdom'. They are honoured by shamans and indigenous peoples for their connection to spirit, and they embody the creative intelligence and intentions from nature.

These essences intend to work with our own blueprints and act as internal guides bringing us back into alignment so that we are able to fulfil our destinies. The human experience is very demanding and oftentimes damaging to the original blueprints we have designed; there is no oasis to go to for realignment so the over-lighting beings assist with the strong intentions and focus through the Dancing Light Orchid Essences.

Imagine a multidimensional blueprint which over-lights and infuses our circuitry with our original blueprints. It takes the struggle out of transformation so one's own intact blueprints are once again accessible and in fact functioning as overlays. Suddenly we can simply realign instead of struggling for ideals of perfection lost.

SSK says that in her experience of the process of co-creating the Dancing Light Orchid Essences:

I surrender my awareness to the subtle energies of the flowers. It is a journey deep into the layers of creation, that are pre-manifest, where the essence of a flower beckons me to follow the energy into the formless, where only my awareness can travel. The consciousness of the essence is my guide, inviting me to follow as deeply and subtly as I am able.

It is through nature and flowers that I live in relationship with the vastness of creation. Their beauty draws me in, closer and closer, until I pass through to the other side, into the un-manifest. I am aware, I am in a space, a not place, where I surrender my awareness to the subtle intelligence of the flowers. Here in the formless layers of creation my being dances with the essences while they envelop me as though we were lovers sharing subtle secrets. In this formless awareness our energies mingle, there is no I. Wordless, thoughtless awareness is direct transmission, pure intention, light and energy.

I hold these precious gifts within so that I may bring them back through the subtle layers of creation and into this manifest realm to share them with you. I focus inwardly to feel with my awareness the gifts I hold within. I do my best to find words to express the essence of the orchids; the energies are pregnant with intentions, alive with unlimited possibilities. This is ho, where etheric essence blends with physical matter, an essential infusion of living, dancing, vibrating light.

The essences are an expression of Mother Nature's compassion for each of us. She showers us with her gifts to nurture our growth on every level. Through the orchid essences she meets us right where we are in any given moment of our personal evolution; like a wise, compassionate mother, if we let her, she not only meets us, she matches our pace then gently teaches, supports and leads us deeper within, while elevating our awareness so that we can open to new possibilities beyond that which we have imagined.

The Dancing Light Orchid Essences beckon us to flow with them into the subtle layers of creation within ourselves. Each essence is a conscious facet of the vastness of creation; with any given essence energy, if followed into the subtle, it could lead one into the infinite awareness within one's Self. Ultimately, essences are our traveling companions for the inward journey beyond the limitations of the ego and intellect and fully into ourselves.

To illustrate, I'll share a bit of my life's journey with the essences up to this point. I was a sensitive child who grew up hearing the subtle communication of the Devas: of flowers, fairies, waterfalls, insects, crystals, fountains, trees, angels, animals and other beings. I also grew up in trauma which was great fodder for needing to do a lot of emotional healing and this is one area in which the essences met and supported me as I grew.

Shifts in consciousness

The essences and I are on a life-long journey which started from a pretty basic need to heal the human self. They have also supported my spiritual expansion through the actual experiences of making essences, with all of the loving wisdom they have imparted through making essences. I have come to understand with each new life challenge I was directed to make new essences; they were exactly what I needed to successfully navigate the turbid waters. As of this writing in 2013 the essences are supporting my very human self as I increasingly learn to surrender to the flow of creation on the path of Self Realization. The path into the Self: Self Realization begins where I am right now, and where I was back then when I had no idea of such things.

I have found that by consistently using essences it is possible to explore the ever-expanding depths they offer; by example: the essence reveals mystery within, when I was very involved in my emotional healing this was a great helper for discovering stuck emotions which were a mystery to me at the time. As the years have passed, it has revealed my inner vastness as that which is yet unnoticed is the mystery within.

The essence Unveiling Self has taken on new dimensions; years ago I learned that my ego needed to step aside to assist my Higher Self. It greatly comforted me while I evolved as it felt like a loving friend walking with an arm around me, reassuring that my ego would not be destroyed but brought along in the evolution. Most recently this essence has been a powerful ally as I progress spiritually. The ego still freaks out thinking it will be annihilated, as the human self transforms, but Unveiling Self has a powerful settling effect and the ego can once again feel at ease and surrender to the flow of creation, while adjusting to the spiritual transformation process. It allows the ego/intellect to gracefully get out of the way so as to not obstruct the flow within.

The Dancing Light Essences

Balancing Extremes (*Paphiopedilum lowii*) Express the truth and radiance of yourself in balance. Has your uniqueness felt misplaced? Why did you go so far out of balance? What did you lose sight of? In the ecstasy, your self will remain grounded; in the Earth plane, you will remember your bliss.

Centred Love (*Bollea coelestis*) This essence embodies heart-centred love. A good essence to use when you want communication to come from the heart. This essence will facilitate heart shifts, for exploring new relationships and new levels within relationships.

Clearing Blockages (*Phragmipedium caudatum*) This essence brings a fresh example of how energy can move most freely through the body. Anything that obstructs the flow of creation's gift of life force energy must go if one is to realize the truth of our inner being. Life force is greater than physical energy and breath; it is awareness of self, the flow of creation's intelligence; another essential companion to use frequently with the ebb and flow of our maturation process. Overall theme: fluidity and flexibility. An analogy in Chinese medicine would be removing blocks to the flow of Qi.

Clearing Energy Fields (Combination essence) Offers energetic support to look within and release. Clears the energies when one feels ready to release, and transform.

Clearing Inner Pathways (*Aeranthes henrici*) My subtle light penetrates and prepares the internal communication paths to enlightenment. An essential companion for realizing self; clearing the inner pathways is essential to knowing the self. We come to feel and know who we are by also realizing what we are not. This essence excels in clearing our inner pathways to allow information and light to travel.

Dance of Creation Blue Orchid (*Vanda coerulea*) I am the soothing essence of exquisite awareness. My purpose is to tickle your mind and the pathways into your heart so you will join in the merry dance of creation.

Dancing Light Spirit Calypso Orchid (*Calypso bulbosa var. occidentalis*) Embody fluidity. Dance between form and formlessness. This essence holds the pattern of fluidity for you to be able to open your perceptions to move between the manifest and un-manifest. It can transform you.

Defining Edges (*Brassia arcuigera*) Create your personal boundaries without creating separation from others. Creating boundaries provides an important part of your definition of self, as well as strength, safety and integrity.

Earth Mother Nurtures (Environmental essence) Earth Mother is a collective of enlightened beings, with a capacity for compassion that is unfathomable. They merge with the form of Earth to nurture all beings who dwell here. They are eager to assist us with our journey towards enlightenment; they know that ultimately we all journey together. This essence is an invitation, a welcoming into the heart of the Earth.

Essence of the Edge (Environmental essence) The Essence of the Edge is for those doing their work at the cutting edge. It is for comprehending the purpose of the edge in your life at present. It is a safety net if you are pushed to the edge of what you can do, understand, cope with and manifest.

Expanding Awareness (*Phaleanopsis* hybrid) This essence creates a wiggle where there is a tiny opening; it wiggles and keeps wiggling, creating an expanding gap, a space for your awareness to expand. You may feel a quickening as this process gains momentum. In the emptiness of the infinite, one has all the space needed to expand in every way; in all the facets of being, expansion illuminates what was once hidden in shadow, where one is confronted with crystallized emotions. As stuck energies as the shadows become illuminated, this is the opportunity to become aware, and then release. This is a natural cycle of Expanding Awareness. A great support in helping one not to resist and allow this natural process of awakening. The flow of Expanding Awareness encourages elevation, expansion, illumination, awareness, surrendering to the flow (or resist, ouch!), feeling the authentic self. If one doesn't resist, the cycle then repeats itself. As we open to deeper relationship with self we become familiar with this cycle of necessary clearing. This essence facilitates going with the flow.

Gossamer Steel/Enduring Love (*Phalaenopsis Texas Star* × *P. Brother Delight*) This essence opens the heart to higher octaves of love. Touch the fine threads of love, let their music resound within. This essence embodies resilience, the strength to endure. This essence is like gossamer steel, born of desire to create the sustainable fineness of love, and to anchor love's higher manifestations.

Graceful Transformations (*Masdevallia coccinea var. harryana*) A caterpillar makes a cocoon wherein it transforms into a butterfly. This essence assists you in discarding unused energies, thought forms and emotional patterns. It helps clothe you with your new forms of manifesting self.

Heart to Heart (Combination essence) This essence assists in attuning to your truest source of navigation, your heart. An energy emanates from your heart that another heart recognizes as true. 'Let your heart be your guide' is an expression based on universal truth of experience and being. Get to the heart of the matter. Let this essence assist you in going deeper within, through the gateway of your heart, to the heart of yourself.

Heart of Nature/Devic Awareness (*Miltonia Jean Sabourin* 'Vulcain') This essence helps you develop an elemental awareness of the life force all around you. The trees, rocks, flowers and other forms are alive with creative cosmic intelligence. Elemental light. Elemental sound. Elemental motion. Elemental breath. Much of this awareness is purely experiential, far beyond thoughts the mind can capture. Let the experience take you; ultimately there will be a story for your mind to know.

Heart Wings Butterfly Orchid (*Psychopsis papilio*) Let your heart fly with the energies of this essence, let the wings of your heart lift you. Perspectives of spirit are unburdened. Feel free, think free, break free and fly free.

Higher Levels (*Paphiopedilum parishii*) Supports transformative growth by helping you release from the accustomed form and allowing movement toward the next higher level of form. Like an energetic lifeline it helps us to move to the next higher level in the flow of life. The physically manifest world around us appears to be solid, stable, able to last through myriad changes with relatively little challenge to its stability. We become mentally/emotionally reliant upon this perception. Quantum physics has proven that matter is mostly empty space. Life flows like a river; there are times when the very foundation we stand upon erodes. When one is required by the flow of life to move away from 'solid ground' into the unknown, it helps with movement so that we move with the flow; the beginning of the movement also allows the next higher level to manifest by the very act of motion.

I Am in My Body/Expansive Embodiment (*Masdevallia ignea*) Assists with the process of full incarnation, bright with the light of spirit being, a new way of experiencing your spirit–body relationship. Imagine your body full of tiny spaces so the light within you shines outwardly like the sun's rays shining through clouds. The source is the sublime within. As one expands, in the natural process of getting to know one's essential self, the body and mind are assisted with expansion and slowly realizing the self. When the body and mind prove to be inflexible here Expansive Embodiment can be freeing. Spirit is not caged inside the body and mind, the limited intellect that prevents you from having full awareness of how vast one is even while inhabiting a body and using the mind. Assists in feeling the expansiveness of embodiment, as well as opening awareness to the spaces between all the particles of the body and the spaces between thoughts. It's in the gap between thoughts where one can feel the energy of the flow of self.

Idiot Glee (*Vanda roeblingiana*) I am the brash youngster, I am the fits of giggles, I am the aches in the face from smiling, I am the tears of laughter. I bring you the most intense, senseless joy that you shall have the good fortune to endure.

I Like Being Me Combination (*Restrepia guttalata and a piece of a granite mountain*) This essence holds a pattern for self-love and acceptance. 'I look to nothing outside of myself for reference as to my self-worth, acceptability, lovability, inner wealth and inner health. I like being me. That which I am is my unique expression of all possibilities. There is no other like me.'

Infinite Patience (*Paphiopedilum rothschildianum*) This pattern of consciousness directly accesses the gaps between your thoughts; drawing on limitless creative intelligence which embodies a deeper level of patience than is generally experienced in life. This is patience to carry one through great and lasting challenges. This is deeper than the patience of the mind; this is like breathing in the infinite.

Light Hearted/Heart Light (*Miltonia* hybrid) This essence supports your emotional body during difficult times so you can avoid falling into the depths of pain and despair, and face your experiences with hope and inner strength.

Lotus Petals of the Heart (*Paphiopedilum* hybrid) This essence helps you open to live life from your heart so you can feel your life more fully; know boundless joy and possibilities that are not limited by the constraints of mind-centred being.

Lucid Dreaming (*Angraecum eburneum var. typicum*) Take this essence to release yourself from emotional terror. It will also assist you with developing lucidity on all levels. A companion for exploring the vast unknown, which is larger than you can ever know, and yet you may go exploring there.

Manifesting Thought Forms (*Paphiopedilum leeanum superbum*) This essence embodies the immanent patterns of the creative process. Intentions manifest gradually at first as they move through the ethers to where you can notice their shadow and then their form. At some point, one's intention is crystallized into physicality. Enhances the creative process.

As one evolves by surrender to the flow of creation and less attachment to the personal 'I', where the mind of the omnitelligence flows through as our intelligence, our ability to participate in manifestation becomes more potent and considers the whole rather than personal gain. Through evolving, one opens up, instructing the intellect/ego to step aside to assist with the flow. The mind is then in tune with the whole mind, thoughts come through the mind as flow and one participates in manifesting that which creation desires to create through one and enjoy how wonderful it feels to play with, and allow ourselves to be played by creation. Imagine being a musical instrument played by a masterful musician who is so skilled, so in tune with every nuance of not only the instrument, but the music, and the breath flowing through it; the music produced by such a master with a finely tuned instrument creates sound so lovely that as it resounds throughout creation all are filled with exquisite bliss.

Imagine the exhilaration of allowing oneself to be such an instrument of the divine. Manifesting Thought Forms essence facilitates just such a way of living at higher levels than individual desires. Let this essence lead, allowing one to be just such an instrument, so that which manifests through one is born of divine will.

Meditative Mind (*Phragmipedium xerophyticum*) How do I learn how to meditate? A quiet mind is like an unusual day of calm flat on the ocean, no waves, just glassy smooth water. A still mind is the diving board from which to jump off into the depths of self, to explore pure awareness beyond thoughts, to simply 'be'. This essence assists you in diving into the deeper levels of the mind in deeper meditative states, where the true treasures of life reside. No words can express pure awareness; by simply allowing oneself to follow the intelligent intentions and go beyond, it is effortless surrender just as sleepiness is so seductive one allows oneself to fall into sleep. Fall into the Meditative Mind, whether sitting meditating or as one gardens, washes dishes or walks in nature, this essence encourages inner stillness.

My Heart Knows (*Paphiopedilum tonsum*) Grace is the quality of fitting actions to the circumstances of the moment: knowing in your heart what to do, and when.

My Own Pure Light (*Paphiopedilum Eagle Peak × Paphiopedilum niveum*) 'The struggle is gone and I am light.'

My Song Calls Me Home (*Phragmipedium amazonica syn. richteri*) This vibration reunites you with lost or disconnected pieces of your self; from reclaiming bits of your playful inner child to soul retrieval. Update: this facet of the essence is a higher octave of the original description. Each is valid as the essence meets us where we currently stand. We *are* the One-Song of the creation that created us. As we expand in realizing ourselves as spirit having human journeys, this essence helps tune and retune our human musical instrument. Light energy flows through our chakras and spines, and we vibrate as subtle sound. A tuning essence which helps to ring true to ourselves.

New Perceptions Leopard Orchid (*Ansellia gigantea*) Keen focus takes place with this essence. It is about shifting paradigms with effortless ease. See, feel, sense, find and utilize abundance and unexpected opportunity.

Purpose Flows Slipper Orchid (*Phragmipedium ecuadorense*) In the heart one finds the wellspring of life's purpose: upwelling, bubbling, spilling over and trickling with the fluidity of water. Let your purpose well up within, let it be your sustaining pool. This essence helps to manifest the unaltered blueprint of purpose flowing freely.

Radiant Strength Slipper Orchid (*Phragmipedium besseae*) This essence supplies the blueprint for increasing radiance. For those who have lived a lifetime afraid of being seen as the radiant, unique and powerful beings they truly are. The stronger your glow the safer you are as you strengthen your energy field by the radiance of your boundless self.

Reading Energy Fields Star of Bethlehem Orchid (*Angraecum sesquipedale*) When auras blend, information is exchanged. You can use this essence to read your own energy field, and the energy fields of others. Whatever others have been holding on to, you will pick up.

Reveals Mystery Within (*Aeranthes grandiflora*) This essence is an invitation to explore the inner mysteries of the self.

Sacred Sphere (*Phragmipedium Sorcerer's Apprentice*) This essence creates a subtle energetic sphere that one can 'be' within, while you engage in your daily activities. It helps you maintain your personal clarity.

Softening the Edges (*Platanthera obtusata*) (a wild Alaskan Orchid) For those who handle delicate situations, precious young creatures and objects to help you have the gentlest of touches. Use this essence if you notice the edges of your personality have become sharp or hardened in reaction to disappointing or painful life experiences. It can help you to release and discard any harsh behaviours that cause yourself and others pain.

Unveiling Self (*Oeonia volucris*) Escape your ego's illusions of self – that is little ego. Recognize that true self dwells in your human form, yet is much greater. Ego is not left behind; it is brought along on the journey of the soul.

Walking Out of Patterns (*Rhyncholaelia digbyana*) This essence is for walking out of the rhythms of old emotional patterning. Feel with your heart, and come into alignment with the purpose of your soul.

Wise Action Blue Sky Orchid (*Cattleya loddigesii var. coerulea*) Use this essence when you want your actions to come from wisdom. It allows you to let the spark of inspiration distil within, so your actions are congruent with your intelligence.

Wondrous Heart (*Vanda javierii*) Have you come to a place in your life where you've lost touch with the sense of wonder you had as a child? This essence will bring you back to that place. 'If you can feel the wonder, you can proceed.'

Combination essences

Acceptance Essence Accept what is. If you are not accepting 'what is' in the present moment, you are resisting. Resistance does not change the present or past, but instead blocks the flow of your life. The gentle vibration of flowers can help you 'just be'. Allowing 'what is' creates acceptance. To create change, accept things for what they are as a first step: then you will know what is real, avoiding illusion and delusion. From there you can make choices and take action according to what is. Acceptance requires pause in action. The essence holds the energy to pause. In the pause, see 'what is'. In the pause accept 'what is'. You will find yourself in a pool of awareness and of acceptance. Pause in this.

Internal Marriage This essence is like taking a walk hand-in-hand with someone: yourself. It is about integrating dualities, complementary opposites, female and male energies within; internal marriage. It is not effort, but creativity.

Letting Go *Wild Alaskan River, Unveiling Self, Walking Out of Patterns, I Am in My Body.* You will come to the time and space repeatedly in life where letting go of past experiences and emotions is required in order for you to move forward in life with clarity, with an open, light, compassionate heart. This essence will help you release your weighty emotions and thoughts, renewing your ability to carry on with a lightened load. Just as solid mountains are eroded away one particle at a time by the elements so too can the embedded charges of body and mental memories be released. Allow yourself to flow into the new days ahead with renewed fluidity and freedom. As mountains are eroded they become lighter, they rise higher.

Stepping Ahead Now You've done the work; now go forth into that which you have prepared. The elements are in place, the atoms and molecules are arranged correctly, in alignment with your intentions. The canvas is ready to receive your brush strokes. Step ahead now. This essence encourages you to do just that.

New essences

Harmony of Heart (*Oncidium 'Sharry Baby'*) In the softness of your heart is the seat of your self. It is common to develop outward protective layers with mental projections so convincing that no one would dare to question, nor breach that well-crafted protective façade. The façade becomes a binding energy constricting authentic and loving expression. No one can see who you truly are even if you may wish them to. This dichotomous incongruence does not allow for authentic visibility nor expression, leaving those in your presence missing the truth of your heart and over time that may even become true for yourself. The gift of this essence is freedom to bring forth the authentic expressions of your spirit Self so that you may freely drop the veils, allowing outwardly harmonious expression sharing the treasures of your loving heart.

Purity Woolly Plantain (*Plantago patagonica*) An Orchid imitator (many Orchids imitate their insect pollinators, some flowers imitate Orchids). Your pure essence may seem as if it were a tiny, quiet part of you that may be nearly unnoticed amidst the loud, bold things that draw and catch your attention. In truth pure essence is infinitely vast, may be noticed and felt in every moment. Purity is the flow of creation expressing itself through you without any hindrance. Look for it – it is always there within you. You and your purity are One. This essence supports your ability to feel it. Your essential being is pure; you cannot lose your purity but you can lose touch with the sense of purity within yourself. Let the essence help you shift from the agendas of the mind and the locomotions of the emotions. Chances are you have already befriended your purity and you just need a reminder that one can tap into it immediately at any time.

Un-Believe (*Spiranthes romanzoffiana*) I can unbelieve my beliefs! I live in awareness. The powerful flow of creation makes me inherently, powerfully creative. My Earth vehicle bows to creation flowing through it. I feel how unbelieving vibrates me, elevating wellbeing. My beliefs are the glue of my reality. My very thoughts and cells are flowing with creative power which can be used to unglue/unbelieve beliefs. Unbounded perceptions are the stuff of my essence, my authentic unlimited self. I can simply *not* believe in something and I can change what I believe, instantly. I can simply unbelieve and live in pure awareness.

The Way Less Travelled (*Paphiopedilum predacious*) The way less travelled is the quiet path that beckons one to follow the ache in the heart to merge, to know oneself as the self, as the One-Song, the universe; to listen to the silence within. This essence is the silent friend who guides with a voice softer than the whispers of a leaf falling; there is the most gossamer of energy to attend; a subtle flow to feel within, nebulous spirit to sense; indescribable bliss to give oneself to.

Magical Me/I Am Infinity (*P. asurescens*) Assists with loosening the tight grip of the intellect as to what reality is; softening the focus of the mind, letting it dilate therefore creating receptivity and in turn, presenting emptiness for unimagined possibilities to enter into awareness; dropping judgement, opening instead to marvel at the play of creativity we are one with.

Focalizing Enhancer essences

These essences were originally developed to enhance a somatic healing process called Focalizing. This healing modality was developed by an expert trauma therapist in New York, Dr Michael Picucci. Shabd-Sangeet sought his help to heal her own trauma, and out of that grew a creative collaboration which resulted in the development of the Focalizing Enhancers. These essences not only support the Focalizing process (which one can learn to do on one's own), but can also be used independently of the Focalizing process. This set of three essences is designed to calm the nervous system, help it release pent-up energies and crystallized emotions in a pleasantly gentle way, while facilitating personal expansion by releasing constriction.

The Focalizing Enhancers work on multiple levels; physically, they immediately enter the olfactory pathways and limbic system putting the cells on alert to a shift, then they begin to facilitate that shift. As conscious humans, we have the ability to use intentional consciousness to focus in on that which has not yet been released from our cells, emotions and energy field. Each of the Focalizing Enhancers have a different molecular structure; with each one, different atoms flood the olfactory and limbic systems in different ratios as they flood the nerves, body and energetic pathways. As the chakras are activated, one is basically playing an energetic and olfactory tune for the body at the quantum level of cellular attention.

The Focalizing Enhancer Essences facilitate the journey inward for healing, illumination and direction. These hand-blended essences come in an organic botanical lotion base with Dancing Light Orchid Essences and pure essential oils.

Edge Excellent essence for dealing with stress and trauma, helping to release frozen, crystallized energy stored in the physical and energetic bodies. It supports living on the cusp of aliveness beyond established comfort zones. It energetically expands any edge you feel inside of yourself, any edge you feel pushed toward. It energetically expands your edge and keeps expanding your edge so you won't go over the edge.

Consenting In permitting you to consent to present existing realities, this essence allows you to gracefully negotiate them. Allows the emergence of the now of personal evolution, thereby reclaiming your personal and robust energies permitting you to move forward with grace.

Vastness Catalyzes emergence of the profound expansive universe within yourself. Helps you ground personal experiences

bringing creativity into your physical world thereby manifesting new realities.

Wild Divine mists

Wild Divine combination essences are effective for shock and trauma for you and your pets (our version of Rescue Remedy) (see also Pets and Animals, section I). They can help to connect you with your smiles, playfulness, inner peace and peace of mind. Wild Divine essences can also help you to unfurl your wings, help you to release stressful energies and are useful for clearing unwanted energies from your spaces.

These combination essences are filled with Alaska's wildness, nature's inspiration, the divine feminine, bits of magic and senseless glee; plus Alaskan flower, tree, rock, elemental, environmental, wild and garden essences; the Dancing Light Orchid and the seven Sister Moon Flower Essences, all to help you create movement in your life, to help you heal, grow and meet life's challenges. They'll help you by uplifting, expanding and nurturing you, and by supporting your inner being and healing. Use them with your pets, plants, kids, friends and especially for yourself in celebration of your life, health and wellbeing.

Alaska is a treasure of purity and wilderness, a vast unbroken web of forests, mountains, glaciers and tundra with moose, bear, caribou, sheep, eagles and, of course, the elements. We can't make essences without including the elements of these very powerful environments. Alaska affects us in powerful ways. Alaska's essence is the life force of the land and it is these powerful energies we are sharing.

Angels' Wings Mist *Filled with the laughter and blessings of angels, fairies and flowers, plus Alaska's Elements, Dancing Light Orchids held in the gleeful scents of Geranium, Orange and Ylang-Ylang.* Helps clear away burdensome thoughts, feeling scared or blue and simply need some cheering up, lifts your spirits to a higher perspective. Nurtures your inspiration and wonder. Mist your feet when your hopes and spirits are low so weighty thoughts won't drag you down. Mist over your head and shoulders to loosen and stretch your wings in preparation to take flight!

Mother's Arms Combination Mist *Contains Alaska Elemental Energies essence and eight very feminine essences for nurturing yourself and those around you, plus Lavender and Blue Camomile essential oils.* Formulated to draw in healing nurturing vibrations of the feminine nature, along with the energetic support to deal with urgent situations. Effective for emergencies, shock and trauma; it also evokes the sense of safety, nurturing and healing. Relax into the cosy embrace of these gentle vibrations, that hold you lovingly as if in your mother's arms, which allows a letting go of trauma in order to settle into being supported by either friends, the capable hands of health-care providers or the sense of safety and healing you feel within.

For fearfulness, panic or terror, stress, or overwhelming feelings; before and after medical procedures to help relieve stress after experiencing fear or pain, due to invasive procedures. Or for children who don't feel safe, are hard to comfort or have trouble with sleep, helps clear your own or your children's emotional energy after frantic escapades. Mist around to allow the flower essences to be evaporated into the aura. Hospitals do not generally allow patients to take any type of remedy by mouth which they do not supply, but often have no objection to a pleasant misting of flower essences.

Protective Shield Mist *Combined from Alaska's Elements, Dancing Light Orchids with Cinnamon, Lemon and Cedar oils.* Helps to provide relief from stressful energies; it envelops you in a protective sphere. Protective Shield is particularly helpful to sensitive people for increasing their radiant strength while helping to clear and define

their personal space in positive ways. It can help them feel comfortable so they don't feel the need to withdraw from people and stressful environments and situations. It is especially helpful for pregnant women whose sensitivity increases as gestation progresses – important for newborn babies and their mother when they re-enter the world together.

For highly sensitive children and adults, and those who are empathic or unable to distance others' emotions from their own. For easing their subtle distress in crowds because they feel the energies of other people's words, thoughts and emotions remaining in their aura.

Sacred Space Mist *This potion is infused with thundering waters, the clearing wind and other forces of nature from Alaska's clean, remote wilderness as well as Dancing Light Orchids blended with purifying Cedar, Sage and Lavender oils.* Designed for cleansing and clearing unwanted energies from around yourself and your immediate environment to help you expand your space, and clear the air around you. Mist when your personal or mental space feels like it is shrinking, to help you hold your ground, expand and define your boundaries and re-establish harmonious flow. Draws in the power of nature to help unblock and reorder the flow of Qi while avoiding chaos during the process. Also useful to release disincarnate beings from very old buildings and landscapes.

Still Mind Mist *Combination of Alaska's Elements, and Dancing Light Orchid Essences; with Marjoram and Tangerine oils.* Invaluable when troubled by thoughts going around in your head, keeping you awake at night. Enables you to be a human being rather than a human doing, allows you to live each day opening to fully experience each moment. Gently touches your body and mind with the stillness found on the high peaks and glaciers in Alaska's wilderness, where the quiet is so profound that the vibrations of tundra flowers seem like noisy chatter. This combination contains the secret wisdom and vibrations from nature to move you into the higher levels of your mind. Here you can live with a sense of inner quiet and emptiness, enabling you to perceive and receive from the sensory to the cosmic.

Young Heart Mist *Contains Alaska's Elements, Dancing Light Orchids and Rose Geranium oil.* Young Heart contains the magic you knew when you were small; it holds vibrational patterns to nurture or rekindle a healthy sense of wonder, angel dust to give lift to the wings of your heart, inspirational seeds for your lofty ideas, and the silent chiming music made by joyful fairies dancing on Scottish Bluebells. Use to rejuvenate your inner fountain of youth. Take it to your work or play place to lift your spirits when things get too serious, too competitive; when you or others around you start to feel and act old at heart. For when you feel weak and tired, disheartened, disappointed, fed up, angry or generally unhappy, or have been sick for a short or a long time. Healing occurs more readily and deeply when the joy and magic of your heart is nurtured.

DESERT ALCHEMY FLOWER ESSENCES (DAL)

The desert is an environment of extremes, with an abundance of heat from the sun and little water. Throughout history people wishing to strengthen their sense of spirituality have spent time in the desert. Key words to describe the energy of the desert are adaptability, individuality, expansion and inner security.

The plants inhabiting this place have evolved amazing strategies for adapting to the formidable climate in order to survive. Some only bloom at night, while others can produce leaves within six hours of a rainfall,

although they can continue to photosynthesize without foliage at all if necessary.

Desert Alchemy was founded in 1983 by Cynthia Athina Kemp Scherer with a view to researching and making essences from desert flowers. The inspiration for making a flower essence from desert plants came to Cynthia while driving through the Arizona desert one day. She found herself in the midst of a whole forest of Saguaro cacti, some standing 15m (50ft) tall with great arms that seemed to reach towards the heavens. She felt as if the Saguaro cacti were communicating with her and giving her a message to make flower essences, though at the time she did not even know what flower essences were.

Out of this experience grew the Desert Alchemy essences, created from 119 individual flowers, which capture the extraordinary qualities of the plants growing wild in this harsh environment. With an emphasis on survival, these essences are perfect for crisis situations, helping us to adapt and cope in extremely demanding situations. They encourage shifts in our perspective which enable us to deal with and embrace any emergency as an opportunity for change and growth.

Agave (*Century Plant*) The 'late bloomer' essence, Agave helps us own our level of mastery and manifest our inner beauty and strength into daily life.

Aloe Cultivates patience and surrender to our healing process. It is excellent if we feel resistance to allowing things to surface, helping us feel supported from within.

Arizona Sycamore (*Platanus wrightii*) For those who experience life or relationships as confining or entrapping, Arizona Sycamore helps us to find inner freedom. It is excellent for those who feel confined or limited by their bodies.

Arizona White Oak (*Quercus arizonica*) Arizona White Oak helps us if we believe that in order to grow we must struggle. It fosters strength through stability and continuity and helps us to feel deeply rested through surrender.

Arroyo Willow (*Salix lasiolepis*) Restoring a consciousness of personal will, Arroyo Willow helps us responsibly create our life experiences while remaining flexibly true to ourselves.

Bear Grass (*Xerophyllum tenax*) Fosters our knowing that no outside influence can overpower our deeply held intentions. It keeps us steadily centred in our hearts.

Big Root Jatropha Excellent for 'growth spurts'. Big Root Jatropha encourages a feeling of security as great inner expansion takes place. It helps us to feel safe enough to allow change to happen without the need to control everything.

Bisbee Beehive Cactus (*Coryphantha vivipara var. Bisbeeana*) Bisbee Beehive helps take us to the core of an issue and feel grace and healing energy at a cellular level. It is very often indicated for recovery of sexual or physical abuse.

Black Locust (*Robinia pseudoacacia*) Those who disregard others around them and insist upon their own way can find a softening effect from this flower essence. It helps balance masculine assertiveness with feminine yielding and nurturing.

Bloodroot (*Sanguinaria canadensis*) Bloodroot is for those who exclude themselves, or feel ostracized, from a group or community, usually because of deep feelings of unworthiness. It helps heal the wounds of rejection and frees us from the bonds of unworthiness.

Bougainvillea (*Bougainvillea spectabilis*) Bougainvillea relaxes the body and deepens our breathing, encouraging feelings of peace and ease. By provoking self-reflection and inner listening, crisis is met with stillness and non-reactivity.

Bouvardia (*Bouvardia ternifolia*) Bouvardia fortifies our will to confront life directly and consciously, changing emotional reactivity and avoidance patterns into positive response and action. An excellent essence for denial.

Bright Star (*Echinacea purpurea 'Leuchtstern'*) Bright Star is indicated when we are unable to say 'No' to an entangling situation or person. It helps us have healthy boundaries by trusting that we deserve what we want.

Buffalo Gourd (*Cucurbita foetidissima*) Buffalo Gourd helps us maintain a deep inner place of healing and calm while participating in external activity. The keyword here is balance, knowing that 'I am the centre'.

Camphorweed (*Heterotheca subaxillaris*) While gently diffusing old patterns, Camphorweed brings a sense of purpose and appropriateness, helping us to stay on track, feel grounded and bring things into manifestation. It is excellent for when we find ourselves caught up in adrenaline-producing situations.

Candy Barrel Cactus (*Ferocactus*) Fostering mental and emotional calmness, Candy Barrel helps us recognize our inner wisdom and uncover long-stored abilities.

Cane Cholla Cactus (*Opuntia imbricata*) Cane Cholla Cactus helps us leap to a new perspective when we struggle with an issue and insist upon defining it in such a way as to block its resolution.

Canyon Grapevine (*Vitis arazonica*) For issues of autonomy, Canyon Grapevine brings appreciation of others as interdependent rather than competing. This essence helps us find a balance between dominance and dependency and encourages us to see obstacles as opportunities.

Cardinal Flower (*Lobelia cardinalis*) This flower essence helps us to redirect sexual energy into other usable forms of energy. It is excellent during menopause, or for those who allow the five senses to dictate their

ponses rather than mastering their bodies and senses.

Cardon Cactus (*Pachycereus pringlei*) Powerful energy is released as repressed feelings
of inadequacy and inferiority are un-
locked. Helps us accept our shadow side
so that it becomes a source of strength and
confidence.

Claret Cup Hedgehog Cactus (*Echinocereus triglochidiatus var. melanacanthus*) Clarity
and focus are the keywords for this hedgehog cactus. This is an excellent essence for
manifestation, meditation or any situation
requiring mental steadiness and acuity.

Cliffrose (*Purshia mexicana*) Cliffrose helps us
unite our will, our intention and the power
to act. It is for those of us who are always
meaning to manifest an altruistic goal but
never quite manage to do so.

Compass Barrel Cactus (*Ferocactus cylindra-
ceus*) Compass Barrel Cactus helps us move
through an emotional state by lightening
up and letting go, trusting our inner wisdom to point the way.

Coral Bean (*Erythrina herbacea*) Coral Bean
helps overcome a drug-like dulling of the
survival instinct. It stimulates focus and
will in facing or recovering from dangerous situations.

Cow Parsnip (*Heracleum maximum*) This essence is for transforming insecurity into a
deep sense of self and surrender to divine
will. It is for an underlying sense of inability to direct our lives.

Creosote Bush (*Larrea tridentata*) Supports us
in releasing what is unexpressed or held in
which is usually at the root of self-imposed
separation from others. It brings us a sense
of being freed. Often used for resolving
the feeling that something is missing in
life.

Crown of Thorns (*Koeberlinia spinosa*)
For those who believe that they must
pay a price for love, or that everything

worthwhile is difficult to obtain, this essence helps us to know that abundance
is our birthright. It is also excellent for
those who are invested in the perspective
of good and bad, or positive and negative.

Crownbeard (*Verbesina encelioides*) For those
with a defeatist attitude, or those who experience the world as unsupportive or hostile, Crownbeard helps us to keep faith and
optimism. It helps us to transmute fears of
hostility and find purposeful expression.

Damiana (*Turnera aphrodisiaca*) When we
feel inadequate, weak, emotionally needy
or detached from the flow of vital life
force, Damiana relaxes and restores our
radiant fullness of energy and sensuality.

Desert Broom (*Baccharis sarothroides*) When
we want to accomplish something but all
parts of our being are not in alignment
with our desire, Desert Broom helps us
to find resolution and readiness to take
the next step. Resolution is the keyword
for this essence, especially when we want
to go deeply into a matter but something
holds us back.

Desert Christmas Cholla Cactus (*Opuntia leptocaulis*) This Cholla Cactus helps
us communicate our limits with humour
and ease, especially if we get caught up
in other people's needs or expectations.
It is wonderful support when we have too
many demands upon us and feel overextended.

Desert Holly (*Acourtia wrightii*) Desert Holly
helps us live in a heart-centred state, opening easily to love rather than working at it.
It is excellent for those who feel stifled by
smothering love or for those who live from
their heads rather than from their hearts.

Desert Jointfir (*Ephedra californica*) Activates our will and our innate healing resources, bringing directedness, vision and
determination. Through confidence in our
self-healing abilities, we learn to escape
potentially damaging situations.

Desert Marigold (*Baileya multiradiata*) When we think that someone else has power over us, Desert Marigold helps us recognize how we actually give the power to them. For taking responsibility and transforming victim consciousness.

Desert Sumac (*Rhus kearneyi subsp. kearneyi*) Desert Sumac helps us transform the pain of loneliness and separation by seeing beyond the superficial differences in people. It is for those who feel they are on the outside looking in in social relationships.

Desert Willow (*Chilopsis linearis*) With Desert Willow, we are supported in feeling respite and in having a perspective of abundance. It is helpful for perfectionism and inflexibility, fostering a perspective of comfort and ease.

Devil's Claw (*Harpagophytum procumbens*) Devil's Claw activates our natural sense of morality. This essence supports us in taking responsibility for owning and expressing who we really are, separate from the projections of others. It is useful if we find ourselves using attractiveness or personal magnetism to manipulate others, or if we try to become who we think others want us to be.

Dogbane (*Apocynum*) Dogbane helps us to access the courage to follow our rebellious instincts, which is an important part of growth and change. For the fear that our rebellion will hurt or damage others, and the fear that we cannot take care of ourselves if we leave home. This is the essence to support self-confidence.

Dyssodia (*Dyssodia pentachaeta*) This yellow flower helps us to assimilate and clarify information, knowledge or wisdom. It helps us to bring things through into consciousness that are felt or sensed but not yet known.

Evening Star (*Mentzelia decapetala*) Evening Star is wonderful for problems of intimacy in relationships due to doubts about our emerging identity. It encourages us in shifting from outer dependence to self-reliance with confidence and quiet surety.

Fairy Duster (*Calliandra eriophylla*) Fairy Duster balances the tendency to swing between high and low energy states. We can use this essence when we have inflated expectations or build castles in the air. It is excellent for nervous excitability and over-reactivity to stimuli.

Fire Prickly Pear Cactus (*Opuntia* sp.) This prickly pear cactus helps us redistribute energy (or focus) if we are concentrating too much attention on one part of our lives (or bodies) to the detriment of the whole.

Fishhook Cactus (*Mammillaria microcarpa*) Fishhook Cactus is for those who hide behind non-communication. It is especially indicated for the fear of risking in communication. It supports us with confidence in public speaking, intimate relationships or for speaking foreign languages.

Foothills Paloverde (*Cercidium microphyllum*) An essence of choice for those of us who are judgemental of ourselves or others, Foothills Paloverde supports us in quieting our minds and finding perfection within ourselves, just as we are. It is also helpful if we feel at the mercy of our emotions.

Hackberry (*Celtis pallida*) Hackberry helps us if we have resistance to feeling grief. Sometimes we have an idea of how long it is appropriate to grieve, but our feelings don't match.

Hairy Larkspur (*Delphinium parryi*) For those with a compulsion or addiction for sweet things, this essence helps us untangle our association of sweet things with a sense of reward. It is excellent for helping us to clarify the difference between desire and self-nurturance.

Hedgehog Cactus (*Echinocereus engelmannii*) Hedgehog Cactus helps us sort out the difference between self-nurturance and overindulgence. It intensifies empathetic perceptions, bringing us closer to nature.

Hoptree (*Ptelea trifoliata*) For those of us who become too easily distracted by the needs of others, Hoptree supports us in staying in alignment with our purpose and remaining focused on what is essential to us. It is excellent for anxiety about boundary making.

Indian Root (*Aralia racemosa*) Do you find yourself trying too hard and making things complex? Indian Root helps us value simplicity. It releases deep-seated fears that block our free-flowing creative expression.

Indian Tobacco (*Nicotiana trigonophylla*) This peace-fostering essence supports us when we view growth processes as hindrances rather than opportunities. It brings a heightened perception of depth and meaning, assisting us to see below the surface of things.

Indigo Bush (*Psorothamnus fremontii*) Indigo Bush helps anchor our spiritually achieved ideas into daily life. It warms the heart and brings the light of clear seeing or inner sight to an area that needs it.

Inmortal (*Asclepias asperula*) Inmortal goes to the core of shame and self-esteem issues. It is excellent for resolving feelings of despair, feeling that problems are insoluble and feeling inadequate. It helps us know the magnificence that we really are.

Jojoba (*Simmodsia chinensis*) For the overly sensitive individual who finds it hard to cope with the mundane, Jojoba brings a sense of ease and security. This grounding essence helps us to participate in daily life and relationships.

Jumping Cholla Cactus (*Opuntia fulgida*) Fostering inner balance, Jumping Cholla Cactus is an antidote for frenzied rushing around. It helps us respond rather than react to life.

Klein's Pencil Cholla Cactus (*Cylindropuntia kleinae*) This cactus essence encourages our creativity and growth in dealing with a relationship that feels stuck. It is excellent for when we stay in a relationship that is not supporting our growth in some way.

Lavender Wand Penstemon (*Penstemon dasyphyllus*) For those who have an inability to deal with emotionally charged issues, this flower essence helps enhance our ability to move into and through difficult issues. It helps bring emotional objectivity and transforms attitudes of struggle and difficulty into ones of confident ease and steadiness of intention.

Lilac (*Syringa*) For those who nostalgically cling to the past or to old ways of being, Lilac helps us to let go. It is a cleansing essence that helps us realize that we are complete or finished with something.

Mala Mujer (*Cnidoscolos angustidens*) Mala Mujer helps the positive expression of feminine qualities, releasing emotional tensions and bringing a lighter, more honest quality to our overall self-expression. It is for when we are bitchy, venomous, shrewish or grouchy. (Guys! This means you too!)

Mariola (*Parthenium incanum*) If we have a false persona, Mariola restores the congruence of our inner experience and outer expression, provoking our essential honesty and enthusiasm.

Mariposa Lily (*Calochortus eurycarpus*) Self-mothering brings joy and freedom, healing separation and alienation. We become receptive to human love.

Melon Loco (*Apodanthera undulata*) Melon Loco helps step down the intensity of our emotions in order to bring us back into our bodies. It helps us have emotional sensibility, responsibility and balance.

Mesquite (*Prosopis* sp.) Opening ourselves to abundance and pleasure, Mesquite amplifies compassion and warmth. This is a great essence for loners and for those who feel an inner barrenness.

Mexican Shell Flower (*Tigridia*) This essence supports our willingness to confront life and its possibilities. It is excellent for 'coming out of your shell'.

Mexican Star (*Milla biflora*) Mexican Star helps us embody strong, self-contained individuality. By knowing that our inner strength is our foundation for survival, we enjoy our uniqueness rather than feeling isolated by it.

Milky Nipple Cactus (*Mammillaria heyderi*) The Milky Nipple Cactus person demands constant attention from others. This 'weaning' essence calms, gives a sense of belonging to the Earth and transforms dependence into self-nurturing autonomy.

Morning Glory Tree (*Ipomoea carnea*) This essence is excellent for becoming conscious of issues of ancestral addictions. It facilitates a conscious chance to change patterns that may be latent or active from our families of origin.

Mountain Mahogany (*Cercocarpus*) Mountain Mahogany provides a gentle but firm push toward our next stage of development. Helpful when we become complacent.

Mullein (*Verbascum thapsus*) Mullein is for when we need to recognize and accept our dark side without feeling overwhelmed by it. We become emotionally self-nurturing, especially when external support isn't available. It brings a sense of security, purpose, protection.

Ocotillo (*Fouquieria splendens*) If we have subconscious or unexpressed feelings that erupt in uncontrolled ways, Ocotillo gives insight into and acceptance of our emotions without feeling victimized by them.

Oregon Grape (*Berberis aquifolium*) When we are never quite satisfied by our performance, the Oregon Grape helps us develop

trust for ourselves and others. An important essence for helping to restore hormonal balance, it supports us in overcoming fear of emotional hostility.

Organ Pipe Cactus (*Stenocereus thurberi*) This cactus helps us survive the dark night of the soul wherein we question our foundations for being. It supports in dealing with mundane aspects of our lives while we allow deep transformation to take place.

Palmer Amaranth (*Amaranthus palmeri*) For those who focus on inessential things rather than getting to the root of the matter, Palmer Amaranth enhances insights as we awaken to a deeper perception of our being. This essence helps us to nourish our roots so we can flower and fruit.

Pencil Cholla Cactus (*Cylindropuntia ramosissima*) For confusion, feeling lost or overwhelmed by details. It helps us focus continually in a specific direction and find steadiness with our intention. It brings clarity and surrender into and through obstacles.

Periwinkle (*Vinca minor*) Periwinkle helps us to integrate and contemplate where we have come from in order to provide wisdom and understanding for the next phase of life. It is excellent when we attempt to forge on ahead into a new project or aspect of our lives without learning from where we have been.

Pink Pond Lily (*Nopalxochia phyllanthoides*) This is an essence to use for self-deception or when we cling to old ways of perceiving ourselves or others. It is excellent for those who have a deep feeling of being unsafe as it fosters total knowing that there is only trust, perfection and safety in being.

Pomegranate (*Punica granatum*) Pomegranate embodies the primal urge to produce, create, procreate and care for. It is excellent for difficulty in giving or receiving maternal support due to a lack of childhood nurturance. It helps when we try hard but get nowhere because our commitment isn't total or right.

Prickle Poppy (*Argemone pleicantha*) This flower essence helps us to be in touch with our natural rhythms and cycles, both physically and emotionally. It is for those who have a taskmaster attitude towards themselves that creates blockages to the natural flow of life energy, and may manifest in joint tension or rigidity. It is excellent for those who are overly controlled.

Prickly Pear Cactus (*Opuntia*) The key word is adaptability. Its qualities help us surrender to the flow of life's events. It is excellent for culture shock.

Purple Aster (*Symphyotrichum patens*) For those whose hard-working efforts create the feeling that they are isolated and that progress is small and difficult, this flower essence changes the feeling of pursuing a goal to feeling as if you are drawn to it. This is the essence of choice for performance anxieties.

Purple Mat (*Nama demissum*) Purple Mat helps us take risks so we can stay true to ourselves and others. For when we secretly harbour our feelings or needs for fear of being rejected or ridiculed if they were openly exposed.

Queen of the Night Cactus (*Epiphyllum oxypetalum*) The Queen of the Night can help us sink deeply into the intuitive root of our being to ground our subtle sensitivities. It helps us open to the qualities of the moon in our daily life, experiencing the blissful perspective of deeper understanding, feeling and sensuality.

Rainbow Cactus (*Echinocereus pectinatus*) Rainbow Cactus is a searchlight to illuminate something dark or held in. Releasing petrified emotion without becoming entangled in it, we emerge bright, free and whole. It is excellent for meditation or regression work as it facilitates easy movement from one state of consciousness to another.

Ratany (*Krameria parvifolia*) If we are pulled between two choices, Ratany enables us to recognize, follow and communicate the truth in our hearts.

Red Root (*Ceanothus azurea*) For those of us who feel guilty because others suffer and we do not, Red Root helps us release enmeshment. It is also for situations in which we are motivated by superstitions or other unconscious forces.

Red-Orange Epiphyllum (*Orchid Cactus*) This essence facilitates grounding of goddess energy into worldly existence. An excellent essence for manifestation.

Sacred Datura (*Datura metaloides*) Sacred Datura facilitates seeing beyond our present view of reality to a more comprehensive, visionary state. When appropriate, it supports us in letting go of a known or familiar reality, such as a relationship or job, without feeling threatened.

Saguaro Cactus (*Carnegiea gigantea*) Saguaro helps us know and trust our inner wisdom and authority. It restores the will to live, to heal and to be the best that we are. It assists us in accessing the perfect inner father who encourages us on in life.

Salsify (*Tragopogon porrifolius*) If we have difficulty in bringing a project or some aspect of ourselves to fruition or completion, Salsify supports us in the maturation process. It is excellent for finding all the vital elements for growth and the expression of our full potential.

Sangre de Drago (*Croton lechleri*) This flower essence helps us to create good psychic boundaries based upon appropriate discrimination and natural morality. It is excellent for those who are afraid of their psychic nature as it fosters the acceptance of sensitive abilities with grounded practicality.

Scarlet Morning Glory (*Ipomoea hederifolia*)
Some of us think about what we will do in the future but never begin to make it reality. For those who have difficulty giving form to their creative impulses, this flower essence stimulates us to get going, making future potential into present reality. It also helps keep us focused if we become caught up in excitement that pulls our focus in other directions.

Scorpion Weed (*Phacelia tanacetifolia*) The strength of innocence and direct confrontation overcomes fear and paralysis. Scorpion Weed helps us with many types of fears: of the consequences of our actions; of our past mistakes; of not being forgiven. It is especially useful when we externalize our fears or when we create monsters out of them.

Senita Cactus (*Cereus schottii*) The grandparent's perspective opens the flow of emotion without pain, without bitterness from the past or expectations for the future. Senita helps us access from within us a soft, sweet support for letting go of old perspectives that keep us locked into unsettled emotions.

Silverleaf Nightshade (*Solanum elaeagnifolium*) Silverleaf Nightshade helps us in recognizing that we have the power to hurt as well as heal. It is used for fear and paralysis created by our minds that keeps us from owning our own power.

Smartweed (*Polygonum hydropiper*) Smartweed is for those who believe that since they were hurt before they will be hurt again. These people hide away and withdraw from perceived dangers of being with others. It encourages openness and willingness to receive love and encouragement from others.

Soaptree Yucca (*Yucca elata*) Soaptree Yucca activates our assertiveness in the expression of our own will or intention, especially if we tend to allow the will of another to dominate us. It helps us to keep sight of our long-term goals with faith, perseverance and endurance.

Sow-Thistle (*Sonchus asper*) Sow-Thistle helps us deal appropriately with obnoxious behaviour, whether our own or that of others. It helps us deal with feeling intimidated by dominating personalities. It is also excellent if we find ourselves wanting a relationship so badly that we don't give the other person the space they need.

Spanish Bayonet Yucca (*Yucca aloifolia*) An excellent essence to help us when we experience indecisiveness, hesitation or fear in facing challenges. It provokes a unification of our will with our intention.

Spineless Prickly Pear Cactus (*Opuntia tuna*) With Spineless Prickly Pear, we discover that all we need for survival is contained within us and that we don't need anything outside of us to 'be'. We find strength in vulnerability.

Staghorn Cholla Cactus (*Opuntia versicolor*) This Cholla Cactus activates our innate capacity for self-ordering and reconstruction after a time of transformation and change. It helps us see that change occurs in harmony with our own unique soul plan.

Star Leaf (*Choisya arizonica*) Star Leaf helps us be simply and purely ourselves, without the need for external approval. It frees up self-expression for those who do not recognize or accept their unique contribution to life.

Star Primrose (*Oenothera primiveris*) An excellent essence for those of us with a poor self-image, Star Primrose is helpful if we blame our negative feelings on an outside source while simultaneously denying such feelings exist. It is also an essence of choice for those of us who are confused about sexuality and spirituality, or who repress sensuality and put energy into occult, mystical or mental pursuits.

Strawberry Cactus (*Echinocereus stramineus*) For those of us who are expecting things to go wrong or be difficult, Strawberry Cactus encourages us to let go and allow our hearts to transmute difficult emotions. We know that there is perfection in each moment and each situation, and we begin to live in joy.

Syrian Rue (*Peganum harmala*) An energetic 'truth serum', Syrian Rue is for all issues of lying, being lied to, betrayal, telling the truth and trustworthiness. It helps us know and trust in our own truth, regardless of external pressures.

Tarbush (*Flourensia cernua*) Tarbush strengthens inspiration and motivation to change something that has been accepted as a limitation or condition of life. It helps us to identify and release deeply imprinted assumptions or beliefs that work subconsciously.

Teddy Bear Cholla Cactus (*Opuntia bigelovii*) A cuddly looking cactus, Teddy Bear Cholla helps with deep fears of intimacy and allowing others close enough to see our perfection. It is also for when we feel impatient with our perceived level of growth or development.

Theresa Cactus (*Mamillaria thereseae*) For those who hide behind serving others, this cactus fosters a deep sense of self-care. It helps us change conditional giving into unconditional service.

Thistle (*Cirsium occidentale*) For those who experience a lack of trust or faith in their spiritual connection, Thistle helps us let down our defensiveness and recognize grace in our lives.

Thurber's Gilia (*Ipomopsis thurberi*) For all types of fears that paralyze us, this is the essence of choice. Also for resolving the frustration of our limitations and the paradoxical fear of living without our limitations.

Violet Curls (*Trichostema arizonica*) Violet Curls helps us release, one by one, congested emotions. It supports us in expressing

our emotions as they arise so as not to create a backlog of them. We lighten up and are able to have a calm detachment.

Violet Soldier (*Elytraria imbricata*) For those who feel defeated and unable to survive a transformational experience, Violet Soldier helps us find a will to live, to heal and to overcome all obstacles. Victory is the key word, victory of the spirit over all possible conditions of external existence.

White Desert Primrose (*Oenothera deltoides*) White Desert Primrose is for those who are overly influenced by what others think is right for them. It helps us see through others' projected images and ideals to realize forms of self-expression that are in harmony with our essential nature. It enhances belief in ourselves and discernment of our own unique soul pattern.

White Desert Zinnia (*Zinnia acerosa*) Those who have a discouraged attitude towards life and who believe that they can never quite get ahead can use this flower essence. It helps bring the ability to laugh at ourselves or a situation and open ourselves to lightness, merriment and renewal.

White Evening Primrose (*Oenothera pallida*) This flower essence has a grounding effect for those who feel disconnected from their sense of spirituality. It helps us to be spiritually receptive by being more present in our bodies and in touch with our childlike sense of innocence.

Whitethorn (*Acacia vernicosa*) Whitethorn helps us be more gentle with ourselves. It brings a sense of optimistic freshness and helps our thinking to move in new, innovative directions. It helps release us from succumbing to old patterns and habits, especially if we have continued to act them out after initially recognizing them. It is useful for calming adrenaline excess.

Wild Buckwheat (*Polygonum convolvulus*) This is the essence to use when you compare yourself to others and set yourself apart from them. When we focus on the differences between us in relationships we isolate ourselves. Wild Buckwheat helps us to find and focus on what we have in common, and helps us to blend and harmonize with others.

Windflower (*Anemone pulsatilla*) When we feel highly energized at one moment and then depleted in the next, Windflower facilitates a more balanced distribution of energy.

Wolfberry (*Lycium pallidum*) Releasing deep sadness from the past, helps us to allow grief to take us to a transpersonal experience. When we experience that something is shifting around inside ourselves but we don't know what it is, Wolfberry helps us to be at peace and allow the process without insisting upon defining it.

Woven Spine Pineapple Cactus (*Neolloydia intertexta*) This cactus loosens old emotional tensions in the body when we are overburdened by the 'shoulds' of life, helping us become our own best friend. For regeneration of energy after exhaustion, burnout, travel or illness.

Zephyr Lily (*Zephyranthes*) This is the essence of choice to use for present or past traumas, whether physical, emotional or mental. It allows deep peace and calm as we heal from shock or trauma.

FLOWER ESSENCE SOCIETY (FES)

The Flower Essence Society has been in existence longer than almost any other flower remedy organization (the exception being the Bach Flower Centre). It was established in 1979 by Richard Katz with a view to gathering together information and research regarding newer flower essences and educating the public through classes and publications. In 1980 he formed a professional partnership with his wife, Patricia Kaminski, and together they not only administer the Flower Essence Society but, through their company Flower

Essence Services, prepare an extensive range of high-quality North American flower essences known as the 'FES Quintessentials'. They are made with flowers wildcrafted from pristine natural habitats in California and other parts of North America, and from organic gardens and wild areas on their 27-acre centre, Terra Flora, located near Nevada City in the foothills of California's Sierra Nevada mountains, a place of granite peaks studded with Golden Quartz and sparkling rivers.

Katz and Kaminski have devoted particular attention to researching their essences thoroughly, using extensive case studies and clinical reports by practitioners, and by studies of the essence plants, including morphological and botanical characteristics. They also conduct seminars and practitioner training and certification programmes, write and publish newsletters and books, including their comprehensive Flower Essence Repertory. Flower Essence Society membership provides a communication network for those teaching, researching and practising in this field.

The FES essences are currently being used by thousands of practitioners and lay people in more than 50 countries around the world. As Katz and Kaminski have said, flower essences are not panaceas, but catalysts which stimulate and energize the inner transformative process, while leaving us free to develop our own innate capacities. Just as food nourishes the body, so can flower essences nourish and heal the soul. They are a harbinger of a new alchemy of the soul, one which incorporates ancient wisdom with a modern awareness of the human psyche and of nature.

Adapted from writings by Patricia Kaminski, used with kind permission.

Professional Kit

Aloe Vera For people who have an abundance of fiery energy but tend to overuse it and literally burn out — workaholics who neglect their emotional and physical needs. Brings a sense of renewal and rejuvenation, restores nourishment. Balances creative activity and centres vital life energy.

Alpine Lily (*Lilium parvum*) For women who have difficulty accepting their femininity, lack of connection, awareness or rejection of female body, who may be susceptible to reproductive and sexual problems. Encourages a radiant and self-assured feminine identity, physical presence grounded in the female body.

Angel's Trumpet (*Brugmansia candida*) For those who fear death, who resist letting go of physical life, and crossing the spiritual threshold. Brings spiritual surrender at death and times of deep transformation or transition, opening the soul to the spiritual world.

Angelica (*Angelica archangelica*) For those who feel cut off, bereft of spiritual guidance and protection feeling like a spiritual orphan. Encourages feelings of being protected, guided and cared for, especially in times of crisis. Good for birthing, dying, festive celebrations and other major life passages.

Arnica (*Arnica mollis*) For deep-seated shock or trauma which may become locked into the body and prevent full healing recovery. For accidents and violent experiences where the soul or Higher Self dissociates from the physical body. Brings conscious embodiment, especially during shock or trauma, and aids recovery. Helpful for treatment of psychosomatic illnesses which do not respond to other treatments, and for dysfunction or latent illness deriving from past trauma or stress. Aids recovery from deep-seated strain, post-trauma or scarring.

Baby Blue Eyes (*Nemophila menziesii*) For those who are unsure of themselves and unable to trust in the goodness of others and the world – defensive, insecure, with a cynical mistrust of the world. Estrangement from higher spiritual authority and lack of support from the father or other masculine influences in childhood. Restores innocence and childlike trust, feeling supported and loved, especially by male figures; and a recognition of goodness in others, the world and faith in the providence of spiritual beings.

Basil (*Ocimum basilicum*) For those who have a tendency to separate the experience of spirituality from that of sexuality. They may be secretive about sex, regarding it as sinful while finding illicit sexual practices attractive and compelling, typically leading to clandestine behaviour, bifurcated relationships or sexual addiction. Integrates sexuality and spirituality into a sacred wholeness.

Blackberry (*Rubus armeniacus*) For those who have lofty visions and desires but are unable to put them into action, concrete or viable activities; often lacking the ability to organize their intentions into specific goals and priorities creating procrastination. Also for poor circulation and sluggish metabolism. Aids competent manifestation in the world, and directs willpower and enables one to take decisive action.

Black-Eyed Susan (*Rudbeckia hirta*) For those who avoid or repress parts of their personality or traumatic episodes from the past, for instance rape or incest, often experiencing emotional amnesia and paralysis, addictive or hypnotic behaviour due to loss of consciousness. Awakens consciousness, enables you to acknowledge all aspects of the self and to achieve penetrating insight.

Black Cohosh (*Actaea racemosa*) For those caught in relationships and lifestyles that are abusive, addictive or violent with dark brooding emotions, congested or toxic psychic forces. Gives us the courage to confront rather than shrink from abusive or threatening situations, transforming the negativity, gaining power and balance in destructive circumstances fostering clear and contained psychic forces.

Bleeding Heart (*Dicentra formosa*) For a tendency to form relationships based on fear or possessiveness; for emotional dependence which leads to a lack of freedom in the relationship, neediness; emotional co-dependency. Sufferers may feel tremendous pain and brokenheartedness by loving someone who is emotionally distanced or no longer present. Brings the openhearted ability to love others unconditionally, and emotional freedom.

Borage (*Borago officinalis*) For heavy-heartedness, depressive behaviour, or lack of confidence in the face of difficult circumstances. For those who feel discouraged or disheartened in times of grief, sadness or other adversity. Uplifts the heart, gives buoyant courage, rekindles a sense of optimism and enthusiasm.

Buttercup (*Ranunculus occidentalis*) For those who feel humbled and lack self-worth, or are self-deprecating and unable to acknowledge or experience their uniqueness and inner light. Brings recognition of the inner light which is a source of healing and peace. Relieves you from the need to judge yourself by conventional standards of achievement and success. Helpful for children who may be physically handicapped or impaired.

Calendula (*Calendula officinalis*) For those prone to being argumentative, who have a tendency to use cutting or sharp words and lack receptivity when communicating with others, verbal abuse. Gives warmth and benign compassion; encourages receptivity in conversations.

California Pitcher Plant (*Darlingtonia californica*) For those who fear their instinctive desires; they may lack strength and physical vigour, be listless, anaemic, with poor digestion or unable to assimilate nutrients properly. Restores earthly vitality,

balancing instinctual desire so these energies can strengthen physical vitality.

California Poppy (*Eschscholzia californica*) For those seeking false forms of light, who become attached to illusion or grandeur, or higher consciousness, 'spiritual glamour' or psychic experiences. Balances the forces of light and love, encouraging more self-responsibility and quiet inner development. Encourages a radiant heart-centred spirituality; strong interior alignment for values and choices.

California Wild Rose (*Rosa californica*) For apathy or resignation, passivity; not wanting to take full responsibility or to experience the pain or challenge of life. For those who recoil from relationships which may involve taking emotional risks or who feel socially alienated. Brings the ability to care for and give oneself to life and to others. Kindles enthusiasm for doing and serving.

Calla Lily (*Zantedeschia aethiopica*) For confusion or ambivalence about sexual identity or gender. Brings acceptance and clarity of sexuality and sexual identity and individualized integration of masculine and feminine qualities. Heals wounding due to cultural gender bias.

Canyon Dudleya (*Dudleya cymosa*) For those who exaggerate the relevance of psychic experiences; attracted to mediumism, channelling and experiences which spark off psychic fantasies; prone to neglecting daily activities. Encourages inner contentment which dispels the necessity for psychic excitement and addiction to trauma drama lifestyle. Balances psychic and physical energies; grounded presence in everyday life; positive charisma.

Cayenne (*Capsicum annuum*) Fiery and energetic, inwardly mobile. For those prone to stagnation, complacency, feeling stuck or immobilized, unable to make any progress or change, caught in a pattern of procrastination and resistance. Ignites and sparks the soul, encouraging our capacity to initiate and sustain spiritual and emotional development and capable of change and transformation.

Chamomile (*Matricaria recutita*) For those easily upset, moody, irritable and unable to release emotional tension, often leading to insomnia and tension that leads to stress in the stomach or solar plexus. Releases tension, encouraging serenity, emotional balance and a sunny disposition. Also good for children's stomach complaints, which are often emotionally based.

Chaparral (also known as Creosote Bush) (*Larrea tridentata*) For disturbed dreams or psychic toxicity when overexposed to violent or chaotic images. Important remedy for modern civilization. Clears post-traumatic stress and physical toxicity due to drugs. Important psychic cleanser which works especially through the dream life to cleanse the psyche. Balanced psychic awareness, deep penetration and understanding of the transpersonal aspects of oneself.

Chrysanthemum (*Chrysanthemum morifolium*) For fear of ageing and mortality, overidentification with youthfulness or attachment to fame and fortune, the material world. For midlife crisis. Brings a shift towards identifying with what is truly eternal, a higher spiritual identity and a transcendent soul.

Corn (*Zea mays*) For disorientation and stress, particularly in urban environments; helpful for those who feel uncomfortable living in congested, chaotic environments, preferring rural or uncrowded areas. Helps you stay centred and in alignment with the Earth, with your feet firmly on the ground.

Cosmos (*Cosmos bipinnatus*) For those who find it difficult to organize their thoughts into words. Unfocused, disorganized, overwhelmed by too many ideas, their speech is rapid and inarticulate. Brings integration

of ideas, harmonizes thinking and speaking patterns to bring more coherency.

Dandelion (*Taraxacum officinale*) For those who have a natural intensity and love for life but who tend to overstretch themselves, overstriving and hard-driving, making themselves overly tense, rigid or stiff, especially in the muscles. Encourages listening to bodily messages. Allows release of tensions from the body and emotions, bringing dynamic, effortless physical energy.

Deer Brush (*Ceanothus integerrimus*) For mixed or conflicting motives, deceiving ourselves by lack of honesty or polite responses not based upon genuine feelings in our relationships with others and in the affairs of daily life. Brings gentle purity, clarity of purpose and sincerity of motive, with actions that are allied with one's true feelings. Helps the soul attain purity so that it radiates truth and harmony.

Dill (*Anethum graveolens*) For when the senses are overwhelmed and overstimulated; for hypersensitivity to the environment, sensory congestion. Enables us to absorb and experience the fullness of life, especially sensory impressions, heightened awareness of taste, touch, hearing, sight, smell, etc.

Dogwood (*Cornus nuttallii*) For emotional trauma stored deep within the body – often springing from physical or sexual abuse or harsh physical living circumstances – which can cause the body to feel awkward and ungainly. Also for those with self-destructive, accident-prone tendencies. Evokes a sense of gentleness, graceful movement, physical and etheric harmony in the body and inner sanctity.

Easter Lily (*Lilium longiflorum*) For those in conflict about their sexual identity leading to an imbalance towards either prudishness or promiscuity, virgin/whore split in psyche. Cleanses the conflict, conferring the ability to integrate sexuality and spirituality; enhancing the inner purity of the soul.

Echinacea (*Echinacea purpurea*) For feeling shattered by severe trauma or abuse, loss of dignity, profound alienation. Poor immune function. Restores a sense of true identity and dignity. Maintains self-integrity and immunity, maintaining a strong sense of self, especially when challenged by stress or disease.

Evening Primrose (*Oenothera elata*) For feeling rejected and unwanted due to past abuse or childhood neglect; avoiding commitment in relationships; fear of parenthood; sexual and emotional coldness and repression. Brings awareness and healing of painful early emotions absorbed from parents; ability to be open, express emotional warmth and presence, and be able to form deep, committed relationships.

Fairy Lantern (*Calochortus albus*) For immaturity, helplessness, dependency – the eternal child, delicate and needy, lacking inner strength to face the world or shoulder responsibility. Brings about a positive integration of child identity and a mature, independent adult. Use during childhood and adolescence for retarded phases of physical or emotional development.

Fawn Lily (*Erythronium purpurascens*) For withdrawal, isolation, self-protection; those who are highly developed spiritually who find it difficult to cope with the stress and strain of modern society and lack the inner strength to participate in community and family. Encourages acceptance and involvement in the world, and the ability to share spiritual, healing gifts with others.

Filaree (*Erodium cicutarium*) For disproportionate worry and those who become too enmeshed in or overly concerned with the mundane affairs of daily life, wasting energy on small problems. Unable to gain a wider perspective in daily life; hyperfocus on small details. Helps give a cosmic overview and puts life into perspective, unleashing inner strength and reserve.

Forget-Me-Not (*Myosotis sylvatica*) For feelings of isolation, lack of awareness of spiritual and karmic connections with others. Loneliness and isolation due to death of a loved one; soul myopia. Encourages awareness of our relationship and responsibility to everyone. Good for maintaining a conscious link with lost loved ones.

Fuchsia (*Fuchsia magellanica*) For hyperemotionality and those who mask their true feelings (such as pain and deep-seated trauma) with false emotions and misdirected psychosomatic symptoms and responses to pain and stress. Brings genuine emotional vitality. Allows expression of deep and intense feelings and enables emotions such as grief, deep-seated anger or rejection to be encountered and transformed.

Garlic (*Allium sativum*) For those who are fearful, weak, due to parasitic influence, or easily influenced, prone to low vitality and tend to be mediumistic by nature. Brings a sense of wholeness which imparts strength and active resistance to adverse influences and a resilient and vital response to life. Good for poor immune response and vulnerability to infection.

Golden Ear Drops (*Ehrendorferia chrysantha*) For those who suppress painful and toxic memories and trauma from the past (especially childhood) which affect present emotional life and identity. Encourages being in touch with one's inner child as a source of spirituality. Stimulates remembrance and ability to understand core experiences that define emotional history; releasing these traumatic memories so the past can become a source of strength and nourishment, wisdom and insight.

Golden Yarrow (*Achillea filipendulina*) For those with a tendency to withdraw from society or artistic involvement due to profound oversensitivity, avoiding the limelight or performance, becoming hardened to cope with vulnerability. Dependence on drugs for protection or social masking. Shields and protects, allowing you to stay open, whilst staying self-contained and balanced without compromising your integrity and health.

Goldenrod (*Solidago californica*) For those easily influenced by family or others, subject to peer pressure or susceptible to social expectations, unable to be true to themselves or to establish their own values and beliefs. Conforming to social norms to win approval and acceptance, such people may one day resort to antisocial or obnoxious behaviour as in adolescence. Encourages a strong, well-developed, secure sense of individuality, greater strength and inner conviction.

Hibiscus (*Hibiscus rosa-sinensis*) For when sexual expression becomes cold and unresponsive – often due to prior sexual exploitation or abuse. Inability to enjoy sexual experience. Particularly for women profoundly affected and offended by stereotyped images of female sexuality. Kindles sexual warmth, vitality and responsiveness, the integration of the soul's warmth and the body's passion.

Hound's Tongue (*Cynoglossum grande*) For those who tend to see the world in materialistic terms, becoming weighed down or dulled by an overly analytical worldly view with the accompanying heaviness or torpor in the physical body. Promotes holistic, balanced thinking; encouraging lively thoughts, integration of imagination and intellect. Restores a sense of wonder and reverence for life. Stimulates the ability to perceive the physical world with spiritual clarity.

Indian Paintbrush (*Castilleja miniata*) For creative people who suffer from low vitality, exhaustion and other forms of physical illness during their work because they are unable to stay grounded and energized, unable to bring creative forces into physical expression. Helps the physical body to be lively, energetic, exuberant and healthy while using creative potential.

Indian Pink (*Silene californica*) For those who take on too many activities at once, becoming tense, emotionally volatile, depleted and unable to see the self as a centre of activity. Whose psychic forces, which are easily fragmented by too much movement, are frayed and overwhelmed during multilevelled activity. Assists in becoming centred and focused even under stress, or high levels of activity; so as to manage and coordinate diverse activities.

Iris (*Iris douglasiana*) For those feeling dull, unable to feel inspiration, lacking creativity and feeling weighed down by the ordinariness of the world. Encourages perception of beauty, making everything seem alive and vibrant, and a deep soulfulness and inspired creativity which is in touch with the higher realms. Brings radiant, iridescent vision in all aspects of life.

Lady's Slipper (Yellow) (*Cypripedium parviflorum*) For those estranged from their inner authority, unable to integrate and align their higher spiritual purpose and direction with real life and work, leading to nervous exhaustion and sexual depletion. Calms and restabilizes the nervous system, helping to regain inner composure and spiritual strength, integrating spiritual purpose with daily work, integration of spiritual vision with vital forces in the root and creative chakras bringing spiritual power into the body.

Larkspur (*Delphinium variegatum*) For those in positions of leadership who are distorted by self-aggrandizement and who feel overburdened by duty or inflated with self-importance, unable to motivate or inspire others. Encourages charismatic leadership qualities, contagious enthusiasm and joy in serving others.

Lavender (*Lavandula officinalis*) For nervousness and overstimulation of mental or spiritual forces which deplete the physical body; for those who are highly strung and wound up, typically suffering from headaches, vision problems, neck and shoulder tension and insomnia. Soothes and teaches moderation. Brings spiritual sensitivity, encouraging a highly refined awareness intact with stable bodily health.

Lotus (*Nelumbo nucifera*) For spiritual pride – those who regard themselves as spiritually correct and who are out of touch with ordinary personality and humble tasks. An all-purpose remedy for enhancing and harmonizing the higher consciousness. Enables an expansive and inclusive spirituality, with the ability to synthesize diverse life experience in service to the spiritual world.

Love-Lies-Bleeding (*Amaranthus caudatus*) For intensification of pain and suffering due to isolation; profound melancholia due to the overpersonalization of one's pain. Brings transcendent consciousness, the ability to move beyond personal pain, suffering or mental anguish by finding larger, transpersonal meaning in such suffering; compassionate awareness and vision of and attention to the meaning of pain or suffering. Helps develop compassionate acceptance of life karma.

Madia (*Madia elegans*) For those who are easily distracted, unable to concentrate and having trouble living in the present, splintering activity so that it is unproductive. Also for seasonal distress, when hot weather can make you feel listless and distracted. Brings precision thinking, disciplined focus and concentration.

Mallow (*Sidalcea glaucescens*) For insecurity in relationships, an inability to trust and paralysis in reaching out to others or radiating warmth, resulting in social barriers. Removes barriers and helps us trust our inner feelings. Encourages warm openhearted sharing and friendliness.

Manzanita (*Arctostaphylos viscida*) For those who have an aversion to their body and feel estranged from the physical world. Often drawn to punishing dietary regimes, such people often feel ill even if they are following perfect health programmes, and have eating and sleeping disorders. Softens attitude to physical matter, encourages a spiritual identity that is fully integrated with the physical body and a positive involvement in the world.

Mariposa Lily (*Calochortus leichtlinii*) For those alienated from their mother or the mothering instinct due to abandonment, abuse or trauma in childhood. Heals the trauma and encourages our ability to nurture and show caring attention to others. Strengthens maternal instincts, warm and positive mother–child bond. Restores the inner child.

Milkweed (*Asclepias cordifolia*) Neediness and emotional regression, dulling the consciousness due to extreme dependency on drugs, alcohol, food as a means of escaping from self-awareness, also creating dependency or sickness to receive attention. Brings independence, strength, self-reliance and a healthy ego; nourishes at the deepest level.

Morning Glory (*Ipomoea purpurea*) For 'night owls' with erratic eating and sleeping rhythms who have difficulty getting up in the morning with an inability to fully enter the body. Feeling hungover, dull and toxic; perhaps making them susceptible to nervous depletion and poor immunity. Also for addictive habits. Encourages attunement with rhythms to restore natural energy and sparkling life force, so that one is refreshed and in touch with life.

Mountain Pennyroyal (*Monardella odoratissima*) For difficulty thinking clearly and making rational decisions because of unconscious absorption on the negative thoughts of others – negative programming, psychic contamination or possession.

Cleanses the mind to promote clear, positive thinking and mental integrity.

Mountain Pride (*Penstemon newberryi*) For fear and withdrawal when faced with challenges, vacillation and lack of assertiveness making us unable to take a stand for what we believe in. Cultivates a courageous warrior-like spirituality and attitude which confronts, takes positive action and transforms.

Mugwort (*Artemisia douglasiana*) For those prone to fantasy or projection, who display irrational, hysterical, overemotional behaviour, who are out of touch with reality. For those who have an overactive psychic life and are unable to distinguish or integrate transphysical experiences. Integrates psychic dreams and balances experiences so we can glean greater insight into the affairs of daily life. Encourages warm and expansive soul qualities.

Mullein (*Verbascum thapsus*) For those feeling weak and confused, unable to tune in to or hear their inner voice and lacking in decisiveness, confused, prone to lying or deceiving themselves and others. Develops a strong sense of inner conscience, truthfulness and moral fortitude.

Nasturtium (*Tropaeolum majus*) For intellectuals who think too much and deplete their life force and emotional verve from too much study. Restores warmth, vitality and radiant energy.

Nicotiana (Flowering Tobacco) (*Nicotiana alata*) For numbing of the emotions accompanied by mechanization or hardening of the body; inability to cope with deep feelings and finer sensibilities. Blunted feelings, shallow breathing. Brings inner peace which is deeply centred in the heart; deep breathing, integration of physical and emotional wellbeing through harmonious connection with the Earth.

Oregon Grape (*Berberis aquifolium*) For paranoid, fearful people who see others and the outside world as hostile and unfair, and have defensive behaviour and antagonistic projection. Helps cultivate trust and positive expectation in the goodness of others. Good for tension and ill will that predominate in many urban environments.

Penstemon (*Penstemon davidsonii*) For those who feel persecuted or victimized, or who pity themselves for having been dealt an unfair hand in life and are unable to bear life's difficult circumstances – they may be disabled or may have lost a loved one, their home or possessions. Develops inner strength, courage and resilience in the face of hardships. Fosters an enduring and persevering attitude.

Peppermint (*Mentha piperita*) For mental dullness and lethargy, craving stimulation or food only to feel sluggish afterwards – unbalanced and underactive metabolism depletes mental forces. Imparts mental clarity and vibrancy and a warm metabolism balanced with cool head forces.

Pink Monkeyflower (*Mimulus lewisii*) For shame, guilt, unworthiness, fear of exposure and rejection, masking feelings and hiding your real self from others. For fear of anyone seeing your pain, possibly due to childhood trauma or abuse. Brings self-acceptance and forgiveness, the ability to let go of the past as well as emotional openness to experience and risk the love and affection of others.

Pink Yarrow (*Achillea millefolium var. rubra*) For those who are overly sympathetic towards others and excessively vulnerable to their emotional influence, with an overly absorbent auric field, dysfunctional merging with others, giving rise to emotional confusion. Imparts appropriate emotional boundaries and greater objectivity and containment, teaching how we can radiate love.

Poison Oak (*Toxicodendron diversilobum*) For fear of intimate contact, being violated. For those who put up a hostile front, protective of personal boundaries; reactive or rejecting in relationships so driving away intimacy. Brings emotional openness and vulnerability so others can make close contact possibly through touch. Especially for men who fear being too open.

Pomegranate (*Punica granatum*) For women torn between career and home life, feeling confused and compromised, especially between values of career and home. Such psychological tension can affect sexual organs. Enables women to see their destiny and choices more clearly, encouraging joyful expression of feminine creativity, active productivity and nurturing.

Pretty Face (*Triteleia ixioides*) For those feeling ugly and rejected because of their physical appearance, such as those born with deformities or whose features are ungainly. Allows inner beauty to radiate within; brings acceptance of our own appearance despite handicaps or blemishes.

Purple Monkeyflower (*Mimulus kelloggii*) For fear of the occult, or of any spiritual experience; fear of retribution or censure if one departs from religious conventions of family or community, apprehension or avoidance of threshold experiences due to fear-based beliefs or ritual abuse. Brings inner calm and clarity when experiencing any spiritual or psychic phenomenon; the courage to trust in one's own spiritual experience or guidance; love-based rather than fear-based spirituality.

Quaking Grass (*Briza maxima*) For those who have difficulty finding their place in the work or family setting. Inability to compromise, overattachment to personal will and desire in social situations. Helps individuals maintain their identity without being subservient or overexerting their ego. Harmonious community consciousness, flexible and receptive in group work.

Queen Anne's Lace (*Daucus carota*) For those who close their eyes to what is really happening, denying the subtler levels of reality. Projection or lack of objectivity in psychic awareness; distortion of psychic perception or physical eyesight due to sexual or emotional imbalances. Helps clear the vision, bringing spiritual insight while keeping both feet on the Earth, integrates psychic faculties with sexual and emotional aspects of self.

Quince (*Chaenomeles speciosa*) Loving strength and firm loving; integration of masculine initiating power and feminine nurturing qualities. Inability to catalyze or reconcile strength and power with affection and tenderness; dysfunctional or inconsistent parenting or leadership behaviour. For difficulty in combining nurturing and gentle qualities with discipline and objectivity. Helps us to use our loving nature in a way that does not compromise our essential dignity and strength.

Rabbitbrush (*Ericameria nauseosa*) For those easily overwhelmed by details; unable to cope with simultaneous events, fuzzy consciousness that is unable to register details. For combining focus and attention to detail with wide-ranging perspective stimulating a lively and alert mental field. Encourages our capacity to integrate details while simultaneously being aware of the total situation.

Red Clover (*Trifolium pratense*) For those whose individuality is challenged by mass consciousness, feeling swept away on a tide of mass hysteria and anxiety, easily influenced by panic around them or other forms of group thought. Encourages awareness of our behaviour, helping us to maintain calm and steadiness, especially in emergencies.

Rosemary (*Rosmarinus officinalis*) For those who tend to be forgetful and absentminded with poor learning ability because their spirit feels insecure about being here, loosely incarnated in body, lacking physical/etheric warmth, with their feet and hands often being cold and devitalized. For traumatic out-of-body spiritual experiences. Brings the ability to feel warm and secure. For feeling vibrant with a healthy embodiment.

Sage (*Salvia officinalis*) For a tendency to see life as ill-fated or undeserved, unable to perceive the higher purpose and meaning in life events. Enables you to learn and reflect about life experience which brings insight, wisdom and inner peace. Helpful during transitions and phases in life when you need to step back and consider the events that are unfolding. Gives wisdom derived from life experience and the ability to assess and understand life process from a higher perspective.

Sagebrush (*Artemisia tridentata*) For those who cling to proof of their existence by overidentifying with illusory parts of the self, needing to purify and cleanse the self and release dysfunctional aspects of the self and surroundings. Encourages us to become more aware of our essential identity, to be true to ourselves – thus capable of transformation and change.

Saguaro (*Carnegiea gigantea*) For rebellious tendencies – conflict with authority – sense of separateness or alienation from the past and reacting against your past. Brings awareness of what is ancient and sacred and an ability to learn from elders and an understanding of your culture, lineage or tradition, in order to embrace and understand the past.

Scarlet Monkeyflower (*Mimulus cardinalis*) Patterns of imbalance: fear or repression of intense feelings; inability to act upon issues of anger and powerlessness for fear of intense feelings/repression of powerful emotions/inability to resolve issues of power or anger/fear of exploding in a blind rage. Needing to be seen as nice rather than real. Gives courage to acknowledge and confront such feelings. Imparts emotional depth and honesty, direct and clear communication of feelings especially anger or disappointment – integration of our emotional 'shadow'.

Scotch Broom (*Cytisus scoparius*) For those disheartened, anxious and depressed by uncertainty and upheaval in the world/ pessimistic and despairing of your role in larger events. Gives tenacity and strength, cultivating hope, a positive view and optimistic feelings of the world's future.

Self-Heal (*Prunella vulgaris*) For those unable to take responsibility for their own healing and wellbeing, lacking in spiritual motivation for wellness and good health, overly dependent on external help. Encourages belief in your own capacity for recovery and an awareness and ability to tap into your own healing potential: a vital and healthy sense of self.

Shasta Daisy (*Leucanthemum* × *superbum*) For overanalytical people who have a tendency to see information as separate pieces rather than parts of a whole, artificial or mechanized intelligence. Gives insight into the larger patterns of mental and emotional experience and helps us to synthesize these patterns into a living wholeness, a holistic consciousness. Helpful for those involved in writing, teaching, research and other intellectual professions.

Shooting Star (*Dodecatheon hendersonii*) For feeling profoundly alienated, not at home on Earth nor a part of the human family; disturbed birth trauma. Obsessed with extra-terrestrial existence. Brings the ability to find the right earthly connection and to be warmed with caring for all that is human and earthly. Humanized spirituality, cosmic consciousness.

Snapdragon (*Antirrhinum majus*) For energetic people with powerful wills and libidos who tend to repress these tendencies – prone to verbal aggression and hostility; sarcasm, lashing criticism, tension around the jaws (teeth-grinding). Misplaced

347

snapping, biting or eating behaviours. Encourages a lively, dynamic, healthy libido and communication which is emotionally balanced.

Star Thistle (*Centaurea solstitialis*) For socially reclusive, lonely people who find it difficult to trust and be generous; those who tend to hoard or guard their material possessions due to a fear of lack, feeling malnourished at a deeper level. For an inability to give freely and spontaneously, miserly or hoarding tendencies. Brings feelings of security and a sense of abundance. Encourages the ability to give and share.

Star Tulip (*Calochortus tolmiei*) For men who deny their softer, receptive side, or women who have built a shell of protection around themselves. For the inability to cultivate quiet inner presence, lack of attunement or soul insight, unable to meditate or pray. Increases sensitivity and receptivity. Encourages quiet inner listening, serene soul disposition, ability to listen to higher worlds, especially in dreams and meditation.

Sticky Monkeyflower (*Mimulus aurantiacus*) For fear and repression of sexual intimacy and contact, often compensated for by seeking superficial sexual encounters. Balanced integration of human warmth, encourages ability to express deep feelings of love in sexual relationships.

St John's Wort (*Hypericum perforatum*) For those sensitive to light/fair-skinned/easily burned/adversely affected by heat and light/prone to environmental stress including allergies/vulnerable to psychic attack at night leading to bed-wetting and night sweats. For psychic and physical vulnerability, deep fears and disturbed dreams. For depression due to lack of contact with spiritual world. Gives protection and strength, illuminated consciousness, light-filled awareness and strength.

Sunflower (*Helianthus annuus*) For inflated ego, arrogance and vanity or low self-esteem and self-effacement resulting from a distorted sense of oneself. Poor relations to father or solar aspects of self. Encourages sense of unique individuality, balancing receptivity and nurturing self-expression, spiritualizing the ego and infusing a sun-radiant personality with outgoing qualities.

Sweet Pea (*Lathyrus latifolius*) For wanderers who have difficulty with caring, committed relationships. For an inability to form bonds with social community. Also for a sense of homelessness which may stem from moving around frequently as a child as well as from living in urban and suburban environments, disconnected from the natural world. Kindles feelings of being at home. Encourages commitment and forming connections with others and the Earth.

Tansy (*Tanacetum vulgare*) For sluggish, lethargic people who are indecisive, prone to procrastination, appearing lazy, indifferent and nonchalant with habits which undermine or subvert real abilities and talents. They may often be exposed to much chaos, confusion, emotional instability and even violence in childhood and respond by withdrawing and restricting their energy. Encourages straightforward responses to others and life. For being purposeful, decisive and goal-oriented.

Tiger Lily (*Lilium humboldtii*) For overaggressive yang forces, hostile, competitive people who strive against others rather than working for the common good. A feminine flower which makes inner peace and harmony the basis for relationships with others, encouraging co-operation and positive social interaction.

Trillium (*Trillium chloropetalum*) For excessive ambition, greed and lust for possessions, power and material wealth. Poverty consciousness that leads to overly materialistic focus. Cultivates altruism, balances energy and brings inner purity. Secure sense of personal welfare and financial wellbeing; brings the ability to serve and give to others.

Trumpet Vine (*Campsis tagliabuana*) For lack of vitality, an inability to be assertive or speak clearly due to feeling intimidated and shy. Also for speech impediments. Encourages articulate, lively, colourful free-flowing speech, an ability to express feelings verbally, dynamism in social situations.

Violet (*Viola odorata*) For those who are profoundly shy, reserved, aloof and lonely. They may long to share themselves with others but hold back for fear of being overwhelmed. They are delicate, have highly perceptive sensitivity, elevated spiritual perspective; socially responsive but self-contained. Allows interaction with others while protecting individuality.

Yarrow (*Achillea millefolium*) For extreme vulnerability to thoughts or the negative intentions of others, overly absorbent of negative influences, psychic toxicity, easily affected by surroundings and depleted and prone to environmental illness or allergies. Protects with a shield of light. Rebuilds vitality and solidity by repairing the aura. Creates a luminous and strong auric field, compassionate and inclusive sensitivity, refined and flexible psychic forces.

Yellow Star Tulip (*Calochortus monophyllus*) For insensitivity to the feelings and the sufferings of others, and lack of awareness of the consequences of your actions. Brings compassion and caring. Encourages empathy with and sensitivity to the suffering of others.

Yerba Santa (*Eriodictyon californicum*) For internalized grief and melancholy, deeply repressed emotions, feelings constricted in the chest, particularly in the heart and lungs. They may appear to be wasting away and are susceptible to chest congestion, pneumonia, tuberculosis, addiction to tobacco. Lightens the heart. Allows the emotions to flow freely, with the ability to harmonize breathing with feeling. Brings the capacity to express a full range of human emotions, especially pain and sadness; positive melancholy and soul depth.

Zinnia (*Zinnia elegans*) For those who are overserious and sombre, too earnest, lacking humour and spontaneity. Workaholic tendencies. Encourages childlike qualities of playfulness, laughter and humour.

Combinations

Yarrow Environmental Solution *Flower essences of Yarrow, Pink Yarrow, Golden Yarrow, Arnica and Echinacea, with Yarrow and Echinacea tinctures, in a sea salt water base.* For exposure to nuclear radiation and other forms of noxious environmental or geopathic stress including radiation from visual display units, X-rays, radiation therapy and other invasive electromagnetic fields. Originally developed in response to requests after the Chernobyl nuclear plant disaster in 1986. Directly counters the destructive effects of radiation on the human energy field by acting as a shield, so imparting powerful vitalizing and restorative properties. Counteracts pollution, or other geopathic stress; residual effects of past exposure; dysfunctional immune response; allergic hypersensitivity. Enhances our physical and etheric vitality, and brings self-regulating and adaptive immune response to environmental stresses.

Self-Heal Cream

This world-renowned skin cream awakens the inner vital forces necessary for healing on all levels: physical, emotional and spiritual. Contains Self-Heal flower essence which is especially indicated for those who have lost belief in their own capacity to be well and is beneficial for those who face great healing challenges, whether physical, mental or spiritual. Self-Heal is an excellent remedy to enhance other flower essences and therapeutic programmes and the inner commitment to be well; it acts as a catalyst in the journey to mind–body health. It affirms the self and draws from the deep wellspring of life, to aid true recovery and restoration. Use alone or add your own essences of choice to personalize your cream. Used for its therapeutic and regenerative qualities, it has an anti-inflammatory property and can soothe the irritation caused by eczema and oversensitive skin.

The Flourish Formulas and the Range of Light Flower Essences are Richard's and Patricia's exploration into new areas of research and development of the Flower Essence Society Flower Essences line.

Qualities for the Flourish Formulas and Animal Relief Formula

Activ-8 Flourish Formula

Positive qualities: Positive activation of the will to accomplish one's goals and complete projects; affirmative leadership; sustained energy and enthusiasm that fires the will; healthy expression of strong masculine 'yang' energy in both men and women.

Patterns of imbalance: Hesitation, procrastination, apathy; inability to engage the will to manifest one's goals, poor leadership skills, flagging energy or distraction, difficulty completing projects.

Fear-Less Flourish Formula

Positive qualities: Calm composure and containment during any threatening situation; ability to move forward with courage and fortitude despite adversity; proactive resolution of any stressful situation; valour and bravery.

Patterns of imbalance: Fear and anxiety; inability to act due to paralysis or numbness; restless agitation or disturbed sleep due to pronounced worry; paranoia, or panic due to extreme fear; nervous tension and distress.

Flora-Sleep Flourish Formula

Positive qualities: Relaxation, restful sleep, de-stressing, nourishing body and soul in sleep, mental and spiritual rejuvenation from deep rest, waking refreshed.

Patterns of imbalance: Difficulty falling asleep or staying asleep, excessive worry and anxiety, restlessness, nervous agitation, inability to release challenging thoughts and feelings before sleep or rest.

Grace Flourish Formula

Positive qualities: Positive relationship to the feminine soul identity in women or men; ability to express and champion feminine values in one's self, family and community; mothering grace, nurturance and sensitive receptivity as active soul virtues; affirmative alignment with biological and cultural milestones within the feminine body and soul.

Patterns of imbalance: Devaluation of feminine values and virtues; degradation or exploitation of women or women's bodies; alienation from feminine roles of mothering and nurturing; trauma due to sexual predation or violence; loss of essential dignity and humanity due to female social status.

Grief Relief Flourish Formula

Positive qualities: Heart balm after painful loss, bringing strength, encouragement, acceptance and a spiritual perspective regarding death, or any adversity.

Patterns of imbalance: Feelings of emptiness or despair after a loss such as death, divorce or disaster, unable to feel whole or to initiate process of rebuilding and revisioning one's life.

Grounding Green Flourish Formula

Positive qualities: Ability to integrate personal identity with a larger awareness of the Earth as a living organism, deeper bonding with living processes, animals and plants, with the ability to see their interrelationships.

Patterns of imbalance: Ego rather than eco consciousness; need for personal wealth, comfort and convenience without awareness of larger consequences for the Earth and other sentient beings; inability to imagine or relate to the Earth as a living organism; lack of integration and harmony of personal lifestyle and larger planetary reality.

Illumine Flourish Formula

Positive qualities: Energized and sustained by a bright flame of optimism and joy for life; ability to maintain equilibrium when challenged by adversity, life transition or seasonal fluctuation; soul capacity to respond to any life crisis or setback as a new opportunity for growth and transformation.

Patterns of imbalance: Lack of resiliency when tested by life challenges; needing to build sustainable structures of soul light that provide strength and sustenance during times of misfortune or hardship; history of depression, despondency or seasonal affective disorder in oneself, family or household.

Kinder Garden Flourish Formula

Positive qualities: Vibrant developmental growth throughout all stages of childhood and pre-adolescence; ability of the child to harmonize interior states of soul consciousness with bodily development; integration of mental forces with emotional learning patterns; soul radiance and exuberance as the foundational identity of the child.

Patterns of imbalance: Developmental challenges, learning impediments, emotional trauma or inappropriate sexual disturbance; loss of innocence, radiance or natural receptivity in the child due to stress or trauma; hardening forces from technology or abstract pedagogical methods that stymie the child's natural curiosity and balanced development.

Magenta Self-Healer Flourish Formula

Positive qualities: Profound recovery from illness leading to deep restoration and rejuvenation; sustained healing capacity and endurance even during severe illnesses, physical accidents or trauma; ability to develop new capacities of bodily resilience and soul insight as an outcome of illness, trauma or disease; core immunity through accessing deeper levels of soul consciousness.

Patterns of imbalance: Lowered immunity and vitality as a result of prolonged illness or disease; bifurcation of bodily and soul forces during illness and disease; inability to bring deeper insight, understanding or positive soul direction when challenged by a devastating illness, physical trauma or disease; loss of self-knowing due to overwhelming medical procedures and related external processes that numb or paralyze the soul.

Mind-Full Flourish Formula

Positive qualities: A vibrant state of mental coherence and clarity; rhythmic and balanced use of intellectual forces; wakeful focus, interest and insight of one's mental forces.

Patterns of imbalance: Scattered or shallow thinking, easily distracted or disengaged; depletion of mental forces due to extreme demand or overuse of stimulants; confused, dull or sluggish mental forces.

Post-Trauma Stabilizer Flourish Formula

Positive qualities: Ability to recover body and soul forces following from any shock or trauma; regenerative and rebuilding forces within body and soul following a crisis, or catastrophe; resilience and reintegration following devastation or loss.

Patterns of imbalance: Numbness, paralysis, disassociation or disembodiment following a shattering life episode; inability to recoup and recover one's body-soul forces after loss or violation of any kind; prolonged shock or paralysis, including fixation on original trauma.

Sacred Heart Flourish Formula

Positive qualities: Integrated heart forces of strength and compassion; beneficial relationships that balance self-identity and receptivity to the other; ability to establish loving boundaries with children, pets or others in one's care; replenishing soul forces after death or divorce.

Patterns of imbalance: Emotional numbness or retreat due to failed or severed relationships; compassion fatigue due to poor boundaries; depletion, emotional enmeshment and merging; lack of trust or healthy vulnerability due to previous relationship trauma.

Animal Relief Formula

Positive qualities: Wholeness and dignity for any animal; ability to form loving bonds with caretaker and other companion animals; capacity to make healthy transitions into a new home or with a new caretaker; responsive and resilient when subjected to any form of stress, travel or relocation.

Patterns of imbalance: Pronounced stress due to abandonment, isolation or abuse; trauma due to natural disasters or other calamities; unable to form nurturing bonds when adopted; mistrust or attachment anxiety due to prolonged absence of caretaker; dysfunction or depression due to death of caretaker or other companion animals.

Range of Light Flower Essences

Almond (*Prunus amygdalus*)

Positive qualities: Ability of the heart to anchor a core structure of life-giving light; integration of physical incarnation and spiritual development; alignment of mental 'light' forces with physical 'life' forces; ability to find self-identity through the integration of physical and spiritual realities (life and light).

Patterns of imbalance: Obstacles to proper physical development such as failure-to-thrive-syndrome; inability to take up earthly nutrition as a form of sustenance for body and soul; imbalances or lack of integration in physical and mental aspects of development.

Alpine Aster (*Aster alpigenus*)

Positive qualities: Body-free spiritual consciousness; ability to realize independent consciousness beyond the body; cultivation of sense-free states of meditation and dreaming; freeing of the spiritual body from the physical in the death transition or other spiritual experiences.

Patterns of imbalance: Fear of death or spiritually transcendent states of consciousness; materialistic identification with the physical dimension; inability to recognize the reality of spiritual dimensions of existence due to overidentification with physical plane or physical body.

Blazing Star (*Mentzelia laevicaulis*)

Positive qualities: Radiant and inwardly vital will forces; masculine soul forces developed from an inner foundation of nurturing life forces; alchemical union of feminine water and masculine fire soul elements.

Patterns of imbalance: Predominance of water element in the body and emotions causing paralysis of the will; inability to catalyze soul fire; bifurcation of soul toward either a strong but rigid will or flowing but weak-feeling state.

California Peony (*Paeonia californica*)

Positive qualities: Celebration of life; healthy instinct for pleasure; cultivation of magnetic and charismatic soul forces through integration with the vital forces in the lower chakras.

Patterns of imbalance: Predominance of passive yin forces, repressed vitality, sensuality or sexuality; difficulty with money and power issues.

California Valerian (*Valeriana capitata*)

Positive qualities: Tranquillity and inner equilibrium; inner confidence for the future due to the soul's understanding of prior experiences; peaceful acceptance of life experiences.

Patterns of imbalance: Shallow breathing due to anxiety about the future; nervous agitation or insomnia; worry and unease when facing future life events that are viewed as challenging; addiction to sleeping pills or tranquillizers.

Cassiope (*Cassiope mertensiana*)

Positive qualities: Soul warmth that rays into the body; appreciation for all creation; the joy of physical existence; warmth as the source of wellbeing.

Patterns of imbalance: Lack of appreciation for the spirituality inherent in the created world and the physical body; aloof or removed from the life pulse in nature or the human body; tendency to use the cold forces of intellect or technology at the expense of the body's warmth.

Cherry (*Prunus avium*)
Positive qualities: Youthful joy and exuberance, feelings of innocence and openness; celebrating the threshold of adolescence; healing and integration of painful experiences in adolescence.
Patterns of imbalance: Toxic blood or related skin conditions such as acne; loss of innocence, hope or youthful outlook on life; traumatic life experiences in adolescence that continue to plague the body/soul identity.

Chocolate Lily (*Fritillaria biflora*)
Positive qualities: Embodiment and acceptance of basic metabolic functions, especially the reproductive and elimination systems of the body.
Patterns of imbalance: Lack of awareness of metabolic functions; aversion for eliminative functions of the body; revulsion for menstruation, lactation; difficulty with elimination, poor intestinal function or blockages.

Columbine (*Aquilegia formosa*)
Positive qualities: Radiant expression of one's unique creativity and inspiration; distinctive individuality as a source of luminosity and radiance for others; inspired acting and speaking in the world.
Patterns of imbalance: Hesitation to express one's creativity and individuality; inability to take social or creative risks; mid-life crisis calling for reconstellation of soul forces and life expression.

Corn Lily (*Veratrum californicum*)
Positive qualities: Developing a positive picture of the ageing process in women; dignity and self-containment; acceptance and celebration of the wisdom and dignity of maturity; celebration of fullness in body and life.
Patterns of imbalance: Feeling old and 'dried up'; despair at the passing of youth and motherhood; difficult hormonal transition in body and soul; false attempt to return to youthful form or identity.

Desert Lily (*Hesperocallis undulata*)
Positive qualities: Ability to radiate beauty, artistry and grace within a mechanized urban environment; rejuvenation of self and others through feminine soul forces of beauty and grace; feminine water element of the soul as balm for fire imbalance in modern technology.
Patterns of imbalance: Feeling oppressed by the invasive ugliness of technological urban culture; sensitivity to environmental disturbances, especially when lacking beauty or harmony.

Downy Avens (*Geum triflorum*)
Positive qualities: Intelligence that is integrated in head and heart; enduring wisdom derived from incremental development of soul forces; patient and progressive cultivation of thinking forces with overall soul identity.
Patterns of imbalance: Precocious development of intellectual capacities with lagging emotional development; easily bored or distracted due to lack of heart attention and imagination; tendency to hyperactivity or Attention Deficit Disorder.

Dune Primrose (*Oenothera deltoids*)
Positive qualities: Connection with a nurturing maternal presence in the spiritual world; soul memory of the spiritual radiance of being born; awareness and gratitude for those beings who have guided the soul's incarnation into Earth.
Patterns of imbalance: Alienation from the mother soul of the world, feeling abandoned by the spiritual world; birth trauma, pregnancy during difficult social circumstances such as poverty, violence.

Explorer's Gentian (*Gentiana calycosa*)
Positive qualities: Renewed strength for meeting one's life purpose and spiritual destiny; transforming crisis and loss into new opportunities.
Patterns of imbalance: World-weariness at midlife; loss of connection with one's spiritual destiny and life purpose; profound health crisis or loss that depletes soul forces.

Fiesta Flower (*Pholistoma aurium*)
Positive qualities: Vulnerability, openness and receptivity in spiritual seeking; flexible yet strong soul structure for core spiritual beliefs.

Patterns of imbalance: Dogmatism, rigid spiritual beliefs that are externally derived; authoritarian social or political viewpoints.

Fireweed (*Epilobium angustifolium*)
Positive qualities: Recovery of vital forces; phoenix-like powers of soul to reconstruct and re-create new life; assimilation of alchemical fire toward new forces of life and rejuvenation.
Patterns of imbalance: Healing for events involving adversity and disruption, 'trial by fire', wounding or disruption due to fire, heat or light and related technology or military weapons.

Glassy Hyacinth (*Triteleia lilacina*)
Positive qualities: Redemption of suffering; transformation of emotional darkness into the light of soul understanding; resurrection forces of soul triumph.
Patterns of imbalance: Profound trauma, sorrow, emotional pain; inability to face evil, or the 'shadow' of humanity; descent into hell.

Green Bells of Ireland (*Moluccella laevis*)
Positive qualities: Awareness of the elemental world in nature; ability to work with elemental nature forces through one's own bodily matrix; nature wisdom acquired through direct sensory experience.
Patterns of imbalance: Overly romantic or mental relationship to nature; lack of physical connection or embodiment in relationship to nature and primal elemental forces.

Green Cross Gentian (*Frasera speciosa Swertia radiata*)
Positive qualities: Courageous soul alignment with the living being of the Earth; hope and resolve for world service and healing despite setbacks or challenges.
Patterns of imbalance: Feelings of overwhelm, despair and defeat with regard to the condition of the Earth; bereft and discouraged when living connection with the Earth is disrupted due to natural or man-made catastrophe; ability to carry the elemental 'cross' of the world.

Green Nicotiana (*Nicotiana alata*)
Positive qualities: Awareness of the heartbeat of the Earth as a sustaining force for humanity; alignment with the breathing pulse of the Earth in one's own soul (such as seasonal rhythms and alternation of day and night).
Patterns of imbalance: Inability to care for life on Earth due to the hardening of heart forces; materialistic, egotistic or militaristic tendencies due to arrhythmic technologies and lifestyles.

Green Rein Orchid (*Platanthera sparsiflora*)
Positive qualities: Ability to feel the life force of the Earth within one's soul being; heart consciousness as a pathway to ecological consciousness.
Patterns of imbalance: Abstract beliefs in ecology or social change that is not integrated as a living presence in body and soul.

Green Rose (*Rosa chinensis viridiflora*)
Positive qualities: Compassion as the doorway of connection to all living beings; love as a form of transcendent embrace and trust.
Patterns of imbalance: Fear, mistrust, defensiveness; fear of being attacked or annihilated and thus developing barriers to other living beings.

Hawthorn (*Crataegus oxyacantha*)
Positive qualities: Strong and vital bodily forces that impart power, courage and bravery; positive assertive forces.
Patterns of imbalance: Overly strong will that depletes heart balance; 'Type A' aggressive, hostile personality; easily agitated or stressed when personal will forces are not satisfied.

Hyssop (*Agastache urticifolia*)
Positive qualities: Body–soul integration of pain and suffering; ability to forgive and to accept forgiveness from others.
Patterns of imbalance: Body-based guilt or shame, self-punishment or mutilation directed consciously or unconsciously at the body; soul memory of previous abuse or shame that degrades body image.

Joshua Tree (*Yucca brevifolia*)
Positive qualities: Individuation of soul forces through conscious transformation of family patterns and related cultural conditioning; enhanced freedom and compassionate insight for family and culture of origin.
Patterns of imbalance: Generational karma which shackles the soul's potential; inability to break free from family or cultural patterns of dysfunction, such as alcoholism, addiction, depression, violence or hereditary illnesses; loss of individual identity and freedom due to lack of insight regarding familial and cultural influences.

Lady's Mantle (*Alchemilla vulgaris*)
Positive qualities: Alignment with the living dew mantle (hydrosphere) of the Earth; ability to catalyze magnetic 'green' forces through hands and heart; plant consciousness integrated as a radiant healing force in the human soul.
Patterns of imbalance: Dry or withered soul forces separated from the life mantle of the Earth; intellectual or technical approach to healing; for the female reproductive system needing nourishment and stabilization when unconsciously aligned with the suffering of Mother Earth.

Lemon (*Citrus limon*)
Positive qualities: Ability to integrate expansion and contraction in mental forces of the soul; mental clarity balanced with imaginative and artistic capacities.
Patterns of imbalance: Mental fatigue or related toxicity in the nervous system; dreaminess; learning disorders, including Attention Deficit Disorder.

Lewisia (*Lewisia disepala*)
Positive qualities: Profound expansiveness of the soul; star-like consciousness radiating exquisite sensitivity; the spirit breath of the cosmos united with the most tender aspects of human love and sensitivity.
Patterns of imbalance: Tenuous hold on Earth forces due to extensive astral forces that do not fully contract; 'indigo' or autistic children who cannot bring their full soul forces into incarnation; protection and sustenance during pregnancy or in early childhood for highly expanded soul types.

Lilac (*Syringa vulgaris*)
Positive qualities: Deep wellsprings of memory that rejuvenate the soul; neurological regeneration through stimulation of memory forces that connect the soul with joy and life meaning.
Patterns of imbalance: Soul amnesia – inability to integrate or be nourished by past experiences of the soul, especially in early childhood; sadness, depression or sense of burden due to feelings of isolation, alienation or abandonment; reduced sensory experience as the precursor of brain disease or dysfunction.

Lungwort (*Mertensia ciliata*)
Positive qualities: Reclamation of soul light in the deepest structures of the body; recovery from depression or addiction with new forces of hope and upliftment.
Patterns of imbalance: Depression registered in the body as physical gravity; listless, languid or drained – often localized in the respiratory system; sense of hopelessness or resignation with resulting depletion of energy; depression and low energy function associated with drug withdrawal.

Lupine (*Lupinus latifolius*)
Positive qualities: Expanded self-identity that is integrated within a larger community matrix; ability to sacrifice or sublimate personal needs or desires for a greater whole.
Patterns of imbalance: Selfishness, greed; intense identification with petty concerns or narrow interests that stymie community welfare.

Madrone (*Arbutus menziesii*)
Positive qualities: Fullness and abundance of the physical body; ability to receive and enjoy physical nourishment.
Patterns of imbalance: Severe dieting, non-acceptance of one's body weight or size; possible history of physical aversion to one's mother; malnourishment or disturbed breast-feeding; absence of physical soul warmth in early childhood.

Monkshood (*Aconitum columbianum*)

Positive qualities: Positive and courageous spiritual leadership; profound capacity for clairvoyance that is well integrated with social and moral values.

Patterns of imbalance: Repression of spiritual capacities due to fear of psychic opening, often associated with traumatic memory of near death or related threshold experiences; paralysis of spiritual forces due to prior trauma or cultic abuse; hidden cultic or sexual behaviour.

Mountain Forget-Me-Not (*Hackelia micrantha*)

Positive qualities: Vibrant and dynamic connection with spiritual teachers and guides; deep soul memory of karmic patterns affecting one's destiny; alignment with soul's life purpose through higher guidance.

Patterns of imbalance: Soul angst and alienation, feelings of isolation due to lack of connection and guidance from the spiritual world; confusion about life purpose and direction.

Ocotillo (*Fouquieria splendens*)

Positive qualities: Positive fire forces grounded and integrated in the core individuality of the soul; charismatic fire as a source of heart radiance.

Patterns of imbalance: Disembodied spiritual experiences not fully owned by the conscious soul; excessive psychic 'fire' leading to emotional reactivity, psychic projection and distortion, or various forms of anger and violence; alcoholism and other drug addiction related to fire-imbalance.

Pedicularis (*Pedicularis groenlandica*)

Positive qualities: Deep mystical forces of the soul; profound soul memory which imparts positive emotional insight and wisdom; connection with ancient sources of Earth wisdom and soul history.

Patterns of imbalance: Pronounced sensitivity or hypochondria leading to seclusion or separation; fits of crying or other water imbalances; excessive emotionality which inhibits deeper

understanding of one's soul pain, suffering or karma.

Pussy Paws (*Calyptridium umbellatum*)

Positive qualities: Physical contact as a source of grace and gentleness in the soul; ability to touch and be touched with sensitivity and sensuality; softening of the soul forces toward greater receptivity.

Patterns of imbalance: Fear of being touched; unable to allow softer side to be recognized or experienced by others; sexual abuse or violence that hardens the boundary of the skin and human touch.

Red Larkspur (*Delphinium nudicaule*)

Positive qualities: Ability to radiate energy through the body as a positive form of leadership; magnetic forces that catalyze and inspire energy in others; positive *esprit de corps*.

Patterns of imbalance: Lack of radiance and physical energy in the body; inability to energize or motivate others to accomplish common goals; lacklustre energy that repels or depletes community or group motivation.

Red Penstemon (*Penstemon rostriflorus*)

Positive qualities: Sense of adventure and risk-taking; positive athleticism at any age; determination and tenacity when facing physical challenges.

Patterns of imbalance: Hesitation to take risks; lack of physical courage; inability to accept physical challenges or to rise to a new level of bodily ability regardless of limitations or challenges.

Redbud (*Cercis occidentalis*)

Positive qualities: Acceptance of the natural cycles of maturation and ageing; body-soul regeneration based on a positive alignment with life cycles of death and birth.

Patterns of imbalance: Overly materialistic approach to the body, desire to preserve the outer form of the body through plastic surgery, drugs or extreme medical technologies that bypass the true cycles of life and death.

Redwood (*Sequoia sempervirens*)
Positive qualities: Stature and majesty in physical incarnation; soul embrace of creative forces for growth and physical vitality.
Patterns of imbalance: Lack of physical strength, stature; hereditary or health issues that deplete vitality; stunted development of physical forces; spinal injuries or other afflictions to spinal health or bone structure.

Rue (*Ruta graveolens*)
Positive qualities: Internal cohesion and containment of psychic forces; activation of appropriate aspects of soul consciousness according to professional and personal responsibilities.
Patterns of imbalance: Scattered or confused psychic forces which deplete immunity and protective boundaries; need for greater clarity and discrimination in the activation of psychic forces.

Scarlet Fritillary (*Fritillaria recurva*)
Positive qualities: Integration of masculine fire forces within the feminine matrix; sexual vitality and reproductive health.
Patterns of imbalance: Exhaustion of vital forces including anaemic tendencies; depletion of physical forces during pregnancy, childbirth and lactation, and early child-rearing.

Shasta Lily (*Lilium washingtonianum*)
Positive qualities: Dynamic and creative expression of feminine soul forces, individuality and internal strength in alignment with core feminine soul values.
Patterns of imbalance: Difficulty balancing feminine grace with masculine strength; overcompensation of masculine traits in order to appear strong or unique.

Sierra Primrose (*Primula suffrutescens*)
Positive qualities: Gratitude for the gift of life regardless of the outer condition of health; joy at the deep wellspring of the soul; physical vitality as the soul basis for enthusiasm.
Patterns of imbalance: Lack of gratitude or reverence for the gift of life resulting in fatigue, boredom or depression; joyless living and habitually dulled response to life.

Splendid Mariposa Lily (*Calochortus splendens*)
Positive qualities: Soul alignment with the Mother of the World; capacity to recognize all members of the human race as having one mother; ability to activate transcendent forces of mothering and mercy for all of the human family.
Patterns of imbalance: Orphan state of consciousness as a root condition of humanity; soul pain and feelings of abandonment due to world trauma and warfare; divisions in the human family due to race, religion, nation, class, ecological disaster or warfare.

Spreading Phlox (*Phlox diffusa*)
Positive qualities: Activation of soul destiny through social impulses and connections; ability to recognize and manifest significant relationships that foster life purpose and destiny.
Patterns of imbalance: Caught in meaningless social circles or false societal expectations; inability to identify new opportunities or connect with groups that are aligned with one's true soul purpose.

Tall Mt. Larkspur (*Delphinium glaucum*)
Positive qualities: Leadership based upon spiritual alignment; ability to hear, see and act in a greater capacity of soul leadership beyond one's immediate personality.
Patterns of imbalance: Inability to receive or trust spiritual guidance; restriction of true spiritual gifts due to lack of dynamic connection to higher dimensions of soul inspiration.

(FES and Patricia Kaminski,
used with permission)

For more detailed flower essence profiles please refer to the Flower Essence Repertory, available in print. An online Repertory with database cross-referencing and plant photographs is available to members of the Flower Essence Society at www.flowersociety.org.

SPIRIT IN NATURE/MASTER'S FLOWER ESSENCES (Ma)
Remedies for inner wellbeing

These essences are made exclusively from the blossoms of flowering fruit trees from local orchards and blossoming plants from vegetable gardens. The ancient yoga teachings explained that the food we eat affects our state of consciousness. Heavy, processed food brings the energy down and creates toxins, which in turn causes fatigue and eventually contributes to bodily distress and illness. Pure, fresh food, such as fruits and vegetables, uplift the consciousness and provide energy.

This is also the philosophy of the world-renowned metaphysician Paramhansa Yogananda (1893–1952, author of *Autobiography of a Yogi*), who came to the United States in 1920 to teach practical, scientific techniques for self-improvement. He taught that food fortifies us on spiritual and psycho-emotional levels and also supplies nutritional benefits. Cherries, he explained, possess a vibration of cheerfulness and raspberries contain kindness. If food has such power, how much more so do the blossoms, containing 90 per cent of the life force of the plant? Commissioned by J. Donald Walters, a direct disciple of Yogananda, Lila Devi developed Master's Flower Essences in the foothills of the Sierra Nevada Mountains just outside Nevada City, California, in 1977, making them the oldest essence line outside the UK. (The tropical essences Pineapple, Coconut and Banana are prepared on the Hawaiian Islands, and Date is made in the desert of Southern California.) Three decades of research, analysis, case studies and direct testimonials, from health-care professionals to lay people, confirm the potency of these 20 essences.

Lila says:

> When we feel distressed by attitudes that block our highest potential, it is natural to want to rid ourselves of them. Even more so do we want to live in those states that are our true nature. Flower essences work by stimulating and encouraging us to manifest those positive qualities which we already possess in our own delightfully unique way. This process is accomplished through the supportive interaction of the essence with our own readiness and willingness to make needed changes in our lives and attitudes. That is their great strength and immense beauty.

She proposes that the essences help people to become 'masters of their own lives'. Spirit in Nature's essences are an excellent first line to work with, because of their simplicity and straightforwardness. A branch of this essence line, Yogananda's Spirit-in-Nature Essences – www.Spirit-in-Nature.com – is becoming nationally known in India. Particularly recommended for children, these essences enhance their clarity of energy and bring forth their unique talents. The Spirit-in-Nature line is especially supportive of the dynamic between mother and child (see pages 440–3). Animals also respond positively to essences (see Pets and Animals, section I).

Almond (*Prunus amygdalus*) Self-control, moral vigour. For the power to rebound vigorously from every setback in life. For calming the mind and nerves. Use when you need to be more inward, less affected by environment and circumstances. Good in times of activity and high demands on your energy reserves. Promotes synchronicity of body/mind/spirit, and restores a sense of balance and moderation.

Apple (*Malus domestica*) Healthfulness. For more inner peace amid life's swirl of activity. To be always 'calmly active and actively calm'. For clarity, receptivity and healthy attitudes. For inharmonious states of mind, including hypochondria, worry and doubt, and recurring negative emotions such as anger and fear. Helps bring clarity, receptivity and joy. Restores a sense of wellbeing to one's thoughts and outlook on life. Unlocks the spring of true health and vitality, providing the motivation to take better care of oneself.

Avocado (*Persea americana*) Good memory. For a retentive mind, important for every kind of success. For the ability to develop mental skilfulness and concentrate wholly on anything you do. Brings focus and recollection of details; inspiration for new projects and challenges for the mind (such as exams) as well as a greater awareness of life's purpose. An attitude of 'Now I get it!' Also for learning from one's mistakes and delighting in the learning process.

Banana (*Musa × paradisiaca*) Humility rooted in calmness. For self-honesty and self-forgetfulness. For projecting your energy outward, away from yourself. For a calm, non-reactive attitude, for perspective and not getting overly involved, especially where emotions are concerned. For objectivity and having a healthy distance from people and circumstances. To be able to let others have the last word and be able to 'agree to disagree'. Excellent for promoting harmony in close relationships.

Blackberry (*Rubus fruticosus*) Purity of thought. To free yourself from every thought that is foreign to your higher nature. Brings kindliness, mental clarity, optimism, and the ability to see the good within oneself and others. Helps us to be inspirational, incisive and direct yet gentle, and supportive of our environment and of all living things. Encourages true friendships and harmony in life.

Cherry (*Prunus avium*) Cheerfulness. For a more light-hearted, less heavy attitude toward life. For being more solution-oriented. A life-brightener! Encourages seeing the good in every situation, being hopeful, inspiring to others, optimistic, positive, light-hearted, even-minded. Helps whenever there is a lack of energy, enthusiasm and interest in life.

Coconut (*Cocos nucifera*) Greater spiritual awareness. For a clearer, more spiritual focus in life. For the energy to endure, or to rise above, every test. For completing tasks, living up to one's highest potential. Helps us to see solutions, and to welcome and offer support for meeting any kind of challenge. Often called the 'walking tall' essence, which means to become aware that you are bigger than any of your tests.

Corn (*Zea mays*) Mental vitality. For being always awake and prepared. Brings initiative to projects, rekindling enthusiasm and, through awakening the will, provides unlimited energy to accomplish anything you desire. For living in the moment, and especially for 'new beginnings' of any kind: a new job, a new home, a new relationship, or starting a new year at school.

Date (*Phoenix dactylifera*) Sweetness and tenderness. To view all living things as our own, including strangers. For overcoming judgemental, negative attitudes or thoughts of separateness from others. Encourages discrimination, receptivity, open-mindedness and sensitivity to others' feelings, allows us to be easy to talk to, welcoming, magnetic and warm-hearted. Good for people who work with the public. Also for self-nurturing when life seems harsh.

Fig (*Ficus carica*) Flexibility and self-acceptance. For the ability to relax, no matter how heavy your responsibilities. To soften too strict a sense of discipline, toward oneself and others. For those too hard on themselves, with unrealistic expectations and difficulty with change. Brings a sense of humour, fluidity, self-liberation, and the ability to go with the flow and be at ease with people.

Grape (*Vitis* sp.) Love and devotion. To awaken the feelings of the heart and to love others spontaneously, whether that love is returned or not. For developing selfless love and all true and noble qualities. Many people, especially in crowded cities, feeling disconnected, alienated and vulnerable, experience the need for this essence through loneliness, isolation or unfulfilling relationships. For weathering the death of a loved one, divorce, separation, neglect and abandonment issues. Brings a realization of the source of love within, loving without condition, demand or expectation, patience with others' shortcomings.

Lettuce (*Lactuca sativa*) Calmness. To have greater calmness and inner strength when confronting the difficulties in your life. Also for clear communication skills and promoting creativity, self-expression and expansiveness. For an inner sense of restfulness and dynamic, energized stillness. For restlessness, inability to concentrate, excitability, repressed and troubled emotions. Dispelling emotional turmoil, replacing it with evenmindedness. Confers the ability to speak one's truth, restores clear communication skills and creates a productive, clear-thinking environment for highly creative people. Freedom to experience the more subtle states of relaxation.

Orange (*Citrus sinensis*) Enthusiasm, hope and joy. Excellent for blasting through obstacles. For 'seeing the light at the end of the tunnel'. For deeply ingrained present and past abuse issues, physical, sexual or emotional, either past or present. Gives a sense of restored energy, resilience, lightness, banishing mild to severe depression and melancholy, and for cultivating an inner smile.

Peach (*Prunus persica*) Unselfishness. For the ability to extend your generosity toward others and include them in your own happiness. Brings concern for the welfare of others, maturity, nurturance, consideration, deep compassion, sensitivity and empathy.

Pear (*Pyrus communis*) Emergency use, creates peacefulness. A 'must' for emergency situations, accidents, trauma, physical and/or emotional shock, or crisis, surgery, childbirth complications, extreme grief and any situation which throws us off balance; uncontrollable thoughts and non-productive habit patterns. Also for balance and harmony throughout the day. For minor to monumental auric disturbances. Restores peace of mind and a sense of rhythm, proportion and balance. For living fully in the present moment; gives an ability to handle crises and awakens our ability to handle life's upsets.

Pineapple (*Ananas comosus*) Self-assurance, for building self-esteem. For those who feel undermined by the criticism of others. Helpful for people in the work world where their identity is reflected back to them by money and job issues. Fosters confidence, prosperity and abundance. For a strong, healthy sense of self that is neither a superiority nor an inferiority complex.

Raspberry (*Rubus idaeus*) Kindheartedness and compassion. Raspberry teaches us that kindheartedness opens the heart and allows us to forgive our own failings. For those feeling easily hurt, touchy, overreactive, insensitive – who lash out, lack understanding and judgement, are clouded by emotions, blame others and feel resentful and bitter. Fosters taking responsibility for our words and actions; for sympathy, benevolence, generosity and the desire to help others heal their hurts; for releasing old wounds.

Spinach (*Spinacia oleracea*) Simplicity. For stress, feeling burdened or overwhelmed and for trust, to replace suspicion. For a sense of wonder, a free spirit, a playful nature and a love of adventure. Helpful for people who are stressed, overworked, or have endured an unhappy or dysfunctional childhood. Allows us to be straightforward, easily understood and uncomplicated, even with numerous responsibilities.

Strawberry (*Fragaria*) Dignity. For centring and grounding and the ability to draw respect from others. For a sense of poise and inner beauty. For those who are guilt-ridden, regretful, self-blaming, undeserving or unsure of themselves. They may have a history of emotionally abusive parents. Also for psychic oversensitivity and for healers who tend to absorb the problems of their clients. Brings strength, stateliness and self-worth. Allows us to leave a dysfunctional childhood in the past.

Tomato (*Solanum lycopersicum*) Strength and endurance. To support you in standing up for your beliefs. Tomato is for fear of any nature, severity and duration, nightmares and also for working on addictions. Allows us to know there is no failure, only another chance to succeed. Encourages belief in oneself, invincibility, psychic protection, and immunity from the effects of large cities, crowds and negative environments.

The Essential Flower Essence Handbook (also in Italian, Spanish and Japanese, as well as in English in India) is also the text for Lila's widely acclaimed home study tri-level comprehensive course.

GREEN HOPE FARM FLOWER ESSENCES (GH)

Green Hope Farm began with a conversation between an angelic being and Molly Sheehan where she was walked through step by step the creation of her first essence, its use as well as its healing qualities. Green Hope Farm with its micro-climate has been created in co-operation with the angelic and elemental kingdoms since 1987 and is specifically designed for the sole purpose of growing flowers in such a way as to obtain the highest vibrational quality of the flower's essence as possible.

The angelic beings are the architects of all form and give guidance season to season as to what grows best and which varieties of plants will be in alignment with the spiritual and climatic realities of any given season. This includes which seeds to order as well as the design mandalas for each garden space. This guidance has resulted in many of the healing gardens holding a specific theme of healing. The flowers from the gardens have become the flower essence combinations. The Overlighting beings have guided every aspect of the flower essence creation.

The elementals are said to take responsibility for manifesting the angelic designs into reality. Elementals help with actually growing each plant, offering endless information about soil, mulch, plant care, down to the choice of which flowers to make into flower essences and on what particular day. The elementals are also responsible for the transfer of the electrical healing pattern of the flowers into the flower essences themselves. Without the work of elementals, there would be no flower essences.

This co-operation and working together of the angelic, elemental kingdom and human kingdom has created beautiful, radiant and healthy gardens and it is through this specific partnership that the unique qualities of Green Hope Farm Flower Essences have evolved. For example, the angels and elementals encouraged them to shift from a brandy-based stabilizer to a Red Shiso herbal-based stabilizer in 1994 which has been key to the vitality of their flower essences. The Red Shiso has a tremendous vibrational quality while also serving as a very strong preservative. At the farm they grow their own source of organic Red Shiso in their completely organic garden beds, which is used as stabilizer across all their essences ranges.

Here is a brief description of each of the Green Hope Farm Flower Essences Collections.

The Green Hope Farm Collection

As the gardens of Green Hope Farm have been planned, planted and cared for in a conscious and co-operative partnership between the people at the farm and the angels and elementals, the essences co-created address the problems that might be difficult for either angels, elementals or people to solve on their own, and therefore can be resolved more easily or avoided altogether. The flower essences made at Green Hope Farm reflect this braiding of divine strengths and hold a very high level of problem-solving wisdom.

Green Hope Farm Combination Collection

The combination remedies offer the collective wisdom of the entire community. More specifically, they build on the angels' and elementals' guidance about flower essences that address various issues as well as their experiences with these essences over the last few decades. Some significant single essences are Golden Armour which aids in protection from energetic dissonance and the Arbour Garden for harmony and oneness. The combination remedies are for such diverse concerns as grounding, birth of the sacred feminine, inner child work, caring for spiritually evolved children, graceful ageing, vitality, release from ego patterns and sanskaras, moving beyond addictions, memory issues and hearing spiritual guidance with more clarity.

The Animal Wellness Collection

This collection reflects more than two decades of intensive flower essence work with literally hundreds of thousands of animals, particularly those living in close proximity to humans. The 22 remedies address a specific challenge faced by animals, but it was noticed almost immediately that these remedies were appropriate for pet owners too; the animals in your life will be delighted you are on this journey with them!

The Bermuda Collection

Bermuda's subtropical environment and long history as an important place for flowers make this collection exuberantly supportive of creativity, physical vitality, spiritual transformation, abundance, alternative healing based on long forgotten wisdom and a playful enjoyment of life.

The Camino Collection

Created in Spain on the ancient pilgrim route to Santiago de Compostela, this line holds the wisdom and spiritual momentum of specific places along this thousand-year-old pilgrimage trail. It supports in the trials and tribulations experienced on our spiritual journeys, offering discernment about the choices we must make about who we travel with, how we travel, what we invest in and what we leave behind.

Camino 2: The Healer's Toolbox

The Healer's Toolbox was made along the vibrant ley lines of the ancient Camino de Santiago and is especially attuned as an aid for light workers, healers or anyone who cares for others as part of their day-to-day lives. These essences remind us of the deep link between the physical body and healing work, and offer support for one-to-one as well as group healing.

The Desert Collection

Rebirth, recovery, healing from abuse, a return to joy, finding contentment with less and experiencing good cheer no matter the circumstances; these are some of the healing intentions of this Desert Flower Essence collection, reflecting its origins in the extreme climate of the deserts of the southwest where less is enough for life to joyously prevail and the human abuse of Earth that often creates deserts is proven to be insufficient to stop Earth and all of us from healing.

The Irish Collection

The Irish Collection offers generous gifts from the ancient elementals of Ireland and connects us to the great wellspring of Celtic wisdom. They lift the veil between ourselves and a more magical experience of reality.

Helps to balance our inner and outer life, and encourage us on the spiritual path when feeling restricted, downtrodden or besieged in any way. Grounds our eternal self and supports us to express ourselves with courage, good cheer, zest for life and a feeling of oneness with all that is.

The Rose Garden Collection

Roses are love incarnate and with their wisdom with infinite generosity are amongst the few most evolved family of flowers on the planet. Their essences are extremely practical and down to earth. The beauty of Roses is echoed in the depth, clarity and power of their essences. They provide support for such diverse issues as feeling safe in the world, holding your light in times of inner and outer turmoil, spiritual housekeeping, finding the courage to do what you need to do and living in a state of grace, joy and delight.

The St John Virgin Island Collection

St John in the Virgin Islands is an oasis of protected land which offers the unique strengths of all seaside flowers with their ability to link the separate worlds of sea and land. Their flower essences show us how to cross similar divides, find common ground between different worlds and people, navigate the ebbs and flows of romantic partnership, solve problems that have defied solution, even pull together and close wounds that have resisted healing. Help to bridge the gap between what we know about ourselves and what we must do to be ourselves. They bring ashore new paradigms of creativity. With St John's feminine nature, the flower essences encourage access to our sacred feminine, one moment at a time.

The Sicily and Santorini Collection

Created from flowers growing in the islands of Sicily and Santorini, who have maintained an unwavering sense of self through experiences of violation, subjugation and explosive events. Their essences help us gain an equally immutable sense of self and anchor us in our sense of eternal identity and soul purpose even when faced with tumultuous situations.

The Venus Garden Collection

The Venus Garden is the most magical, high vibrational spot at Green Hope Farm where each year a different mandala of flowers is planted. The flower essences created are the cutting edge of Green Hope Farm's entire collection and akin to taking an advanced course of spiritual study, allowing the freedom to heal and evolve in unexpected, dynamic and surprisingly joyful ways.

The Wildflower Collection

As wildflowers live their lives somewhat apart from the human community they have more freedom in contrast to cultivated flowers, to pursue their own spiritual purpose and full expression of their divine identity. Hence they offer a very direct and strong energetic wisdom about spiritual growth and self-realization. Their essence holds a clear unwavering route to divine self-identity.

Arrowhead Helps to find a purity of response in muddy times.

Blackberry Extremely versatile remedy, improves all rhythmic body functions, eases depression as well as any fear of death, helps us feel closer to God.

Black Cohosh Helps us balance our male and female energies into sublime use of our wisdom and power.

Black-Eyed Susan Shows us a way to unconditional love by embracing us with its complete love.

Bloodroot Shines a clear beam into even the most murky river to illuminate the family's divine wisdom, offers unequalled support for reclaiming this divine wisdom so we can use these strengths for good and leave the family's ego detritus behind once and for all.

Boneset Helpful information about healing broken bones, bone health, how to move more energy through our bones and integrate spiritual shifts that affect our bones and core experience of self.

Bottle Gentian All issues of vision, helps to see our situation clearly, hold our power, feel serene amidst chaos and resolve trauma as it affects our eyesight.

Burdock Holds wisdom about the blood including oxygen transport, extremely restorative during any healing crisis, helps with cellular discernment, getting to the bottom of a situation, bringing the core issue to light as well as composing a template for healing.

California Poppy Especially useful during spiritual awakenings as it helps us assimilate what we are learning and settle questions of motivation by grounding us in our heart's chalice.

Cardinal Flower Essence of consecration, wonderful for when we move into a new house, follow a new calling, begin a new relationship or in any way deepen our commitment to our spiritual path.

Celandine Improved information transfer, better cell-to-cell connection as well as person-to-person communication, helps us make a crystal clear, indelible impression as well as improve our health.

Chicory Helpful for sustaining momentum on our spiritual path, helps us towards self-lessness.

Coltsfoot Information about bone, muscle and orthopaedic health as well as spiritual flexibility.

Daisy Focus, heart-centred wisdom when we are scattered or unable to understand or appreciate our situation.

Dandelion Wisdom about physical vitality and purpose at all stages of life, helps us go with the flow, release emotional tension in muscles and navigate spiritual transitions with greater ease.

Fireweed Spiritual breakthrough, helps to make the connection when inability to create change has prevailed.

Goldenrod For opening and keeping clear the third eye of the sixth chakra, also helps us have a backbone and be true to ourselves in the face of peer, family or social pressure.

Hardhack Enduring complete love for self and others.

Indian Pipe Elementals peace, the balance of the four winds and four directions, reveals peace as an enduring reality within us, one that permeates all reality.

Jewelweed For all irritations, rashes or poison ivy, helpful when we feel thin skinned or impatient.

Joe Pye Weed Helps to lay down our burdens to God so we can feel totally supported by God.

Ladies' Bedstraw Helps us sleep well as it creates a protective cushion around our etheric field so sleep is deep and unchallenged, also helps us assimilate new information as we sleep.

Meadowsweet Takes us towards a gentle view of self so we know we deserve to receive love.

Milkweed Helps us bring an inspired idea into form just the way we first envisioned it.

Motherwort Support for the creative wellspring of the feminine, support for mothers to know their pivotal irreplaceable role in the world and to help them stay clear about what they need to do for themselves and their children.

Niella Cleanses, aligns and balances all chakras. Can reverse chakra direction when appropriate.

Nodding Ladies Tresses Unknotting of problems. Angels call it the detangler of flower world.

Orange Hawkweed Constructive management and flow of creative energy, helps children channel their abundant energy in the often stressful challenges of structured situations such as school.

Partridgeberry Helps to experience our partners as spiritual equals and part of a common divinity, illuminates common ground and helps partnerships bear fruit.

Purple Flowering Raspberry Passionate essence that helps us explore life's mysteries and the unexplored wilderness of our soul, excellent for dream work.

Pyrola Elliptica Dream work, brings unconscious into conscious focus.

Queen Anne's Lace Dismantles illusions of powerlessness, pulls the threads of a divided situation together when we feel scattered or face conflict within or without.

Rattlesnake Master Shows us the way to rebuff negativity wilfully directed at us, as well as move through poisonous situations with serenity and calm.

Red Clover Helps to calm emotional body and defuse reactions of panic, fear or hysteria in times of stress or emergency.

Self-Heal Helps us clear out illusions that prevent us from knowing our full healing power.

Silver-Rod Master essence for the chakras. Works particularly with the pituitary gland. During electromagnetic shifts in the Earth, helps us make the necessary adjustment in our chakras especially the sixth and seventh chakras and ride out all disturbances in our energy field.

Skullcap Enhances our ability to heal and get the most from healing sessions, helps to ground the new energies in our crown chakra and anchor these higher energies at certain places on Earth.

St John's Wort Helps to be more conscious of our protective golden armour.

Swamp Candles Support during dark night of the soul experiences.

Teasel To seal leaks or weak spots in our chakras, helps keep all inappropriate energies out of our energy field, the excellent essence for Lyme disease, a very powerful healing ally.

Thistle For clarity about boundaries if we tend to have our privacy invaded or are not sure what is or isn't our business.

Titan Practical information about owning our own power and living in an evolving light body.

Trillium Echoing the configuration of the Star of David, promotes a balance of learning and grounding and an experience of centred peace.

True Wood Sorrel Support to stay centred and know our own value in the face of excessive emotion, fanaticism, frantic behaviour or any extremes that might normally knock us off balance.

Vetch Helps us follow the spiritual thread in everything that happens to us.

White Baneberry Blood health, especially white blood cells.

The spiritual significance of deserts and their wildflowers

Many deserts are the result of humanity's abuse of the natural world. They are landscapes that have borne so much mistreatment in previous eras that they have scarred over into what appears to be dead zones. As humanity confronts the need to change course and save Earth from more depredations, it is important to look at deserts for the messages they carry. Angels note, 'We come to tell you that the messages from the deserts will cheer you.' The messages are ones of hope. Even in the suffering desert landscape, a place that appears beyond salvage, there is an upwelling of life in the blossoming of wildflowers. To visit the desert wildflowers is to be bathed in hope and vibrations of recovery.

Desert wildflowers embody the possibility of renewal, the truth that no landscape or person is beyond the grace of a new life and healing of old wounds. Wildflowers in the desert not only heal abused landscapes but their electrical patterns are part of the healing process.

When we separate self-care from planetary care, and have the 'I must get what I need at the expense of everyone and everything else' attitude, this creates deserts and reflects the illusions of separation and otherness. At heart we know caring for ourself is care of all creation. It is a collective of human hearts working in harmonious oneness with nature that will heal the deserts and other damaged places on Earth.

When desert wildflowers bloom they give to their landscape, to themselves and whatever life populates their realm, as they know themselves to exist in oneness with all creation. Their vibrational gifts are for *all*.

In order to blossom in an abused landscape, a desolate place of extremes, little physical nourishment and rare precipitation, desert wildflowers evolve an ability to find the goodness and sustenance that is available in their environment. They learn to seize any given window of opportunity that allows them to thrive and express their radiant selves. They learn how to transmute a situation of abuse and flourish. How to accomplish this triumph over adversity is the vibrational wisdom they give as flower essences, showing the abused places within us how to likewise heal and flourish anew.

The original Desert Wildflower Essences were made in the Sonoran Desert and Rio Verde Valley, Arizona, by Catherine Barritt and Jayn Bi. Recent Desert Flower Essences were made in Death Valley, the Mojave Desert, and, in the case of the White Flower from Druid Rock, in the Sierra Nevada near Bishop, CA, by Elizabeth Sheehaner.

Essences in the Desert Collection

Arizona Lupine Making the most of available resources, finding win-win solutions in situations where a scarcity model has ruled the day.

Brown Eyed Evening Primrose For healing from abusive experiences, especially childhood abuse, helps us leave bitterness behind when it no longer serves us.

Chapparral Zesty self-expression for the shy or retiring, restores joyful vitality after illness or times of dormancy.

Chia For increased vitality, life force and stamina.

Claret Cup Cactus Heals any divide between body and soul, helps us experience our physical bodies as whole and holy.

Desert Chicory For those who have experienced childhood abuse, helps to know healing will prevail without us 'pushing the river' or trying to scrub our experiences from our energy system, offers deep support to relax and trust that the flow of life will naturally take us towards healing.

Desert Forget-Me-Not Helps us remember ourselves before difficulties left their mark, reclaim our joy and delight in the world and our sense of the world as a gift unfolding before us, not a punishment to be endured.

Desert Garden For finding the vast spiritual nourishment available in even the most inhospitable situations and reclaiming our wholeness and holiness.

Desert Gold Confidence in the abundant flow of the generous universe even in times of apparent scarcity or lack.

Fremont Pincushion For those whose core experience of self is of being unwanted or of no value. Helps us move through traumatic experiences that have degraded our self-esteem to experience once again our infinite unwavering value and place in the world.

Palmer's Penstemon Gift from the fairies to help us dive into happiness.

Pebble Pincushion Support for the beleaguered and those who bravely shoulder their burdens, helps us quietly and cheerfully bear what we cannot change.

Purplemat Help to know less can be more, help to experience contentment with what is.

The Three Phacelia Sisters Help to mend the etheric wounds caused when we are repeatedly mistreated by human communities and help to release any mistaken ideas that we deserve this.

White Flower from Druid Rock Support to find the immense strength needed to birth a new life.

Woolly Easter Bonnets Support to find the divine gift of cheerfulness when our daily life is difficult.

The Bermuda Collection

Abundance

Long known as the Garden Island, Bermuda is a landscape of flowers, some cultivated and many wild. The island was so covered in flowers during the last two centuries that sailors knew they were nearing Bermuda, even before land was in sight, because of the fragrance of Orange blossoms on the wind. Bermuda's history as the site of the Atlantean flower research station is one reason for this continuing abundant flower population.

Bermuda was long the garden where angels, elementals and people created new flowers and new methods of healing with flowers. Flower essences were, of course, a vital product of the co-operative efforts.

Flowers and their essences defy humanity's illusory view of the world in which scarcity is the order of the day. Flowers are found in abundance everywhere people live. Even the Arctic has its spring deluge of generosity from the flower kingdom and the desert has its flood of spring flowers. Flower essences embody generosity in their incredible ability to stay fully potent even when diluted. Flowers and abundance are practically synonymous ideas.

This truth is particularly evident on the island of Bermuda. The flowers and flower essences made on this island have a strong predilection to do their work with total, abundant generosity.

As we explore the flower essences coming from Bermuda in the present day, we are called to remember what we once knew. Abundance is the offering of the Bermuda flower essences. We need only remember that we deserve this garden of abundance. Having long wandered in the wilderness, Bermuda's flowers remind us it is time to go home.

Molly loved Bermuda immediately and for years went on trips a couple of times a year and would wallow in aquamarine seas, sun on pink sand beaches and make fabulous flower essences.

Agrippina Rose Improves our skills as healers and the efficacy of other healing modalities, helps us heal with precision and finesse.

Allamanda Helps us heal trauma linked to hearing so we hear better, especially good for hearing our inner guidance better.

Aloe Ciliaris Helps us find harmony on the cellular level.

Aloe Vera Soothes internal and external inflamed tissue, a true physic for all healing situations.

Anthurium Balanced and creative use of masculine life force energy in relationship to feminine energy.

Asclepias Radical support to unleash our healing gifts and take our relationships and creative talents to a whole new level.

Avocado Helps us process and release strong emotions, such as anger and bitterness, generated from challenging interpersonal drama. Helps us physically heal when we've held on to these emotions to the detriment of our third chakra area, especially the liver.

Banana A versatile remedy useful in a wide range of situations including overly yang behaviours including male machismo, issues of the teeth, gum, jaw and mouth and problems with sugar cravings.

Bignonia Life force! Helps us live with more robust enthusiasm, fire energy, joy and vitality.

Bird of Paradise Helps with issues of synthesis and flow in our creative efforts, promotes the combining of unlikely elements into a unified whole.

Bottlebrush Excellent cleanser that also aligns physical and subtle bodies and increases our physical vitality.

Calliandra For the circulatory system as well as related emotional issues, helps us break up, release emotional and physical blockages resulting from heartbreak, violation or betrayal.

Cedar Strong cleanser of mental and etheric body which in turn opens the spiritual 'Gate of Remembrance' so we can access information about our divine purpose; a lovely additional benefit is how it improves hair health.

Chinese Fan Palm All palms offer our central nervous system much useful information; with this palm, the information is about healthy nerve ganglions.

Chinese Hat Plant Helps us find balance in situations creating a lack of equilibrium, imbalance, disorientation or change; good for motion sickness.

Clitoria Helps us manage spiritual awakenings and strong surges of spiritual energy including kundalini energies and move these energies up the chakras to our heart chakra.

Clivia Helps our creativity bear tangible results.

Coffee Support to break free from habits and unconstructive patterns of behaviour and thought.

Coral Aloe Helps cool down any heated situations, drama, heated arguments, burnout, high octane stress or firestorms.

Cotton The essence for wisdom about healthy hair.

Date Palm Ancient powerhouse offering wisdom about our DNA.

Dombeya Wallichii Sheltering love for those who shelter others as well as those who need comfort for any reason.

Frangipani Helps those who live in their feminine energy of knowing to assert themselves in wise action.

Gardenia Intimate friend and ally, a mysterious but powerful essence that helps us pierce the veil of illusion.

Ginger Helps us release our worldly concerns, avoid overextending ourselves or scatter our energies. 'Yoga in a bottle.'

Grapefruit For the relief of mental tensions including those that cause headaches.

Heavenly Bamboo Aligns main chakras and keeps us grounded to our divine identity during spiritual growth spurts.

Ice Plant Helps us warm up and find our sense of joy, humour and bliss, also excellent for all issues of poor circulation such as cold extremities.

Ixora Helps us make life-affirming decisions about our sexual choices, boundaries and partnerships.

Lemon Mental clarity, decisiveness, intellectual acumen, the 'Mr Clean' of the flower essence world, good for breaking up scar tissue.

Lime Superb cleanser, amplifies other healing modalities, assists healers to know their own strengths and move more healing energy, also assists those working with a healer or healing modality to get the most from this support.

Locust and Wild Honey Replenishes us when we are spiritually thirsty and helps us find spiritual community and kindred spirits.

Loquat All issues of digestion including the digestion of our life circumstances.

Mutabilis Rose As we adapt to changes in the planetary vibration, this one helps us mutate harmoniously and without fear.

Old Blush China Rose Helps us feel safe, especially when things fall apart. The angels suggested after 9/11.

Orange Helps us de-escalate highly charged emotional situations, explosive interpersonal dramas or polarized debates especially about sexuality.

Papaya Linked to sense of touch, helps bring clarity and peace to issues of sexual identity and partnership. Helps resolve relationship issues when both partners take Papaya.

Passion Flower Helps us feel the divine safety net that is there as we move towards self-realization, this in turn helps us both relax more deeply into the process and also release any cultural and religious rules of engagement that no longer serve us.

Pink Tecoma A comfort essence bringing a reassuring vibration of love and comfort much like a security blanket does when we are small.

Pomegranate The essence for female power, vitality, freedom, creativity and choice.

Rain of Gold A favourite for abundance.

Red Hibiscus Supports constructive and gentle release of abuse memories, especially sexual abuse, as well as the healing of the emotional scars.

Royal Ponciana Calms heated debate, promotes polite and civil dialogue, helps us see the divine in each other.

Sago Palm Profound, life-altering essence that helps us align with our physical body's divine blueprint.

Screw Pine For healing support during explosive or chronically irritating situations including allergic reactions.

Shrimp Plant Help for our bodies to work in an integrated manner, help to feel the unity of our lives and selves instead of experiencing life as a disconnected series of events.

Solandra Support to lay down our burdens, especially good for those of us who are overachievers, perfectionists, workaholics or those who believe they must be a human doing not a human being.

Spanish Bayonet Information about cellular cleansing.

Spider Lily For the improvement and discerning use of telepathic skills.

Star of Bethlehem Helps us confidently and joyfully let the old order go and give birth to the new.

Summer Snowflake Promotes adaptation to unexpected or radical changes in fortune, life directions, location or climate, especially good for travel or for uncomfortable extremes of temperature.

Tuberose A crown chakra powerhouse that will kickstart your spiritual journey if stalled, better align all your chakras and help the light of God pouring into your system in a coordinated and thorough manner.

Turnera Helps improve our daily rhythms about such things as receiving and acting on inner guidance and finding a regular rhythmic sleep pattern.

Vanda Orchid Help to get to our core healing issues; from this place the turnaround can be profound.

Vitex Information about assimilating the most of minerals in the foods we eat.

Water Hyacinth Going with the flow especially in regards to processing emotions.

White Hibiscus Support to heal from experiences of abandonment by making our relationship with our divine inner mother more real to us.

White Sweet Clover Support for sweet people to know the strength of their position and be able to express themselves without apology even to cynical audiences.

White Water Lily Helps us surrender with confidence and joy to the perfect geometry of divinity's unfolding plan for each of us.

White Yarrow For energetic protection especially in regards to computers and other technologies involving electromagnetic fields.

Wild Iris Helps us more closely align our creative processes with healing.

Wintergreen Helps us shine, especially when we've been doormats for others and haven't had much chance to express our inner zest.

Yellow Mullein We deserve the stars and this essence helps us know it.

Yellow Water Lily Helps us feel anchored and sustained by our Creator as all the old security blankets unravel and fall away.

Combination essences

All of the Green Hope Farm Collection combination flower essences are mixes of many individual flower essences.

All Ego Contracts Null and Void Helps to release habits, patterns of behaviour, personality choices or relationships that no longer serve us.

The Arbor Garden An essence greater than the sum of its parts, helps us feel connected, consoled, in sanctuary, soothed and safe no matter the circumstances.

Babies of Light To calm, protect and balance the electrical systems of the children coming to Earth right now, especially indigo children from the seventh root race, also useful for all sensitive souls.

Beautiful Skin Much-loved mix for all skin issues.

Carry Less Helps to remove the filters of ideas, opinions, impressions and sanskaras that limit our direct experience of life.

Centered Birth Much-loved combination for before, during and after birth for the mother-to-be and baby.

Cherokee Trail of Tears The Grandmothers, Native American sacred wisdom keepers, created this combination essence to support us on our own Cherokee trails. Just as on the original Cherokee Trail of Tears, the suffering of our individual trails takes us on a journey from our minds to our hearts, beyond the mind's ideas of duality towards a greater experience of oneness with our Creator. This encourages and comforts us on these difficult journeys and helps us harvest the gifts of these journeys.

Emergency Care For electrical support during any situation of stress, illness, emergency, ongoing chronic health challenge or trauma.

Ethereal Fluidium Super Glue Helps to keep the etheric body and connection between physical and etheric body clear and strong. This positively impacts the movement of life force or *prana* into the physical body and helps keep degenerative diseases from entering the physical body.

Golden Armor Protection from the discordant sound vibrations and electromagnetic dissonance of the modern world. The angels ask us to take this and give it to the animals every day; also good for other sorts of protection from resistance to viruses to rebuffing negativity of any sort.

Green & Tonic *The* mix for plants.

Grounding A mix containing many tree and other deeply rooted flowering plants that supports us to be fully in our bodies and in the now.

Hesperides' Gift For healers of every sort to help with burnout and other stresses of their lives and work, help for all of us to reclaim our divinity.

Inner Child To support the healing of our inner child's wounds so that we are more fully present in our daily lives and more cognizant of our power, wisdom and ability to solve our own problems.

Memory All memory issues.

Pack Leader Support to anchor in our own inner authority and find within us the calm and confident assertive energy necessary to handle the animals and the people in our life with appropriate boundaries, clear expectations and from a place of emotional balance.

Precious Blood A mystical powerhouse of all our red flowers and all our flower essences vibrationally linked to blood or bloodlines.

Purify Part of our Purify, Restore and Inspire trio, this is a cleanser that helps us to leave any addictive pattern behind.

Restore Part of our Purify, Restore and Inspire trio, this one helps us to find equilibrium and renewed strength when we leave any addictive pattern behind.

Inspire Part of our Purify, Restore and Inspire trio, this one helps us set a new course for ourselves after we leave an addictive pattern behind.

The Sacred Feminine Helps us individually and collectively receive, contain and birth new paradigms, new visions and new life for the transformation of humanity towards an embodiment of our sacred wisdom.

The Sacred Masculine Support to protect and transform the wisdom of our Sacred Feminine into right action.

She Changes Support for navigating the changes of menopause and perimenopause.

To Hear the Angels Sing Support to hear our heart's voice more clearly and all the spiritual guidance available to us.

To Thine Own Self Be True Rock-solid support for being true to ourselves.

Vitality A energetic kick in the pants that reminds us to go to our hearts for grounding, strength, direction, connection to God and everything else.

Watch Your Back Powerhouse of Palms and all other Green Hope Farm flower essences carrying information about the spinal column, the back and the health and wellbeing of the all the chakras. Also offers gifts of protection.

HAWAIIAN GAIA FLOWER ESSENCES (Haii)

Hawaii is renowned for its wonderfully exotic subtropical species of flowers, many of which were reputedly introduced by the migrating Polynesians when they discovered the islands and settled there some 1600 years ago. Inspired by the beauty of these islands, some suggest they may be the remainder of ancient Lemuria/Oceania, a mythical land that is said to have existed some 50,000 years ago. They speculate that some of the endemic Hawaiian flower essences such as Koa and Hawaiian Sandalwood have properties which help to enhance spiritual awareness, and these species could date back to these times.

The Hawaiian people traditionally turned to herbs for healing wounds and easing digestive problems. Internal illness was believed to be induced by evil spirits which weakened the *mana* or spiritual life force in a person. Their medicine men or *Kahunas* treated illnesses by holding a ceremony called a *ho'oponono* in which they used herbal potions with rituals to clear psychological disharmony within the family and so appease the spirits. The Hawaiians as a race of people recognized and were respectful of the spirit of life present in the plants, trees and rocks, referred to in the Western world as fairies or devas.

Natural medicine came into Cathie Welchman's life in the early 1990s when she was cured of a chronic allergy to wheat. Becoming interested in complementary medicine, she trained in crystal therapy, reflexology, aromatherapy and hypnotherapy. She became intrigued by gem and English flower essence making, which she still does. However, there is a certain something about the inspiring and magical atmosphere that draws Cathie back to Hawaii repeatedly.

The plants on Hawaii grow super-abundantly, due to the subtropical climate, the rich volcanic soil and the magnetic power rising from the still active volcanoes. These 62 essences have been gathered from amongst over 50,000 tropical plants on the main Hawaiian islands of Oahu, Maui, Big Island and Kauai. Many of the flowers used for the essences, such as Noni, Sandalwood, Ti and Koa, come from plants that were traditionally used by the native *Kahunas* for healing

disease, wounds and mental afflictions. The essences have absorbed and now embody the islands' magnetic healing qualities. The original mother essences were made with Hawaiian mineral water, drawn from deep artesian wells sunk beside the highest volcano, Mauna Loa, on Big Island.

The Hawaiian essences come from the lava desert, high altitude grasslands, tropical jungles, tree parks, the beachside and water sites. Cathie found the essences both potent and reflective of the primal forces of nature or *mana* which have been absorbed and reflected by plants. They offer a simple, safe way of returning us to health and happiness, resolving stress, despair and confusion, communication, vulnerability and relationship issues.

Aloe (Panini-awa 'awa) Aura repair. This essence protects one from lower astral interference, and helps to close holes in the etheric body caused by the effects of psychotropic drugs.

Angel's Trumpet (Nana-honua') (*Brugmansia candida*) Calling spirit. Stimulates reintegration on all levels of the personality. For those people who have lost touch with their intuitive side and focus only on the physical side of existence, and have a great fear of death, or anything otherworldly.

Banana Poka (Passion Flower) (*Passiflora bryonioides*) Lack of control. Stimulates co-operation and brings a sense of calm to those exhibiting wild, hyperactive or out-of-order behaviour, such as toddlers or teenagers. Dietary advice should also be sought.

Blue Ginger (*Dichorisandra thyrsiflora*) Fear of known things. Stimulates courage and strength in nervous people to be able to face their everyday fears. These include fear of the dark, spiders, needles, animals, heights, strangers, etc.

Bougainvillea (*Nyctaginaceae bougainvillea*) Enthusiasm. Encourages inspiration, purposefulness and enthusiasm. Discourages feelings of anxiety, fear or guilt.

Chenille (*Acalypha hispida*) Severing emotional ties. Cuts emotional ties formed through duty, base desires, programming or emotional blackmail, that bind one to an unhealthy, negative or harmful relationship.

Chinese Violet (*Asystasia gangetica*) Keeping it all together. Gives those who habitually overstretch their energies the wisdom of knowing when to say no, and to act on the need for rest, pleasure and holidays, despite the pressures of work and others' demands and neediness.

Cotton (Ma'o) (*Gossypium tomentosum*) Fearing the worst. Stimulates the ability to anticipate the future in a positive manner, and meet future challenges with courage and optimism. Lessens negative expectations, fear and apprehension of what might happen.

Crepe Myrtle (*Lagerstroemia indica*) Speak out without fear. Essence encourages those who are shy or nervous to state their needs, and speak up for themselves without fear or embarrassment.

Crown Flower (*Calotropis gigantea*) Independence. Instils courage and inner strength in those who are afraid of being on their own. This essence helps people to overcome the need to use emotional blackmail and states of ill health to maintain their overdependence on others.

Cup of Gold (*Solandra maxima*) Fear of the unknown. Opens the heart to bring deep inner calm and security in the face of constantly perceived danger. Decreases fear of fear.

Hau (*Hibiscus tilliaceus*) Calming extreme nervous stress. A calming, soothing and balancing essence for those overcome by extreme negative emotions.

Heliconia (*Heliconia caribaea*) Attention-seeking issues. Encourages acceptance of others' needs and talents, without feeling jealous, inferior or of lesser value.

Hibiscus Releasing memory of abuse. Realigns and restores emotional balance in those who are frigid or unresponsive in intimate relationships, due to past trauma from sexual abuse or exploitation. Heals soul loss and spiritual shocks.

Hina Hina Ku-Kahakai (*Heliotropium anomalum*) Empowered lady. Restores self-esteem, self-worth and the ability to make choices for one's own needs. Especially helpful for those women who have given up their lives and wishes completely to follow the desires of their spouse or children.

Ili'ahi (*Santalum*) Releasing stuck energy. Stimulates mental and emotional flexibility. It also amplifies the effect of other essences. For those with rigid, inflexible ways, that lead to escalating levels of stress, and difficulty in being able to unwind at the end of the day.

Ilima (*Sida fallax*) Dispelling illusions. Releases narrow-minded tendencies and hostility towards the spiritual views of others, due to cultural programming or religious dogma.

Impatiens (*Impatiens wallerana*) Calming anger. Encourages patience and tolerance in those who get easily annoyed and aggressive with others and the little problems of everyday life.

Ixora (*Ixora* sp.) Accepting change. Encourages interest and enthusiasm in present circumstances. Helpful for those who find it difficult to adjust to changing circumstances because they want to keep living in the past.

Jacaranda (*Jacaranda mimosaefolia*) Focus. A magically calming essence that stimulates decisiveness, clear-headedness and the ability to focus. Good for ditherers and those who constantly change their mind.

Jatropha (*Jatropha integerrima*) Spirit of fairness. Restores self-esteem and an ability to assert one's individual rights. Helpful for those whose kind and gentle natures have led to them being bullied, abused, unappreciated and used as scapegoats.

Kamani (*Calophyllum inophyllum*) Cleansing negative energies. Strongly positive essence for protecting a person or sacred place from profanity, or ignorant, negative or insensitive people. Neutralizes negative energies.

Koa (*Acacia koa*) Feeling fulfilled. An inspirational essence that promotes optimism and contentment at the deepest level of being. It eases the state of inner emptiness and deep pain and depression that people suffering from a lack of childhood nurturing or soul loss can't help returning to whenever life becomes temporarily more difficult.

Kukui (*Aleurites moluccana*) Emotional support. Promotes calmness and understanding. It dissipates emotionally charged situations, agitation and deep-seated, subconscious fears. It is particularly helpful for toddlers, children and teenagers going through stubborn phases, or experiencing 'growing-up' difficulties or hormonal changes.

Kou (*Cordia subcordata*) Maintaining personal boundaries. Stimulates strong personal subtle boundaries around those who are easily affected by the negative energies of others, especially when in crowds or bars.

Lani Ali'i (*Allamanda cathartica*) Making the right decision. Instils inspiration, willpower and wisdom for making important decisions. Helpful for those in authority who are unnerved by their responsibilities.

Mai'a (Banana) (*Musa paradisiaca*) Balancing male sexual energies. Encourages balance in male libido. Also helps to overcome tendencies towards sexual obsession or perversion.

Mango (*Mangifera* sp.) Lightness of spirit. Increases one's ability to utilize cosmic rays for energy needs, and lessens the desire for dense foods such as meat.

Milo (*Thespesia populnea*) Self-esteem. An essence to restore self-worth to those who have been held in a restrictive environment for some time, such as a mental institution or prison. Essence increases the ability to be able to act in an independent, positive and decisive manner within the human community.

Morning Glory (*Ipomoea tiroides*) Revitalize. Rebalances the natural pattern of sleep and daytime alertness. Essence breaks the vicious circle of repeatedly stimulating more instant energy with addictive substances such as coffee, cola or sugar, which then leads to a feeling of tiredness and irritability upon awakening.

Mountain Apple (Ohi-a-'ai) (*Myrtaceae*) Vulnerability. Stimulates the ability to overcome a weakened immune system through increasing the strength and determination of the mind's powers.

Naio (*Myoporum sandwicense*) Balancing appetite. Guides the soul to satisfy true inner needs instead of mollifying the outer symptoms of an emotional problem. Increases willpower to break addiction to comfort food.

Naupaka-Kahakai (*Scaevola taccada*) Moving on. Helps one to seek inspiration in the present and future, whilst gently encouraging release of the past. For those who want to move forward, but haven't been able to achieve closure or peace of mind due to personal injustices, bereavement problems or unfinished relationship issues.

Noho Malie (*Thevetia peruviana*) Calming agitated minds. Instils peace and calm in those who quickly become fearful and agitated for the smallest of reasons.

Noni (*Morinda citrifolia*) Faith in yourself. Stimulates invincible self-confidence and faith in yourself, particularly when you are being undermined by people who are gossiping behind your back. The essence prevents easily overwhelmed people from being pressured into acting against their will.

Nui (Coconut) (*Nucifera*) Perseverance. Helps sensitive people to develop a protective outer shell, so that they can reach their greatest potential. For those who lack endurance, or find it hard to meet challenges or to make tough decisions.

Ohai-Ali'i (*Poinciana*) Empathy. Encourages a greater awareness and understanding of the feelings of others. Helpful for people who are so self-involved that they don't listen to anyone, and are out of touch with those around them.

Ohia Lehua (*Metrosideros macropus*) Facing challenges. Helps one to master new skills and face challenges. Brings resilience, determination and an increased resolve to those who give up too easily. Helps to overcome addictions.

Orchid Tree (*Bauhinia*) Change. Stimulates the impetus to make necessary changes. Assists those who do not know how to change, even though they want to, and know they should.

Papaya (Paw Paw) (*Carica papaya*) Clear head. Helps in the assimilation of information, even where there is prior fatigue present. Stimulates the clarity of mind needed for taking exams or making big decisions.

Pa-Nini-O-Ka (Night-Blooming Cereus) (*Hylocereus undatas*) Light in the night essence helps to balance night and daytime energies. Alleviates fear of the dark or the sunlight.

Pink Ginger (*Alpinia purpurata*) Hugs. A wonderful essence to revive warm interactions with others. Especially helpful for those who never share their feelings with others. Also for those who have become emotionally cold and insensitive, due to past trauma.

Pink Waterlily (Day Blooming) (*Nymphaea odorata*) Feeling safe. Reinstigates trust in oneself, and releases apprehension in intimate relationships. Releases old patterns of feeling inherently unsafe that have been instigated by past experiences.

Plumbago (*Plumbago auriculata*) Family issues. Restores love, empathy and respect to family relationships. Reduces animosity or lack of caring between family members.

Pohuehue (*Ipomoea pes-caprae*) Mother issues. Puts those who have been hurt by their mother's behaviour in touch with their own deep inner self, where love always resides.

Protea (*Protea* sp.) Openness. Encourages openness of emotions and expression, especially in those who are unable to fully express their feelings, even with those closest to them.

Pua-Kenikeni (*Fagraea berteriana*) Overcoming hedonism. Releases psychological cravings for sensual overindulgence or dips into directionless apathy, restoring a balance and purpose to life.

Pua Male (*Stephanotis*) Marital harmony. Enhances co-operation, communication and compromise in close relationships. Instils respect for each other's differences.

Pua Melia (Frangipani/*Plumeria*) TLC. Empowers, motivates and strengthens resolve to look after your own health and personal needs. For those who put everyone else's needs and demands before their own, eventually resulting in a breakdown of their own health and wellbeing.

Pukiawe (*Styphelia tameiameiae*) Zest for life. A revitalizing essence that decreases apathy, and encourages the desire to improve your quality of life.

Red Ginger (*Alpinea purpurata*) Increasing sexuality. Enhances a healthy interest in sensual pleasures. Increases libido in both sexes by opening the base chakra and deepening a sensitivity in bodily desires.

Rose Apple (Ohi'a loke) (*Syzygium jambos*) Inner compromise. Instils an inner acceptance to be content with what one has. Helps those who think true happiness can only be found through money, partners, homes, career or other external things.

She Oak (Ironwood) (*Allocasuarina* sp.) Mother instinct. Promotes an emotional balance needed for optimum fertility in both sexes. Clears any feelings of inadequacy, lack of confidence or other subconscious emotional blocks. Promotes the need for adequate hydration. Take 2 or 3 drops of essence in a glass of water twice daily for at least three months.

Spider Lily (*Crinum asiaticum*) Childhood issues. Works on the inner child to help release damaging emotional programming learnt during childhood. Especially helpful for children or adults with painful memories instigated by parents or those in authority.

Spider Orchid (*Brassia*) Emotional blackmail issues. Stimulates respect and understanding of others' needs and kindness. Increases give and take, and lessens the need to bully, threaten or use emotional blackmail tactics.

Star Jasmine (*Jasminum multiflorum*) Overperfectionism. Essence encourages an inner acceptance and contentment with what talents and abilities you have. Helpful for those who make themselves unhappy by being overcompetitive, too perfectionist and highly critical of themselves and others.

Stick Rorrish (*Stenogyne caliminthoides*) Confusion. Restores communication between the mind, body and subtle bodies. Use for personality integration and soul loss problems.

Strelitzia (Bird of Paradise) In crisis. Offers support and inner strength on a day-to-day basis to those who are exhausted, traumatized and at the end of their tether.

Ti (*Cordyline fruticosa*) Banishing negativity. A powerful essence to remove negative energies or neutralize curses. Also for over-stimulation of the mind by circumstances or external environment.

'Uala (*Ipomoea batatas*) Releasing trauma. An essence to restore communication in a child or adult who has suffered a trauma, and is unable to express their feelings of shock, grief, frustration or helplessness.

Yellow Ginger (Awapuhi-melemele) (*Hedychium flavescens*) Releasing the past. A magical essence for gently releasing knots of disharmony in the subtle bodies or subconscious mind, which have become stuck there due to repressed or unhealed present and past-life traumas. Essence also links with liver issues. Helps to restore the sensitivity to the senses.

Wiliwili (*Erythrina sandwicensis*) Lessening autocracy. Brings in wisdom, altruism and understanding. Dissolves selfish motives. Helps to release a superiority complex. Helps those who have a tendency to be arrogant, bossy and insensitive.

17 new additions to the original 62 Hawaiian Gaia flower essences

A'Ali'i (*Dodonaea eriocarpa*) – Healing the Heart. Heals the heart of those who have been hurt through deep personal disagreements or betrayal in love, leading to the lack of trust in anyone. Helps one to pick up the pieces, cope positively with any backlash from the past, and regain a positive attitude towards others.

Akia (*Thymelaeaceae*) – Make Life Fun. Releases the feeling of being utterly overwhelmed by the everyday problems and never-ending demands of life. Enables one to see the bigger picture, concentrate on the most important things in life and still have time for some fun.

Amazon Swordplant (*Echinodorus tenellus*) – Freed Emotions. Dispels emotional blocks that are due to past or present trauma, the suppression of emotions, negative cultural programming or a lack of nurture and love experienced in childhood. Improves self-esteem, deters self-denial and encourages harmony within relationships. It encourages one to release deep-felt emotions in a safe environment, without fear.

Bamboo Orchid (*Arundina bambusifolia*) – Life Purpose. Helps to promote a sense of inner direction towards one's life purpose, especially when one has become frustrated with not knowing what special skills one should focus on. It stimulates confidence and trust in one's abilities and talents.

Guava (Wild Strawberry Guava) (*Psidium cattleianum*) – The Value of Mistakes. Overcomes learning difficulties and instils the ability to accept and learn from mistakes, without feeling inadequate or stupid. It helps those who won't try anything new, in case they make a mistake or a fool of themselves. It eliminates the need to constantly prove oneself right, due to fear of being seen as a failure. Links to physical flexibility and fluid balance.

La'Au Aila (Castor Bean) (*Ricinus communis*) – Calm in a Crisis. This essence instigates the ability to remain unfazed by the crises of life by balancing the yin and yang aspects of one's being. Helps one to maintain an undisturbed inner peace no matter where you are, or what difficulties arise. Particularly useful as a calming agent and inner strengthener for those who have become oversensitive to their own and others' emotions and fears.

Lotus (Pink Lotus) (*Nelumbo nucifera*) – Pure Harmony. Opens the crown and heart chakras to encourage harmony and balance in every aspect of life. It can be used in meditation to calm the mind and improve focus. Purifies the emotions and helps to release deeply ingrained experiences that no longer serve one's highest good. It provides a support structure for any healing activity, and amplifies the effects of other essences. Links to imbalances in the crown chakra.

Macadamia (*Macadamia integrifolia*) – Love of Co-Operation. Liberates those who feel stuck in a situation or lifestyle because their willpower and desires have been stifled by others. Helps to clear delinquent patterns of behaviour, due to being dominated or suppressed in childhood. Instils order and understanding, as it disengages repetitive thought patterns that cause reactionary and destructive behaviour.

Mamane (*Sophora chrysophylla*) – Clarity. Links one to the Higher Self, to resolve conflicting belief patterns, especially religious ones, that have negatively influenced one's life. It improves understanding and tolerance of others' beliefs, and brings a sense of inner contentment.

Melastoma (*Melastoma dodecandrum*) – Forgiveness. Releases paranoid thoughts of being wronged, victimized or belittled. It encourages trust in new relationships, and releases grudges, feelings of revenge and 'chips on the shoulder'. Vitality and wellbeing are restored, as knots of resentment lodged in the etheric body are dissolved. Particularly appropriate for those who are overcoming stress-related illnesses.

Mexican Creeper (Coral Vine) (*Antigonon leptopus*) – Love of Appreciation. Boosts sense of self-worth and acceptance of individual uniqueness. Heals emotional wounds where one has continually felt the need to take the victim or underdog role, and encourages one to outgrow the role of victim or masochist in personal relationships. Restores confidence to those who feel inferior, downtrodden or used following the breakdown of a relationship.

Night-Blooming Water Lily (*Nymphaea 'Emily Grant Hutchings'*) – Sensuality. Enhances emotional and physical enjoyment of lovemaking, dispels worries about sexual performance and improves intimacy between couples.

Panama Pacific Water Lily (*Nymphaea 'Panama Pacific'*) – The Freed Mind. Encourages optimism and releases cynicism, bitterness and kill-joy attitudes. It overcomes feelings of envy, resentment and pessimism in those who are jealous of others' happiness, because of their own lack of positive life experiences.

Passion Flower (*Passiflora mollissima*) – Christ's Love. Bestows an inner calmness as it helps one get through trials and challenges in life. Stimulates the heart chakra to revive spiritual energy, and instils the determination to succeed. It initiates self-love and a faith in one's body to heal itself. Lessens pain memory resulting from past-life traumas.

Pa'u-O-Hi'Iaka (*Jacquemontia sandwicensis*) – Spiritual Protection. Stimulates powerful spiritual white protection, when encountering dark forces. Connects one with angelic and higher guidance in times of stress and danger, by opening a channel to higher realms to gain any assistance needed. Reclaims the soul, as well as restoring protection for those who may have been harmed by dark forces.

Pua Pilo (*Capparis sandwichiana*) – Get-Up-and-Go. Promotes a 'get-up-and-go' attitude to life. It releases those who have become stuck in a state of lethargy, that prevents them from doing anything with their life. Helps to overcome a weight problem, that has arisen from a feeling of

apathy and helplessness, due to a negative self-image.

White Ginger (Awaphi ke-oke'o) (*Hedychium coronarium*) – Integration. Hawaiian flower essence combination of White Ginger (*Hedychium coronarium*), White Lotus (*Nelumo 'alba grandiflora'*), Yellow Ginger (*Hedychium flavescens*) and Thunbergia (*Thunbergia battiscombei*). Specifically for encouraging the return and harmonious integration of lost soul parts from any lifetime, any realm and any dimension, whether the cause is physical trauma, mental imbalance, genetic manipulation, deprivation, emotional or mental abuse, torture, curses or black magic.

PACIFIC ESSENCES OF CANADA (Pac)

These are the first Canadian essences and are made by Sabina Pettitt from the plants and marine life of the Pacific Northwest.

On moving to Vancouver Island, in the Canadian province of British Columbia, Sabina was excited to discover new kinds of plants, and began making some of them into vibrational medicines. The Arbutus trees of the west coast of Canada were among the first to catch her attention. The Arbutus essence acts as a spiritual tonic; one of the qualities it promotes is wisdom.

Sabina is a Doctor of Traditional Chinese Medicine and for nearly 25 years has been researching the essences in the context of their specific resonance with the meridian pathways with which each essence interfaces. Because each of the meridians has specific physical, mental, emotional and spiritual correspondences (or signs and symptoms of imbalance), using essences in conjunction with this ancient knowledge impacts on the whole person and produces remarkable healing effects.

In 1983 Sabina formed Pacific Essences and proceeded to research the plant energies that attracted her. By 1985 she had researched 24 wildflower remedies and 13 spring flowers and to date has developed 48 flower essences in her range.

One day when she and Michael, her husband and life partner, were walking along a sandy beach Sabina came across a Sand Dollar, a round flat shell with five petals etched on its top surface. Simultaneously Michael and Sabina heard a message to make the Sand Dollar into an essence for a friend who was suffering from some rare form of skin cancer. The results were astounding and in fact 30 years later that friend is alive and well and working with other cancer patients to help them explore the core issues underlying their disease. To capture its essence they placed the Sand Dollar in a glass of seawater and left it under a pyramid in the sun. This incident marked the beginning of her work with essences from the ocean, from which a whole new realm of energetic medicine began to unfold.

Michael and Sabina are credited with making the first sea essences on the planet and introducing this whole new range of healing frequencies to the vibrational medicine pharmacopoeia and there are now 24 sea essences in the Pacific Essences Repertory.

Sea Essences are about transformations in consciousness and are indicated for major breakthroughs, for they help us to contact the basic rhythms of the universe when we are going through change. Sabina's sea essences differ from her flower remedies in that they come from salt water, which is very similar in composition to our own blood plasma and seems to have a special affinity for the body. In Chinese medicine the water element is related to reproduction, growth and maturation. At the level of the spirit it is linked to Qi or psychic strength, which leads us through obstacles to growth. It is also the symbol for the unconscious.

Sabina proposes that, by their very nature, sea essences reveal the unconscious and strengthen consciousness in order to move forward towards a unique unfolding. Each essence is very precise and powerful and usually has quite noticeable and immediate results.

In conjunction with Michael, a gifted energy healer, she has also researched the essences in relation to their impact on the chakras. These are the *prana* vortices of energy at specific locations on the physical body which literally act to download the life force into the physical. Each of her essences (wildflower, spring flower or sea essence) have been researched in relation to the particular chakras of Ayurvedic Medicine and Pranic Healing.

In developing the understanding of energy as both preceding and affecting matter, a clear sense of how essences can impact on physical conditions became apparent for her. Like Dr Edward Bach she sees that it is fundamental that we treat the patient and not the disease. She trains her students to really listen to the patient and to be open to what their body/mind wants rather than having preconceived notions of which essence should work based solely on symptoms. Involving the patient in the cure is fundamental to work with essences. We cannot practise Energy Medicine® in the same way as chemistry-based medicine.

Native wildflowers – Kit 1

Bluebell (*Endymion non scriptus*) For giving up constraints, releasing old programmes, opening the channels of communication, engaging in what is fulfilling. Helpful for emotionally caused speech disorders, autism. Combats shyness. Boosts low energy, combats fatigue, alleviates fear, strengthens the will and ability to breathe during panic or anxiety attacks. Chakra: throat. Meridians: lung and kidney.

Blue Camas (*Camassia quamash*) For acceptance and objectivity. Balances the intuitive and rational, unifies and balances the left and right brain. For the creative person who is impractical, and the down-to-earth person unable to access his or her intuition. Also for dyslexia, learning disabilities, inability to learn from experience. Releases stored memory from past lives. Chakras:

solar plexus and throat. Meridians: kidney and bladder.

Blue Lupin (*Lupinus rivularis*) For clear and precise thinking. Links the pineal gland (organ of spiritual perception) with the pituitary gland (organ of metabolic control and balance). Also for toxin-related headaches and digestive disorders. Eliminates confusion about who we are. Alleviates depression, frustration and despair. Focuses attention and simplifies issues. Chakra: base/root. Meridian: liver.

Easter Lily (*Erythronium oreganum*) Truth, purity, integrity. Helps to integrate different aspects of our personalities, allowing open and honest self-expression. Eliminates social masks. For bypassing acquired personas of illusion, duplicity and dishonesty. Also effective for premenstrual syndrome and gynaecological imbalances. Chakras: heart, third eye and crown. Meridians: kidney and bladder.

Fireweed (*Epilobium angustifolium*) For realizing the abundance of love, both within and without. For emotional experiences recorded in the heart. Eases a broken heart, clears emotional wounds, coldness and the inability to feel. For embracing new relationships without residue from past ones. Loving, surrender. Improves circulation, softens muscle fascia in chest and upper back. Chakra: heart. Meridian: heart.

Goatsbeard (*Aruncus sylvester*) For meditation, creative visualization and the power to visualize oneself in a deep state of relaxation, being calm and relaxed in stressful situations. Resolves tension by creating inner alignment before action. Activates thymus to deal with stress. Strengthens immune system, white blood cell production. Helps to rejuvenate our body's chemistry. Chakra: third eye. Meridians: small intestine and spleen.

Harvest Lily (*Broadiaea coronarisa*) Community, relationships, social interaction.

Encourages expansion and awakening. Supports group energy and the ability to see another's point of view. For problems linked to reproduction, elimination, digestion, absorption, respiration and heart. Chakras: solar plexus and crown. Meridians: triple warmer and heart protector.

Hooker's Onion (*Allium cernuum*) For freedom, inspiration, spontaneity. Replaces blocked energy and heavy feelings with being refreshed and light-hearted. Nurtures creativity. Remedy for the spirit. Potential for releasing birth traumas and resolving the emotional attachment between mother and child. Chakras: all. Meridians: all 12.

Orange Honeysuckle (*Lonicera ciliosa*) Inner direction, expression and identity. For crises of personal identity and related physical tension. Releases creative blocks, diffuses anger and frustration. Evokes peaceful creativity. Useful for the turmoil of the teenage years. Also a powerful tonic for digestive disorders. Chakras: hara or sacral and solar plexus. Meridian: triple warmer.

Plantain (*Plantago major*) For releasing mental blocks and drawing off negativity. Purifies and cleanses the effects of poisonous thoughts, attitudes and resentment. Also for blood and liver disorders; any physical toxicity resulting from emotional or mental poisons, such as migraines and indigestion. Chakras: hara or sacral and crown. Meridians: liver and gallbladder.

Salal (*Gaultheria shallon*) For holding grudges or resentment. Releases power to forgive yourself and others; to let go. Clears stress and allows you the freedom and joy to experience the embodiment of the spirit in mysterious ways. Chakra: heart. Meridians: heart and small intestine.

Snowberry (*Symphoricarpus albus*) For accepting life as it is at the moment, dissolving resistance to what is – even when it is painful. Being here now. Also helpful for chronic fatigue and seasonal affective disorder. Chakras: crown and heart. Meridians: kidney and bladder.

Native wildflowers – Kit 2

Arbutus (*Arbutus menziesii*) Spiritual tonic – enhances qualities of depth and integrity. For homesickness or abandonment. For hanging on tightly while letting go lightly. Also benefits the lungs when their energy is depleted by sadness. Chakra: crown. Meridians: lung and liver.

Candystick (*Allotropa virgata*) Physical tonic – releases pelvic tension and promotes pelvic alignment. Releases blocked energy surrounding the experiences of abortion, miscarriage, birth, sexuality. Transforms self-anger and frustration to honour of self despite trauma. Survival and free will. Also for injuries to the sacrum and pelvic girdle, any insult to the reproductive system. Chakras: hara or sacral and throat. Meridians: kidney and bladder.

Chickweed (*Stellaria media*) 'For clear and precise thinking' and acknowledging and experiencing timelessness, being fully present and able to respond. Allows free and easy expression. Works on gallbladder channel to release tension and give up resentment and control. Useful for losing excess weight that is caused in part by old emotional baggage. Good for health practitioners. Chakras: throat and base or root. Meridian: gallbladder.

Death Camus (*Zigadenus venenosus*) Spiritual rebirth: awareness of spiritual connection with all life, for new beginnings, transformation and change. Alleviates stress and worry in times of transition. Helpful for new jobs, relationships, adventure. Assists self-cleaning efforts such as fasting, examining beliefs. Chakras: hara or sacral and heart. Meridians: lung and kidney.

Grass Widow (*Sisyrinchium douglasii*) Releases old beliefs and limited patterns, and the fear of being judged by others. Challenges mental structures and beliefs (linked to family, work, religion) that are not working for us. For fear of letting go. Also helpful for digestive problems and food intolerance. Chakra: heart. Meridians: stomach and large intestine.

Nootka Rose (*Rosa nutkana*) For expressing love, laughter and joy. Kindles enthusiasm. Reminds us that the life of the soul does not begin with birth or end with death. Excellent for spiritual crisis, abuse, abandonment, psychic, emotional or physical assault. Reintegrates the psyche after assault, heals fragmentation after years of self-abuse – such as with drugs, alcohol. Chakras: all. Meridians: all 12.

Ox-Eye Daisy (*Chrysanthemum leucanthemum*) For vision and the visionary. 'Total perspective; for being centred.' Brings a greater perspective when we cannot see the woods for the trees. Dissolves the blockage of fear which prevents clear sight. Develops better vision. Benefits the eyes and ears. Chakra: third eye. Meridians: heart protector and kidney.

Pipsissewa (*Chimaphila umbellata*) For making decisions. Clears ambivalence and indecisiveness. Releases worry and confusion around choices in life. Benefits the area of the brain involved in choice. Chakras: solar plexus and throat. Meridians: spleen, liver and kidney.

Poison Hemlock (*Conium maculatum*) For letting go, moving through transition periods without getting stuck and holding on to old structures and beliefs. Dissolves emotional, mental, physical paralysis arising from periods of major change. Releases rigid feelings, ingrained thought patterns, no longer relevant unconscious thoughts. Also beneficial for constipation, fluid retention, weight problems, paralysis of the physical structure or nervous system, stalled labour during the birthing process. Chakra: crown. Meridian: gallbladder.

Salmonberry (*Rubus spectabilis*) A physical tonic – for spinal alignment and structural balancing. Works on bone, muscles and fascia. Helps chronic misalignments of physical structure due to injury. Chakra: third eye. Meridian: bladder.

Twin Flower (*Linnaea borealis*) Acceptance and compassion. Clears judgement and a critical attitude towards everything. Teaches discernment to make choices without criticizing others. Fosters optimism, humility, and peace of mind and heart. Chakras: base and heart. Meridians: liver and gallbladder.

Vanilla Leaf (*Achlys triphylla*) For affirmation and acceptance of oneself. Replaces self-loathing with self-esteem. A grounding remedy of exuberance, joy, acceptance. For skin disorders and any problem rooted in self-denigration and lack of self-love. Chakras: third eye and crown. Meridians: lung and large intestine.

Spring flowers – Kit 3

Camellia (*Camellia sasanqua*) A catalyst for opening up to new attitudes which reflect one's true inner nature. Replaces guilt and shame with openness and flexibility. Stimulates expansion and vision beyond self-inflicted limitations, and expression of our uniqueness and inner power. Releases cell memory of earlier experiences in this life. Accesses self-trust and creates shifts in attitude. Chakra: solar plexus. Meridian: large intestine.

Forsythia (*Forsythia suspensa*) Catalyst for change. Provides motivation for transforming old useless thought and behaviour patterns which may be self-destructive (such as addictive and self-destructive habits: mental, emotional and physical addiction, especially to alcohol, drugs and tobacco).

Liberates dysfunctional relationships. Detoxifies the liver. Chakra: crown. Meridian: gallbladder.

Grape Hyacinth (*Muscari racemosum*) For times of external shock, despair and stress. Allows one to step back from the situation while harnessing inner resources to meet the challenge. Replaces shock and trauma with balance. Dissolves hopelessness, despair and depression. Eases stress felt in the stomach and aids breathing in times of stress. Also for bumps, bruises, accident shocks and all forms of trauma. Chakra: third eye. Meridians: stomach and lung.

Lily of the Valley (*Convallaria majalis*) For freedom of choice by discovering the simplest form of behaviour. Replaces sophistication and overcontrol with innocence. An emotional tonic that helps us to see with simplicity through the eyes of a child. Used in Europe as a cardiac tonic. Brings inner radiance and vitality. Chakra: throat. Meridian: heart.

Narcissus (*Narcissus pseudonarcissus*) For identifying and resolving conflicts by going to the centre of the problem or fear. Slays internal dragons, calms butterflies in the stomach and alleviates worry. Clears obsessive thinking, connects us to the impulse for survival, assists in feeling grounded. Also promotes digestion and eases digestive disorders (such as excess stomach acid, ulcers, gas). Chakras: base/root and hara/sacral. Meridian: stomach.

Periwinkle (*Vinca major*) Helps us to be responsible for our own depression and thereby dispel it. Lifts the dark cloud of depression, moves us to a place of inner knowing. Calms the mind and clears confusion and the memory. Also for hypertension, haemorrhaging, nervous disorders especially anxiety and seasonal affective disorders. Chakras: hara/sacral and crown. Meridian: heart.

Polyanthus (*Primula × polyanthus*) Dissolves blocks to abundance and transforms attitudes of inadequacy into those of worthiness and willingness to receive. Increases sense of self-worth, abundance and gratitude. Also benefits the respiratory and elimination systems. Chakra: base. Meridians: large intestine and lung.

Purple Crocus (*Crocus tomasinianus*) Enhances ability to tune in to all aspects of pain, grief or loss in order to release and resolve the tension and restriction associated with these feelings. For embracing issues; beneficial for those who turn their blocked energy against themselves after grief, or heartache causing life-threatening disease. Helps tension in the upper back and shoulders, releases the heaviness related to loss and grief. Also assists the lungs. Chakra: throat. Meridian: lung.

Purple Magnolia (*Magnolia soulangeana*) Promotes intimacy and non-separateness, enhances all the senses. Replaces withdrawal, coldness and frigidity with open intimacy. Elevates sexuality to its fullest potential for intimacy and non-separateness. Benefits the senses of smell, touch and feeling. Also a remedy for the spirit. Chakras: solar plexus and crown. Meridian: heart protector (circulation/sex).

Snowdrop (*Galanthus nivalis*) For letting go, having fun and lightening up. Combines enthusiasm and joyful exploration of life. Embodies qualities of personal power and leadership. Dissolves energy blocks and personal holding patterns that prevent the free flow of energy or Qi. Strengthens the will to dissolve paralyzing fear, attracts hope and release. Physically good for paralysis problems – arthritis, multiple sclerosis, poliomyelitis, cerebral palsy. Chakras: base, solar plexus and crown. Meridians: kidney and bladder.

Viburnum (*Viburnum carlesii*) Strengthens our connection with the subconscious and our psychic abilities. Excellent aid to channelling, meditating or centring. To hear and trust the intuitive voice within. Clears self-doubt and insecurity. Fosters clarity of sight. Affects the ears and ability to listen. Helps relax the nervous system. Chakra: third eye. Meridians: spleen and triple warmer.

Windflower (*Anemone pulsatilla*) A spiritual tonic providing grounding and inner security. Provides the security necessary to express our spiritual being, allowing the soul to dance. Balances scattered and spaced-out feelings. Also for stomach disorders, both physical and emotional – for nourishment on all levels. Chakras: throat and heart. Meridian: stomach.

New flowers – Kit 6

Alum Root (*Heuchera micrantha*) The power of the small; manifestation of 'godness'; ability to move in a pattern without having to do it 'your way'; willingness to choose 'to be'. Clears conflict and power struggles in relationships, moves a judgemental attitude to easy-going acceptance, creating trust, grace and beauty. Chakra: heart. Meridians: heart protector.

Douglas Aster (*Aster subspicatus*) Endless expansion while maintaining our centre; savouring life experience, living fully and consciously connected to our source, promotes courage and adaptability. Releases attachment to the ego, attracting expansion, generosity and radiance. Helps with staying centred, whatever turbulence is encountered, and in the face of many demands. Chakra: heart. Meridians: kidney, governing vessel.

Fairy Bell (*Disporum smithii*) Light-hearted release from murky thoughts; expands willingness to follow one's guidance; eases depression. Helps through the pain of a healing crisis emotionally and physically, sometimes has a mild sedative effect. Thaws frozen feelings and frozen body patterns. Physically frees the lungs and eases breathing. Can be used to assist the newborn to take its first breath, and help others breathe through the feelings of despair. Dissolves ambiguity and resistance bringing a lightness of being. Chakra: third eye. Meridian: lung.

Fuchsia (*Fuchsia* × hybrid) For recreation, letting go of dysfunctional patterns; being the change we wish to see in the world. Helps the slow phlegmatic types to 'lighten up' and move, and the fast, busy, overdoing types to slow down, 'chill out' and relax. A remedy of balance which peels the layers of programming of acceptable behaviour patterns and attunes to our own inner rhythms. Behavioural shifts occur as a level of self-actualization is experienced. A constitutional remedy for the water element, tonifies and nourishes the kidney and bladder channels. Chakra: sacral. Meridians: kidney, bladder.

Indian Pipe (*Monotropa uniflora*) Reconciliation with others and making peace with oneself with reverence for all of life. Allows standing alone in closeness, to be able to be fully in a relationship whist maintaining and expressing our own unique qualities of being. Fosters self-respect, banishes negative self-talk, feelings of worthlessness, so that we can find and live our life purpose. A constitutional remedy for the metal element, aiding self-expressing in the world, and gives the ability to recognize and claim what is valuable. Chakra: root. Meridians: lung, conception vessel.

Pearly Everlasting (*Anaphalis margaritacea*) Commitment and lasting devotion; opening to the mysteries of life; transformation through service. Deepens connections with another, reminding us that when connected on the soul level it is easy to remain beautiful in the eyes of the beloved. Shifts and transforms anger and brings the earthy 'stuff' into perspective. Encourages us not to throw the baby out with the bathwater

in relationships. Helpful for those unwilling or unable to make deep and lasting commitments. Chakras: third eye, navel. Meridians: liver, gallbladder.

Poplar (*Populus tremuloides*) For contacting spirit; for the ability to transmit healing energies; to improve choice-making; attunes to the gentleness of nature. Connects with the triple warmer channel, harmonizes the energy flow spiralling upwards from hara through the heart to the crown and tunes the physical body to a higher frequency. Chakras: throat, back neck. Meridian: triple warmer.

Red Huckleberry (*Vaccinium parvifolium*) To experience the power of introspection, to be able to withdraw from the madding crowd, the rush and business of daily life, allowing ourselves to go within with ease, reminding us of the power of nourishment when taking time to digest, and the wisdom of regeneration contained in hibernation. For being not doing, attuning to the cycles of nature on the planet and in our body. Helpful for preventing seasonal affective disorder, by resting in the winter months. Chakra: solar plexus. Meridians: gallbladder, stomach.

Silver Birch (*Betula pendula*) Enhances the ability to receive and to conceive; softens the need to control; dispels suffering and develops humility. A catalyst for balancing the female energy, strength in yielding. Physically for healing the reproductive organs. Emotionally and spiritually helps with conception when there are mental and emotional blocks that stand in the way. Also can be used to eliminate power struggles in relationships, especially when one person needs to be in control, and trying to play many roles simultaneously, clears self-sabotaging behaviour, making it easier to create agreement and harmony. Chakra: heart. Meridian: spleen.

Wallflower (*Cheiranthus*) For hopelessness, endurance, preparedness; attuning to our own inner rhythms. Dispels the sense of hopelessness when feeling misunderstood and can help us find the right means to make ourselves understood. Helps us to honour and delight in the many manifestations of divinity in form. The medicine of saints and mystics, it fosters an appreciation of the individual who can step to the beat of a different drum. Wallflower essence enters into the solar plexus chakra; it cleanses the imprint of old emotional pain resulting from feeling like 'the ugly duckling'. For sensory deficits and autism. Chakra: solar plexus. Meridians: stomach, spleen.

Weigela (*Weigela florida*) For integrating experiences on the physical and emotional planes. For realizing that others are both our teachers and mirrors who reflect our own negative and positive energy patterns. Clears disassociation, fosters trust and integration. Also for accidents and unexpected physical/emotional traumas. Chakras: throat and third eye. Meridians: liver and gallbladder.

Yellow Pond Lily (*Nuphar polysepalum*) Allows us to float free of emotions and attachments; fostering a secure sense of self, feeling strong and secure in one's path; blesses relationships. Through the bladder channel grants the ability to see things anew, to release emotional patterns so we are able to move forward fearlessly without being at the mercy of our feelings. Connects the throat chakra and allows us to express ourselves purely and without artifice, helps us to centre and perceive differently and act on our new information. Chakra: throat. Meridian: bladder.

Sea essences – Kit 4

Anemone (*Anthopleura elegantissima*) For acceptance of ourselves and others by helping us to take responsibility for our own reality, allowing us to be organized by

the universe. Aligns the mental body with higher soul purpose. Empowerment versus victim mentality. Releases karmic blockage in the solar plexus. Also for physical pain, allowing movement through pain rather than resistance to it. Helps eye problems. Also for overcontrolling both emotionally and mentally; for those prone to tension, muscle spasms and injuries. Chakra: solar plexus. Meridian: liver.

Barnacle (*Balanus glandula*) For attuning with the feminine aspect of the self in order to develop complete trust. Embodies wisdom, nurturing, fertility and abundance. Also for the female reproductive system, especially cysts and fibroids. Regulates hormone production and release. A powerful birthing remedy. Chakra: heart. Meridian: small intestine.

Brown Kelp (*Nereocystis luetkeana*) For shifts in perception leading to clarity. For those who get in their own way because of fear and confusion. Balances energy between the base/root and crown chakra. Also dissolves back tension, helps bladder infections and ear problems – especially fluid imbalance of the middle, inner ear. Chakras: base/root and crown. Meridian: bladder.

Jellyfish (*Aurelia aurita*) A birthing and rebirthing essence. Dissolves resistance that causes pain, helping us to be fluid and flexible and let go into the experience rather than be rigid and stuck. Spiritually connects us to the rhythms of our own being. Helps self-expression and depression. Also works against arterial plaque and hardening of arteries. Dissolves bitterness and hardness on the mental and emotional level before physical manifestation of disease occurs. Chakra: throat. Meridians: heart and heart protector.

Moon Snail (*Polinices lewisii*) Cleanses the mind and lets in light. Eliminates physical toxins which cloud the mind. Helps cultivate innocent wonderment instead of rigid thought structures. A helpful tool for meditation, illumination and inner journeys. For mapping unconscious territory in order to harness and explore creative expression. Chakra: hara/sacral. Meridian: triple warmer.

Mussel (*Mytilus edulis*) For releasing the burden of anger, enabling one to stand up straight. Transforming anger, it allows creativity and inner radiance to shine through. Excellent for a 'victim consciousness' that prevents our alignment with inner power and strength. Resolves irritability, frustration and anger. Also relaxes neck and shoulder tension and eases headaches and dizziness. Helpful for whiplash; promotes the flow of bile and aids digestion. Chakra: hara/sacral. Meridian: gallbladder.

Pink Seaweed (*Corallina vancouveriensis*) A grounding remedy for the patience needed before new beginnings, to harmonize thought before action. Helps us to move out of our 'comfort zone' into the new and challenging. Softens and allows change to occur with grace. Helpful when beginning new jobs, schools, relationships and experiences. Physically strengthens the bones and teeth; aids constipation. Chakras: hara and solar plexus. Meridian: heart protector.

Sand Dollar (*Dendraster excentricus*) For 'coming to your senses', awakening to reality versus illusion. For positive thinking that helps us to overcome the underlying cause of disease in the physical body. Effective for bronchitis, asthma, throat problems and self-expression. Chakra: throat. Meridian: lung.

Sea Palm (*Postelsia palmaeformis*) For breakthroughs in consciousness. For those who hurry for no reason, who are busy, preoccupied and controlling but not really allowing themselves just to be. For activity, being busy and preoccupied, which is a hindrance to success and meaningful relationships. For those who crave nurturing and emotional/physical nourishment. Also

helps digestive problems and eating disorders. Chakra: heart. Meridian: stomach.

Starfish (*Pisaster ochraceus*) A grief remedy. For willingly giving up the old and allowing the experience of being empty and releasing attachment. For appreciating our own unique soul path. Helps us to remember that 'to everything there is a season and a time for every purpose under heaven'. Stimulates a deep spiritual connection with those we love. Chakra: crown. Meridian: large intestine.

Surfgrass (*Phyllospadix scouleri*) For courage, strength and power rooted in stability and flexibility. Encourages integration of opposites by embracing paradox. Brings us the courage to be. For achieving goals that reflect our life's purpose, not our ego's desires. Alleviates fear and integrates courage. Strengthens will and gives a second wind. Also benefits kidney disease, infections, calcifications, inflammations. Balances the adrenal glands, enabling adrenaline to be used in a life-supporting way: stress without distress. Chakra: heart. Meridian: kidney.

Urchin (*Strongylocentrotus purpuratus*) For safety and psychic protection. For charting unknown territory, such as past-life regressions. A spiritual essence that expands the mind to access stored memories from early childhood or a previous life. Also for the effects of childhood abuse which have created self-abuse patterns (e.g. alcoholism, eating disorders, suicidal tendencies). Helps to dispel panic attacks, and respiratory problems that arise from feeling unsafe. Chakras: crown and solar plexus. Meridian: spleen.

Sea essences – Kit 5

Chiton (*Mopalia muscosa*) For gentleness which serves to break up and to dissolve blockages and tension. Rigidity, promotes gentleness and flexibility. Primarily a physical remedy, helps us to live softly in our bodies instead of tightening up under stress. Remedy for whiplash or other neck injuries, also for dysfunction of the thyroid gland causing holding patterns in the body, for ecample, excess weight. Helps us to be more flexible within our body/mind structure. Useful before going into a situation where emotional distress exists. Helps move beyond limitations of cultural conditioning and rigid beliefs, encouraging the full creative expression of the liver channel. Allows you to receive new information, perceiving something in a new way and change course acting on this insight. Chakra: throat. Meridian: liver.

Coral (*Pocillopora meandrina*) For living in community; respect for self and others. Allows us to retrieve ancient memories, lost connections with the Earth and how to be human. Helps us to remember we are not enemies, only those who have agreed to play roles in our own script of learning and evolution. Cleanses old 'stuff' held in the solar plexus so we are not held back by emotionally charged memory patterns. Connects with the kidney channel and is potent for the brain and the central nervous system; the kidneys are where the inherited Qi resides. It affects physical growth and mental potential and is appropriate for central nervous system disease such as post-polio syndrome, Parkinson's, multiple sclerosis, etc. Also encourages cell adaptability, so with those who have lost part of their brain function, the viable cells will be able to take over the function of the missing cells. Chakras: solar plexus, throat. Meridian: kidney.

Diatoms (*Amphipleura pellucida*) Repatterning cellular memory; letting in the light. To be used when the purpose of a cell has been forgotten, as in cases of cancer and degenerative disease, helps to enlighten the cells and assist with its return to normal if that is the soul's intent. Chakra: heart. Meridian: heart.

Dolphin (*Stenella longirostris*) Appreciation for all that is, brings a playful, light-hearted, dancing energy. Dolphins are considered water creatures' manifestation of angels. For those who feel profound alienation and loneliness with a sense of deep loss and abandonment. A remedy of the heart and mind, expansion and transformation and connects with the limbic system where we experience pleasure and joy. Opens the heart, moving energy through the crown to the higher dimensions in order to expand consciousness. Chakras: sacral, solar plexus, heart, throat, third eye, crown. Meridians: spleen, heart.

Hermit Crab (*Pagurus granosimanus*) The ability to enjoy 'aloneness'; contentment and sensitivity. For help through the dark night of the soul when our aloneness feels overwhelming. Aids understanding and reconnection with our soul whose journey is always alone, individual and unique, which brings freedom and easy self-integration physically, emotionally and mentally in all situations. Diminishes fear, and those so insecure that they are unable to enter or maintain authentic relationships. Quiets the mind, and helps feeling comfortable with the self wherever we are. Chakra: throat. Meridian: stomach.

Rainbow Kelp (*Iridaea cordata*) Alignment of front and back brain, that is, reactivity and sensibility; alchemical transformation. A remedy for depression, mental confusion, helps to release, relax and attune to a higher perspective and connect to our light source. Connects with the third eye chakra and hara, the adrenal glands, 'the fight or flight response' and fear states. With its affinity with triple warmer channels it balances all the other meridians and regulates the body temperature. Harmonizes the extrovert and introvert and therefore has an impact on social relationships. Chakras: navel, third eye. Meridian: triple warmer.

Sea Horse (*Hippocampus*) Energizing the spine and central nervous system; accessing the 'wild one' within. No matter what physical form we have chosen, this remedy allows us to express unique talents and abilities and let go of notions of how men and women 'ought' to be. Physically for disease or dysfunction of the cental nervous system, communication between the brain and motor or sensory function. Benefits the lungs, assisting utilizing of *prana* or Qi whilst breathing. Good for athletic and physical endurance. Resolves stiffness of the spine through the effect on the governing vessel which also allows dispersion to all other meridians as needed. Chakras: root, sacral. Meridians: lung, governing vessel.

Sea Lettuce (*Ulva lactuca*) Embracing and healing the shadow; for dispersal and elimination of toxins. Affords the ability to recognize, heal and transform those faults, flaws of the ego that we hide even from ourselves. Known to Native Americans as the 'eater of filth', Sea Lettuce detoxifies, purifies and releases, acting as a blanket which soothes and heals the lower abdomen as well as being useful for the reproductive organs or bowels. Resonance: purification. Chakra: solar plexus. Meridians: small intestine, stomach.

Sea Turtle (*Chelonia mydas*) For persistence, grace, commitment. Benefits the spleen and assists in its functions of transformation and absorption of nutritive Qi. It helps those who tend to be 'spaced out' and underground to reconnect with solid Earth energy, to get out of their heads and into being in their bodies and living on the Earth. At the spirit level helps find the 'spark of divinity' in our souls and connection to the source. Chakra: heart. Meridians: spleen, heart protector.

Sponge (*Myxilla incrustans*) Everything is unfolding in perfection; nothing happens to me without my consent. Filters impurities from the mind and spirit so freedom can be experienced. Helps us to let go and embrace life fully and gives the ability to dance between the two polarities of attachment and detachment. For those who tend to absorb the energies of others and have no way of transmuting them. Connects with the stomach channel, assists with digestion and absorption of emotions and ideas. Connects with the bladder channel by maintaining energy reserves and fluid balance and by maintaining the position of active participation and passive observation. Chakra: crown. Meridians: stomach, bladder.

Staghorn Algae (*Lessoniopsis littoralis*) Holding ground (sense of self) amidst turbulence and confusion; accessing higher consciousness. An aid to reconnecting with our own divinity when feeling lost or alone. For attunement and perception and is beneficial for the eyes. Awakens spiritual clarity, promoting steadfastness and gentleness. Works on the gallbladder channel and physically on tight and painful shoulders. Improves coordination, mentally aids clear thinking, decision-making when making life-supporting choices which benefits physical and emotional health. Chakra: root. Meridian: gallbladder.

Whale (*Globicephala macrocephalus*) Enhances ability to communicate through vibration and sound; expansion of human consciousness; ability to contact the record keepers. A remedy for healers, an aid to expanding, enhancing and transmitting the healing ability as well as receiving and interpreting subtleties of nature revealing knowledge of our roots, path in life and future possibilities. Physically a general tonic, that tonifies the circuit of Qi in the governing and conception channels which directly influences all the other meridians as well as the mind/body connection. Chakras: third eye, crown. Meridians: conception vessel, governing vessel.

18 + Good Vibrations™ Combinations: Abundance®, Balancer® and Heart Spirit®

While doing the early research on individual essences three combination formulas emerged – Abundance, Balancer and Heart Spirit balancer. These combinations address moving through stress, acting from grace and ease, and attracting prosperity.

Sabina created the Abundance Program, a 22-day journey of using the essence with specific intention. Heart Spirit gifted us with healing for the heart at all levels. The ancient Egyptians had an image of a person's heart being weighed against a feather on a set of scales at the door to the next life. Only if your heart is lighter than the feather can you proceed into the next world. This is the gift of Heart Spirit.

These combinations have been one of the most exciting additions to the Pacific Essences repertory. Their gift is that they work at so many levels. When a number of essences are combined in a formula the whole becomes greater than the sum of the parts and the impact is far bigger than when they are used individually and at the same time they become a unique individual vibration.

Abundance® Discover your inner connection with the source of all that is and manifest your heart's desire in any area of your life. Abundance essence connects us to the source of all manifestation, allowing use of the principle of creation in our daily life so that we are 100 per cent responsible and accountable for the reality that we experience. Helps to tap into the potential that 'I create my own reality' and reinforces the understanding that we are each the author of our lives instead of the audience in our lives. Aligns body, mind, emotions and spirit to act in a unified manner to achieve individual goals while forging a connection with the larger flow of all of life. It is an essence of transformation of consciousness.

The **22-day Abundance Program®** consists of two Abundance essences, an Abundance oil, an instruction booklet for undertaking the 22-day journey and a CD with four guided meditations on it. The Abundance Program is a commitment to yourself. Its purpose is to create a new framework for manifesting abundance at any and all levels of your life. Choose your focus, whether it is money, relationships, work, family, health or any area where you are experiencing lack or scarcity.

Each exercise is designed to release 'stuff' which no longer serves you, or to assist you in creating a particular experience of abundance in your life. Essentially the programme, coupled with that of the Abundance essence and oil, will repattern cellular memory so that you can experience your own inner power to manifest exactly what you want.

Heart Spirit® Embrace life wholeheartedly – with joy, compassion and generosity. Dissolves old heart pain, encourages us to truly embrace the 'spirit of the heart'. The 'spirit of the heart' is love, light, laughter and joy. It is peace, allowing, embracing, acceptance, comfort and enthusiasm. The primary effect is to raise the vibrational frequency of the heart centre to its highest level, promoting self-worth and lending new meaning to the dignity of being human, allowing us to interact with each other with grace. It is much needed at this time. Heart Spirit is an essence, oil and spray.

Balancer® Maintains centre in stressful situations. Restores balance and harmony. The Balancer essence harmonizes the body/mind in any situation of psychic, emotional or physical overload. It allows us to shift our attention, regaining perspective and balance. It resets homeostatic mechanisms in the physical body, calms the mind and dissolves turbulent emotions. It feels like immersing yourself in a cooling, soothing waterfall and emerging rejuvenated and refreshed. A powerful adjunct to a first-aid kit, Balancer offers immediate, safe and effective results. It balances excess or deficiency in any of the channels or chakras. Balancer is an essence, oil and spray.

Nine synergistic formulas

As a result of the phenomenal success of these first three combinations, Sabina introduced nine new synergistic formulas in 2003. These combinations are designed to be 'user friendly' for people who know little or nothing about essences. Already they are proving to meet a growing need on the planet for gentle medicine.

Being True Worth® Recognizing who we are with the freedom to express who we are in our daily lives and relationships. Transcending cultural programming/ brainwashing. Physically nourishes lung and large intestine, and enables the receiving of new vibrant energy and the release of old toxic energy. Emotionally welcomes new feelings, releasing old emotional patterns that don't serve. Mentally embraces new thoughts and attitudes, dissolving crystallized thought forms, and spiritually brings grace.

Cellular Memory® Supports and enhances the innate intelligence of each cell, coaxes each atom to perform impeccably to maintain balance and harmony to survive, and to contribute to the survival of the whole. Reminds each cell of its *dharma* (purpose) and unique contribution to the whole being. Physically restores memory of cellular purpose, activates and enlivens our own unique DNA blueprint. Emotionally dispels discouragement. Mentally brings inner peace and knowing that it is all unfolding perfectly. And spiritually it embraces the divine.

Fearlessness® Ability to move into love and the heart centre; what is not love is fear. Encourages the ability to stop time, shape shift, broadcast energy from the heart instead of adrenaline and fear vibes. Physically nourishes adrenals, supports kidneys. Emotionally promotes non-attachment. Mentally creates clarity, and spiritually awakens consciousness.

Forgiving® Gives the freedom to disconnect from any and all 'old and painful' stuff by letting go of any blame or shame that we might attribute to ourselves or others. Forgiving is the ultimate gift to ourselves and restores our own sense of self-empowerment and self-direction. For 'control freaks', it is the ultimate and optimally healthy form of control. Physically cleanses every cell memory of any perceived harm from others. Emotionally dissolves bitterness, resentment, fear and hostility. Mentally erases resentment, and spiritually frees our soul to dance the dance we came here to perform.

Kids' Stuff® For all the fears (imagined and real) and dramas and traumas of childhood when we can't get into bed at night until we are sure there is nothing or no one hiding under the bed or in the closet. For when we think the 'sky is falling in' or 'it is all our fault' when parents are fighting or when one of them gets sick, when 'bad stuff' happens. Restores innocence and harmony and 'acceptance of what is' with calm detachment and light-heartedness. Physically tickles the heart with a feather. Emotionally restores innocence, brings joy and delight. Mentally dispels seriousness, promotes spontaneity. Spiritually helps us to know the spirit within, nourishes inner security and self-referral.

Optimal Immunity Strength and protection for body/mind/spirit: physical, emotional, mental and spiritual safety. Physically strengthens spleen, increases white blood cells. Emotionally protects against psychic and/or emotional attack. Mentally prevents toxic thought patterns and eliminates old ones. Spiritually fosters safety and protection at all levels of being and a warrior spirit.

Optimal Learning Helps to access and decode information with ease and promotes the ability of the brain to function holistically and to access more of its potential. Practically assists with learning disabilities like dyslexia and Attention Deficit Disorder (ADD) and in the bigger picture it can help those of us who repeat the same mistakes over and over and over again. Physically promotes wholeness and integration in the brain. Emotionally destroys fear and restores self-esteem. Mentally promotes mental acuity and perception, and spiritually is a reminder that the incarnated soul is here to learn.

Radiant Beauty Switches on the light of our inner beauty and illuminates the body and mind so that through whatever the shape, size and physical features of the 'vehicle' we are driving in this lifetime, we appear beautiful to all who perceive us and perhaps mostly 'we accept and appreciate who we really are'. Physically enlivens the *Shen*, and nourishes spirit. Emotionally dissolves and erases 'ugly' emotions. Mentally catalyzes 'beautiful' thoughts. Spiritually balances among the five spirits – *Shen*, *I*, *Po*, Qi, and *Hun* – allowing us to connect with the divine; accepting, expressing and allowing others to see who we really are.

Super Vitality For rejuvenation and revitalization of body/mind/spirit. Enhances stamina and promotes peak performance. Useful for athletes to encourage peak physical performance or for anyone whose natural vitality of the sex chakra is diminishing, and for anyone who is feeling the effects of ageing. Physically it is revitalizing. Emotionally it is harmonizing. Mentally it restores optimism and optimal neurological function. And spiritually it is renewing.

The five elements of traditional Chinese medicine
1. Fire

- expression of consciousness
- ability to deal with shock and trauma
- connection with others
- expression of the light within
- love, purity, protection, communication
- joy, laughter
- inspiration, expression
- communicator, wizard.

Physical circulation, body temperature, toxicity. **Emotional** enthusiasm, passion, spontaneity. **Mental** equanimity, presence. **Spiritual** consciousness.

Harvest Lily For healthy relationships and co-operation among people, unification of group energy, promotes community.

Hooker's Onion Sparks the fire of creativity and removes blocks to creative expression, assists us to come from inspiration instead of memories.

Nootka Rose It is in the experience of loving that we experience our highest potential; releases and heals the heart from damage of trauma.

Purple Magnolia Nourishes sensuality and sexuality; helps us to experience the fullness of all our senses in a good way, so that consciousness has opportunity for maximum experience in the physical.

Rose Quartz Promotes love and compassion for self; nourishes gentleness and vulnerability.

Snowberry Being in present time is like being an impeccable spiritual warrior, a master martial artist; being fully present allows us to use our fire energy in wise and constructive ways.

2. Earth

- ability to digest experience
- ability to have clear boundaries
- groundedness and connection to the earth
- ability to discern what is nourishing and life supporting
- satisfaction, safety
- worry/pensiveness, sighing
- intellect, needs
- peacemaker, mediator.

Physical digestion, immunity. **Emotional** sympathy, hypersensitivity. **Mental** worry, overthinking. **Spiritual** embodiment.

Amethyst Allows us to feel safe and protected; dissolves guilt and fear and purifies the body/mind.

Fireweed Helps us to restore and replenish perfect health after attack and crisis; dissolves feelings of separation from self and others while maintaining our own unique and individual integrity.

Hermit Crab Being 'at home' wherever we are and in whatever circumstances we find ourselves. Promotes the feeling of contentment and the ability to be alone.

Narcissus Dissolves worry and incessant thinking; helps us to feel grounded, nourished and secure.

Urchin For safety and psychic protection; dissolves obsessions and compulsive behaviour.

3. Metal

- receptivity to life force energy via lungs
- letting go of toxins via large intestine
- having courage and conviction to express who we are

- balance between control and flexibility
- receiving, letting go
- grief, weeping
- vitality of Qi, values
- artist, alchemist.

Physical breathing, elimination. **Emotional** sadness. **Mental** melancholy. **Spiritual** instinct.

Bluebell Helps us to release constraints and promotes self-expression; allows us to give up judgement and the fear of being judged; fortifies courage to 'follow our bliss'.

Citrine Promotes clarity of thoughts, feelings and intention; augments happiness, prosperity, generosity, confidence and stability.

Death Camas Spiritual rebirth and transformation, especially empowering when we are faced with unexpected challenges; helps us to feel connected to the eternal web of energy that is life.

Grass Widow Grants us the gift of letting go and releasing the past, supports us to question and evaluate structures and beliefs.

Purple Crocus Provides a safe environment in which to experience grief; allows us to fully embrace whatever experience we are in.

4. Water

- DNA blueprint
- determination
- courage, fearlessness
- finding our way through trusting inner wisdom
- faith, trust
- fear, groaning
- will, direction
- sage, philosopher.

Physical hydration, purification. **Emotional** fear, anxiety. **Mental** shyness, timidity. **Spiritual** vital essence.

Brown Kelp Encourages leaps of faith which brings us back to our centre; promotes hydration and dissolves fear and confusion.

Easter Lily Helps us to integrate different aspects of ourselves; allows us to express ourselves openly and honestly – without artifice or pretence.

Plantain Dissolves toxicity in the mental and emotional bodies; resolves frustration and resentment.

Salmonberry Nourishes the physical structure and aligns the spine; erases thoughts and feelings which keep us in a state of holding, tightness and chronic misalignment.

Smoky Quartz Helps turn our wishes, dreams and desires into reality; teaches us to simplify our lives and to live in a sacred manner; grants us the gift of discernment.

Sponge Filters impurities from the body/mind and allows us to experience our lives and ourselves with hope and wonder; promotes inner peace.

Tourmaline Fosters willingness to be guided and nourishes inner radiance; balances and energizes the channels of light energy in the body – chakras and meridians.

5. Wood

- expression of the potential within
- energy and physical capacity to fulfil our life purpose
- competitiveness to achieve our personal best creative expression of who we can be
- action, vision
- anger, shouting
- spiritual purpose
- visionary, pioneer.

Physical movement, action, muscles and mobility. **Emotional** anger, frustration. **Mental** belligerent, aggressive, competitive. **Spiritual** soul.

Anemone Grants us the gift of being 'able to respond' to what is and to trust in the infinite wisdom of who we are and why we chose this particular incarnation.

Candystick Helps us to appreciate free will at the level of the soul; supports our life purpose.

Pearly Everlasting Promotes openness to the mystery of life and devotion in relationships; seeing self in other.

Twin Flower Grants us the gift of compassion for others and mostly for ourselves; fosters optimism, humility and peace of mind.

Quartz Amplifies all experience; promotes expansion and dissolves uncertainty.

Being Peace Finding peace within; tapping into the Root of Compassion; practising loving kindness, good will and the will to do good.

Physical makes our bodies temples of harmony. **Emotional** supports mindfulness. **Mental** being compassionate. **Spiritual** supports our commitment to the peace we want to experience in our world.

Detox Gentle cleansing of toxins at a cellular level; clearing away cellular debris whether it is physical, emotional or mental; revitalizes the body/mind.

Physical cleanses at the level of the cells. **Emotional** cleanses toxic thoughts. **Mental** cleanses toxic emotions. **Spiritual** allows who we really are to sparkle and shine.

New Attitudes Removes difficulties and to 'switch on' commitment to transformation; to do whatever is necessary to make changes in our behaviour; to feel empowered to let go of addictions.

Physical assists with weight loss, smoking, and other physical habits which are not life supporting. **Emotional** supports new and positive thinking around our ability to make changes in our behaviour. **Mental** releases guilt and shame related to past failures. **Spiritual** reminds us to ask for help and to rely on our guides and helpers.

Shielding Protection against radiation; protection against EMFs (electromagnetic frequencies); syncing the energy systems of the body/mind.

Physical acts as a physical protective shield against radiation and EMFs. **Emotional** supports life-supporting thinking in the face of electromagnetic toxins. **Mental** dissolves fear of being harmed. **Spiritual** reminds us that who we really are is absolutely safe and protected.

PEGASUS ESSENCES (Peg)

Fred Rubenfeld, the owner of Pegasus products, was introduced to the world of vibrational healing when he went to work in the diamond industry in New York. While surrounded by gemstones and crystals he began to learn about and experience the healing effects of the stones he worked with. In 1983 he was among the first to open a mineral and crystal store, selling gem elixirs in New York. He then expanded into the world of flower essences when he took over the Pegasus company. Fred has now created a phenomenal 'remedy bank' which offers a vast range of more than 500 flower essences and more than 300 gem elixirs, as well as star light elixirs from the stars and planets.

The Pegasus range is made up of contributions from all over the world: Lily from Africa; Holy Thorn from Glastonbury; Creeping Thistle from Scotland; and many flowers from Tahiti, etc. The company is based in the Rocky Mountains in a town called Love Land,

near Boulder, Colorado, a sparsely populated area with an abundance of wildlife and rich Gold and Quartz deposits. Geographically it is the centre of North America. People living here seem to derive a great deal of energy from the land, which is conducive to good health.

Fred believes the secret of making good essences and elixirs is to welcome participation from all kingdoms – floral, mineral, elemental, planetary and extraterrestrial – while detaching ourselves mentally and emotionally from the process of making essences.

To make his flower essences he uses a special quartz crystal bowl and sunlight that is filtered through xenon gas before hitting the water. The gas acts as a filter, reputedly eliminating any harmful effects of the sun's rays.

The essences are potentized by a geometric shape called a metaform, an Aquarian pyramid filled with crushed quartz. This process is carried out after the essence is made, again after it is bottled and once again prior to shipping, to clear any negativity and ensure a safe journey and long shelf life.

At this particular time these essences aim to deal with and provide the energy needed to cope with issues, destruction, change and disaster. Flowers and crystals in particular, Fred Rubenfeld maintains, can assist with these issues. He feels there is something quite unique about the urban flowers that push themselves up through the sidewalks/pavements of New York. They show a determination to move through obstructions, a strength of spirit that is appropriate for dealing with the issues of today, and indicative of the tenacity needed to work through the kinds of obstacles we face daily. He also feels that at this time there is greater awareness of the higher realms, as there was in biblical times and even earlier. At a time when so much life on Earth is in jeopardy, flowers and gems are providing some possible solutions. For example, elephants are now being saved thanks to the discovery of a new substance that comes from a bean plant and can be worked to look like ivory. Its qualities are captured for the first time in Fred

Rubenfeld's Tagua Essence. Here are some of his vast range of flower essences as well as his Roses collection.

Agave Yaquiana (*Maguey lechuguilla*) Affects the unconscious decisions people make based upon deep-seated beliefs about separation, loneliness, aloneness, etc., that are often the legacy of past-life information and experiences. When taken repeatedly it helps loosen the hold of these hidden or unconscious belief-patterns.

Aloe Eru (*Aloe camperi*) Helpful in closing holes in the etheric body due to other entities and, to a lesser extent, due to an individual's own experiences. Soothes after severing an association with a negative entity.

Alyogyne Huegelli (Blue Hibiscus) Increases the capacity of the crown chakra to assimilate and work with information. For accessing the 'cosmic computer'. Can increase understanding of the nature of kundalini energy as it moves through the spine.

Bird of Paradise (*Strelitzia*) For understanding flight, movement. Brings a realization of the interconnectedness among people and communities. Useful in people-management and for the appropriate use of new technology and its impact on freedom – for humour created around relationships and freedom.

Blazing Star (*Liatris* sp.) Can awaken expressive energies felt as a build-up of energy in the heart which then pours through the hands and fingertips, especially the middle finger. Useful in utilizing the energy of love for healing.

Blue Witch (*Solanum umbelliferum*) Has the ability to create energy shifts in chakras 4–9 (the eighth and ninth chakras reside in the subtle bodies), beginning at the heart and extending upwards before returning. May provide a deeper understanding of the higher dimensions.

Butterfly Lily (*Hedychium thyrsiforme*) For attuning to the process of transformation as symbolized by the butterfly; increasing awareness of this transformation for the human race. For those involved in group work when they are faced with insurmountable obstacles. Brings encouragement, strength of purpose and the ability to let go of stress.

California Baylaurel (*Lauris nobilis californica*) Opens the mind and gives a feeling of flexibility to the mind and nervous system. Helps overcome rigid mindsets, ideas and body armour, bringing wisdom. Soothes and relieves.

California Buckeye (*Aesculus californica*) Strengthens one's ability to understand and work with vision. May provide attunement to one's purpose as well as to ecosystems, agriculture and nature spirits. Increases third-eye abilities.

Calypso Orchid (*Calypso bulbosa*) Helps one climb through several spiritual levels simultaneously. Enhances the ability to communicate with the Higher Self or one's guides; encourages teachers to be drawn to you. Cleanses and opens the crown chakra.

Cape Honeysuckle (*Tecoma capensis*) Can bring coordination between the physical body and chakras 4–8. May intensify psychic abilities and a shift in the emotional body. Balances the energies of grief, loneliness and other difficult emotions.

Caterpillar Plant (*Phacella mutabilis*) Brings encouragement to access and receive spiritual gifts of which one is not aware. Makes it easier to assimilate and integrate psychic abilities when they start to appear.

Choke Cherry (*Prunus virginiana*) Brings illumination to a lack of clarity in ourselves and our relationships. Sheds light when we need to see the problem, chasing away the darkness, ending confusion and clarifying motivations.

Clarkia (*C. purpurea*) Brings some affiliation with the energies of forgiveness, especially in relation to physical aspects and the influence of our genetic structures. Brings greater awareness of genetic structures and our ability to work with them.

Coralroot (Spotted) (*Corallorhiza maculata*) Brings greater awareness of the role of disease in our lives, the need to recognize and understand the lesson of disease on subtler levels so that the disease no longer needs to manifest physically. It may reduce the influence of antibiotics which can last for a long time after taking them.

Creeping Thistle (*Onopordum acanthium*) Produces tendrils of light and energy from the seventh chakra, causing a temporary blending or bringing of new energies in many different forms and directions. Can make a bridge from the seventh to the heart to the base chakra. Brings clear internal healing energy to the physical body and steps up vibrational transference from other subtler levels to the physical, which can be a joyful experience.

Curry Leaf Tree (*Murraya koenigii*) A catalyst for things already happening in one's life. Spiritual practices become clearer. Encourages synergy in relationships, especially within the family. Brings playfulness and a sense of relaxed purpose.

Dayflower (*Commelina*) Allows access to greater light, which is especially helpful for the physical body and those using light therapy, and for a greater awareness of the connection between the sun and the Earth. Benefits those seeking to reduce their food intake and increase their attunement to light.

Desert Barrel Cactus (*Ferocactus alamosanus var. pottsii*) Assists those seeking to understand boundaries, where they begin and end, where their relationship to someone begins and ends, where and how they relate to the whole of humanity. Helps us to confront the sadness and separation sometimes felt during our spiritual journey between ourselves and our soul family.

Dragon Flower Cactus (*Huernia macrocarpa*) Assists the capacity to apply spiritual principles to the physical realm. For balancing the physical aspects of the body properly. Especially helpful in movement and exercise.

Dutchman's Breeches (*Dicentra cucullaria*) Enhances the release of emotional residues into the aura which can then be cleansed easily by movement, water or air. Can also clear away residues from negative environments.

Easter Lily Cactus (*Echinopsis multiplex*) For deeper attunement to chaos and the balance of perfect symmetry. Improves communication through gesture and movement.

Elephant's Head (*Pedicularis groenlandica*) Creates a vibrational link to the energies of the angelic kingdom and those associated with humanity's own development. Strengthens the ability to perceive and work with Earth energy. For deeper attunement and awareness of angelic or spirit guides; for wisdom.

Everlasting (*Antennaria rosea*) Helps to moderate a shift in consciousness which contains repressed memories from childhood or past lives. Increases self-esteem and self-recognition of spiritual progress. Encourages positive energy.

Gardenia (*G. jasminoides*) For emotional shifts from accepting one's consciousness in a new way; greater attunement to knowledge received in the recent past. Excellent for student/teacher relationships. Creates a sense of peace, caring and compassion.

Gentian (*Gentiana simplex*) Improves the ability to communicate on many levels. Improves speaking abilities for deeper insights and connection with others. For future expression.

Gilia-Scarlet (*Ipomopsis aggregata*) Gives deep strength to those seeking an understanding about how they populate the Earth and share it with others. Enhances the possibilities of the spiritual aspects of sexuality. May assist in treating mysterious skin complaints. Enhances empathy with the plant and animal kingdoms. Encourages harmony.

Green Gentian (*Frasera speciosa*) Awakens psychic gifts of an expressive nature. Working with the sixth chakra, these gifts can project mind-energy. The accelerated and enhanced ability to project energies of love from a group to many beings will assist the Earth at this time.

Green Rein Orchid (*Habenaria sparsifolora*) For seeing the continuity of patterns of emotions – a common thread running through lifetimes – particularly for understanding one's parents and early upbringing. Benefits both therapist and patient when used for depressive states or co-addictive energies.

Heliconia (*H. flava*) Creates energy spirals which can influence the left and right balance of the subtle bodies. The brain and spine are positively affected. Helps to gain ideas and put them into form, accepting the results and making the necessary internal changes. Strengthens the seventh to tenth chakras.

Holy Thorn (*Euphorbia milii*) Opens the crown chakra, bringing a greater willingness to work with a universal energy connection. Allows a deeper attunement to any particular spiritual avenue. It is best to have a specific being or ideal in mind when taking this essence. Forms a bond with the essential energy behind the spiritual idea or ideal. Best used by itself.

Hooded Ladies' Tresses (*Spiranthes romanzoffiana*) Maintains higher states after peak

experiences, catalytic change or catharsis so they continue in a constant but less intense fashion. Brings a slight strengthening of psychic gifts.

Hydrangea (Green) (*Hydrangea macrophylla*) Works in many ways to combine energies of the chakras, balancing them and allowing them to intermingle and transmute energies in useful ways. For visualizing and awakening the different chakras.

Indian Pipe (*Monotropa uniflora*) Balances the flow of energy between chakras, so enhancing movement. For establishing a clear contact with higher vibrations in channelling. Releases stress/strain in the back.

Kinnick-Kinnick (*Arctostaphylos uva-ursi*) Allows one to connect consciously more easily to others and to break any unnecessary connections. Assists one to move with ease and more freedom and to alleviate unwanted past-life connections.

Lemmon's Paintbrush (*Castilleja lemmonili*) May bring a deeper level of connection to our higher energies. Especially useful in creating a deeper understanding of our interaction with society or communities. For social interaction.

Leopard Lily (*Lilium parvum*) Strengthens our ability to improve self-image. For expressing ourselves clearly and allowing our inner nature to shine through. Especially helpful for public speakers and writers who have an alternative viewpoint.

Lobivia Cactus (*L. aracnacanthus*) For attuning the heart to an awareness of the Christ principles manifest in your relationship to the Earth. May bring a feeling of deeper groundedness and awareness of another, enhancing the interchange of energies between you both.

Milkmaids (*Dentaria californica*) Dissolves critical attitudes towards oneself and others. Brings sweetness, love, acceptance and self-esteem. Helps the heart understand and appreciate goodness and positive qualities so one can let go of judgements and move back to spiritual love.

Mock Orange (*Philadelphus lewisii*) Increases the ability to coordinate in deep states of relaxation and meditation. Useful in forming new ideas. Reduces stress.

Monkeyflower (*Mimulus aurantiacus*) Helps emotional clearing, especially with issues of denial and addictive states. Enhances ability to absorb light directly, providing deep nurturing for the second and third chakras.

Monvellea Cactus (*M. spegazzinii*) For attuning to and understanding the symbolism of the breast and genitals. Brings attunement to moonlight and the unconscious.

Mountain Misery (Kitkitisi) (*Chamaebatia foliolosa*) Increases the ability to stick with a task. To modify old ways so new energies can be brought in. Assists in discovering additional inspiration and deeper understanding of a project.

Mountain Pride (*Penstemon newberryi*) Brings awareness of base chakra energy and understanding of the emotional connection with spirituality. May bring greater acceptance of sexuality and sexual feelings. Restores a clearer sense of one's connection to the Earth energy.

Myrtlewood Tree (*Umbellularia californica*) For projecting healing capacities across long distances. Useful in transferring information about healing work.

Neoporteria Cactus (*N. paucicostata*) Strengthens your higher potential by assisting a deeper contact of the soul with incoming energy. Clarifies and focuses the soul's energy for understanding how to put this into action. For overcoming procrastination and getting going when you see where you wish to go. May create a deeper

and stronger connection to and awareness of your soul group. Enhances motivation.

Noble Star Flower Cactus (*Stapelia nobilis*) For blending of love energies and an awareness of the consequences of eating meat. Assists in giving up meat and adopting a lighter, vegetarian diet out of love and willingness to assist all animals. Brings a sense of love and compassion for the animals that are consumed for food.

Old Maid (Pink/White) (*Catharanthus roseus*) Brings greater understanding of and clarity about what is truly important in life. For working with the inner child. Brings acceptance and forgiveness of parents and of older plaguing patterns. Increases our connection with all things.

Orange Flame Flower Cactus (*Notocactus horstii*) Assists in understanding and releasing anger, to enable us to see how it can improve relationships by creating greater enthusiasm. For understanding our deliberate attempt to be alone and separate in ways that are self-forgiving. Aids an understanding of the differences among people and brings a willingness to release negative attitudes.

Owl's Clover (*Orthocarpus purpurascens*) Brings out joy and an appreciation of artistic expression and talent. Endeavours to develop self-expression, especially those of the dream state. Brings optimism to those out of touch with, depressed about or lacking confidence in their artistic expression.

Pegasus Orchid Cactus (*Epiphyllum*) For evolving a new creation of destiny and purpose which affects this life and future lifetimes. May bring a shift in the way we create new kinds of relationships, which allows the chance for a deeper connection and intimacy between both partners. For future relationships.

Pine Drops (*Pterospora andromedea*) For a clearer perspective on the entire nature of difficult relationships. To realize the higher aspects within any relationship. For increased understanding of the genetic structure and code for individuals. Combines well with alternatives to antibiotics.

Plumeria (*P. obtusa*) Brings a deep awareness of one's roots, connection to the human family and attunement to one's ancestors. Useful in group meditation, especially across great distances, in world peace meditation and harmonic convergence.

Prickly Poppy (*Argemone polyanthemos*) Increases the ability to love in the face of various obstacles, creating a love bond that transcends time and space. Enhances past-life recall in those consciously seeking it. Can increase forgiveness of our own past-life actions and those of others. Assists absolution of those creating war, famine and disease.

Protea (Pink Mink) (*P. neriifolia*) Helps to focus energy in one particular direction. Aids in receiving information from past lives, especially concepts and ideas, integrating them into current ways of thinking. Increases telepathy.

Purple Nightshade (*Atropa purpurata*) Calms and relieves irritation, especially that brought on by trying too hard. Soothes jangled, burned-out nervous states and relieves the emotional disturbance brought on by coffee and other stimulants.

Rattail Cactus (*Aprocactus flagelliformis*) Enhances the capacity to reach into multidimensions, across time and space to extract information including a new knowledge relating to one's cultural heritage. Assists in transcending time and creating a deeper connection to time-flow in the future.

Rattlesnake Plantain Orchid (*Goodyera oblongifolia*) For issues relating to aggressive or male-orientated tendencies. Helps men deal with anger and aggression. Helps women seeking a greater male/female balance in their manner of speech, approach

to men, how they are seen and the way they see themselves.

Red Ginger (*Alpinia purpurata*) Brings the ability to spiritualize many physical characteristics. Opens the base chakra to spiritual energy. Deepens understanding and acceptance of the male/female balance within. Useful for martial arts and dance. Enhances sexuality, Tantra and Taoist, the union of male/female with the Earth.

Red Mountain Heather (*Phyllodoce breweri*) For improving the ability to perceive and work with different forms of sound such as music. Brings greater attunement to the inner voice and vibration of all kinds. Enhances our capacity to love and recognize ourselves in all things. Brings a deeper attachment to all forms of vibration.

Shasta Lily (*Lilium washingtonianum*) Speeds up the etheric bodies. Promotes greater awareness of one's role in serving to heal the Earth. Helps in understanding and utilizing the energies available in different power spots, such as the site of the Joshua Tree and Sedona, which have in the past been a source of revelation to many.

Sierra Rein Orchid (*Habenaria dilatata*) Has an excellent capacity to transmute emotion, so that deeply buried or denied feelings can surface. Especially effective for depression or sadness.

Snowplant (*Sarcodes sanguinea*) Creates a deeper understanding of incoming light and energy, especially for hands-on healers. Strengthens the aura and subtle bodies; supports changes in one's life: new job, new home, new relationships.

Spider Lily (Red) (*Lycoris radiata*) Increases ability of the nadis to reach other dimensional areas. Helps the nadis in the base of the spine to transform and transfer energy from the interdimensional regions, especially the etheric body. Improves the ability to open and close the chakras at will, for taking in what is useful and rejecting that which is not beneficial. Benefits those seeking to strengthen the digestive organs, the sexual reproductive organs, the kidneys and skin.

Starflower (*Trientalis latifolla*) Assists those working with others to understand the truth better, even when it is blocked in their consciousness. Stimulates the second chakra.

Star Thistle (*Centaurea solstitialis*) Helpful for radiating energy. Useful for therapists working with patients, encouraging a higher spiritual awakening in both. Activates the ninth and tenth chakras.

Sulcorebutia Cactus (*S. arenacea*) Creates a vortex of energy within an individual to increase one's focus and alignment with one's own capacities – those associated with the soul, centre of the universe and universal purpose or earthly manifestation. Helps remove obstacles from one's path and may be useful to those who respond poorly to certain holistic treatments.

Swamp Onion (*Allium validum*) Brings a powerful cleansing, usually beginning at the top and working down through the body, from head to toe. Creates an awareness of higher energies associated with such cleansing – a powerful universal energy pouring lovingly through you. Especially useful for cleansing the subtle bodies of things like psychic debris which stand in the way of greater evolution.

Sycamore (*Ficus sycomorus*) Eases stress and overcomes problems of too much or too little discipline. Gives us a handle on life, so we know when to let go.

Tagua (*Phytelephas macrocarpa*) Encompasses the beautiful aspects of elephant ivory in plant form. Brings a sense of great power, longevity, increased memory, strength of purpose, kindness and a deep awareness. Allows direct connection to higher realms. For being aware of how we can release old ways and come to new ones.

Tree Opuntia (*O. consolea falcata*) Assists in maintaining a willingness to change, even when we are comfortable at certain levels of existence. Reminds us to shift and offers us the physical energy for the rapid change necessary at this present time.

Trillium Red (*Trillium rubrum*) Assists in amplifying and grounding our natural healing abilities. Enhances our ability to understand another's life lesson, to recognize what may be beneficial to his or her change and how it may be our own learning experience. Assists those who are bored in their jobs, bringing new ideas into form.

Waikiki Rainbow Cactus (*Epiphyllum*) For seeing our own self-expression act as a deeper connection to others. Enhances self-worth.

Washington Lily (*Lilium washingtonianum*) Increases our innate ability to love unconsciously and universally. Creates a deeper understanding and acceptance of spirituality in its different forms in those approaching difficult spiritual change in life. Strengthens the etheric and astral bodies. Brings spiritual perseverance.

Woolly Sunflower (*Eriophyllum lanatum*) Benefits those working with the sun's energy. Represents the gentler, subtle, female-related aspects of the solar principle. Strengthens the third chakra.

Roses

Fred has further developed a range of roses and feels that of all of the plants that contribute to humanity on Earth, the Rose family is at the apex of the potential healing available for most people. They sit at the top of the flower essence world much in the same way that diamonds offer the greatest healing in the mineral kingdom.

Long ago, in Lemuria times it is said that the Rose family was being worked with by many guides and helpers to ensure their healing attributes were available to humanity in the future. Legend has it that a primary light being, *Cha-a-ra* was instrumental in this group work. In acknowledgement of this, greater healing energy has been brought through the Rose family.

Angel Face Rose (rosy purple) Appreciation. This rose is utilized to deepen appreciation of beauty, the opportunity to awaken higher chakras, and infuse positive helpful energies into people. It acts as a conduit; in appreciating the beauty of this rose, higher vibrational qualities will be enhanced for most people, awakening those spiritual principles in their lives and putting them into action. A natural contact with guides and helpers occurs.

Beauty Secret Urban Stress. This rose essence helps to ease stress and stimulates balance in city environments.

Bella Portugaise Rose (light salmon, pink, peachy and creamy shades) Grace and Beauty. Confers aspects of grace, inner confidence and kindness to those who do not necessarily work with such energies normally. It was especially developed for men to ward off or shift energies that would eventually give rise to the utilization of powerful harmful technologies for war on the planet. Helps to find inner courage and strength, to bring ideas to create a more peaceful society, a way of co-existing and learning from each other. When people are trapped in busy schedules, too much to do, drawn in different directions, it helps to find an inner sense of calm in the busy schedule.

Buff Beauty Urban Stress. This Rose essence stimulates the intellect to better deal with city pressures. It will open the heart, allowing people to adjust to urban living at the heart chakra level.

Cabbage Rose (*Rosa centifolia*, medium pink) Intimate Relationships. Helps change in attitudes towards sexuality, aids understanding the intimate relationship between love and sex. Encourages a new deeper appreciation of the physical bodies, enhancing sexual performance, whilst releasing unconscious shame, guilt and various energies associated with negative sexual patterns from the past. When planning to marry, it helps to dispel previously held belief patterns and find new ways of loving and accepting each other.

Charles de Mills (rose/purple flowers) Humility. This Rose induces courage within people to reveal their true nature. An obvious application is in the acting profession, particularly with method acting, where one utilizes past-life experiences, early childhood experiences, to help shape character. As one's true nature is revealed, it is possible to step back and look at oneself in a new light. Reminds people of their own inherent beauty, allows them to forgive and love others. The result is the emergence of a true humility, and to understand one's place in the universe and receive the highest wisdom from the true source.

Green Rose (*Rosa chinensis viridiflora*) Psychic Balance/Channelling. Enhances all psychic abilities. Develops spiritual healing. One can become a conscious or trance channel. Improves emotional stability, especially for psychics.

Koenign Van Daenmark (*Rosa alba*) Left/Right Brain. The etheric, mental and spiritual bodies are aligned, making it easier to make decisions and recognize destructive elements within the physical body. The left brain is stimulated so that mathematical, computer and language skills are activated. Excellent for use with colour therapy.

Old Blush China Rose (blush pink) Wisdom and Mercy. This rose derives from many naturally occurring blends, and has its roots in ancient Chinese history. In recent times, its focus has been to gain greater wisdom and awareness on how to direct and utilize love for the highest good in society. In Confucian times, wisdom was tempered with mercy and deeper levels of understanding. It helps to recognize past lives lived in ancient China, connect and draw on the wisdom from these lives, making this available at a positive and helpful level for those individuals now alive in China. Tuning into past lives associated with China, with awareness of balance and beauty, helps to see how this energy might be appropriately utilized to assist others, in a caring way.

Reine des Violettes Rose (cerise then violet) Loving Will. A fascinating plant providing interesting and stimulating qualities to connect to higher levels of consciousness and develop a deep understanding of God, directly from one's heart. Assists in creating a powerful loving presence and helps to connect to others, plants and animals. It allows a sense of forgiveness to manifest in the heart. Powerfully energizes and strengthens many characteristics in the physical body. Clears issues based on scarcity, struggle or various habit patterns from humanity. Enables one to switch off and receive energy from a spiritual force, a guiding light or a true path of awareness and awakening.

Rosa Alba (Maiden's Blush, blush pink) Releasing Shame. Helps develop a deep sense of self, and ability to allow the higher energies to make their way into the human consciousness. This rose strongly stimulates the astral body; past-life connections and blocks may come up, relating to shame and aspects that have prevented a deeper awareness of subtler energies being available. With repeated use this confers a deep sense of lovability, and acceptance of love within. It is extremely helpful to take this flower essence just before going to sleep, and invite a dream in which you might feel and sense God's true nature in relation to you.

Rosa Alba Semiplena (white) Deep Forgiveness. Creates a deeper sense of compassion

and the ability to forgive and to have a deep sense of caring. When releasing sadness in deep emotional cleansing, tears may result. These tears can carry away toxicity, and deeply buried energies, such as pesticide, metals, various hormonal imbalances. To cry cleansing tears can be a very powerful healing experience.

Rosa Arkansana (bright red) Acceptance. Provides a newfound ability to love where love previously was denied due to a past-life experience. Allows an individual to accept that love is present deep within, and that it has always been there to draw on. An obvious application is inner city places where there is little exposure to nature. Inspires bringing nature into the city or urban environments, and finding ways in which this most naturally and easily can be introduced. In addition, as one begins to open a more conscious love, the deep levels of sadness can be healed. Helps one understand the entire process of accepting deeper love.

Rosa Banksia Lutescens (yellow) Divine Intellect. Opens the intellect to the divine. Activates the solar plexus chakra and enhances mental faculties.

Rosa Beggeriana (white, N. Persia) Increased Intuition. Stimulates intuition and psychic sight. Increased insight into personal issues.

Rosa Brunoni (Himalayan Musk Rose, white) Higher Purpose. Brings the capacity to enhance spiritual wisdom in humans. This encourages a conscious awareness of the need for deeper spiritual connection and contemplation of the important attributes within spiritual teaching or spiritual wisdom. Brings dogged persistence and a willingness to address issues. As shifts occur awareness of higher purpose on Earth comes through; simultaneously a wonderful positive joyful feeling occurs. As the individual surrenders to divine purpose, it fosters awareness of one's place in the universe and the sheer joy of being.

Rosa Californica (pink, California) Outgoing and Friendly. This elixir can be very useful for introverted personalities, helping to overcome problems and phobias around small, enclosed places.

Rosa Canina (Dog Rose) Enthusiasm. For those who need a change and more interest in life. And those who have lost the spark, and have become resigned to their lot. Helps positive change.

Rosa Carolina (Pasture Rose, rosy pink) Family Forgiveness. For self-forgiveness, where it relates to family matters. Relieve the need for revenge or retribution, so deeper acceptance of the soul family can result. Families tend to travel across the karmic landscape in groups, frequently reincarnating to work on issues, to heal them and change them. Many issues will be brought into greater clarity and it will be easier to have the patience to allow these issues to unfold naturally. Brings a sense of forgiveness for all of the buried aspects in one's family, so that memories of earlier childhood incidents are cleared.

Rosa Centifolia Cristata (pink) Enhanced Love. Combines emotion and the understanding of universal love. For the increase of consciousness so deeper states of meditation can result in the better understanding of religious concepts. Emotional difficulties and blocked feelings dissipate. This is likely to give individuals far greater ability to love. One may experience a natural release of emotional blockages, and a tendency to open the astral body. This opens, when it is fully cleansed, so understanding of the future, not always conscious, but as a gut feeling, can occur.

Rosa Centifolia Parvifolia (pink, violet, Europe) Divine Purpose. Helps to open the crown chakra to assist in understanding one's divine purpose. Positively stimulates the dream state.

Rosa Chinensis Mutabilis (flowers opening yellow inside, orange outside, becoming coppery-salmon on the second day, then crimson as they age) Higher Creative Force. Integration of higher subtle bodies; the mental into the astral, to some extent into the emotional. However, there is a higher component, sometimes found in the astral body and the mental body, strengthened by the mental functioning. Producing a sense of deep relaxation felt in the neck and shoulders, eases tensions, and positively affects the gallbladder and bladder meridians.

Rosa Chinensis Minima (Fairy Rose, rosy pink) Devic Perception. Associated with the devic orders, the fairy kingdom, and the devas working with small plants and fungi. It allows individuals a deeper sense of the joy in connecting with this realm. When welcoming and attuning to this energy it enables engaging with the childlike self and to be able to see with the eyes of the child, and recognize energy in a more fluid, open way.

Rosa Chinensis Serratipetala (red, pink in cooler climates) Universal Love. Creates a deep sense of fearless love, when entering into dangerous situations; finding love in ways that they would not normally be available. Where society has taught to hate, dislike, shun or judge. When releasing prejudice, it shows the interconnectivity amongst all; as one recognizes how much alike we are. Then we are able to love, honour, appreciate other cultures, particularly helpful when travelling. Awakens the root chakra, fourth or heart chakra, and the ninth chakra.

Rosa Cinnamomea (pink, purple, Eurasia) Mental Insight. Balances philosophical issues. The intellect is stimulated to transcend the mundane, for example, if someone felt that the philosophies of the East and West were incompatible, this essence would generate the intuitive insight to show the compatibility of these teachings.

Rosa Complicata (brilliant pink with a white centre) Easing Fear. Unconsciously eases fears, helping you to acknowledge them. In relation to self-image, to demonstrate how ideas about oneself can leave one vulnerable to fears of others when fears are transferred. This often takes place unconsciously in childhood; it is natural that children will tend to absorb the fears of their parents. Valuable for becoming more aware of your own fears or habit patterns, and how they may be unconsciously transferred to your children.

Rosa Coriifolia Froebelii (white) Higher Manifestation. Stimulates and opens the crown chakra allowing stored childhood energies into our consciousness, draws in higher energies to be received at the appropriate chakra level, relieving stress that develops as a result of the sense of this communication not made clear enough.

Rosa Corymbifera (white/pink, Asia) Calm/Peace. Releases stress stored in head, neck or shoulders. Better understanding of spiritual, religious or philosophical ideals occurs.

Rosa Damascena Bifera (pink, Europe) Addictive Personality. For the addictive personality and for overcoming addictions. Opens the third chakra.

Rosa Damascena Versicolor (white/pink, Europe) Thought Addiction. Enhances telepathy, and other intuitive processes are better understood and utilized. It can lessen overreliance on thought, logic and reason in one's life.

Rosa Ecae (yellow, Asia Minor, Turkestan) Astral Balancer. This flower helps to overcome philosophical prejudices or preconceptions, which naturally increases intuition and insight. It can be a strong balancer for the astral body.

Rosa Eglanteria (bright pink) Opens Heart. Awakens the heart energy connecting it to higher spiritual wisdom. Some people may be pushed to states of despair as they feel a powerful love inside. Helps us recognize that as love increases, wells up or strengthens it creates focus, and the need for the person to be useful or valuable. Springing from a deep awe of many aspects of life, it focuses in the heart to awaken deeper levels of acceptance of God's energy in all things. Forgiveness for mistakes made in life occurs, breaking habit patterns and finding new ways to struggle less with habits. At the higher vibrational level, it provides a sense in individuals of deep appreciation of many aspects of the world, a sense of sweetness or benefit to life.

Rosa Farrerii Persetosa (pink, China) Artistic Ability. This elixir opens the heart and the crown chakras, stimulating artistic ability.

Rosa Fendleri Woodsii (pink, white, United States) Overcomes Shyness. Helps overcome acute introversion and fear of meeting people. It will also improve one's insight, and enhance one's negotiating skills.

Rosa Foetida Bicolor (yellow/orange) New Aesthetic Sensibilities. Encourages a sense of beauty in art, shifts consciousness because of seeing with new eyes, and seeing in ways not previously seen before, making new associations. When overstimulated it is helpful for brain fatigue and difficulty with assimilation of new knowledge. Applicable when seeking to develop a new aesthetic sense, deepen understanding, shift judgement. Brings the ability to re-evaluate, re-prioritize and let go of judgements. Aids perceiving beauty, art or magnificence of life, musical and dance forms, and graphic arts. Helps to transform landscape, urban or rural, change various living conditions by working with Feng Shui and a sense of balance.

Rosa Forrestiana (pink) Creative Imagination. Engages imagination, perceiving and exploring new areas. Imagination without constraint. Encourages an abundant source of inspiration and creativity. The uplifting energies of creativity are valuable and useful to help people to feel excited about life, and feel a sense of accomplishment leading to new ideas, new ways of relating to others. A light-hearted playful essence.

Rosa Gallica Officinalis (red, France) Spiritual Rejuvenation. Promotes mental and emotional balance. Powerful opening of the heart chakra. Stimulates joy and spiritual rejuvenation.

Rosa Gymnocarpa (Little Woods Rose, pink) Psychic Function. Helps blend different parts of the personality, accepting them in a loving way, and allowing psychic abilities and paranormal abilities to naturally blossom and strengthen. Especially for those with a clairsentience ability or those who work with psychometry, or kinaesthetic abilities. Develops acceptance of the buried hidden abilities, the shadow self and the willingness to blend these aspects with other parts of one's life. Encourages self-acceptance as well as the loving self, the judgemental self, integrating these aspects that have previously created disharmony or stress.

Rosa Hardii (yellow, Europe) Inner Joy. Can attune individuals to their own inner awareness, light and energy. Brings a greater connectedness to life, the sun and the fairy kingdom. Also brings a greater understanding of the need for joy, and an awareness of the light and joy around and within.

Rosa Horrida (white, Europe) Universal Love. Cleansing of spiritual sadness. Brings an awareness of humanity's struggles and helps show how they can be overcome. Helps achieve forgiveness for the human condition.

Rosa × Harrisonii (Harrison's Yellow Rose, Yellow Rose of Texas) Honest Communication. Pioneering, finding freedom, accepting personal responsibility and a willingness to share this with others. In the revelation of truth, finding ways to be more honest with oneself and sharing this with others, even if this causes some temporary disharmony. Encourages clarity within finding areas of denial so that a way of deeper honesty can be revealed. Confers a level of warmth, as the devas associated with this Rose share loving energy, encouraging people to find a way of being clear in their communications with each other.

Rosa Helenae (white) Higher Truth. Devas associated with this plant are very adaptable and are programmed with information from the Lemurian times; helps to adapt to many different energies. At the subtle level, it is important for humanity to draw in new concepts to work with as needed, and having gained sufficient knowledge, find the next level of awareness. Aids the understanding of different absolute truths and relative truths. Helps to ascertain the specific aspects of truth in your life, and is helpful for understanding and growth, and letting go of past-held belief patterns.

Rosa Hemispherica (yellow, Sulphur Rose) Energy Generation. Aids blending of different energies within, at the physical and etheric level. The blending together of the male and female aspects of the self results in many different approaches in life, and different ways of being. This enables flexibility. It is valuable for self-healing, to integrate and work with energies of all different types, and bring a sense of self-love and the capacity to assist our own healing throughout life.

Rosa Hugonis (yellow, China) Visions. This elixir helps to stimulate visions as well as literary and linguistic skills.

Rosa Kamchatka (red, Siberia) Perseverance. It activates the ability to focus and persevere and strengthens the will.

Rosa Laevegata (Cherokee Rose, white) Enhanced Healing Ability. Encourages and strengthens the sixth chakra, opening the third eye, bringing a deeper sense of clarity, and at the same time, an awareness of an inner silence, and the capacity to receive energy from many levels. Hands-on healing or energy work will be accelerated and assisted. With repeated use, a deeper sense of connectedness and understanding of humanity and its role on Earth develops. As adaptability increases, the capacity to fit into other societies, learn other languages, and adapt to their customs develops which can assist multicultural bridging or capacity to expand horizons.

Rosa Longicuspis (white, Himalayas) Creativity. This essence will open the brow and crown chakras and the kundalini. It activates creative and artistic sensitivities.

Rosa Macrantha (light pink, Europe) Energy Blocks. Use it to release blockages in the meridians and nadis.

Rosa Macrophylla (red, Himalayas) Greater Love. This is the most powerful Rose essence on the planet. Opens the heart chakra. Native to the Himalayas.

Rosa Maximowicziana (white) Shifting Boundaries. Using this Rose can assist individuals in understanding themselves better, where they have walled off or allowed various aspects of their own personality, consciousness or things that they are interested in to become segmented, to become in some sense denied or unavailable. To make such an energy more available in a loving, welcoming, accepting fashion is likely to be enhanced for nearly everyone using this flower essence.

Rosa Moschata (Musk Rose, white) Improving Relationships. Awareness of compassion, caring and the love felt in the Higher Self. Clears self-blame, in which an individual is unaware of how they are creating a deeper separation by holding judgemental beliefs. The heart begins to open in new ways, in order to incorporate love from one's Higher Self.

Rosa Moyesii (pink) Life Purpose. This flower can energize the evolutionary process, either of reincarnation, or the process of successive levels of self-awakening that a soul goes through. Gives one the concentration to overcome many earthly distractions in the accomplishment of one's life purpose. Reawakens a sense of joy in being on the Earth, having the capacity to do good in the world.

Rosa Multibractea (light pink) Life Purpose. Enhances the ability to have a sense of one's own sacred work, and appreciate what we are here for and how work can be of maximum utility and value to others. Typical flashes and awareness of this higher purpose will tend to occur early in life, perhaps at age three or so; then as a more defined purpose, focalizing around age 28. A deep sense of forgiveness and love must be felt and at the same time a deeper sense of joy.

Rosa Multiflora (white) Earth Sensitivity. Creates a powerful connection to Mother Earth, and the ability to assist our life path through a deep self-love. As the heart is opened when working with these energies, a deep sense of peace or calm develops, a sense of timelessness and patience develops when waiting to see how things will unfold. Enhances psychic awareness of Earth changes, the properties of plants and animals. Brings attunement to the weather, and encourages the ability to perceive the weather before it manifests. Produces a healing effect that can be transmitted to others, stimulating the healing abilities through the use of sound or working with sound from the human voice.

Rosa Multiflora Carnea (pale pink variety) Unconditional Love. The Lemurians developed and worked with this flower. It holds the energy of unconditional love that is an aspect or manifestation principle of the Earth's energy. If we resonate with this sense of Earth's unconditional love, it awakens unconditional love within.

Rosa Nutkana (pink, United States) Self-Denial. Useful in bringing forth denied emotions. Aids in creating more loving relationships. Promotes greater intergenerational understanding and bonding.

Rosa Odorata (white, pink or yellow) Integration. Awakens the root chakra with energy that bubbles up through the rest of the body. Shows how integration can occur, brings energies from many different sources, learned from past lives, this life, integrating and utilizing it for the problem at hand, giving rise to new possibilities and new applications. Helpful in group activity, corporations or wishing to change what is established, especially when struggling with bureaucracies, and seeking to understand systems as they are. It is helpful in order to be patient and to see things from other people's point of view, then find the right steps to take in order to deal with the situations. Also brings joy and strength to gardeners, to those who wish to work with Roses, through attunement.

Rosa Paulii (white, clove scented) Shifting Ego. Allows a deeper sense of love and humility. For those who wish to help others, but don't want to be in a position of obligation or constant interaction. Releases the desire or need for appreciation. Encourages a deep understanding or appreciation of God's energy, not asking anything in return, allowing opportunities on many levels which can lead to all kinds of pleasurable and wonderful aspects in life.

Rosa Pendulina (*Rosa Alpina*) (pink to purple) Risk Taking. Allows people the opportunity to take risks more easily, share energies with each other in ways they have not previously. Opens us to new ways of loving, feeling and working, with love as a result. Risk taking can be pathological in some individuals, with the addiction to dangerous sports or activities that risk life and limb. Helps to modify these practices, see them in a different perspective and find ways of achieving the same sense of thrill or life-awakening, without bodily danger.

Rosa Primula (pale yellow) Spiritual Healing. Accelerates the development of spiritual wisdom when applied to healing, and counselling that comes from the heart, where a deeper loving energy is established. This can shift consciousness to awaken the Christ-like principles. Discovering an inner Christ-knowledge depends on people's own particular perception. It awakens the crown chakra; connecting through the body into the heart, allows a deeper fuelling of heart energy from incoming energy through the crown chakra. But this energy must have some point of focus or some particular quality of assistance, either to assist or help someone.

Rosa Pterogonis Group Healing. Develops a deeper sense of group identity and a sense of that group being loving and helpful to others. Useful to teams who seek healing or give assistance to others, in esoteric or practical healing: a hospital staff or a group of hands-on healers. Those who are studying and working with healing energy of any kind may find a level of unconscious competition between the members. Helps to relieve this, bringing people to a state of harmony as they work together. At the gross physical level provides rapid healing from surgery, other forms of interventions in the body, and ways in which the healing would be speeded up.

Rosa Roxburghii (pink, Japan, China) Meditation Enhanced. This is to be used for enhancing meditation and all right-brain type activities.

Rosa Rubrifolia Interpersonal Relationships. Imparts greater conscious will in one's ability to manifest love in the world. Stimulates the heart on the etheric level.

Rosa Rugosa Alba (white, China) Isolation. This is to be used for getting through periods of isolation, such as when in retreat with fasting or meditation.

Rosa Sericea (white, Himalayas) Spiritualizes Intellect. This elixir will open up the kundalini, the crown, heart and base chakras. It also clears blockages from the meridians. The intellect is spiritualized, and there is more communication with one's Higher Self and guides.

Rosa Sericea Pteracantha (white, Wingthorn Rose) Higher Purpose. Gives a deep understanding of the principle of tough love. This can be the capacity to love in a way that can produce dramatic change, such as installing new habit patterns, modes of thinking and feeling. Some individuals who go through a shift around the age of 28 experience deep levels of sadness and lost opportunity. This essence gives an innate sense of joy, strength and awareness of greater possibilities. Develops an intuitive sense of what is appropriate in our life, what we are here to learn and do, and who we are here to meet, but have for some reason denied or unconsciously avoided. Simply becoming aware of that pattern can be of tremendous value to individuals and save them a great deal of time and effort.

Rosa Sinowilsonii (white, China) Clairaudience. Activates psychic hearing (clairaudience).

Rosa Spinosissima Altaica (white) Interconnection. Utilized in assisting individuals with deep transformation and their ability to connect to other people, to feel a sense of commonality or bridging at a heart level. For people who find themselves isolated, separate, alone, perhaps in a place of darkness and struggle, it encourages understanding and receiving of the energy from this flower. As a flower essence it encourages a sense of camaraderie, shared oneness, loving energy between people. Works with the issue of loneliness, to help the individual to understand that they are inherently connected, that they are not alone.

Rosa Stellata (mauve) Vibrational Reception. Encourages communication with guides and helpers, to allow new sources of coherent, well-integrated information to be better transmitted, as if one's antennae are strengthened. Creates the release of inherent belief patterns blocking these energies. Fears will be eased, and better understood. For fear of intimacy. Enables speaking personal truths regardless of the consequences; and results in enhanced telepathy, and contact with other beings, guides and helpers. Allows vision from a higher perceptive; has a profound effect in helping an individual to see issues which they had previously held back.

Rosa Sweginzowii (bright pink) Higher Group Interaction. Shifts the nature of love people experience, making it more physical. Helpful in relationships of all types – business, personal or family. Creates clarity in one-to-one and group interaction.

Rosa Villosa (pink/red, Eurasia) Creative Visualization. This can stimulate dreams, astral projection and creative visualization.

Rosa Virginiana (pink, United States) Inner Calm. Assists individuals in projecting an inner sense of stillness and calm into their words as they speak them. Charisma will be encouraged and amplified.

Rosa Webbiana (pink, Himalayas) Earth/Angelic Attunement. Use this major essence to attune to the Earth's crown chakra. Stimulates the super-conscious and rapport with angelic realms. Opens the heart chakra and psychic abilities, especially channelling faculties.

Rosa Woodsii (Mountain Rose, pink) Energetic Connection. Enables better personal contact, communication and awareness. For most individuals, this energy extends from the navel area, integrating energies of the second and third chakras. Relates to emotional connection, specifically in relationship to business or pleasure, and the ability to see yourself in someone else. At a higher vibrational level, one can perceive the good nature in another, and see it as intrinsically lovable. This helps with negotiation, to see somebody else's point of view, understand their consciousness, desires, needs; and then be able to meet them halfway. Perceiving this deeper level sometimes involves letting go of aspects of yourself in order to truly see the other person as deeply lovable, as well as yourself.

Rosa Xanthina (golden yellow, N. China) Creative Visualization. For creative visualization, meditation and hypnosis practices. It will help healers remove negativity, and it also opens the heart.

Seven Sisters Rose (*Rosa multiflora platyphylla*) Youthfulness. There is a natural affiliation between this Rose and the star system of the Pleiades. As people work with these energies, they discover all kinds of shifts, sometimes a reminder of an ancient lifetime associated with the Pleiades. Shifts at a physical level will reduce the ageing effect, resulting in greater youthfulness, inherent strength and other energies of a positive helpful nature.

Sterling Silver Rose (Silvery Lavender) Law of Reflection. Helps with working out issues in relationships, especially understanding more deeply and consciously the law of reflection. Allows seeing things from different points of view, and perspectives, helps in holding a dualistic vision. Awakens higher consciousness, and the awareness that love can bridge apparent opposites. Encourages a deeper acceptance of oneself.

White Bath Rose (*Rosa centifolia mucosa alba*, White Moss Rose) God Awareness. Develops a deeper understanding and awareness of past lives, and the last intermissive period. Promotes connection to God and awareness of God's love. This energy connects with the heart and higher spiritual reality. Above all else it is a direct awareness of God's love.

PETITE FLEUR ESSENCES (PF)

The Petite Fleur essences are created by Judy Griffin, a fourth-generation flower essences maker on her Italian mother's side; she is a master herbalist and professional gardener who has already written five books on these subjects. She is a scientist with a PhD in nutrition from the University of Alabama who has also spent time studying various disciplines with Chinese, Indian, Native American and Mediterranean peoples.

These essences were developed in response to Judy's recognition that 80 per cent of disease prevalent in Western society is related to stress. This brought her to the realization that any treatment which focuses on just one aspect of illness will always be incomplete. A more holistic approach is needed which addresses mind, body and spirit.

The Petite Fleur Essences are used internationally by progressive medical and chiropractic physicians as well as health-care practitioners. The original 60 wildflower essences affect the attitudes connected to our emotions and fears and their related endocrine responses. The Native Texans strengthen the essential character – a form of fine-tuning – and clear inappropriate models and, together with wildflower essences, focus on enhancing the immune system by correcting unstable emotional signals which trigger the 'fight or flight' stress response. Essences in the Antique Rose collection enhance the nervous system, while the Master essences awaken consciousness by aiding personality transitions and helping us to focus on the here and now so we can fulfil our destiny. They also work to harmonize all chakras. These can be used as enhancers in association with the Native Texans and Antique Roses.

In the words of Judy Griffin: 'Mother nature awaits with open arms to transcend physical, emotional and mental limitations as we expand our conscious awareness and oneness with the Eternal Life Force.'

Judy has continued to develop the range and brought out the New Native Texans which address immune system issues and the New Antique Roses which expand their work with the nervous system.

In her work with hospitals and hospices she has shown how supportive the Petites can be with cancer (see pages 108–109). She has also created special blend combinations appropriate for common-day problems. Judy has also designed Feng Shui sprays, especially to cleanse, harmonize, balance and enhance life and the environment as well as attracting positive and abundant energy.

African Violet (*Saintpaulia* sp.) Promotes nurturing, love from within and the release of endorphins which bring feelings of elation and ease pain. Helps heal wounds.

Amaryllis (*Hippeastrum l.*) For anxiety about the future. Brings clarity about the future, helps overcome fears of what may lie in store and enhances intuitive abilities. Also treats parasites.

Anemone (*Coronaria coccinea*) For when life is hard, a struggle and you cannot experience pleasure. Also helps regenerate tissue damaged by scarring or burning.

Azalea (*Rhododendron oblongifolium*) For those who are left-brain dominated and wish to be more creative. Enhances creativity and visualization, bringing forth latent talents.

Babies' Breath (*Gypsophila paniculata L.*) For those who reject new ideas by thinking 'it won't work'. Encourages childlike faith and innocence. Eases congestion in the lungs; benefits asthma and emphysema.

Bachelor's Button (*Centaurea cyanus*) For those who keep looking back and are afraid to release the past. Brings beginner's luck and an ability to complete projects. Helps release suppressed tears and eases oedema.

Bamboo (*Chamaedorea erumpens*) For those who are not sure what to do next. Helps in planning career, setting goals, learning to have fun. Eases intestinal upsets, lack of colonic acidity.

Basil (*Ocimum basilicum*) For critical people, high achievers who feel they are not good enough. Encourages self-nurturing habits. Helps purify the blood.

Begonia (*Begoniaceae odorata*) For having a belief in limitations. Encourages letting go and the realization that even global problems can be solved. Acts as a diuretic for the kidneys. Helps the sensory nerves.

Bouquet of Harmony (blend) For uncontrolled thoughts and emotions when the imagination runs riot. Helps discipline the mind, focusing attention and bringing a sense of direction.

Bougainvillea (*Nyctaginaceae glabra*) For guilt, fear of reprisal. Helps others enjoy life and fulfil their desires. Eases local aches and pains.

Chamomile (*Anthemis nobilis*) For those who swallow their hurt, feeling misunderstood. Brings counsel. Good for indigestion and a sluggish gallbladder.

Crepe Myrtle (*Lagerstroemia indica*) For those who are afraid to speak their mind or of seeming foolish by expressing themselves incorrectly. Brings the realization that rage often underlies such fears. Fosters the ability to release this anger in a creative way and to speak only words of kindness.

Crossandra (*C. infundibuloiformis*) For people who are insecure and fearful of new ideas or any major changes in life, not wanting to rock the boat. This personality is prone to gastrointestinal stagnation and toxicity, and also to catarrh. Helpful in any new situations over which we have no control – such as having a baby, moving to a new job or environment. Encourages you to 'go for it'.

Daffodil (*Narcissus naegelia*) For quiet, timid, shy people who try to please everyone, placing themselves under constant tension and anxiety which causes symptoms like heart palpitations. Their aversion to anger and angry scenes may stem from being intimidated by explosive or violent parents. Helps you to feel more at ease with yourself and others, not needing to appease others all the time.

Dianthus (*Caryophyllaceae chinesis*) For apathetic people who claim they 'don't care', feeling uncared for and separate from humanity, uninterested in life and having nothing to look forward to. They are withdrawn and often anaemic. Helps us to view life in a brighter way, rekindling enthusiasm and self-nurturing.

Garden Mum (*Chrysanthemum morifolium*) For critical, bitter thoughts which often affect the liver and gallbladder. Aids the flow of bile. For those secretly wishing the worst for everyone else and always looking for a scapegoat. Enhances love for mankind, and acceptance of people as they are. Brings compassion.

Iris (*Pallida*) For mental strain that stems from being overanalytical and logical, left-brain dominated, having an explanation for everything, prone to violent behaviour. Releases latent creative abilities, allowing us to feel carefree and humorous. Encourages carefree feelings, promotes a sense of humour. Helps regulate blood pressure, temperature and breathing.

Japanese Magnolia (*Magnolia verbanica*) For women who are unhappy, feeling dependent on men, vulnerable and used. Also for sufferers of premenstrual syndrome, headaches, fluid retention. Brings a sense of

independence, equality and security. Eases physical problems.

Jasmine (*Jasminum nudiflorum*) For loners, those who rebel against authority and find it difficult to get on well with others. They may be prone to accidents such as bone fractures due to a weakness in skeletal structure. Eases bursitis and cartilage/bone/tendon disease. Replaces feelings of alienation with diplomacy. Helps you to find peace in your environment.

Lantana (*L. camana*) For those who are quiet, artistic, oversensitive, easily hurt and shy. They may be sensitive to allergens – hay fever sufferers. Helps us to become more independent and assertive, feeling less threatened. For commanding respect.

Lemon Grass (*Cymbopogon citratus*) For those who need nurturing, often rejected by parents, feeling that love hurts and being drawn to painful relationships. Eases pain and promotes self-nurturing, learning to trust and reach out to love. Enhances the absorption of vitamin A.

Ligustrum (*Oleaceae privet lucidum*) For an inability to be assertive or express anger, leading to apathy or haughtiness, fatigue and lack of spontaneity. Also for energy leaks from the aura, internal bleeding, liver toxicity, weak eyes, immune deficiency, hypothyroidism. Releases repressive feelings, rekindles optimism and encourages self-expression. Eases physical symptoms.

Lilac (*Syringa vulgaris*) For those with a tendency to hold grudges. Also for tumours, growths and cancers. Helps forgiveness of self and others, releases the past.

Lily (*Lilacea longiflorum*) For those who are anxious about the outcome of everyday affairs and the future, fearful of not being in control of their destiny. Typically such people bite their fingernails or demonstrate other compulsive behaviour. Also for colds, flu, autotoxicity, skin diseases and allergies. Releases anxiety and fear. Helps to boost the immune system.

Magnolia (*Magnolia grandiflora*) For those lacking self-appreciation or belief in themselves, feeling undeserving. For problems with the assimilation of nutrients and protein. Increases self-confidence and boosts self-image, so you can prosper and grow.

Marigold (*Tagetes patula*) For guilt about sexual permissiveness, sexual guilt, confusion about sexual role or identity. For impotence, hormone imbalance, prostate problems, sterility and frigidity. Balances male and female aspects of the self so we can accept both sides of ourselves without feeling threatened.

Morning Glory (*Convolvulacea*) For those deluding themselves with the idea of a golden past, romanticizing better times and making the present seem unpleasant. Also for uric acid accumulation and bowel problems. Helps us to find faith in ourselves and in the future. Aids circulation and eliminatory systems.

Moss Rose (*Portulaca floreplens*) For those feeling they need more of anything – money, possessions – giving rise to anxiety and the feeling that they lack something. They may also be prone to weight problems. Also helps problems of pancreatic function, irregular glucose absorption, poor digestion of starches and fats, and proteolytic enzyme production. Enables a change of outlook, seeing yourself as sufficiently providing for your needs.

Mushroom (*Shiitake*) For feeling insecure about changes in life, leading to procrastination and resistance. Also for discomfort in the feet, ankles, calves, spine and neck. Helps you to become more independent and adaptable.

Narcissus (*N. cyclamineus*) For those who are withdrawn and introverted, living in their own world and reluctant to share themselves with others. Prone to migraine,

tension and neuralgia. Enhances feelings of pleasure and security, promoting warmth and affection.

Onion (*Allium cepa*) For those who are narrow-minded, holding one-sided opinions and becoming critical of others' views and habits. Cultivates tolerance, compassion and the ability to listen. Also helps treat viral infections and fevers.

Orchid (*Onchidium sphacelatum*) For those (often high achievers) who silently punish themselves for past failures. May suffer from numbness and nerve degeneration. Helps us to become less workaholic and more interested in loved ones and the community.

Pansy (*Viola tricolor*) For those experiencing a deep-seated sense of grief over the loss of a loved one. Affects adrenal and kidney function. Brings transcendence over grief, pointing the way to new outlets for our loving nature and generosity. Helps in the elimination of toxins.

Penta (*Pentas lanceolata*) For selfish, self-reliant people who are inconsiderate of others, withholding love and thinking that love hurts. They often suffer from low blood pressure. Also for vertigo, lack of oxygenation. Eases pain and promotes feelings of wellbeing and self-love, making for a more delightful partner or spouse.

Peppermint (*Mentha piperita*) For those who live in fear of losing loved ones, possessions, health, security, of having little control over their emotions. May suffer inner conflict related to an incomplete relationship with their mother. Builds confidence and a sense of control; fosters the ability to visualize a future in which their desires are fulfilled, making life feel safer. Also aids protein digestion and treats gastric ulcers.

Periwinkle (*Vinca rosea*) For clearing past experiences. Clarifies goals, affords a greater overview of life and boosts energy levels. Heals and regenerates.

Pine (*Pinus sylvestris*) For those who only remember mistakes of the past, experiencing guilt, punishment and pain. For fatigue brought on by poor absorption of nutrients; for aches and mood swings. Cultivates inner strength and perseverance, so we can learn positive lessons from past misfortunes.

Pink Geranium (*Pelargonium* × *hortorum*) For those who appear tense, suppressing their anger and intense emotions. Linked to spastic colon, liver/gallbladder trouble and muscular spasticity. Eases emotional pain, bringing laughter and enjoyment of life.

Pink Rose (*Rosa chinesis*) For those with a 'fat' complex, always trying the latest diet, rejecting themselves. Also for those who are genuinely overweight or plagued by cellulite. Promotes a better self-image and a perspective that acknowledges and focuses on what can be changed.

Poppy (*Hunnemannia*) For demanding, selfish people who can be jealous and covet others' belongings. Also for mucoid colitis, constipation and tuberculosis. Cultivates generosity and service to others.

Primrose (*Primula vulgaris*) For those rejecting love as not being good enough, having a romantic and idealistic view of what 'love' should be. Physically manifests as diabetes, hypoglycaemia. Cultivates an appreciation of relationships and an acceptance of love.

Ranunculus (*Asiaticus*) For mental instability, imbalance in the brain expressed as schizophrenia, violence, rage, psychosis. Sufferers may have been abused in childhood and/or deprived of tender loving care by their mother. Also for premature birth, epilepsy, poor muscle tone and immature nervous system. Restores a balance of energy to the pleasure centres of the brain.

Red Carnation (*Caryophyllacea rosa*) For those with an inferiority complex, feeling unworthy and lonely, unable to accept success. Prone to lymphatic congestion, swollen glands, skin afflictions, hair loss and baldness. Enhances self-image and feelings of worthiness.

Red Rose (*Rosa chinesis*) For gloominess and occasional depression. Replaces negative thoughts with enthusiasm and joy.

Rose of Sharon (*Althaea officinalis*) For those who are idealistic, straightforward, honest, highly creative and successful but sometimes feel burdened by responsibilities and want to escape from reality. Indicated for heart action – angina pectoris. Attracts just rewards for creativity.

Salvia (*Salvia coccinea*) For self-dislike and feeling ugly. Brings constructive changes to one's self-image. Improves acne, warts, moles, birthmarks and other blemishes, and skin diseases.

Shrimp (*Beloperone guttata*) For those who are dissatisfied with themselves, disliking and feeling lumbered with their lifestyle, keenly aware of others' achievements and assets. This attitude upsets the immune system's ability to handle everyday stress. Also for combating the ageing process. Speeds the process of change and allows creative ideas to flow.

Stock (*Matthiola incana*) For tense, nervous, hyperactive types – dependent on nicotine and other chemicals – susceptible to physical exhaustion and mood swings because they are unable to pace themselves. Slows down and balances out energy, enabling completion of projects.

Sunflower (*Helianthus annuus*) For those feeling separated from the universal spirit, rejected and left to fend for themselves – persecuted, fearing death, feeling suicidal. Brings a sense of responsibility for actions. Integrates the personality and soul/spirit.

Tiger's Jaw Cactus (*Faucaria tuberculosa*) For those who like sitting and watching others do the work. Essentially immobilized by fear of failure to the point of apathy and laziness. May be spoiled and inconsiderate or a 'non-participant' (out of hypochondria). Brings the motivation to be confident and productive.

Vanilla (*Vanilla planifolia*) For those overwhelmed by negative energy from others and themselves, feeling tired, depressed and irritated for no apparent reason, needing to withdraw from a situation or individual. Also for neurological overload or psychic attack. Offers protection against such influences, helping you stay clear and in control of your individual environment without unnecessary interference.

Verbena (*Verbenaceae*) For inner turmoil, frustration, impulsive action. Induces a meditative feeling of inner peace. Allows mind and body to relax and regenerate.

Wandering Jew (*Setcreasea purpurea*) For those who are easily discouraged, lacking discipline, giving up easily. Prone to inflammation or neuritis/shingles. Helps us to achieve greater confidence and self-discipline so projects can be completed; to learn patience and tolerance.

White Carnation (*Caryophyllaceae*) For those who are stubborn and headstrong, resulting in constant anxiety, tension and mood swings. Adrenal hormone upsets (the fight-or-flight syndrome). Eases fear of failure, balances desire and releases anxiety. Brings contentment.

White Hyacinth (*Hyacinthus*) For shock and trauma, especially that of birth which is linked with feelings of uncertainty and insecurity. Nervous exhaustion. Releases the shock of emotional and physical trauma (e.g. accidents, operations and violence). Enhances sense of self-reliance.

White Petunia (*Solanaceae*) For those who have difficulty making decisions and acting on them, unable to synchronize thoughts, concentration and body movements. For dyslexia, stuttering – and also

past negative programming. Aids coordination and the synergy of right and left brain function.

White Rose (*Rosa alba noisette*) For those attracting negativity from others, feeling undefined fears. For 'psychic attack', and also loss of memory. Offers protection from negative thought-forms; cultivates self-confidence and ability to feel comfortable with anyone.

Wisteria (*Wisterea macrostachya*) For those who are unaware of loving feelings, not feeling love at all. Opens us up to receive and give unconditional love. A heart tonic for enjoying everyone.

Zinnia (*Zinnea elegans*) For those feeling unloved, hurt and angry, critical of themselves and others, bitter at being deprived of nurturing attention. Often affected by arthritic or rheumatic pain. Heavy metal toxicity. Encourages self-nurturing, releases bitterness and cultivates generosity.

Native Texans

Aster (*Callistephus*) Promotes strength within and gentleness without. Increases powers of concentration and encouragement to promote loyalty and honesty in others. Stimulates the immune system to cleanse the internal environment of toxins in cases of disease.

Carrot (*Daucus carota*) Enhances initiative for developing healthy disciplines and organizing priorities so that ambitions are realized through natural rhythm and cycles. Improves the properties of mucus in respiration and reproductivity, enhancing fertility.

Christmas Cactus (*Schlumbergera*) Lends psychological support to help us focus on what is right for ourselves and others. Reinforces strengths and helps healing of others from the heart. Supports genetic strengths and natural talents to enhance wellbeing. Compensates for inherent character weaknesses.

Columbine (*Aquilegia skinneri*) Enhances ability to think and act independently, dropping role models imposed by others. Helps an infant to become independent of its mother's immune system, increasing antibody efficiency and destruction of bacteria.

Dill (*Anethum graveolens*) Releases fear of abandonment and death. Clears self-alienation and denial of feelings. Allows effective thinking and channelling of our 'self'.

Echinacea (*Echinacea pupurea*) Purifies thoughts, clarifies visions, refines judgement and understanding. Enhances resistance to viral toxicity.

Gaillardia (*Pulchella*) Enhances determination to succeed by overcoming obstacles. Lightens the personality through the joy of overcoming. Boosts immune system, enhancing resistance to viruses and toxicity.

India Hawthorn (*Rhaphiolepis indica*) Works with group karma, dispels confusion, accents impersonal love by expressing this through deed and example. Loving all as one.

Knotted Marjoram (*Majorana hortensis*) Enhances clarity of thought to work out details when change is needed. For avoiding premature action, aiding a calculated transformation. Enhances immune system's defence mechanisms.

Kalanchoe (*Blossfeldiana*) Helps correct ingrained illusion of opposites, such as good and bad consciousness, creating dualism, polarity in personality and separation. Mends this fragmentation so we can see our blind spots.

Meadow Sage (*Salvia clevelandii*) Aids expression of strong emotions such as anger without transgressing or being vindictive. Allows us to express emotions and feelings without being controlled by them.

Mexican Oregano (*Poliomintha longiflora*) Enhances ability to understand quickly and respond to new situations correctly, teaching by example and drawing to one experiences that develop character. Helps lubricate and cleanse the skin.

Rose Campion (*Verbascum thapsus*) Strengthens the body's natural defences when there is a congenital weakness which is karmic. Develops character by uprooting old, ingrained patterns that prevent movement forward. Creates liberation in the subconscious.

Silver Lace (*Polygonum aubertii*) Aids contemplation and learning from set-backs, seeing them as a potential for growth rather than failures. Helps us to ride the waves and know when to advance or to retreat. Aids synthesis of interferon, the body's antiviral agent.

Snapdragon (*Antirrhinum majus*) Increases perception and discernment. Helps us to recognize what brings us into alignment with others and define guidelines so that we can clarify and refine plans with reasonable expectations. Enhances internal and external judgement, raising consciousness of the immune system.

Antique Rose collection

Alfredo de Demas Assists command over body and mind to affect constructive habits. Tunes the mind with the environment. Affords clarity of perception and grounding for those who are 'air-headed'.

Fortuniana Aids realization and penetration of universal truths. Leadership qualities emerge, inspiring co-operation in others by integrating the universal soul's desires with personal desires. Enhances intuition or sixth sense.

Lady Eubanksia Expands inner awareness. Brings integration of mind, body and spirit — the expression of all talents in a

415

new and unique way. A previous reclusive person will realize goals through others, emerging as a teacher of wisdom and understanding.

Old Blush Enhances stamina, catalysing inner strength and the ability to keep going. Allows creativity to be expressed and adapted to every aspect of life and health, so that we accomplish more in life than seemed possible. Strengthens willpower to integrate motor pathways and neural systems to initiate muscular contraction.

Viridiflora Helps those who are extra-sensitive to their environment by maintaining alignment of their personal power centres. Enhances grounding and personal power, feeling centred and integrated by clarity of purpose.

Master essences

Bluebonnet (*Lupinus texensis*) For those awakened by the call of their own destiny, the quest for one's true identity revealing great powers within. Increased inner awareness creates important changes (e.g. career, relationships and health) that foster our service to humanity.

Gardenia (*Rubiaceae jasminiodes veitchii*) Integration of personal life with future goals. Encourages long-range planning; awakens teaching, writing and speaking talents so concepts can be translated into reality. Dreams come true. Nourishes creativity, inspiration and achievement, encompassing home and family as well as the environment and career.

Indian Paintbrush (*Castilleja*) Brings the source of spirit and light into daily life, so that every challenge is met with a consciousness of success. Confers wisdom and a positive attitude, transforming and illuminating health, career and relationships. Makes every day a miracle.

Yellow Rose (*Rosa c.* × *floribunda*) For the reformer who has chosen the life of service, who desires to serve society unselfishly. Helps us to be attuned to the times and environment, so that our good works benefit and improve the established order and are an inspiration to others. 'Love isn't love until you give it away.'

New Native Texans essences

The Native Texans are varieties of flowers from around the world that have naturalized in the extremes of the Texas climates. They are of benefit in the communication of the immune system.

Anise Hyssop (*Hyssopus anisum*) Enhances public speaking and teaching abilities, alleviating 'butterflies' in the stomach before a performance. Indicated for those who have chronic headaches, dizzy spells or stomach aches with stabbing or fluttering pain. For overcoming a speech impediment, combines well with Daffodil and Silver Moon.

Borage (*Borago officinalis*) Aids those who feel they must be self-sufficient and stand alone in their career or personal life. Indicated for those with structural difficulties with feet, ankles and hips. Combines well with Viridiflora and Mushroom to enhance balance and agility.

Catnip (*Nepeta cataria*) Brings people closer together enhancing friendships and common bonds. Indicated for those who feel socially inhibited or in unfamiliar social situations. It softens perceived boundaries, eliminating apprehension, promoting contentment.

Cinnamon Basil (*Ocimum basilicum*) Fortifies those who buckle under adversity, or feel they can't go on under present circumstances. Indicated for those who suffer from weak knees and lower back pain. To enhance new potentials and personal growth, combine it with Gaillardia and Madame Louis Levique.

Curry (*Helichrysum italicum*) Aids those who have to think on their feet. Enhances new potential by freeing the mind of linear thought patterns. For those who want to figure their life out in advance or lack spontaneity. Combines well with Christmas Cactus and Mexican Oregano. It is indicated for migraine headaches resulting from tension and decreased circulation.

Daylily (*Hemerocallis aurantiaca*) Helps planning major changes in personal life or career. Indicated when one's job affects the future of others. Can help the process of brainstorming to overcome social, economic and political problems. It is beneficial for sufferers of chemical sensitivities and environmental pollution.

Delphinium (*Delphinium cultivars*) Aids focus or completion projects. It helps those who suffer from low blood sugar affecting attention span and memory. Eradicates the effects of parasitic infection when combined with Amaryllis. Also combined with Alfredo de Damas for hand to eye coordination problems.

Bronze Fennel (*Foeniculum vulgare*) Helps overcome limitation affecting the imagination and planning centres. Aids those who want to create; enhances visualization. Bronze Fennel strengthens mental and psychic abilities, enhancing clarity and direction. Combines well with Azalea, Autumn Damask and Echinacea to enhance creative pleasures.

Foxglove (*Digitalis purpurea*) Attracts fulfilling personal relationships, enhancing compassion and sensitivity for others. Indicated when the heart beats out of control or poor circulation is indicated. For cardiovascular congestion or irregularity. Combines with India Hawthorn and Wisteria to attract good working relationships.

French Lavender (*Lavendula reverchon*) Helps us appreciate and focus on the blessings in our lives. It also releases the need for more or bigger and better. Combine French Lavender with Christmas Cactus, apply to temples for headaches or the outside of the ears to decrease congestion.

Iberis Candytuft (*Iberis sempervirens*) Encourages regeneration and self-healing by activating the light inherent in each cell. It enhances a balanced mineral pattern within the cell, allowing the tissues to be bathed with nutrients. Works well with Crossandra to facilitate transition and lifestyle changes.

Lobelia (*Lobelia inflata*) Teaches us to create boundaries with others. It is for those who have difficulty saying no. Combine with Snapdragon for discernment and with Country Marilou to reduce the need to please others or be liked by peers.

Mexican Brush Sage (*Salvia leucantha*) Enhances our ability to be unique. Indicated for those adversely affected by peer pressure. Gives us permission to be who we really are, combining well with Aquilegia Columbine to help drop the roles others give to us. It is indicated for red itchy skin; combine with Salvia.

Mexican Hat (*Ratibida columnifera*) Brings prosperity, combining well with Indian Paintbrush for a success consciousness. Fimbriata and Fairy Rose will help fulfil our needs.

Purple Garden Sage (*Salvis officinalis purpurea*) Helps focus on what is valuable and true in love and relationships. It is indicated when relationships are tested by external conditions. Helpful when sinusitis, viruses and profound sweating or heat flashes occur. Combine with onion and thyme to counteract viral complaints.

Rain Lily (*Cooperia pendunculata*) Reconciles lovers and rifts in relationships. It is indicated when one feels slightly left out in relationships. Combine with Marquis Bocella to encourage long-term relationships.

Red Malva (*Malva slyvestris mauritanica* × *hibiscus rosa sinensis China*) An essence that helps us to stay centred and in tune to receive guidance and channelling. This guidance will be focused on spiritual development. Combine with Dill and Verbena to calm the desire to withdraw from others or isolate.

Rosemary (*Rosmarinus officinalis*) Encourages an endorphin release associated with pleasant memories and releases past painful memories when combined with Bachelor's Button and Morning Glory. When others misunderstand us, Rosemary will bring out the best in us.

Salad Burnet (*Poterium sanguisorba*) Overcomes depression from unfulfilled desires in relationships. When the romance fades, it is time to surrender to the nurturing this essence provides. As melancholy lifts, nutrient uptake and dispersion increases, enhancing blood volume and neuromuscular response. Combines with Fortune's Double Yellow, Daffodil and Chamomile as an anti-inflammatory heart tonic.

Soapwort (*Saponaria officinalis*) This essence opens the channels for inner hearing to increase the inner wisdom of the 'still small voice' within. It detoxifies fatty deposits, affecting cardiovascular health and lymphatic drainage. Combines with Pink Rose to reduce cellulite or feelings of heaviness.

Spike Lavender (*Lavandula latifolia*) Aids those who need to practise the art of co-operation instead of domination. It helps to reduce lung congestion and bronchial spasms and is indicated for frequent sighing and a heaviness in the chest.

Sweet Annie (*Artemisia annua*) Benefits those who wish to enhance their public image. Indicated to draw out the best in personal appearances especially when unexpectedly in the public eye when it is not natural to be in the limelight. This essences also aids ageing gracefully.

Tansy (*Tanacetum vulgare*) Tansy protects the aura of the spiritual warrior. Indicated for those affected by environmental chemicals and pollution. This may include emphysema, pleurisy and bronchitis. Combined with Old Blush and Verbena it enhances energy and muscle tone.

Texas Dandelion (*Taraxacum officinale*) Frees the psyche from fretful dreams and those who wake up with a feeling of falling into their body. It enables one to receive answers in dreams and to remember dreams.

Thyme (*Thymus vulgaris*) Draws all those that inspire, aid and encourage our greatest achievements. This essence attracts unseen beneficial elementals such as griffins, devas, nymphs and fairies. Combines with Onion and Sage essence to guard the immune system against viral invasion.

Wild Wood Violets (*Viola odorata*) This essence helps the personality choose endeavours that benefit society. The path of modesty and non-interference allows the mind to enter the wholeness of the universe and predict the evolution of events to follow.

Wild Oats (*Avena fatua*) Enhances and develops a sense of humour. We can let go and laugh our way past inhibitions holding back our natural growth. Also indicated for the 'blues' and for children who are sad. Combined with Dianthus, Red Rose and Fimbriata to let the good times roll.

Yarrow (*Achillea millefolium*) Used to potentize the Petites. Add 2 or more drops to an essences combination to receive the benefits of the 10,000 Lotus petal flowers within. It reduces auto-immune reactions and inflammatory responses adversely affecting the immune system and central nervous system.

New Antique Rose essences

Archduke Charles Enhances intimacy, allowing us to feel safe when touched. May help those who withdraw or push people away who get too close. For those who avoid total commitments, always finding a reason to move on. Touches the heart where true intimacy grows unhindered by intellect and desire. In the body, it encourages the structural stability of the skin, arterial and stomach lining.

Autumn Damask Helps develop constancy in faith. For those who have experienced many disappointments in past relationships, now hesitant to become involved again. This essence helps with learning from past disappointments and in becoming more discerning in relationships. This will attract fulfilling relationships, as well as enhance nutrient uptake in the body cells.

Cecil Brunner Encourages those who withdraw or hold back from entering new relationships. It helps overcome fear arising from new challenges. Beneficial for those who are easily persuaded to define boundaries creating realistic goals in relationships. Creates security in reaching out and connecting with others. When ability to love is unhindered, it attracts those who will assist with achieving the highest goals.

Champney's Pink Cluster The Rose of integrity, teaches us to love through respect rather than passion alone. We connect with others by recognizing and honouring the love that created each person. Seeing through the eyes of love allows us to accept ourselves as we are as well as others. Through acceptance we are transformed. Forgetting about changing others we share love in the best way possible. Enhances the resting potential of the nerve cells, encouraging muscles to relax and regenerate.

Cherokee Rose This essence opens the crown chakra to stimulate creative ideas.

It enhances the endocrine balance of the pituitary, pineal and hypothalamus to regulate menstrual cycles and reduces fluid retention and female complaints. For men it enhances protein metabolism and muscle strength as a new vision of oneself is created.

Country Marilou This rose unlocks inner joy to promote vitality and regeneration, releasing inner strength and security which is ageless. Helps to release uncomfortable feelings and perceptions from the body. Beneficial for those who form nodes of neuronal tissue and neuritis affecting healthy neuronal tissue.

Fairy Rose Promotes passionate connection with every life form, links the first and seventh chakras. A transpersonal experience witnessed in a dreamlike state. Nature spirits may be seen enabling the experience of learning to think, feel and seeing life as nature does. Bloom with the roses or fly like an angel, but your life will never feel ordinary again. Indicated for those who tap Mother Nature's power to heal others.

Fimbriata Encourages a passion for life. Indicated when the need is to release nonproductive relationships. It opens the mind and heart to new possibilities activating the law of attraction. Even in friendships it enhances contagious enthusiasm, forming new alliances with those of like mind. May also encourage pathways enhancing the synergistic harmony affecting organ function.

Fortune's Double Yellow This essence calms excessive desires and attracts our greatest good, gently reminding us we always have what we need. It discourages envy and feelings of lack. Aids a tendency for hypertension and tension headaches, nurtures those separated from loved ones by distance. Soothes an aching heart with a feeling that time is on our side.

Gruss an Aachen Encourages us to withdraw from partnerships and relationships that require us to settle for less than the best. Quality, not quantity, will open the heart to fulfilment. During transition time, frequent awaking at night or food craving may be experienced. It encourages us to walk with a good heart and run with success.

Louis Philippe Offers hope to those who feel love has passed them by. Overcoming hopelessness by surrendering to the love within. Affirm truth and call on the heart to receive its greatest good. Encourages growth of receptor sites activating cardiovascular flow, enhancing the feeling of love. This warmth not only provides new life for the blood, but also new love to bless your life.

Madame Alfred Carriere Encourages prophetic dreams, for seeking answers in dreamtime. Enhances parasympathetic responses to stimulate the body to heal itself, transcending time and difficulty. As dreamtime dispels opposites, the subtle body is able to function without inner conflict. The spirit seeks freedom like a bird seeks flight, and this Rose invites you to allow your intellect to rest and seek answers from the depths of your subconscious.

Madame Louis Levique This essence increases the desire for service and devotion, surrendering the need to be in control. Helps to neutralize toxins blocking the free flow of Qi. By letting go, we also let go of insecurities behind control issues. As we learn to be part of nature we will better serve it. Surrender to the present moment of grace.

Maggie Helps to see the truth in situations before it becomes apparent. Hidden aspects can only be seen and felt from the heart. Your heart will guide you as it has the capacity to 'see' and feel what is best for you. The seat of the soul is in a peaceful heart, content with all things, lacking none. Maggie calls on our greatest capacity

to see through the masque of the personality to the soul level.

Marie Pavie Encourages following the heart's desire in love for when thoughts deny what the heart knows is right. It can ignite the flame in burnt-out relationships. Also for recovering from deep disappointments in family relationships causing a feeling of loss and grief. Encourages recovery from post-viral syndromes and symptoms of aching and malaise.

Marquis Boccela The constant bloom of perpetual love encourages long-term relationships building intimacy through trust. For when one is searching but not attracting kindred spirits to share joy with. In the body, this essence affects the subtle energy inherent in the nervous system. The energy communicates sensory messages to the subtle body and impacts the sensory organs. Especially useful for those stressed by a busy schedule, replenishing vitality and increasing acuity.

Silver Moon Subdues a restless mind, obsessive thoughts, fearful dreams and constant mind chattering. From a quiet mind pure awareness emerges. Restless energy often affects the heart chakra causing stuttering and an increased need for personal attention and admiration. An imbalanced fire element can exaggerate the sense of importance and the need to be 'different'.

Rose Oil Petite Fleur essences
Combinations and sprays

The Petites provide a combination of aromatherapy and their special qualities and properties to encourage healing, releasing underlying sources of stress. They gently encourage us to let go of past and present pain, while gaining wisdom from each experience. Petites open the heart by reconnecting the inner joy and harmony within the body. They encourage self-esteem and release energy by reducing emotions created under stress and expectations. Specific blends have been created to address particular general day-to-day challenges.

The Rose Oil Combinations have been designed over the past 26 years for hospitals, pain and therapeutic clinics in the United States, Europe and Canada. The blends (described in *Country Living* magazine, June 2000) are made from organically grown aromatic herbs and Roses, distilled on site, and hand separated without chemicals to produce the purest products. The blends have been used at Baylor Hospital's Healing Environment Program in Dallas, Texas, since 1999, the Bone and Joint Hospital in New York City and many hospitals and clinics in the United States and United Kingdom, and now are available in sprays for topical use.

Abate Anger (*Onchidium sphacelatum*) Reduces pent-up anger, road rage, disappointment, outbursts and tantrums. Beneficial for stress-induced hypertension, headaches and tense shoulders.

Allergy (Echinacea – *Echinacea purpurea*) Reduces sensitivity to allergic reactions. Use daily for seasonal allergens, asthma and environmental reactions. Reduces symptoms of sneezing, wheezing, runny nose, itchy eyes and sinus drainage.

Cold Flu (Periwinkle – *Vinca rosea*) Antiviral, antibacterial essences and essential oils prevent and reduce symptoms of viral cold and flu.

Cravings (Gaillardia – *Pulchella*) Reduces obsessive compulsive habits and addictive behaviour. Apply two times every day or as often as needed. Add Harmony blend two times daily; add Self-Image to increase self-worth two times daily.

Deep Sleep (Madame Alfred Carriere – *Rosa chinensis*) Promotes better sleep patterns, reduces fretful dreams and insomnia. Apply at bedtime and rub 2 drops on each earlobe to increase REM (rapid eye movement) time and wake up refreshed. Repeat as needed if awakened during the night.

Energy (Old Blush Rose – *R. chinensis*) Increases mental and physical stamina and alertness during long workdays and workouts. Feel the power. Enhances stamina.

Fatigue (Geranium – *Pelargonium* × *hortorum*) Reduces mental stress and chronic fatigue, fibromyalgia and mild depression, achiness and jet lag.

Female Balance (Japanese Magnolia – *Magnolia* × *soulangeana*) Reduces menopausal and premenstrual tension symptoms, dark moods and crankiness.

Harmony Blend (Antique Roses) Reduces anxiety, nausea, physical and emotional trauma, and welcomes peace of mind. Used by cancer patients before and during treatment of chemotherapy, bone marrow and stem cell transplants, and anxiety disorders.

Inner Strength (Red Malva – *Malva sylvestris mauritanica* × *hibiscus rosa sinensis China*) Develops strength during challenging and adverse times. Enhances personality development and maturity, increasing motivation and self-actualization. Used in clinics and hospitals to increase flexibility and mobility for bones, spine and joints, bone density, and structural correction.

Learning Skills (*Delphinium cultivars*) Increases alertness, focus and concentration for adults and children. Apply before school and study.

Male Power (Basil, Lime, Curry (Immortelle) and Peppermint) Increases self-worth, enhancing the determination to put ideas into action. Creativity and vitality increases as the soul's purpose is expressed through the personality.

Manage Pain (Country Marilou – *Rosa 'ausmary'*) Reduces symptoms of chronic and acute pain, neuralgia and inflammation.

Used in pain clinics and hospitals for neuropathy, sickle cell anaemia symptoms, joint pain, rheumatoid arthritis, shingles and auto-immune symptoms.

Maternity (White Jasmine – *Jasminum nudiflorum*) Enjoy the thrill of a child of your heart growing within you. Adjust to the many physical and emotional changes during pregnancy. Prepare for a joyous birth. Used for gestational diabetes and difficult pregnancies.

Passion (Morning Glory – *Convolvulacea*) Enhances productivity; increases attraction for passionate and like-minded relationships. Used in clinics to reduce depressed low energy and apathetic symptoms.

Recall Memory (Texas Bluebonnet – *Lupinus texensis*) Enhances cognitive functions, study habits and sensory perception.

Recovery (Sunflower – *Helianthus* sp.) Enhances the body's wisdom to catalyze innate healing after acute or prolonged illness. Emphasizes strengths rather than character weaknesses. Used for chemically dependent support after treatment; after chemotherapy, radiation, antibiotic and antiviral drug therapy.

Reduce Stress (Verbena – *Verbenaceae hortensis*) Reduces physical, emotional, environmental and mental triggers of stress. Used in clinics to reduce herpes virus symptoms.

Regenerate (Tiger's Jaw – *Faucaria tigrina*) Reduces tendency to scar, regenerating cell growth in tissue.

Self-Esteem (Magnolia) Enhances self-appreciation and success consciousness: self-esteem, self-worth and self-satisfaction.

Stop Smoking (Stock – *Matthiola incana rosa*) Reduces compulsive urges, breaking habits and addictive patterns, benefits hyperactivity and Attention Defect Disorder.

Weight (Vanilla Orchid – *Vanilla planifolia*) Reduces compulsive behaviour and the need for 'comfort food'. Beneficial for those who perceive themselves as heavy.

Feng Shui sprays

Petite Fleur Feng Shui sprays are a combination of flower essences made by a steam-distilled and hand process method with purely organically grown flowers and herbs specially formulated to catalyze potentials and enrich the mind, body and soul. The flower essences are mixed with essential oils to produce sprays for specific conditions designed to promote balance in your environment and enhance peace of mind.

Attraction Spray Encourages opportunities to enhance and nourish career, family and love relationships. Spray on clothes, in family and meeting rooms.

Clearing Spray Dissolves negativity, upsets, disappointments, procrastination and electromagnetic build-up. Spray rooms, work areas and yourself.

Enhancement Spray Increases prosperity, knowledge, health and career recognition. Spray study areas, doorways and corners of rooms.

Harmonize and Balance Spray Reduces stress and anxiety. Harnesses beneficial energy to recharge stagnant areas. Spray inside car and elsewhere to encourage peace and quiet.

STAR PERUVIAN ESSENCES (Peru)

In the Vilcabamba Sacred Mountains in and around Machu Picchu, Peru, grow many species of Orchids that have within their matrix the ability to affect global consciousness. They resonate to a frequency which can be directly translated by the vibrational bodies of all who encounter them.

Traditionally Orchids are considered the most evolved species of the plant world carrying in their DNA the information of all the other plants. One of the main purposes of the Andean Orchid flower essences is to assist us in balancing our energies as we go through shifts into expanded consciousness.

Growing wild and free in nature's laboratory, at an altitude of 10,000ft, the Andean Orchids are well adapted and very happy in their environment. They are growing on energetic ley lines, at the sacred centre of Machu Picchu, and they have a strong energetic field.

Created by Star Riparetti and Roger Valencia in 1994 the Andean Orchid flower essences open and expand our hearts. Love is a magnet which draws all things to it. Star's passion is vibrational medicine; she was chief technician and director of the school of Nuclear Medicine at the cancer foundation of Santa Barbara before working with essences. Roger is an avid botanist who was born in Cuzco, in Peru, and with his passion for wild Orchids, along with the fact that he is fluent in Quechua, the language of the indigenous population of Peru, he was instrumental in the creation of the Andean Orchids Project with Star.

Andean Orchids of Machu Picchu

Ancient Wisdom (*Lycaste longepetalia*) Discover Soul Purpose. Enhances awareness and openness to the wisdom of the ancients that is returning now to Earth. This is an important dream essence. Apply to the back of the neck as it aids in opening the chakras so that we can remember ancient truths and also remember who we are. It assists in discovering soul purpose, and awakens us to our divine potential.

Anchoring Light (*Sobralia dichotoma*) Grounding Planetary Light Work. Useful when we are consciously serving as a divine instrument for anchoring light, connecting ley lines and healing the planetary grids. This essence lubricates the pathways so that energy can flow, enabling us to be more effective conductors of the new frequencies entering the planet. Good to use when feeling overenergized, as it brings grounding energy. Apply on head to bring energy in, or on feet to ground and anchor energy.

Balance and Stability (*Habenaria*) Emergency Remedy. Harmony. A broad spectrum essence. It helps us to feel balanced in our environment. For any kind of stress or emergency situation and when feeling out-of-balance. Brings stability throughout. Assists in adapting to the new high planetary frequencies. For working with planetary healing and disharmonic energy patterns.

Divine Child (*Ponthieva montana*) For Sensitive Children and Adults. This essence is especially effective for the very sensitive beings that are being born now. Also, for reconnecting with gifts that were suppressed in the past. It is now safe to be sensitive and to stay in the realm of delight and express our divine brilliance. Good before and during pregnancy, to connect with the soul of the new child. It is especially good for the newborn. Put a drop on pulse points and the third eye.

Divine Goddess (*Masdevallia veitchiana*) Intuition and Deep Issues. Aids in birthing, attuning to the divine goddess energies, acknowledging the feminine as the source of creativity. Helps in developing intuition and building self-esteem. An extremely powerful essence for deep issues. On a physical level, this essence is useful for shifting premenstrual syndrome and hot flushes; while the heat may still be there, what shifts is your attitude to it.

Eternal Youth (*Epidendrum ibaguense*) Rejuvenation and Regenesis. This is called the Wiñay Wayna orchid, which means forever young in Quechua. Promotes rejuvenation, by retaining our cells to remember the optimum frequency of life, and by raising our resistance beyond disease and ageing into super-health and youthfulness. This essence can be put on the skin and can help with the effects of premature ageing of the skin. Use every day and add to all your creams, lotions and potions.

Faith and Courage (*Odontoglossum*) Protection. This essence creates a protective frequency around us, rather like having a powerful, yet gentle watchdog at the edge of our energy field. It helps us to wake up to our inner courage. Take it when you feel vulnerable, in order to build up a field of protection, or when you need more faith and courage. Excellent for use in hospitals. It also helps to protect from all the X-ray and negative electromagnetic frequencies.

Freedom/Libertad (*Xylobium with 24 carat gold*) Manifestation. For freedom on all levels, especially to express ourselves, and freedom to manifest our truth. It assists in realigning us to our original divine blueprint. The frequency of gold added to the Xylobium works synergistically and assists in opening dimensional doorways. Regardless of what other essences we are taking, Freedom/Libertad is here to assist us as we cross the threshold and take the first steps of ascension.

High Frequency (*Peurothallis*) Meditation. Heart and Lungs. A high-frequency essence. Aids in opening channels to the highest dimensions. For meditation, flower essences facilitate your highest conscious and unconscious desires. This essence is also useful for issues around heart and lungs and it can lift us out of grief and sadness.

Nature Communion (*Trichoceros parviflorum*) Connection to Nature. Enhances your level of consciousness and your connection to the nature kingdom and your connection to your physical body. It is also good for fertility. Use when working in the garden or walking, as it assists us in communing with nature. It synergistically enhances herbal preparations. It is also useful

when you have been inside too long or in front of the computer.

One Heart (*Epidendrum cuscoense*) Acceptance, Love and Unity. This essence is about oneness, unity, unconditional love. Connects us to the heart frequency for unification and acceptance. One Heart is great for balancing male/female energies within oneself, for increasing telepathy and non-verbal communication. This is an excellent essence to share with groups.

Red Union (*Maxillaria*) Oneness. Addresses integrated, sacred sexuality. A catalyst to move us to a new level of union, with ourselves or with a partner. Rejoice in fulfilment conjoined to make one soul. This love in itself is an instrument for peace in the world. Use alone for tantra. It is for taking sexuality to a higher level.

The Higher Chakra Trilogy

This trilogy of essences, Gold+Silver/White, Zeal Point and Awakened Thymus, is useful in preparing for the activation of the higher chakras. These essences can be used on their own or in any combination. Using all three of them, and doing numeric harmonic sequencing, can be very powerful.

Magenta Zeal Point Chakra (*Epidendrum federicci guillemi*) Expression through the Voice. Assists in opening, balancing and releasing the Magenta Zeal Point chakra, which is located at the base of the skull. It balances the body, mind and emotions and assists in moving kundalini energy through the body. It opens us to the next level of initiation. Zeal Point Chakra helps us to speak our truth. The colour magenta indicates it is an entry point into a new evolution.

Gold+Silver/White Chakra (*Sobralia setigera*) Balanced Light Body. Peace, Serenity Harmony. This Orchid essence encompasses two chakras. The gold chakra is like a halo above the head. The wisdom of the gold chakra is love and acceptance. This chakra cascades out to the silver/white chakra encompassing the luminescent light body. This Gold+Silver/White chakra essence contains the new energies for us to access the space where truth and peace flow out of our hearts. Assists our subtle bodies in sustaining balance, tranquillity, peacefulness, divine contentment.

Awakened Thymus (*Erythrodes simplex*) High Heart, Graciousness. This essence is useful for telepathy, and connecting the third and sixth chakras. The thymus empowers loving communication and is also called the high heart. Useful when healing with voice and sound. The thymus receives spiritual life force energies and transforms them for use in the etheric, subtle body and physical vehicle. The essence will strengthen and nourish it.

Peruvian flowers

About Face (Dandelion – *Taraxicum officinale*) Facing Issues. Helps us face issues we have been avoiding, keeps us on track and it alleviates procrastination. Addresses actual physical problems such as acne on the face. Add Eternal Youth and About Face to a cream or oil. It is also good for liver balance and detox, especially if alcohol has been used to numb feelings. Allows us to face ourselves as we are and continue to grow.

Bushilla Good for female issues, especially reproduction at any stage. This essence is made together with Arbildo Murayari Mozombite, a shaman from the Pulcalpa Jungle, a vegitalista, curandero and perfumero, who has said it is also an important and valuable essence for men.

I Am Generosity (Chijchipa – *Tagetes multiflora*) Grand Fortune. This essence is a treasure. It is about prosperity consciousness and manifestation, affluence and abundance. We are also reminded to give generously.

I Am Gratitude (Yuyu/Mustard – *Brassica*) Holy Grace. This essence reminds us of the rich rewards, and of our holiness. This essence magnifies the higher octave love energy and we are filled with gratitude. The essence was made in Peru (Chaska Land).

Inocencia Coca (Coca – *E. coca*) Shifting Patterns. Stamina. The Coca leaves are used extensively for ceremony and healing in Peru and are multifaceted. It is invigorating and used to increase stamina. It balances appetite and metabolism, in addition to shifting addictive patterns. Use for dieting, rejuvenating and raising the metabolism. Coca helps strengthen the will and intent. It aligns us with our source of joy, passion and effectiveness, and our true service. Aids psychic ability. It is also very good for altitude sickness.

Integration (Mutuy – *Cassia hookeriana*) Open and Clear Mind. Balances the mental and emotional bodies, works with the pancreas. Sweetness, self-esteem. Useful for integrating shifts, during chaotic times. According to Maximo, the 87-year-old medicine man who helped make the essence, it helps soothe your head when you are scared.

Mango Paradise (Mango – *Mangifera*) Celebration of Life in the Physical Form. This essence is about robust sexuality, sensuality. It is about jubilance and enthusiasm. It is also primal, uncomplicated and earthy, free of belief systems. This essence is a gift and a celebration of life in the physical form.

Master Teacher (*Chiri Sanango*) Expansion. Considered a Master Teacher plant in the jungle. It can connect us with the deva of healing. For expansion, and about temperature regulation. People have reported that hot flushes have disappeared after using this essence. Cold extremities warm up as it regulates temperature, and supports the blood and bones.

Purification (*Muòa* – High Andean Mint) Sanctify. Cleanse. Assists connection with our guides, and in passing through the veils of the other dimensions. Use it for balance, especially during purification. Good for cleansing and clearing. Use this essence to sanctify and purify in a multitude of ways. Also good for altitude sickness.

Strength and Qi (Fava – *Vicia faba*) Wellbeing and vitality. The essence facilitates all functions of brain activity, including memory, energy and sense of wellbeing. It is useful for balancing hormones. Strength, energy and radiant vitality come from being in balance. Good for menopause, supports a parasite cleanse. Creates and sustains balance in your subtle bodies.

Sublime Chocolate (Cacao – *Theobroma cacao*) Balance Metabolism. This essence balances metabolism. Excellent to use when you crave chocolate. Good for women during their menstruation. Helpful for remembering dreams and stimulates psychic abilities. Provides energy after meals. Etheric endorphins. Assists in clearing ancient DNA. Assists connection to Mayan and Incan cultures, awakening and getting in touch with the ancestors. Chocolate correlates with pleasure, enjoying a rich history.

Wild Feminine (Wild Potato – *Solanum diploide*) Uninhibited. Spontaneous. Nourishing. The Wild Feminine brings all of our aspects together whether our gender is male or female expressing our unique diversity as we choose. It also has a nurturing feminine quality to it. It helps to anchor important feminine aspects of us in a new way.

13th Gate (Cantu Flower – *Cantua buxifolia*) Open Portals. The 13th Peruvian essence. This essence carries hummingbird medicine and has been found to be a very pleasant and peaceful essence, smoothing edges during these interesting accelerated times. Helps with changing frequencies. Made at the sacred Lake Titicaca, from the Cantu flower, which is the national flower of Peru. It helps us navigate through the portals, octaves and gates that we are moving through.

Santa Barbara Flowers

Be Nurtured (White Ceanothus – *Ceanothus leucodermis*) Soothes the soul. Called Mother's Milk, as it is filled with the Divine Mother's energy. Feel safe and nurtured. The essence is especially good for children and babies. We are surrounded with an abundance of love from a higher realm, feel nurtured by nature.

Creation/Focus (Jacaranda – *Jacaranda mimosaefolia*) Creative Vision. Assists our ability to hold the energy to dream the new dream. Supports creative vision and staying focused. Stimulates new ideas. Great when working on computers. Helpful for studying. Creation/Focus was made as the comets were entering Jupiter – in a super force-field of meditation. It was a second bloom in one season for this tree – the Jacaranda very strongly offered itself during this time for this important essence.

Dance (*Bougainvillea*) Grace, beauty and brilliance. Gives assistance for flowing through life gracefully. It gets us moving. Good for all forms of sacred movement, especially dancing. Take it for dancing through life gracefully. Also, use it in relationships, which are dances of harmony and perfect rhythm. Dance the journey into the self, and then this is the cosmic dance. Try dancing at dawn with your eyes looking east. Activate your imagination and awaken. Experience spontaneity, and naturalness. Feel good for no particular reason – or any reason!

Deep Breath (Eucalyptus – *Eucalyptus niphophila*) Divine Inspiration. This essence is about breathing. It opens and expands the chest and the lungs, and makes sure you remember to breathe. Breathing connects all systems in our bodies. Inspires us to breathe air/life into the soul. The best way to get more air is to exercise outside. Do complete inhalations and exhalations to eliminate the carbon dioxide. Mastery of breath is mastery of health. This essence will assist in the journey.

Early Bloomer (Oxalis – *Oxalis stricta*) Family Harmony. Trust. This essence assists in adapting to accelerated, early growth and maturity. Use our advancement to awaken to our divine potential and become a positive instrument. Great for children and teenagers who are advancing at an accelerated rate.

Emancipation (Tobacco Flower – *Nicotiniana*) Physical and Emotional Wellbeing. Freedom from anything that has power over us. Liberation. Release cravings gracefully (especially nicotine and marijuana). Tobacco is grounding and good for travelling between worlds. The Tobacco Flower essence cleans the meridians. If you are choosing to quit smoking, this essence assists with grace and ease.

For Giving (Acacia) For Giving and Receiving and Worthiness. For giving and receiving gracefully. This essence reminds us to give and receive from the heart to assist in moving into the frequency of forgivingness and for forgiving ourselves. Know that you are perfect. Also useful when working with allergies. For release. Give, and you receive. It is time to transcend the need to forgive anyone for anything.

Full Moonlight (Lavender – *Lavandula*) Full Moon Energy. Excellent for addressing full moon sleeplessness or feeling out of sorts. This essence helps to balance full moon energy so it can be harnessed and used beneficially, creatively and peacefully.

God/Goddess Unity (Banana Flower – *Musa × paradisiaca*) Masculine Balance. For merging of the male/female and bringing unified oneness in our sexuality. This essence assists gender healing at very deep levels, and balances the first chakra. Banana flower essence is useful for dealing with sexual issues in relationships, enabling us to view them from a higher frequency.

Graceful Shift (Fennel – *Foeniculum vulgare*) Change with Ease. An excellent essence when you are going through great changes. Useful for balancing physical energy when going through dimensional shifts. Should an influx of light cause discomfort, this essence will address it. Excellent for grounding. Fennel addresses nausea, and butterflies in the tummy.

Initiation of the Heartlight (Pink Lotus – *Nelumbo*) Openheartedness. Reach a new level of openheartedness. This essence will help us to recognize any judgement we may still have. Sometimes you will feel warmth in your heart after taking the essence. In ancient Egypt, the Lotus is associated with resurrection, rejuvenation and eternal life. It is said to have mind-altering capabilities. The Pink Lotus is also associated with Lakshmi, the Hindu goddess of spiritual wealth, spiritual abundance and spiritual evolution.

Inner Guru (Purple Sage – *Salvia leucophylla*) Inner Guidance; Higher Self; Individuality. The Purple Sage essence helps access that part of us that knows the answers; the sage within. Be your own guru. Knowingness. Omniscience.

I Remember (Rosemary – *Rosmarinus officinalis*) Remembering; Clarity. This essence deals with remembering on all levels. 'I remember who I am, I remember my gifts, I remember what I came here to do, I remember how to manifest.' (I even remember where my keys are.) Excellent for clarity in all realms. Certainty of self.

427

Creativity, inner peace that creates prosperity, to heal oneself and to be one with spirit. It also strengthens the immune system. Awakens the full memory of our own potential. When we remember what we are really supposed to do in life, it can restore our health. When we remember what all of humanity is supposed to do, we can heal the world.

Let Go and Trust (Oregano – *Oreganum vulgare*) Release. Helps us let go of attachments. Release with ease the things that no longer serve us. It is good for use during a cleanse. It is excellent for birthing. It is also like an etheric colonic; it gets rid of gunk in our auras. Space is created for something new.

Light Navigator (California Pepper Tree – *Schinus molle*) Interdimensional Journeys. The Molle tree is a Peruvian native plant. This essence can take us to places where we are connected on the inner planes. It helps us to know our direction. It lights the path, and is good for meditation. Take it alone, or in combination with other essences. There is a very strong grandmother connection with this essence. Inner vision lights the path to know our direction. It is a direct portal to Peru. It assists in time, and interdimensional travel.

Magic Healer (Plantain – *Plantago lanceolata*) Accelerated Healing. A catalyst for healing the body, especially the skin. It aligns body, mind and spirit. Use alone or to boost other healing modalities. It works like magic to accelerate healing. Use on plants to balance insect population.

Male Strength (Agave – *Agave americana*) Power; Virility; Enhances Masculine Aspects. This essence speaks for itself. There are positive reports about this essence's effectiveness. It is also useful for women who wish to be more in touch with their masculine aspects. Addresses issues of power and virility.

My Passion (Passion Flower – *Passiflora bryonioides*) In the Moment; Compassion. Teaches us to be in the moment and love that moment, then it becomes our passion (e.g. studying, lovemaking, artistic endeavours) and brings out its highest aspects. Expands awareness and ability to recognize magic. Receives, circulates and broadcasts energy.

Open Mind/Future Vision (Mugwort – *Artemisia vulgaris*) Dreams; Visionary. This essence has many qualities. For clairvoyant dreams and divinatory acuity; it increases our visionary capabilities and insights. Heightens openness and spiritual perceptions. Mugwort is good on pressure points and meridians. Stimulates and expands our sensibilities.

Pure Joy (Orange Blossom – *Citrus sinensis*) I Am *So* Joyous! Renewed Enthusiasm. This essence takes us an octave higher. Brings excitement and enthusiasm. Gives us a boost in conjunction with other essences.

Solar Power (Sunflower – *Helianthus annuus*) Heart Opening; Personal Power; Sovereignty. The flower of the Incas. It brings forth our personal power at its highest level and brings strength through an open heart. Reminds us to stand up straight. Assists with father and fathering issues. It reflects the solar energy.

Soul Family (Blue Ceanothus – *Ceanothus thyrsiflorus*) Precious Connection; Births and Deaths. This essence helps to unify soul groups, or tribes. It is especially good for hospice work and for individuals during the death process, and those assisting them. It will guide the dying person out of the crown chakra when they are ready to leave their body. So they may go directly into their soul group at the moment of transition.

Sweet New Beginnings (Pink Jasmine – *Jasminum polyanthum*) Clarity and Ease with New Things. Useful for remaining balanced during these new, ever-changing times and energies. Take it each time you feel a shift to another octave. Helps us remain connected to the Divine as we expand. With this essence, we can go through change from a clear vantage point, because it provides clarity.

Zania (Zinnia – *Zinnia elegans*) Fun; Playful; Lighten Up; Be Zany. This essence helps us relax and open up and be less serious. We can see things in a brighter, more colourful light. It encourages relaxation and fun.

Combinations

Attention Formula Focused and Peaceful. This essence is said to be of great value to children and adults with Attention Deficit Disorder and Attention Deficit Hyperactivity Disorder. It assists in staying attentive, focused, relaxed and peaceful. Helps concentration. Some children have been able to stop prescribed medication completely.

Brilliant Student Studying. We have taken our broad spectrum anti-stress, stabilizing essence, Balance and Stability, and added Faith and Courage and Clear Quartz to amplify the effects with universal love. Works like magic. The rescue remedy for the new millennium. Use whenever you are off-balance. Good for everyone, kids, pets, plants, adults and teenagers. If you can't decide what essence to take, then take this one. Put 7 drops in a glass of water and sip it during acute situations. If you only have one essence, keep this one with you.

Radiant Sensuality Love. A magical Star Flower and Gemstone Essence blend that encourages a loving atmosphere. Take this ecstatic, synergistic combination to enhance your romantic mood. It covers a beautiful range of sexual vitality and sensuality. Marvellous for drawing your beloved to you. Put 4 droppers full in your bath.

Immerse yourself in the essence. Cherish yourself, and each other.

Shield of Light Safe and Protected. Creates a protective vibrational frequency around you. Valuable for healers. Use when working with computers. Useful for travelling in cities, and around high tension wires and airports. It is especially valuable to use (for patient and visitor) in hospitals. Also on the perimeters of the house, yard, office, etc. (inside and out) to build a shield of light.

Soul Purpose Dreams. Take when you have questions regarding direction, and divine will. Your dreams will help determine your direction and choice. Discover what contributions you have for the world and, by listening for the answers, find your purpose. Have clarity, and make clear choices. Physical healing often comes about when you discover your soul path. This essence helps you direct and remember your dreams.

Super Immune Wellness and Purification. A combination of flower and gemstone essences and the powerful rose-coloured salt from the Sacred Valley of the Incas. Good for any physical healing and for strengthening the immune system via the electrical system, allowing the body to concentrate full time on the physical – thus speeding up recovery time. Take when the first symptom appears. It is useful for radiation exposure and protection on any level: diagnostic, therapeutic, accidental or employment-related. It will enhance and accelerate any healing modality.

Travel Solution Airplanes and Altitude. Helps adaptation to the changes that take place while travelling. This super balancing essence helps with altitude and jet lag, and assists with flying trepidation. It protects from electromagnetic radiation and strengthens coping abilities. Helpful to start taking a day or two before you leave, and continue during your journey as necessary.

Sprays

Angel Rejuvenation Spray Facial Spray, Aura Cleanser, Room Clearing. *Ingredients: Eternal Youth and essential oils of Frankincense, Lavender and Geranium.* Angel Spray lifts the spirit to a higher vibration, brings immediate clarity and positivity. It feels really good; use it often for rejuvenation.

Cool Flash Spray Make Menopause Merry. Spray Your Face and Body. *Ingredients: Balance and Stability, Divine Goddess, Freedom/Liberation, Graceful Shift, Master Teacher, Strength and Qi, Sublime Chocolate, Wild Feminine, Moonstone and Pink Tourmaline. Essential oils: Clarysage, Lemon and Geranium.* This spray can facilitate a light, gentle, easy, graceful and empowering menopause. The essences and oils in it have been known to balance metabolism and temperature. Considered to be beauty oils, bacteria, hormone regulators and morale boosters. Excellent for the skin and keeping wrinkles at bay. They can improve sleep and dream recall in this deeply profound, powerful time of life.

Crystal Clear Spray Spray Your Hands and Face and Your Space. *Ingredients: Rose-coloured salt from Maras, Peru. Essential oils of Lavender, Frankincense and Mint. Flower essences include: Balance and Stability, Faith and Courage, Purification, Freedom/Libertad and Be Nurtured.* Crystal Clear Spray is great for clearing crystals. Deeply cleanses our aura leaving it radiating and pure and is excellent for clearing energy in a room. Brings one in touch with their light body and the anchoring of the Higher Self into the physical body. Spray your hands after doing healing to clear the energy.

Fab Spray Focused. Awake. Brilliant. *Ingredients: Ancient Wisdom, Creation/Focus, Faith and Courage, I Remember, Inner Guru,* *Inocencia Coca, My Passion, Kyanite and Purple Tourmaline. Essential Oils: Lemongrass, Peppermint and Rosemary.* Use this spray while you are studying or need to focus. Use it to help clear your head. Promotes alertness when driving and beginning to feel foggy. This combination is effective in many dimensions.

Super Immune Spray Purify and Protect. *Ingredients: Balance and Stability, Faith and Courage, Freedom/Libertad, Magic Healer, Master Teacher, Purification, Strength and Qi, Emerald, Pink Coral, Red Coral, White Coral, Dark Green Aventurine, Yellow Agate and the powerful high-vibration Rose-Coloured Salt from Maras, Peru. Plus essential oils of Eucalyptus and Oregano.* Super Immune Spray is good to have when an immune boost is needed. It is especially good when those around you have colds or flu. Take it and spray it around if you are in the hospital, whether you are staying or visiting.

Another area of exploration and research in the same realm as those producers who have created dolphins and whale essences are butterfly essences

BUTTERFLY ESSENCES (Bfy)
What they are and why they have come now

In almost every indigenous culture butterflies are known as a symbol of transformation, and it is said that the energies that they emit actually bring about transformation.

Butterflies 'channel' the most divine iridescent colour energies into the physical dimension, and have an uplifting, transformative effect on us all, enhancing the quality of our lives in many ways. They can help our development and personal process by opening us up to the greater potential and freedom of life.

Obviously the essences are not made from butterflies themselves, but in a shamanic way of old. Erik is another one of these extraordinary producers with a very intimate connection with devic beings.

His journey with essences began some 25 years ago when he encountered a being which he calls OM and was requested to start doing hundreds of analyzes of flower essences with the devas (or angels of the flower energies) who taught him what essences were, how they worked and their quality and frequency. He was guided to go to flower essence world conferences to talk about what he had discovered and gain feedback from flower essence makers – thus consolidating his knowledge of essences. In 1996 he connected with beings in the spiritual world, that which Erik calls the Solar Colour Beings, for the first time and from this point onward he was able to make butterfly essences.

Erik recalls they were made as a result of a divine empowerment – and are directly energized in a very focused, conscious way and in a potent form as they are the actual energies that butterflies emit, which resonate with the very light frequencies that compose our subtle bodies, so they are completely natural and self-adjusting in their action.

NB, Erik has also created a set of sea essences in co-operation with the Sea Devas and there are 84 in all. Please see the Useful Addresses section on page 519.

Butterfly Essences – Group One

1. **Mio Pea** – Deep Purple/Magenta – de-traumatizing, total wellbeing, Spirit Healing. A healer for our spiritual self and heart/emotional centre. Deep peace and restoration of true inner wellbeing are some effects from using this essence.

2. **Wio Lio** – Red – activation of soul consciousness. This essence brings an enhancement of spirituality and an activation of 'higher consciousness'. It can help to initiate a deeper spiritual process in us, bringing transformation and major life changes.

3. **Peo Tio** – Orange – vitality, angelic joy. An elixir of eternal youthfulness, vitality

and restoration of total wellbeing. There is an intensification of the senses, greater freshness and vitality in all things. We resonate with the joy of angels, for greater happiness.

4. **Via Sio** – Gold – divine wisdom, Om resonance, problem solving, true leadership. Brings infinite expansion of the soul body into the OM resonance with a strong resonant connection with divine wisdom. For wisdom and balance in leadership and deep harmony at all levels, especially with sound/chanting/mantras.

5. **Mea Kio** – Coral – divine sensuality, appreciation of sensual beauty. Produces a deep softness and sensuality of being with a very fine resonance and attunement in 'lovemaking'. For a blissful appreciation of male/female beauty with inner balance.

6. **Hea Hio** – Rose Pink – divine femininity. An enhancer of higher femininity bringing incredible softness and tender caring for all Beings. Helps us to manifest the beauty of the Divine Mother in the physical world, with a blissful attunement to angelic love.

7. **Wio Rea** – Pink – divine love and caring. To help us manifest divine love with true caring and compassion for others. A deep attunement to divine love helping us bring a harmonious order to our life. For positive relationship transformation.

8. **Gio Kia** – Pale Pink – soul restoration and alignment with divine unconditional love. A healing for our soul body to restore complete proper functioning from some types of damage. divine/angelic love attunement.

9. **Fia Dio** – Yellow – divine radiance and bliss. Brings an inner radiance like the sun, which is 'higher' than joy – it is the 'root of happiness'. An attunement with the 'inner joy' of our Creator emanating a soft blissful peace.

10. **Deo Ria** – Pale Yellow – inner clarity and focus, inner sight, creative visualization

booster. Stimulates a very light joyfulness. For greater clarity of consciousness and spirit to appreciate the 'inner nature of things' and to get to the 'core of problems'. Can stimulate clairvoyance in some, and clearer mental focus.

11. **Jio Hea** – Lemon Yellow – divine humour, laughter with angels, objectivity in relationships. For clearer sight and the ability to see the light within all things. To become one with the light in the eternal dance and symphony of life.

12. **Lua Kou** – Olive Green – divine compassion, divine cleansing from hurts, pain and fear. A deep healing for conflicts, pain and abuse in relationships – for oneness with others in perfect balance and harmony.

13. **Vio Tea** – Green – unity with the divine heart, effortless integration with all things. A blissful essence to unite our consciousness and spirit with all things and all beings in love and harmony, which brings a conscious state of unity with all.

14. **Lia Deo** – Pale Green – interdimensional integration, inner freedom to move between dimensions of light with ease and joy. Helps us assimilate guidance and experience from other levels and integrate these into our daily life, with a child-like playfulness.

15. **Nio Kia** – Emerald Green – heart attunement with angels, heart alignment to the consciousness. An essence to access angelic support and love for all 'affairs of the heart'. Brings inner strength and balance between being and doing. For those needing a more heart-centred consciousness.

16. **Mio Goa** – Turquoise – Reconnection with divine creativity, receptivity to higher creative inspiration. For finding our true 'inner teacher' for our creative expression in the world. To find clear creative focus and accessing divine/angelic inspiration.

17. **Eoa Ora** – Pale Turquoise – interdimensional communication accessing 'higher world' technology and innovation. A key 'New Age' tool for manifesting many new modalities into our daily lives and linking with beings at many other levels of creation.

18. **Kio Koa** – Blue – cosmic relaxation and peace, dissolving of stress, responsiveness to angels. For bringing the peace of God and the angels down into our daily lives – for deep harmony, relaxation and perfect resonance throughout the whole being. Helps to link us to angels, to work as a team in 'New Age' projects.

19. **Lia Mio** – Pale Blue – alignment with divine will, complete trust in the divine source, peace. An essence to resolve all levels of conflict and disharmony, and bring all into a resonant attunement with OM. Brings very deep peace and trust, with faith in justice.

20. **Ria Sea** – Royal Blue – calm and inner strength, spiritual healing, confidence and relaxation. Deep wellbeing for the whole self comes with the power and confidence to apply where we need it. Like an 'angel in the night' this essence is a true divine protector to help with all challenges and problems.

21. **Lio Meo** – Indigo – telepathy, spirit communication, opening of the 'third eye'. A key essence for the mind, this enhances and extends 'higher mind' abilities. For those who 'connect' with spirit it facilitates accurate information reception and it enhances all intuitive communication between people.

22. **Lia Dio** – Violet – Divine Breath connection. This clears disharmonies, strengthens the life force in us and improves wellbeing through easier breathing and a stronger connection with the Divine Resonance. A powerful meditation tool for connecting with the Divine Realms of Light, as well

as improving our physical being through better breathing – liquid yoga!

23. **Quo Dia** – Pale Violet – angelic bliss, very high meditation energy. A very special energy connection with the finest light resonances and energies of the angels, to produce an indescribable, blissful state of consciousness and wellbeing. A tool to help in the deepest meditations.

24. **Kia Kei** – Purple – inner transformation, enhanced sight. A deeply transformative energy which can raise our whole being to a divine frequency, raising all the individual vibrational frequencies within us – this is true transformation! All aspects of inner and outer sight are enhanced.

25. **Mia Kio** – Lilac – appreciation of divine beauty, purification with the love of angels. Our whole vibration is raised by this essence to attune to the incredible beauty around us – both internal and external. There is a deep angelic purification of being through love, beautifying and harmonizing us.

26. **Kio Nia** – Magenta – oneness with OM, divine attunement. An essence of pure bliss for which there is no description. An amazing tool to discover the essence of 'what *is*'; it is impossible to predict the effect of this essence as that depends on the individual relationship we have with the 'source'.

27. **Sia Soa** – Silver – soul illumination. The highest light frequency in our creation, for illumination and purification at all levels. Through this process some may attain 'samadhi' or enlightenment. Brings about an intense quieting and harmonizing of the whole being, and a raising of our being to the highest resonances.

28. **Rainbow Angel Butterflies** – ecstasy with angels, soul liberation, celebration, joy and fulfilment. A fabulous elixir manifesting a rainbow of colour in our soul, and boost to the whole being. True soul food for spiritual seekers and an incredible

support for those who are 'lightbearers' in the world today.

Butterfly Essences – Group Two

1. **Sinninia Rommala** – Pale Golden Yellow – alleviation of frustration, angelic wisdom. Intense peace and harmony comes to the consciousness as mental frustration and irritability are dissolved. Wisdom permeates the consciousness, so solutions to problems and challenges can be more easily found.

2. **Sissinka Soseino** – Silver – clarity in consciousness and perception with true discernment, dissolves illusions. This energy clears distortions and confusion in consciousness, helping us see everything as it actually is. Brings clear focus and flexibility to our thinking, for greater mental achievement and clarity of will.

3. **Tiyan Riyalla** – Lilac – deep caring through focused perception. Our senses and perception of the world are purified and sharpened, and we can effortlessly focus our attention on just one person (good for relationships). The perception of beauty and deep caring associated with Lilac can easily be mentally applied now.

4. **Mikia Kilhima** – Pale Turquoise – attunement of the mind to spirit communication. Attunes the consciousness to the communication frequencies of high spirit Beings, to facilitate better contact and work with other levels of being. Can help clear blockages relating to this, especially coming from past lives.

5. **Rialiki Ninila** – Blue – freedom and expansion of all possibilities. An empowerment for the consciousness to see and realize many new possibilities in our lives. Helps to dissolve our self-imposed limits within the mind, so we expand our consciousness to see that anything is possible, and we have the will to do it as well.

6. Tikia Solaria – Deep Indigo – restoration of brain function, new patterns of consciousness. Helps to restore full brain functions after accidents, shock or trauma working energetically through the brain nervous connections. Can initiate completely new ways of thinking and improved patterns of consciousness.

7. Winia Ririaka – Deep Coral – physical and social harmonization. It has strong relationship enhancing properties as well as harmonizing our relationship with the physical world, through the colour frequency of Deep Coral. For greater harmony and love in our day-to-day lives improving our work, family life, friendships, etc.

8. Sinhema Takia – Rose Pink – female dignity, beauty in femininity, divine female consciousness. A highly supportive energy to the femininity of any woman or girl, this enhances the whole consciousness of being female, improving dignity, self-esteem, confidence and freedom to be yourself. Opens us consciously to true beauty in all dimensions and expressions, and the awareness of the Divine Mother.

9. Isiaki Rillika – Warm Olive – conscious empathy with wisdom, love in action. Expands heart-centred consciousness to embrace others in love. Brings wisdom to apply our love practically in all situations with discretion, and with real empathy for other people's problems.

10. Rillenka Mamakia – Pale Indigo – Greater consciousness in our perceptions, alignment with the higher universal consciousness and stimulation of the higher mind. This essence expands the mind to its highest potential helping anyone with a mental or conscious impairment. Helps us to connect to divine, angelic and spiritual consciousness to access what we need.

11. Winnolia Vimmala – Pink – clarity in integrating relationships with balance.

This is an enhancer of mental love helping us to handle relationships in a better, clearer and more effective way. Helps us to be more objective in our own relationships, to be more successful in them, and improves our ability to help others; for example, counselling, marriage guidance, support services, etc.

12. Sisia Kikala – Deep Blue Violet – doorway to the inner worlds, greater ability to explore our own subconscious mind. A fascinating essence for opening up our subconscious mind to explore who we really are and to delve into past lives, and other aspects of our psyche. For finding answers within.

13. Vivia Lasaya – Deep Yellow Gold – conscious happiness, 'Sunshine of the mind'. An uplifting, harmonizing essence for our consciousness which brings greater wellbeing, positivity and optimism. A mental antidepressant which enhances creativity and wisdom.

14. Ristiya Tashisi – Deep Royal Blue – greater clarity and focus for our will, greater motivation and achievement. A power essence, which brings clarity to the mind and motivation to the will. Helps us to achieve successful results in challenging circumstances. To be clear about what we want.

15. Sasia Shalanka – Pale Orangey Red – renewal of consciousness, transforming negative patterns from the past into positive ones. Helps us to break bad habits and release negative patterns of behaviour, and replace these with positive and productive consciousness.

16. Xifia Kirrana – Deep Mid Blue – empowerment of self-expression, integrating and balancing left/right brain. A great help for anyone with communication difficulties and a confidence booster for shy and insecure people. This improves our abilities to express ourselves in many different ways, balancing left/right brain activity for more fluent easy communication, for example, for stammerers.

17. **Wiaka Sossinka** – Golden Coral – harmonizing our conscious relationship with the world. This is a great social enhancer, which will help all types of group activity and co-operation with other people. It brings real harmony and love into all relationship interactions at a conscious level, so we can put love into practice with wisdom.

18. **Yoninia Tirikra** – Deep Azure Blue – universal communication healer. A wonderful energetic support when relationships have broken down and need healing, as it stimulates communication and reconciliation in difficult circumstances. Energetically it helps us to access real support from our environment when we need it, for example, from the dolphin beings.

19. **Tulka Zennekia** – Pale Lemon Yellow – integration of feeling and thinking with clarity. For clarity about what we are feeling and thinking *in ourselves*, and integrating this with the world we are in, as well as *with ourselves*. A fine tool for knowing ourselves and bringing this into practical benefit for our relationships. Clarifies our senses and our interactions with everything.

20. **Vonia Yinnoka** – Deep Emerald Green – improved ability to express our heart to others. For courage and an enhanced ability to connect to and attune our heart energy to the heart energy of others. Helps us to overcome fear of being vulnerable and expressing our heart to others. Enhances oneness with others.

21. **Ishiani Rolia** – Pinkish Violet – conscious attunement with 'spirit', integration of our personality with spirit. It integrates the personality with the spiritual aspects of life to produce deep peace, effortless wellbeing and a positive state of mind.

Can help many states of mental imbalance, helping the mind be united with the whole and not compartmentalize itself, for example, as in 'schizophrenia'.

22. **Positha Tisika** – Deep Mid Turquoise – merging consciously with experience, unity with sound/music. This essence is a consciousness transformer, which has the property of merging the experiencer and the experience, so the two become one. It is especially exciting for musicians as it opens up all dimensions of sound equally, to initiate incredible creativity and experiencing.

23. **Timika Sommolia** – Green – freedom, integration of the spirit with situations. An important Lemurian energy, the Green 2 essence helps the spirit feel completely free in any situation. It does this by fully integrating our spiritual being with that situation, so the spirit fully accepts it.

24. **Mimika Sommala** – Pale Azure Blue – improved awareness, perception of energy movement in the environment. This essence brings a much greater sensitivity and response in us to others, and the demands of the environment. We can get greater control of our thoughts and actions and harmonize these better with other people. Good for work and relationship situations.

25. **Reloa Hikimia** – Gold – harmonizes mind and will together, mental clarity. Gives us greater energy with more harmony and focus, by harmonizing the will and the mind together so they do not pull in different directions but work as one together. Good for working situations, especially as the Gold 2 also helps us solve problems with increased wisdom.

26. **Cegia Giakala** – Aquamarine – enhances heart-centred communication, conscious expression of the heart. It brings a great peace and softness to our being, helping us to feel what other people are thinking and feeling about us. Relationships are

improved as it enables us to share their heart-space much more easily. Integrates head, heart and will beautifully.

27. **Kimia Kelhira** – Mid Indigo – restoration of mental functioning, clearer and stronger thinking. Restores the mind to full and proper functioning if it has been dysfunctional for any reason. Our emotions also become clearer and more harmonious, and our thinking processes are boosted. Good for all mental challenges, e.g. exams, business meetings, etc.

28. **Nikia Goagada** – Magenta – spiritualizes the consciousness, aligns the mind with OM, uplifts the being. It frees the mind from earthly burdens by uplifting it to the very resonance of the mind of the Creator – in this consciousness there is no time, no disharmony, no pain, no situations – only eternal bliss. A total transformer of painful Earth-bound consciousness.

Butterfly Essences – Group Three

1. **Xifa Vissislion** – Deep Purple/Magenta – the butterfly essence is renowned to have the potential for instant support when a sudden need arises, for example, trauma. It can be a very calming, nurturing and supportive effect in many instances of emotional or spiritual distress.

2. **Rono Simaron** – Red – grounding, centring and energizing essence for wellbeing and harmony. Can bring forth a connection to the Earth and our fellow inhabitants. Good for connecting with new people and new places with ease.

3. **Nola Marilion** – Orange – a refreshing, revitalizing energy for restoring a dynamic sense of direction and fun. May alleviate depression, restoring joy, direction and drive. Could be helpful in spiritual shock situations. For restoring vitality. And wellbeing.

4. **Simi Parillion** – Gold – a harmonizing, balancing, clarifying and enriching energy

for connecting to 'abundance' in all things. For finding the Hero inside ourselves. A great problem-solving essence which helps in the access and assimilation of wisdom.

5. **Kana Yinarron** – Coral – enhances sensuality, boosting imagination, stimulating the senses and beautifying expressions of love and creativity. Can increase our co-operative ability and awareness of interdependence.

6. **Suma Mimarilion** – Yellow – brings warmth and 'sunshine' into our relationship with others. A good antidepressive essence for loneliness. An uplifting essence bringing a new sense of vitality, joy and emotional wellbeing.

7. **Kimi Pinirion** – Pale Yellow – brings delight – real lightness and joy. It brings a very refined and pure sense of happiness. Artistic abilities such as dance may be helped, and real inspiration is enhanced, stimulating the creative process.

8. **Timi Mokariron** – Rose Pink – a beautiful strong female energy – helping, caring and cherishing. There is a connection with Divine Mother and Earth Mother together, giving real support to women, in pregnancy for example. Sexuality and sensuality can be boosted.

9. **Kaya Ninilion** – Pink – a universal love energy bringing balance and harmony in relationships. This enhances love in many different ways and it may enhance social cohesion, peace and a positive relationship with the natural world.

10. **Tema Visiron** – Pale Pink – helps to cleanse and harmonize many levels of our being, bringing the vibration of real caring. For divine, unconditional mother love. Can support delicate and sensitive beings with the nurturing of the mother – enhances caring, renewal, relaxation and self-acceptance.

11. **Solo Tisillion** – Lemon – a strong antidepressant which can bring joy and happiness. Enhances positivity, optimism and wellbeing, helping us to develop a very positive outlook in our whole life. Helps us to attract the best to our life.

12. **Wima Pilliron** – Olive – a releasing energy which frees us from fears and negative emotions. Empathy, feminine leadership, compassion and solidarity with others are enhanced. An essence to help bring equality and a deeper, more loving connection with others.

13. **Yisa Summaron** – Green – integration is the keyword for this essence with clarity, space and direction. Boosts the growth of plants, and activates the heart chakra to bring love, creativity and wellbeing. Helps to bring us together after stress and traumas.

14. **Sola Vikerlion** – Pale Green – helps to support our inner freedom, imagination and enhances personal creativity. Can enrich the 'inner child' giving greater lightness and playfulness and it connects us directly with the 'little people' in their energy and joy.

15. **Wira Tentaron** – Emerald Green – increases inner strength and courage. The heart is harmonized and balanced, and the flow of Qi energy around the body is enhanced. Practices such as yoga and Tai Chi are helped. Leadership qualities improve, such as calmness, strength and decisiveness. Good for work with plants and animals.

16. **Tira Winirion** – Turquoise – can bring enhancement to all levels of communication, relationship and socially expressed creativity (e.g. acting and music). Enjoyment of music and all sound resonances increases, as well as creativity in performing music. Deeper connections with others become possible.

17. **Mala Linilion** – Pale Turquoise – communication with angels, spiritual beings and elemental beings is enhanced by this essence. This reconnects us to our soul being consciously and energetically, helping effortless and intuitive communication with spiritual beings. Enhances work with crystals and 'higher energies' for wellbeing (e.g. essences).

18. **Nori Ristillion** – Blue – can bring relaxation of stress, and restoration of wellbeing. Improves responsiveness to others to improve our communication and balance with them. A wonderful relaxer and restorer of mind and body together.

19. **Lina Sinlinlon** – Pale Blue – for bringing forth inner peace, trust, freedom and alignment with the Divine Will. Can help to balance power and love to bring perfection and happiness. Restores faith in Divine Justice and connects us to the Father Being of God.

20. **Tori Sommarion** – Royal Blue – a strong enhancer to our will and personal power. It improves our control over events in our life, bringing a powerful relaxed ease to all of our activities. Physical wellbeing can improve and we can be strengthened and feel more confident.

21. **Vima Tokaron** – Indigo – A strengthening essence for our thinking and mental functioning. This essence can help us to access universal consciousness when we need to, and improve our ability to accurately bring higher knowledge down to Earth. Telepathy improves.

22. **Puma Tosaron** – Violet – brings an effortless integration between spiritual awareness and earthly activities bringing improved meditation with deep peace and effortless wellbeing. For conscious connection to our soul plan to help to make clear our true service to the world.

23. Wina Simarion – Pale Violet – the keywords for this essence are 'angelic healing', and this is an incredibly beautiful essence for working with the angels and the spiritual world. Sensitivity, receptivity and consideration can be enhanced with deep stillness. Deep meditation essence.

24. Zila Sissilion – Purple – a very creative essence for artists and those who appreciate the visual arts. This essence can enhance eyesight attuning us to beauty and creativity in the visual world. We can see the 'inner beauty' of people and the world and respond creatively to it.

25. Yova Tirillion – Lilac – for cherishing ourselves and others. An energy of deep transformation and connection with angelic love. Opens us up to heavenly beauty on this Earth linking us deeply with the angels in love and care.

26. Vaza Risiron – Magenta – for transcending our earthly experience and entering a heavenly one. We can connect effortlessly to spirit and earthly problems dissolve. There is a very special connection to the heart of divine mother and in meditation we can explore the 'higher worlds'.

27. Nina Sirion – Silver – unity can be experienced through this essence possibly bringing a deep understanding of 'core' issues. We can connect with divine light for cleansing and greater knowledge and learning. Good for all sorts of cleansing, especially crystals. For connection with all levels.

28. Rainbow Butterflies – Enhances our energy on every level – this can bring a 'feast' of colour and wellbeing to us, opening us up for real divine health and joy. All chakras are stimulated and open together with the help of this essence for our greater good and happiness.

G.

SHAMANIC ESSENCES

JAGUAR SHAMANIC ESSENCES "JAGUAR IS CALLING" (JAG)

My mother is a Shamanka, Medicine Woman and Healer of both the North and South Native American traditions, and after teaching in one of her workshops the instruction came through to me that we should make Jaguar Essences designed for her and any other budding shamans (flower shamans included) for use during their healings and ceremonial practices. There are now new categories of essence ranges emerging that are purely energetically downloaded from Spirit. In line with the ancient Shamanic practices of the medicine men of the Amazon Rainforest, who are able to call and communicate with the spirit of plants, animals, mountain Apu's and over-lighting energies of sacred places, the Jaguar Essences were made in this tradition with techniques I learnt whilst in the Amazon.

This has proved to be a very succinct and powerful set of essences of which I am sure there are more to come.

1. The Spirit of the Jaguar Circles the path of truth. Walks the road of power and integrity. Works with direct perception, focus and intent.

Jaguar speaks: I process heavy hucha for humans and Mother Earth, I am a clearer of paths and in circling the road of truth I make way for empowerment.

2. Red Condor Circles the path of vision. Sees truth behind the vision – illusion.

Condor speaks: Call on me for illuminations. I am the guardian that circles the sacred citadel of Machu Picchu and I hold the memory of the ancient seed.

3. Machu Picchu Awakens the path of consciousness.

The spirit of Machu Picchu speaks: I am the vortex of light built on the double helix of light itself. I connect human kind with the ancient seed race that lies in their DNA.

4. Mountain Apu Awakens the path of power and strength.

The Overlighting guardians spread light through power.

Mountain Apu speaks: We hold the matrix of life – itself, we are fierce challengers of human intent and integrity.

5. Double Helix Holds the balance for consciousness's shifts.

The spirit of Double Helix speaks: I am the stream of consciousness that holds the double helix in balance, I work with the DNA-change conditioned consciousness giving opportunities for change and growth, and hold the balance during major shifts in consciousness.

H.

ESSENCES FOR BABIES AND CHILDREN

Many of us remember a childhood that was simpler than today, when we were satisfied with inventing our own games, creating something out of nothing, and what was expected of us was clearer and more defined. The major change has been in the speed of communication, the exchange of information that has dramatically accelerated, resulting in us all having to step up a gear in order to assimilate and process this more rapidly in order to cope.

Although children become familiar with this faster pace of life, the extra stresses and strains of contemporary life demand new ways of handling the problems with which parents as well as children are increasingly confronted. Here it makes sense to use the flower essences for both the parent and child with emphasis on mother, baby and child, as the first few years are when the patterns of response to the world become set.

Purely Essences have created remedies for mother and newborn baby and Lila Devi, producer of the Spirit in Nature/Master's Flower Essences, has also addressed this special relationship between mother and children.

SPIRIT IN NATURE/MASTER'S FLOWER ESSENCES FOR MOTHER AND CHILD (MA)

Most mothers know the more stressed they are, the more the child reacts and the less likely she is to be able to handle situations calmly. What creates more tension is the knowledge that she is not doing it right, giving her the feeling of not being 'a good mother', so flower remedies tailor-made for such moments are invaluable.

As parents we realize the more we are able to interact with our child in an understanding and intelligent way, the better equipped they are, by example, to grow into emotionally balanced, assured adults. This is where the Spirit in Nature/Master's Flower Essences come into their own.

This beautiful range of essences from the blossoms of flowers, fruits and vegetables is based on the principle of the metaphysician Yogananda that 'You are what you eat'. Created in 1977 by Lila Devi to enable becoming 'masters of our own lives' by manifesting those qualities that we already possess in our own unique way, these essences are recommended for families and are exceptionally supportive of the unique dynamic between mother and child. It is this important interrelationship that has led Lila to research for solutions within the Spirit in Nature/Master's Flower Essences range.

As these essences lend themselves to this special interaction, it is beneficial for both to take essences simultaneously as it not only clears any difficulties the child is experiencing with coping with life but helps the mother understand more fully how to help so that she is part of the solution and not part of the problem.

Almond (*Prunus amygdalus*)
Mother: In control, balance and moderation. For being spread too thin, overindulgence in food, substances, activities, etc. Helps to find the middle way, calms mind and nerves, syncs the mind/body/spirit.
Child: Out of balance. For excess, feelings of being out of control. Balances emotional extremes, helps find inner balance, the middle way. Beneficial for pre-teens.

Apple (*Malus domestica*)
Mother: Healthy mindset. Clears worry, doubt, toxic emotions such as anger, jealousy or fear, cultivates a positive outlook, a nourishing and abundant attitude.
Child: Healthy and happy. Good during illness or when the thought of illness is present, especially when emotional upset creates physical symptoms. For periods of discouragement. Helps to maintain wellness when overwhelmed by emotional issues.

Avocado (*Persea americana*)
Mother: Clarity, absent-mindedness, forgetful and feeling dull and flat, without direction, brings clarity and focus, sense of purpose, learning from past mistakes. Feeling alert and alive.
Child: Learning, focus and concentration. For the child who forgets his or her chores, manners, etc. Helps with school work, homework, exams, sharpens concentration, fosters a love for learning, enthusiasm about homework and aids creativity and the development of musical or artistic endeavours.

Banana (*Musa paradisiaca*)
Mother: Oversensitivity, stepping back, observing, a non-reactive attitude. Clears anxiety, being overwhelmed, loss of perspective, not seeing the wood for the trees or being caught up in others' negativity.
Child: Going bananas, calm and thoughtful, gaining perspective and for the child who needs to centre less on him or herself and be more caring, relating better with family, siblings and friends.

Blackberry (*Rubus fruticosus*)
Mother: Positive thoughts. Clears negative thinking, unkind thoughts, fault finding, bluntness or pessimism. Brings purity of thought, optimism and compassion, seeing the good in oneself and others.
Child: For worry and negative thoughts and behaviour. For the child stressed by exposure to negative influences often through the media such as disturbing movies or TV programmes or people, nightmares, thoughts of uncleanness. Good for the 'terrible twos'.

Cherry (*Prunus serrulata*)
Mother: Cheerful, optimistic, positive and light-hearted, clears moodiness, feeling contrary, somewhat out of control emotionally. Brings inspiration and seeing the good in life.
Child: Happiness, brings a happy mood, for the child who is prone to periods of withdrawal and sadness. For disappointment. Helps to heal the trauma of divorce or separation, imminent or past. Aid for bedwetting.

Coconut (*Cocos nucifera*)
Mother: Uplifted and determined, clears lack of endurance, escapism, giving up, making excuses, avoidance, helps completion of tasks, living up to highest potential, determination, ready to take the next step.
Child: Being positive, helps deal with sibling rivalry, challenge or struggle in school or peer dynamics. Develops maturity and ability to make healthy choices in difficult situations and in life.

Corn (*Zea mays*)
Mother: Energy and vitality. Clears blocked energy, sluggishness, resistance, procrastination and lethargy. Aids enthusiasm, joy, living in the present, initiating projects, saying yes to life's challenges and new beginnings.
Child: New start. Alertness, helpful for new beginnings, new school year, new friends, moving house and home, gives encouragement for periods of procrastination and

bursts of energy for 'study blues'. Aid for car sickness.

Date (*Phoenix dactylifera*)
Mother: Tolerance and receptivity. Open-minded, easy to talk to, self-nurturing, clears intolerance, irritation and the tendency to be critical. Develops a warm, welcoming nature.
Child: Sweet nature and tenderness. For the child who can be overcritical and judgemental of other children or siblings. Fault-finding, whining and sometimes clinging. Brings sweetness and ease. Encourages self-nurturing when life seems harsh. Date brings out the tender side in children who tend to be whiny or clingy.

Fig (*Ficus carica*)
Mother: Self-nurture and flexibility. Helps with going with the flow, being at ease with self and others. For those who are too hard on themselves, prone to self-judgement, unrealistic expectations, trying too hard, and who are tense and overextended and finding it difficult to change. Encourages relaxed healthy self-nurturing, boundaries and energy to move forward.
Child: It's OK for the child who is too hard on him or herself or tries too hard, unsatisfied with accomplishments even when noteworthy. Good for nail-biting and thumb-sucking; helps children develop a positive overview about themselves.

Grape (*Vitis* sp.)
Mother: Love and compassion. Patience with others' shortcomings. Clears strong negative emotions, jealousy, resentment, feelings of abandonment, grief and vulnerability due to separation, divorce or death. Helps to find forgiveness and that inner source of love.
Child: A loving nature. Great for tantrums and any attitude that is not loving. Clears stubborn, self-willed moods and any bullying tendencies or attitudes. For the child who keeps saying no!

Lettuce (*Lactuca sativa*)
Mother: Calm and clear. Inner quiet and ability to speak one's truth. Clears restlessness,

nervousness, excitability and agitation, crowded thinking, lack of concentration and indecision. Unblocks creativity, self-expression, success in undertakings. Aids sleep.
Child: Settled and chilled. For children who are too wound up, running on nervous energy, prone to restlessness, agitation and sleeplessness. Helps them to play or study constructively, good for exam nerves to calm and steady the mind. Dislike of salad.

Orange (*Citrus sinensis*)
Mother: Joy. Banishes depression, hopelessness and despair, any past or present emotional/physical abuse trauma, headaches. Renews hope, helps to resolve conflicts and endure difficulties. Cultivates an inner smile.
Child: Smile. For the child who can be sad and moody, dispels discontentment and periods of depression, helpful during teething. Good for emotional issues resulting from accidents to the head and for conflict resolution between family and peers, for restoring a sense of excitement.

Peach (*Prunus persica*)
Mother: The mothering essence. Concern for others, empathy, nurturing from wholeness rather than from neediness. Clears overinvolvement and tendency to smother. Balances mothering, equilibrium of response.
Child: Sharing and co-operation. Promotes the sense of sharing and co-operation with other children, for example, with favourite toys and prized possessions. Excellent for helping the weaning process be a positive experience for infants.

Pear (*Pyrus communis*)
Mother: Emergency rescue remedy, for any kind of crisis, physical or emotional. Being thrown off balance during traumatic events, accidents, illness, childbirth and postnatal depression. Clears shock, and fear, giving peace of mind, and stability during major changes.
Child: Shock remedy. Rescue for accidents, sudden illness and crisis situations. Helps with toilet training, learning of new positive habits. For the fidgety and restless child who has a hard time listening in school or at home.

Pineapple (*Ananas comosus*)

Mother: Brings self-esteem and assurance, and feelings of confidence and empowerment. Clears dissatisfaction. If you are unhappy with your job it helps you to match your career with your talents. For strong identity, clarity with money issues and the ability to attract abundance.

Child: Shyness and confidence, helps the child to 'untie the apron strings'. For being singled out by peers for being different in some way. For the painfully shy child, gives self-esteem.

Raspberry (*Rubus idaeus*)

Mother: Brings kindness, generosity, forgiving and willingness to turn the other cheek. For the easily hurt and touchy who take things too personally, and tend to overreact. Releases old emotional wounds. Promotes understanding and generosity of spirit.

Child: Easily hurt, oversensitive and reactive. For the child who is easily hurt especially for youngsters who in reaction can hurt others. Nurtures a kind and giving nature.

Spinach (*Spinacia oleracea*)

Mother: Simplicity and trust. For mothers who are stressed out, overwhelmed, worried and distrustful. Brings a childlike sense of joy, clearing dysfunctional childhood patterns. Bringing a carefree spirit and *joie de vivre*.

Child: Stressed out. For the child who is too grown up, overly serious. For times of stress, exhaustion, feeling over-responsible, distraught and overwhelmed. Restores innocence and a sense of fun.

Strawberry (*Fragaria*)

Mother: For dignity and a grounded, quiet strength and sense of self. Dissolves guilt, feeling unworthy and undeserving. Clears history of emotionally abusive, dysfunctional childhood. For those who are psychically oversensitive. Brings poise, grace and feeling comfortable with one's body.

Child: Good self-image. For children who have trouble letting go of being a baby. Nurtures a deep sense of self-worth, and brings clarity of a positive self-image. For the child dealing with divorced parents.

Tomato (*Solanum lycopersicum*)

Mother: Makes you into Superwoman, knowing no failure and seeing all challenges as only another chance to succeed. Self-belief, invincibility, courage. Clears fears, nightmares, defensiveness, addictions, defeatist attitude, others' negative energy, and the stress of city life and travelling.

Child: Brings an 'I can do anything' attitude, mental strength, courage, helps to dissolve fears, nightmares. Encourages a child to move forward in their life when anxious, nervous, hesitant or unwilling.

BLOESEM FLOWER ESSENCES AND THE CHILDREN VORTEX

The **Children Vortex** is an especially powerful and important essence for children and also useful for adults. An essence for the times we live in, it is created from the energy of a vortex, and presence of angelic energy. It helps in receiving and integrating the support and love from the angelic realm. Opens one to the magic of being alive and awakens the inner child.

Created from the following gemstones:

- Fluorite: gives protection and self-confidence; opens the door to the unconscious releasing of stuck limitations and habits. Removes negativity and aids understanding of emotions.

- Celestite: connects with the angelic realm, brings a deep peace and spiritual evolution. Helps with resolving conflicts, giving faith in the infinite wisdom of the divine.

- Aquamarine: calms and protects, helping release the responsibility of the thoughts of others. Aids understanding of emotions and old problems through interpretation of one's own thoughts and feelings.

- Halite: clears the soul, dissolves old patterns, negative thoughts and stuck emotions, releasing the feelings of abandonment and rejection.

- Morganite: has a strong heart energy, awareness of the existence of pure divine love. Connects you with the higher light frequencies and the angelic realms. Releasing and transforming, the stone of change, strength, hope and the feminine.

- Rhodolite: gives energy, restores and clears the chakras. For serenity and passion, an important gem in a crisis, because it provides courage.

- The amethyst: a powerful, spiritual gem that enhances the mental capacities, brings wisdom and calm. Balances highs and lows, expels anger, grief, fear and worries. Helps one cope with loss. For spiritual wisdom and love of the divine.

- Petrified wood: is important for grounding, especially for the sensitive new world children.

The Children Vortex clears all trauma, pain and grief from childhood, such as trauma from being beaten up, but also for those not allowed to play outside, who had to work, and felt imprisoned by duties. For when the joy of playfulness has disappeared and the heart is a place of pain. When there is an attempt to do something enjoyable, the feeling of old obligations and old pain returns, stopping enjoyment of life.

This essence integrates the qualities that obstruct the evolution of the (child) soul. Renews the memories to the cellular level, reconnecting with the original qualities of the soul, before it incarnated. It integrates newly gained knowledge and old universe knowledge, making it possible to live without the restrictions of the earthly existence and to feel connected with the universal light. Be who you are, beyond all restrictions. Opens the heart for the evolution of love and the realization of all one's universal qualities of light, love and the awakened consciousness of the here and now. Gives the star child both security and protection from the angelic world and connects it with his or her original strength, making it possible for the star children to be here on Earth with an open heart.

NATURE AND NURTURE
The teenage years

I've found that in my practice the Flower Essences of Australia remedies are most acceptable to this age group as mostly anything with an Aboriginal connection is considered cool! Flower Essences of Australia's Blackboy is especially designed for those donkey years when teenagers really don't know how to handle themselves or really what's happening. The boys especially can become day-dreamy, procrastinate, sleep till lunch time, or be aggressive or rude with communication going out the window. For girls when reaching puberty and developing their curves, Woman Balance Essence taken with Blackboy works wonders for this delicate stage.

For the pressure of exams, a combination that's stood the test of time with all exams is Learning & Focus, which has helped them sail through, with great results. It clears learning problems and helps with assimilation, integration and focused thinking, especially when distracted, scattered and feeling overwhelmed. Also invaluable for accident-prone teenagers, at the clumsy stage when hormones are playing havoc with their emotions.

Environmental and electromagnetic pollution

This is a more recent phenomenon; in our age of rapid technological advances and wizardry, childhood has radically changed. Most children, especially teenagers, are totally computer literate, mobiles double up as cameras, virtual reality and cyberspace are part of their everyday existence. The health implications of this increasing exposure to radiation and electromagnetic energy on developing brains is just beginning to register, as our children spend more and more time in front of the TV, or playing with their PlayStations, surfing the net, researching school projects, emailing, communicating via Facebook or just chatting or texting with their friends on their mobile phones. More evidence of the possible link to cancer with the use of mobile phones is coming to light, so it seems important to protect the health of our children.

Flower essence producers, parents themselves, have been concerned about this growing problem and have developed combinations such as Electro-guard, Eclipse Spritz, Radiation Cactus and T1 to protect against and clear the side-effects of electromagnetic pollution.

A return to nature and childlike innocence, by Peter Tadd

The most significant change in the flower essence world in the last decade is the growing appreciation that using essences as remedies for specific ills is also an entry into deepening our relationship with nature. This is the very reason that environmental essences are finding their way into the sets of a growing number of essence makers. These essences put us in touch with the 'spirit of the place'. I focus on nature because in this context we are speaking not of natural beauty alone but invisible intelligences. As adults becoming more aware and more capable of sensing these subtleties, we are in fact returning to a state of childlike innocence.

Being in a state of awareness, being present, calm and in harmony with our environment is a most worthy goal. Yet in this same time period, life has become more stressful because we are surrounded by greater numbers of disharmonious forces, environmental hazards, and unnatural electromagnetic and microwave forces which invade our auras. We are looking at visuals made up of square fragments, which no longer offer the etheric light bridge to our eyes, but digitalized pictures

that interrupt this subtle life-giving flow. Therefore, essences are more than ever important for us. But what about our children?

One recent and exciting development in the essence world has been the recognition that today's children are in need of help, perhaps more than ever before. They are more vulnerable than adults to the stress factors mentioned above. Indeed, many children are suffering from greater and greater academic demands that challenge their right to be children, open and curious. This pressure is magnified for very creative and gifted children. Some essence makers, such as Lila Devi and Sabina Pettitt, are now including essences in their lines which meet the specific requirements of children, such as Lila Devi's Spinage, Flower Essences of Australia's Blackboy essence and Sabina's Pacific Essences' Kids' Stuff.

Lila Devi's Spirit in Nature/Master's range has designed essences for the special dynamic between mother and child and mothers and their babies. One other maker, Ann Callaghan, has also devoted her essences entirely to children: Indigo Essences.

Why should we consider essences for children and how do they operate differently than for adults? Children are very open to the subtle energies of etheric forces found in homeopathic remedies and in flower essences. Their etheric bodies are not so dominated by rigid mental states, nor weighed down by years of emotional scarring. Thus the results of homeopathic and flower/mineral/animal essence treatments are more easily or dramatically seen in children. This is to say that the auras of children are more easily imprinted – in the same way that some children remain open to 'invisible friends' and some see fairies.

Let us take a moment to look at the aura of a child. A young child's aura is undeveloped. The chakras are not fully opened in the lower three centres. Children are their surroundings, and up until the age of seven they have not yet constructed a mental optic by which to observe life.

Thus certain aspects of a very young child's aura are very open to spiritual dimensions. In an infant the crown chakra is aligned to the divine, as it is unfettered by self-denial or authoritarian belief systems. If a child can remain open to the light through to the age of nine the likelihood for continued access to spiritual realms is very strong. This is to say that the child knows that he or she is a 'being' or a soul. The material world is the stage or playground but they retain this essential identity of self.

This is in part due to interplay of the chakras in these developing years. There exists in the area of the hip sockets two very important minor chakras. These are the eyes of the child. They combine with the solar plexus and the third eye chakras and provide the integration of hormonal and ego development, socialization skills and visual and psychological perspectives. As the child grows, this integration can continue with unbroken direct contact with the kingdoms in nature and of the heavens. This is rare but in the cases when children have access to nature and are allowed to wander outside and to wander inside – daydream that is – they retain this ability to be at one with all that is natural. It is actually this fluidity of movement that most resembles the spiralling patterns found in nature, its whirlpools in streams, cloud patterns, rock flows that form the very basis for the now-acclaimed modern chaos theory. This freedom of nature in the child aligns them to the intelligence in nature and to their own creativity. Where this is not the case then an intervention is needed and that can direct us to including the root chakra in our treatment protocol.

Ann Callaghan's Indigo Essences are one of the few lines, as well as Lila Devi's Spirit in Nature/Master's Mother and Child range, to have appeared on the horizon specifically designed for children. They are as effective for adults working with the inner child (see Ailment Chart, Appendix 1). There are many to choose from in the global flower essence world which help us to reconnect with our inner self as well as that innate state of child-like wonder.

What I like about the Indigos is that they have a unique effect on the root chakra because they are not plant derived. The root chakra has two placements, and one is in the perineum aligned with the mineral element. This point is vital to our sense of 'grounding' or for the child incarnating. The fact that this essence line is created from stones and crystals uniquely can help some children feel 'OK in their bodies' and, more than that, these essences strengthen the white light or vital sheath of the etheric body. Moreover, this can mean many things but it gives the child a sense of solidity and clarity.

To sum up, technology is pushing our families and us in one direction. The benefits of the IT world are obvious; the negatives are not always so evident. Essences can be of the greatest value to us, as a way back home, as a means to bring our children back to their birthright as sensitive creative beings. Nature awaits and is never far away.

Peter Tadd is known for his clairvoyant skills, analysing essences for makers and developers worldwide and his role for many years as the quality control person and lecturer for I.F.E.R. (my original flower essences company). His present work is a further study and teaching of how essences enhance the aura and chakras, including and especially the transcendental chakras.

I.

ESSENCES FOR PETS AND ANIMALS

An important area in many of our lives is the relationship with our pets and how bonded and fond of them we can become. They provide companionship and can be a positive source of unconditional love. Many of us have an intuitive communication with our cats, dogs or horses, for example in the way they seem to know how we feel and the exact time that we will be arriving at home. We feel drawn to keep them healthy and happy, especially as they can often take on our negative emotions and need to be cleared and protected from this in order to maintain their balance. My Angora Turkish Van cat, Picchu, often alerted me to the fact that my aura needs cleaning by intensely looking around my aura and, whilst vocalizing her observations, flicking her legs in sequence to suggest shaking off the negative energy. She is only satisfied when we have both been spritzed. This is where flower essences come very much into their own.

SPIRIT IN NATURE/MASTER'S FLOWER ESSENCES FOR PETS (Ma)

Spirit in Nature/Master's Essences are also invaluable for treating pets and animals. Pets and animals, who are free from the mental interferences that often plague the human mind, also respond quickly and dramatically when given flower essences. Case after case shows that animals, possessing a rich

instinctive nature and a wide range of emotions, are able to adapt more easily to a life of domestication with the assistance of these essences. Lila Devi's book *Flower Essences for Animals* elucidates her essence line and provides the text for her widely acclaimed bilevel pets and animals course.

Almond (*Prunus amygdalus*) For pets who are confined, who pace or display repetitive behaviours.

Apple (*Malus domestica*) For pets who were the runt of the litter or who tend to pick up worrisome attitudes from their owners.

Avocado (*Persea americana*) Helps pets with alertness, training and responding to commands.

Banana (*Musa × paradisiaca*) Good for pets who are easily agitated or who tend to bully other pets in the home. Also to reinforce the positive behaviour of an already calm animal.

Blackberry (*Rubus fruticosus*) For pets who are ill or older and can no longer care for themselves. It is good to spray this essence in the litterbox area for cleanliness.

Cherry (*Prunus avium*) For pets when they get grumpy, or act listless and uninterested in their surroundings (be sure to rule out medical causes).

Coconut (*Cocos nucifera*) For ageing pets who are adapting to limited movement or range of physical abilities and for overcoming any difficulties in adjusting to domesticated life.

Corn (*Zea mays*) For older pets, Corn helps them to act younger again and supports recovery from illness and surgery.

Date (*Phoenix dactylifera*) Helps pets express their natural sense of friendliness and, for those who are domineering, to be more accepting of other household pets.

Fig (*Ficus carica*) This essence aids pets in training and also helps them overcome bad habits. Good for pets who have had multiple homes or been confused by inconsistent training.

Grape (*Vitis* sp.) For pets who have been abandoned, or who feel threatened by other animals in the household; for strays and feral animals. To ease territorial disputes, dominance issues, and helping animals who are jealous or possessive.

Lettuce (*Lactuca sativa*) Good for pets, especially younger animals who are easily riled or who bounce off the walls, especially with strangers or guests.

Orange (*Citrus sinensis*) For pets who have lost an animal or human companion, are nearing their own time of passing or are dealing with ongoing physical pain. Orange is imperative for grieving animals who have been unnaturally altered, such as declawed or debarked (not including spaying or neutering).

Peach (*Prunus persica*) Good for pets who are demanding or unusually needy, and for animals who were weaned too early and tend to chew or suckle on clothing.

Pear (*Pyrus communis*) Good for pets any time their regular routine is disturbed, including vet visits, car travel or nearing their time of passing (especially good for their owners at this time as well). This is a good essence to keep on hand at all times.

Pineapple (*Ananas comosus*) For pets, especially show animals, to take pride in their accomplishments, and for multi-pet households, as well as for the runt of the litter.

Raspberry (*Rubus idaeus*) For pets who are extremely sensitive and seem to be good listeners. Also for pets who tend to feel slighted. This remedy is especially helpful for inappropriate urination (as opposed to spraying) and soiling problems.

Spinach (*Spinacia oleracea*) To restore a pet's youthfulness, good for post-surgical procedures and for any kind of stress in the household.

Strawberry (*Fragaria*) To support pets in their growing expressions of likes and dislikes, the flourishing of their personalities and their innate charm. Helps with the imminence of their passing.

Tomato (*Solanum lycopersicum*) For pets who cower or retreat, especially from any loud noises. Also for animals who have been previously mistreated, including those with an unknown history.

SUN ESSENCES FOR ANIMALS (Sun)

Sun Essences for Animals is based in Cromer, Norfolk, close to where Dr Bach lived and worked. Since the 1980s, Jane Stevenson, an experienced flower essence practitioner, has provided individual consultations for people with emotional problems, and discovered this pure and natural remedial method to be extremely effective and rewarding. Jane also found that she was increasingly treating animals with flower essences. Her love of flowers and affinity with animals culminated in the development of a unique collection of flower essence blends, designed to alleviate the key emotional and behavioural problems experienced by animals.

As a co-founder of 'Sun Essences' making a range of flower remedies (see page 244), with her passion for helping animals it was Jane's wish that they all also have the opportunity to benefit from flower essence therapy. A natural result was the creation of 'Sun Essences for Animals' and Jane feels privileged to continue this important work so close to the original roots of Dr Bach, who felt that every household would benefit from his Bach Flower Remedies.

Jane is currently dedicated to helping animals and works closely with vets, trainers, animal sanctuaries and the RSPCA (Royal Society for the Prevention of Cruelty to Animals).

The natural way to happy, healthy pets

Anyone who has a pet or works with animals knows that animals can suffer with emotional as well as behavioural problems. They can experience the same range of emotions as us: fear, rage, sadness, anxiety, jealousy, etc. The flower essence blends can help by promoting calm, balanced and well-adjusted behaviour. Flower essences are frequently used to help alleviate emotional problems because they can gently soothe an animal, without masking their true nature. Veterinary clinics, training clubs and rescue homes use flower essences as an effective way of helping animals with emotional and behavioural problems. It suggests that these natural products can be used alongside other treatments and have no known side-effects. Natural, simple and safe to use – just add to food and water.

Apathy Natural help for animals who are lethargic, miserable or weary. Useful for when an animal's disposition seems low, down in spirits, miserable or apathetic. Also consider during times when the animal may be overtaxed and an extra tonic is required, for example, pregnancy, lactation, old age, during convalescence, etc.

Distress Natural help for animals who are: frightened, anxious or alarmed. Use for alarming or distressing events, as it can initiate a calming process. Can also be used to relax an animal prior to, or during, particularly upsetting situations, for example,. accidents, emergencies, travelling, thunder storms, fireworks, 'show' nerves, visits to the vets or farriers, etc.

Dominant Natural help for animals who are impulsive, stroppy, stubborn. This blend has been developed especially to help balance the nature of headstrong, stubborn or bossy animals. Also suggested for jealous, impulsive, unmanageable and possessive behaviour.

Highly Strung Natural help for animals who are boisterous, frisky or scatty. Blended specifically for overactive, scatty, frisky, boisterous and excitable animals. Other indications may be restlessness and attention-seeking behaviour. This blend can also be helpful for training animals who display erratic behaviour.

Pining Natural help for animals who are relocating, alone or bereaved. For pining and lonely pets who are left 'home alone' (e.g. while the owner is at work) or for unhappy or bereaved pets who may have lost an owner or animal companion. Also use for 'relocation', for example, adjusting to a new home, kennel accommodation, 'separation anxiety', etc.

Timid Natural help for animals who are submissive, ring-shy, nervous. Helpful for animals who may be generally fearful, sensitive, frightened, spooked or insecure. Also indicated for low confidence, nervousness or withdrawn and submissive behaviour.

Dosage for Timid; Dominant; Highly Strung; Pining; Apathy

Large animals (horses, goats, etc.): 12 drops three times daily.

Medium animals (dogs, cats, etc.): 7 drops three times daily.

Small animals (rabbits, guinea pigs, birds, etc.): 3 drops three times daily.

Dosage for Distress Blend

Large animals (horses, goats, etc.): 12 drops every 10–30 minutes until calm, then three times daily if required.

Medium animals (dogs, cats, etc.): 7 drops every 10–30 minutes until calm, then three times daily if required.

Small animals (rabbits, guinea pigs, birds, etc.): 3 drops every 10–30 minutes until calm, then three times daily if required.

Use and administration

The essences should be added to food, treats or water. They can also be rubbed onto gums or the drops can be shaken onto fur to be licked off. For birds (particularly), the essences can be put into a spray mist bottle and sprayed onto the feathers.

Only use one blend at a time, except in certain 'emergency' situations – for example, if the animal is frightened during the firework season, thunder storms, a sudden traumatic experience, show nerves, etc. In this instance the Distress Blend can be used alongside one of the other blends – use every 10 minutes, if required.

If the animal isn't already taking a blend during the firework season it is advisable to give them the Distress Blend three times daily for up to two weeks before 5 November or New Year's Eve, and for a few days after, until the fireworks season is over.

NB, flower essences are not a substitute for correct veterinary care.

DANCING LIGHT HAPPY PET (DL)

Happy Pet is a blend of Alaska's Elements, and Dancing Light Orchid Essences Gentle first-aid support for animals large or small, to assist with emergencies, shock, trauma, fear, injuries, trips to the vet, pregnancy and birth, sickness, death, sadness, recovery from abuse, wild animal rescue and rehabilitation, and other transitions. Keep several bottles on hand as the unexpected is bound to take place. Using Happy Pet yourself when you give it to your pet may help you both feel more relaxed, trusting, bonded and a bit cosier together. When helping a new pet to adjust to new people and surroundings, mist the areas where your pet will sleep and play.

Alaskan Animal Care Combination *Alpine Azalea, Black Tourmaline, Chiming Bells, Cotton Grass Horsetail, Jadeite Jade, Lady's Slipper.* Animal Care is intended for use in animal rescue work, although it can be given to any animal in need. It is most valuable when it is integrated into the initial care provided to any animal that arrives at an animal shelter, treatment centre, veterinarian clinic, or sanctuary. This formula is also a must when adopting a 'rescue' animal.

Use Animal Care for domestic animals who:

- live in large cities, are restricted from normal contact with nature and are alone for much of the day;

- have been voluntarily given up to an animal care shelter because their owners can no longer care for them;

- have been abandoned and then rescued off the street after a prolonged struggle for survival;

- have lived in conditions where the care given them was inadequate, the living environment toxic, and the relationship with their humans abusive; are exhibiting self-aggressive behaviour.

Use Animal Care for wild animals who:

- are brought to a clinic because they have been injured or their habitats have been damaged or destroyed;

- are agitated, irritated and exhibiting aggressive behaviour, which may be endangering themselves, other animals or humans;

- have lived for some time in pet shops, and subsequently in the homes of people, in isolation from other members of their own species;

- must be kept in captivity in a shelter, sanctuary or zoo, because their injuries cannot be fully healed, and need to be handled in order to receive treatment;

- are suffering from 'toxic' interference from their contact with the public and need to release this energy so they can be released back into the wild.

Animal Care Spray Animal Care Spray contains small amounts of organic Lemon Grass and Roman Chamomile essential oils. These enhance the calming effects of the formula and add their refreshing qualities to the spray, which can be misted around the animal, on its bedding and in its immediate environment. This spray is particularly useful when working with injured animals or those behaving aggressively.

STAR PERUVIAN ESSENCES

Happy Pet Spray *Balance and Stability, Be Nurtured, Faith and Courage, Nature Communion, Clear Quartz and Kyanite. Lavender essential oil.* Animals (wild and domestic) respond well to vibrational essences. This combination is effective for all kinds of pet upsets including moving, any accidents and travel. Use to speed the recovery process. Spray their bed or their space. Spray your hands and pet them. Add the drops to their water or put it on their paws. Put it directly in their mouths or on their fur.

BLOESEM REMEDIES NEDERLAND

Animal Freedom *Red Henbit, Snowdrop, Trumpet Vine, Alternanthera, Rue, Smooth Hawksbeard, Foxglove, Clematis and Sensitive Weed.* This combination remedy helps to free the soul of the animal. It releases the animal from the problems and sufferings it has taken on from its owner, as well as also releasing animals from the problems and suffering inflicted on it by humans, both conscious and subconscious. Many animals' problems are related to the owner's tensions and stress. Gives the animal the feeling of freedom, helping it feel calm and at ease. Connects the animal to its original strength and sense of being, so that it can live out the original purpose of its life. It has given good results in cases with epilepsy.

J.

ENVIRONMENTAL AND SOUND ESSENCES

There is a growing awareness that taking responsibility for our environment is very much part of our stewardship as cohabiters on this planet. Essences created from the energy of the environment, the elements and sacred places are a new departure in the development of essences. I first became fully aware of the powerful energy held within a sacred place when in 1996 I spent a full moon night in the sacred mountain city of Machu Picchu, in Peru.

In preparation the whole day was spent in ceremony with the guardian and shaman of the sacred city and that night, whilst making an essence on the ancient temple altar, I was left in no doubt about the existence of the mountain Apu (spirit) who made its presence very clear to me. There was no way that the essences would have been made had I not approached with respect and asked for permission and co-operation. This essence is included in the Eclipse Spritz from the Sound Wave Essences range.

Recently on return to my childhood home of Uganda, I was inspired and instructed to make waterfall essences at the source of the White Nile at Lake Victoria, Murchison Falls at Lake Albert and high up in the mountains of Mount Elgon at Sipi Falls, a magical place with three revered waterfalls. The trilogy of essences have proved to be an extremely powerful essence.

Steve Johnson also has been guided and explored the energy and power of environmental essences and created a range.

ALASKAN ENVIRONMENTAL ESSENCES (Ask E)

The creation of these essences begins with the identification of specific elemental qualities in the environment with which we wish to enter into a co-creative healing agreement. An attunement from our hearts communicating love and blessings to the devic and elemental beings that represent these qualities is the start of the process. When requested, the energies are transferred into the bowl of prepared water, and the environment responds, resulting in a totally unique essence, where the vibrational qualities it contains can never be duplicated in exactly the same way.

How the Alaskan Environmental Essences work

When taken internally, these essences stimulate and support change and transformation at the most basic level of the energy system. They are very catalytic in their actions and are often indicated when a strong, cleansing energy is needed to awaken or bring vitality to someone who is not responding to other therapies or modalities. They also provide a strong base of support for our healing work with flower essences, lending energy and vitality to the healing processes catalyzed by the flowers.

The Alaskan Environmental Essences are very effective tools for space clearing. This process involves cleansing and releasing old energies from our living and working environments and then recharging and revitalizing these spaces with fresh, clean energy from nature. Space clearing with Environmental Essences is an especially useful process for those living in crowded and polluted urban areas where the natural elemental forces have been weakened or dissipated altogether.

Environmental Essences can also be used to provide balance and stability for those involved in emergency situations such as natural disasters where the environment itself is in transition.

Chalice Well Made in the Chalice Well Gardens of Glastonbury, England, with water from the Chalice Well, this essence connects us to the profoundly personal and eternal support that is constantly available from the angelic, elemental, plant and mineral kingdoms. It reminds us that we are not alone – we are a part of the entire web of life and all that is, and we can draw upon this matrix of support whenever we are struggling and need help to take the next step on our life path.

Full Moon Reflection This essence was made on a cold, clear, full moon night, in a canyon overlooking Kachemak Bay. An essence of reflected light – the sun's light reflected by the full moon off the water of Kachemak Bay and into the snow-filled canyon. This essence penetrates deep into the subconscious to bring forth that which lies unresolved beneath the surface. It offers us an opportunity to let our shadow-self be illuminated by the light of our conscious awareness.

Glacier River An essence of solarized water prepared below the terminus of the Gulkana glacier in the central Alaskan range. This water emerges from the base of the glacier carrying suspended particles of ground-up rock from mountains eroded by the constant pressure and movement of glacial ice. This essence embodies the process of perpetual release from form. It helps us release patterns of feeling, thinking and

doing that have become rigid and unyielding.

Greenland Icecap An essence of solarized glacier water prepared on the Greenland ice sheet over an area where two of the Earth's continental plates come together. The Greenland Icecap essence contains the intense energy of convergence, the energy of the natural movement of the Earth's crust translated upwards through thousands of feet of ice. This essence helps us remain flexible and feel supported as we move through deep inner change.

Liard Hot Springs This essence was prepared from mineral hot springs water on a clear −35°F day at Liard Hot Springs in northern BC, Canada. An essence of cleansing, re-creation and renewal that brings us back in touch with the innocent truth of who we really are – spiritual beings who have come to this Earth to learn.

Northern Lights This essence was made on a windy subzero Arctic night under a swirling green display of Northern Lights. An essence of reaching beyond ourselves into the fundamental creation forces of the universe. For cleansing and repatterning our energies, at a very deep level. Helps us release energies from the heart which have been allowed to obscure our original life patterns.

Polar Ice This essence was prepared on the Arctic Ocean ice pack near the North Pole. An essence of transition and the completion of cycles; for achieving a more patient understanding of the subtleties of time; helps us stay present in a place of pure waiting, with no anticipation of what is to come.

Portage Glacier This essence was prepared on the banks of Portage Lake near the terminus of Portage Glacier in south-central Alaska. A powerful and catalytic energy that helps us release what is unnecessary and inappropriate in our lives from the mental, emotional, etheric and physical bodies. Use it to revitalize and balance the entire energy system.

Rock Spring Prepared from a spring high in the Talkeetna Mountains of south-central Alaska, the water from this spring emerges from the centre of a sheer rock face and cascades down to a pool at its base. Rock Spring is an essence of hope and miracles! It embodies the constant proof that everything is possible. It is an essence that can help us find our way through seemingly insurmountable obstacles with infinite patience and never-ending trust.

Solstice Sun This essence was prepared on the 'night' of 21/22 June, as the midnight sun danced along the peaks of the Brooks Range in the northern interior of Alaska. Solstice Sun catalyzes our ability to access and circulate a stronger current of light energy throughout the physical body. It opens the heart and the energy pathways of the body in preparation for a 'peak' experience, and helps a person integrate such an experience after it has taken place.

Stone Circle Prepared within a naturally occurring circle of stones located high in the Talkeetna Mountains of Alaska. The formation of energy created by this circle of stones has immense healing power. Stone Circle introduces a highly balanced and protective energy into the aura that invites us to relax, rest and replenish our vital forces. This essence is especially helpful for those doing energy balancing work with people and spaces, as it will enable them to maintain their openness and sensitivity without absorbing or 'taking on' any of the energies they are being asked to clear.

Tidal Forces This essence was prepared with creek and seawater on Kachemak Bay during a full 24-hour, 22-foot tidal cycle. An essence of rhythm and balance, of loss and gain, of adapting ourselves to the swiftly changing currents of life. Helps us release the old and receive the new with constant

and unyielding fluidity. Soothes and balances overly emotional, fiery states of being; washes away mental resistance to change; helps us accept what is in the present moment.

SOUND WAVE ESSENCES (SW)
Exploring the nature of sound

Essential to our nature, sound gives us a sense of space, depth and form, and like colour, adds richness to life and our world, and a feeling of interconnectedness with others and the environment we find ourselves in.

Sound is significant in creation myths and puts one in mind of Christian mythological legends of the beginning of creation, where it is stated that: 'In the beginning was the word'; this is also echoed in Aboriginal mythology where it is believed that their ancestors sung the worlds alive, calling the flowers and trees into being with sacred words that wrapped the planet in a web of song, and tells of how they walked the 'song lines' to keep the world alive!

In particular, harmonious sound has a profound healing effect on our systems, engendering us with a sense of being and wellbeing; even in nature, bird song stimulates seedlings to open their pores in order to encourage the absorption of nutrients and therefore ensure profuse growth.

The DNA role

In esoteric science and mythology it has been said that the DNA within each cell has its own harmonic note or song, every atom, molecule and cell in the body has its own frequency, and that the cells sing the vibrational patterning of the body alive into its own dance of frequency into the chakras and beyond. Altogether this creates such a synthesis of vibration that the body has its own unique individual frequency, hum or song.

We understand that all sound is vibration, which travels from one source to another as waves, each with their own frequency and pitch; as each person vibrates at their own unique frequency, it is important that the balance within this frequency is maintained. The Aboriginals, with their instinctual understanding and grasp of the importance of sound, and its effect on our physiology, feel that the point at which we feel most out of tune is the moment we have forgotten how to sing our own song.

We all know what a powerful force sound can be. Different sounds have different and profound effects on us, both destructive as well as healing and transformative; some may irritate us, causing dissonance, while others will please us, creating harmony. A glass can shatter when a perfect C note is held long enough by the human voice; equally a fractious baby is soothed and falls asleep when sung a melodious lullaby.

Research into the effect of sound on DNA

Carl Sagan, the American astronomer and astrophysicist, writes that most of our genetic information (about 97%) is unused DNA. This allows tremendous room for growth and expansion. DNA has also been found to be extremely sensitive to sound frequencies and the latest research carried out by biochemists finds them now using the frequency 528Hz to repair human DNA. It is interesting to note that it is not the regular C note (which vibrates at 512Hz) that we know today, but the C of 528Hz that has been discovered to be most effective and is used in DNA repair. This note was part of an ancient scale called the Solfeggio Scale, part of a six-tone scale sequence of electromagnetic frequencies, which is not the diatonic scale do, re, mi, fa, so, la, ti, do, that we know and hear often on the airwaves today.

The difference in the scales existed because of different tuning methods that were utilized in ancient times and can best be heard in Ancient Gregorian Chant, the Higher Renaissance sacred music of the 15th century where the Flemish composer Josquin Desprez was

master of the polyphonic vocal style (the interweaving of many voices). A good example is his 'Gaude Virgo'. This was further developed by the Italian composer Palestrina, who studied the sacred texts to shape the music and sound in order to express spirituality; an excellent example is his 'Excelsis Deo' composition, which was believed to impart tremendous spiritual blessings and upliftment when sung in harmony. This was especially enhanced when sung in churches due to the caustic qualities of the churches and cathedrals of the time. It is said that these tones can assist all the channels in staying open and keep the life force (the chi) flowing through the chakra system smoothly and quite freely.

Dr Leonard Horowitz in his book *The Healing Codes of Biological Apocalypse* describes this original Solfeggio Scale, of which the six-tone scale sequence of electro-magnetic frequencies is a part of, to be an ancient scale. These particular frequencies were rediscovered by Dr Joseph Puleo, who received them in a wonderful almost mystical experience and also reports that these frequencies are not something new, but they are something very old. The six Solfeggio frequencies each have qualities associated with each note as they progress up the scale, which indicate they can initiate a process of transformation.

The six Solfeggio Frequencies include:

UT – 396Hz – Liberating Guilt and Fear

RE – 417Hz – Undoing Situations and Facilitating Change

MI – 528Hz – Transformation and Miracles (DNA Repair)

FA – 639Hz – Connecting/Relationships

SOL – 741Hz – Awakening Intuition

LA – 852Hz – Returning to Spiritual Order

The frequency 528 relates to the note MI on the scale and derives from the phrase *MI-ra gestorum* in Latin meaning 'miracle'. Stunningly, the C note referred to above is the exact frequency used by genetic biochemists to repair broken DNA – the genetic blueprint upon which life is based!

Sound researcher and musician Fabian Maman's recent book, *Medicine for the 21st Century*, also offers amazing photos and information from laboratory research on the positive effect of musical tones on human cells and haemoglobin (Maman 2011). Fabian shows how he uses sound to affect damaged cells, to disrupt their caoitic frequency and to heal and repair discordant and damaged cells.

Sound, vibration and form

For more than 200 years, researchers have been validating the connections of sound and vibrations on physical form. In 1787 the German scientist Ernst Chladni was first to make that connection, detailing his research in his pioneering book *Discoveries Concerning the Theory of Music*, and explaining ways to make sound waves generate visible structures. He detailed how a violin bow, drawn at a right angle across a flat plate covered with sand, produces shapes and distinct patterns. These shapes and patterns are called Chaldni figures today. Following up on Chladni's discoveries, mathematician Nathaniel Bowditch concluded that the conditions that allowed these designs to arise were the frequencies, or oscillations per second, being in whole number ratios to each other.

The study of wave phenomena, the ability of sound to organize and re pattern matter, is called cymatics. John Beaulieu, in his book *Music and Sound in the Healing Arts*, preports that 'form is the more elusive component of sound. Sound forms can be seen by subjecting mediums such as sand, water, or clay to a continuous sound vibration' (Beaulieu 1995). Latterly the eminent quantum physicist Professor David Bohm said, 'Space is not empty. It is full, a plenum as opposed to a vacuum, and is the ground for the existence of everything, including ourselves. The universe is not separate from this cosmic sea of energy' (Bohm 1980).

Sound, vibration and water (frequency + intent = healing)

Frequency + intent = healing
Mr Emoto's research on water's ability to record or hold a frequency truly demonstrates the reality of this formula (Emoto 2002). Remember that water comprises more than 70% of a mature human body and covers the same amount on our planet. Water is the very source of all life. The fact that the molecular structure of the water can be affected by our consciousness, our intent and our sounds is extremely important and may have great implications for the future of personal and planetary harmony and healing.

Sound and flower essences supporting the transformational process

In her book *Molecules of Emotion*, Dr Candice Pert describes energy and vibration as reaching the molecular level, and the effect on the 70 different receptors on the molecules when vibration and frequency reaches them; they begin to vibrate and touch and tickle each other, play and mount each other (Pert 1999). It is this whole energetic dance ritual, at the cellular level, that opens the chromosomes and exposes the DNA to the frequencies; at this DNA, molecular, cellular level, it seems that sound gathers and collects and focuses the cells' individual song. Through sound, these tones can assist all the channels in staying open and keep the life force (the *chi*) flowing freely through the chakra system. Using sound can be a way to direct energy for transformational purposes.

Not only are the six electromagnetic frequencies able to accomplish this but given that water is able to record frequencies, and store memory molecules, sound essences can be made. When water is specially used as a vehicle to capture sound waves and its frequency is stabilized, mother tincture can be made from sound waves, as with flower essences.

In the case of the range of Sound Wave Essences, the first inspiration and concept came to me when working in a session on Being, Vibration and the Nature of Original Sound in 1992, with Beautiful Painted Arrow (Joseph Raele), a Native American visionary. I was inspired to make an group essence, by intoning the ancient word-sound for Woman (with the women toning only) and ancient word-sound for Man (men only), both of which hold within their frequency the essences of what it is to be male or female. Simultaneously, during her dreams and work as a therapist, gifted healer and good friend of mine Colette Prideaux Brune was also listening and absorbing the original teaching of sound. Both of us have trained extensively with shamanistic medicine men and women of Central and South American traditions.

But it was not until 1993, after I was inspired to make a sacred site essence on Machu Picchu, and Colette made an essence at the sacred site of Palenque in Mexico, that together we created Sound Wave Essences from two sets of crystal singing bowls in the beginning of 1996–7.

They were created in Star House, a building built on the principles of sacred geometry, designed by Keith Critchlow, a master of Sacred Architecture, with the ancient sound of 'OM' built into its very structure. Each crystal bowl is tuned to its own chakra, and the essences were produced by each specific sound frequency being encapsulated in water held at the apex of the emitted tone. We produced two sets of sound essences: the Moon Essence Set (receptive principle) energies were made over a year during significant phases of and at the point of the full moon and reflects the feminine aspect. The Sun Essence Set (active principle) were made in a day on the solstice, at the high point of the solar eclipse and works with the masculine aspect of vibrational energy.

The essences were created with both the light of the sun and energy of the moon and relate to the seven major chakras of the body plus an eighth chakra above the head.

The sun by its nature is naturally expansive and the moon by its nature is naturally reflective, giving the essences these inherent qualities. Sun essences help on the conscious level with:

- processing the changes in patterns held within the mental and emotional levels

- accessing information held within the body at a cellular level, repatterning cells and shifting consciousness

- intensifying creativity, imagination and intelligence

- atimulating and waking up the chakras into action and reaction

- helping to access silent knowledge within so we remember who we truly are.

Moon essences help the subconscious level with:

- lighting up awareness of our dreamtime

- reflecting back our original blueprint

- switching on cellular intelligence

- activating the inner ear so that our soul's message is audible

- heightening all of the senses.

Everyday living causes the colours of the chakras to become dull, and stress, shock or trauma can leave toxic residues behind. These dense energies clog the chakras and stop them vibrating in their pure frequencies, causing more rapid ageing. Not only transformative, the sound essences help to restore the spin and vibration of the chakras so that they can shine with their pure colours once more.

The liquid sound essences sun and moon

Heart of the Earth – base chakra. This gateway connects us directly to the heart of Mother Earth, the feminine principle. Roots of energy travel down the legs into the ground, creating stability and security. This forms a solid foundation for the luminous energy and chakra system to anchor itself into the body. The doorway to the heart of the Earth simultaneously grounds and protects us whilst enabling us to deal with the unique relationship to our tribal roots.

Sacred Void – sacral chakra. The void is not empty but contains both elements of the sacred fire and water. Alchemically blended, these two vital forces create a state of dynamic balance that provides the fuel to empower our dreams, reconnecting to the waters of life; it renews, refreshes and deals with issues around our own birth, returning us to that sacred place of innocence.

Warriors' Path – solar plexus chakra. Strengthens the inner core, the column of light that embodies the principles of solar light. Connects us to the universal warrior's energy, the vehicle for both the solar and lunar qualities inherent in the male and female form. When in balance it allows access to the courage that abounds in the universe, and reflects back our unique interaction with all life, enabling us to move forward with empowerment along our true path.

Listening Heart – heart chakra. To walk the path of the heart is to walk the path of the soul, hearing the inner whispering of our soul's voice. Circulating its wishes through the compassionate spirit of the heart, the soul reveals the nature of its true self. This is the key to opening the doorway to the heart of the universe, whilst simultaneously hearing the imperceptible teachings of the cosmos.

Divine Purpose – throat chakra. The instrument of speaking one's truth and trusting in the clear expression of our soul's journey. Enables us to call back the threads of our timelessness and reconnects us with our lives on the planet. Opens the doorway to the divine purpose of the universe.

Perceiving Spirit – third eye chakra. To perceive the web of life as an indivisible matrix that holds the blueprint of all time. The awareness of spirit behind all things cuts through illusion and opens perception to the space between the worlds.

Universal Present – crown chakra. Eminessence, essence of spiritual consciousness, in the present, is the moment that holds all time. The portal to the heavens, illuminating and guiding our passage towards who we are becoming. Aiding the mastery and transcendence of time.

Star Traveller – eighth chakra. The golden orb of spinning light held in the luminous energy field above the head contains the imprint of our next incarnation waiting to be born. To become a star traveller through time and space, journeying to the union with our original source.

Liquid sound essences when especially combined and formulated together harmonize the energies of all as well as specific chakras and hold the dynamic balance and integrity within the chakra system as a whole. They were also developed in order to balance and adjust the subtle energy system, assisting with its stability and realignment.

We then developed the Sun and Moon Chakra Rebalancers.

Sun and Moon (Male/Female) **Chakra Rebalancers** are combinations of all eight sound wave essences – one comprises the sun sound wave essences and the other the moon sound wave essences. The **Sun Rebalancer** particularly restrengthens and nourishes, while activating what we are aware of in the present, at a conscious level, whilst the **Moon Rebalancer** reflects what is going on at the subconscious level. By using both combinations, the two aspects of inner and outer (male and female) are brought together in an alchemical Dance of Light. Any disruption in the coordination of this alchemical dance within ourselves creates an instability that contains within it the seeds of disharmony and disease. These sound rebalancers activate the cell's innate ability to re-coordinate itself, re-adjusting to hold the correct dynamic pattern, as we move through the discord of daily life.

The **Integrate** and **Transmute** combination essences were the next stage of development.

Since the earthquake in Japan 2012, many of us are experiencing difficulties in regaining our balance. This is as a direct result of the Earth wobbling on its axis and parts of Japan shifting by as much as 13ft.[1] As our usual point of reference has shifted, it is important to reset our vibrational patterning to a new matrix, with this in mind Integrate and Transmute were developed – for times like these not only specifically developed after the Japanese disaster but for future events.

Integrate This combination essence is a blend of the sun and moon sound wave essences, especially designed in a sequence in order of the essences chosen, a blend that encourages balance and integration of the male and female polarities, both physically and within our psyches.

When this alchemical balance occurs within the cellular structure of the body, and as the ancient male and female archetype guidelines are dissolving, there is a need for a new perspective and envisioning on how these energies are intermingled and consequently ultimately expressed. It is important in this time of transition that this delicate alchemical balance is achieved without getting caught by the limitations of previous traditional concepts. It is vital that this happens with mutual respect and honour whilst maintaining the integrity of both polarities. The Integrate essence maintains one in a state of dynamic balance whilst completing this transformation process and helps us to discover the divine purpose of our soul.

Transmute This combination represents the interwoven energy of the male and female fully harmonized and integrated with the finer vibrations of the higher chakras including the eighth higher dimensional chakra situated above the crown. It facilitates the transmutation of the cellular structure into the matrix of the subtle levels. Now equal in balance and strength a sacred marriage can occur between the male and female energy. This fusion ignites the spark of the soul and creates momentum to move the soul forward.

The Integrate and Transmute essences can be used separately or together. The Rebalancers create a solid foundation to anchor the male and female energy; Integrate weaves them together in an alchemic dance and Transmute creates a dynamic fusion which results in the sacred marriage within the soul.

Eclipse Clear and Protect aura body spritz

A further development was this unique blend of Sound Wave frequency essences, essential oils and sacred site essences, we designed it to clear discordant and electromagnetic energy. It uplifts and refreshes, fine tuning and raising the overall vibration of the body and subtle anatomy.

It was made during a total solar eclipse – incorporating essences made at world sacred sites such as Machu Picchu (in 1993), Palenque and the Pyramids of Guimar – with crystal sound bowls.

We then blended it with Lotus and Pink Lotus flower essence and essential oils of Pink Lotus, Ylang-Ylang and May Chang oil from China to create a cleansing, uplifting and refreshing effect on the aura and subtle bodies

1   http://news.nationalgeographic.com/news/2011/03/110316-japan-earthquake-shortened-days-earth-axis-spin-nasa-science

as well as clearing negative atmospheres in rooms and workspaces.

This spritz clears the subtle body's electromagnetic field, protecting and allowing you to move smoothly and cleanly through the day without picking up the residue and negativity that usually clings to the subtle anatomy through daily interactions with discordant energies.

Leaving one feeling clean, centred, protected and in control of one's personal space, it facilitates clarity of thought and emotional calm. This spritz also aids by shifting the vibrational patterns of the body, fine tuning its frequency, generally raising its overall vibration, aiding in meditation and attunement to one's higher self.

Ways the essences can be used

Place on the chakras: Put the bottle onto or close to the relevant chakra.

On the skin: The energy of the remedies can be absorbed through the skin and can be applied to anywhere you feel you need it, for example, on a chakra, lips, forehead, wrist, soles of the feet or palms of the hands.

By mouth: Dilute 10 drops to 2 tablespoons of pure spring water or take 7–10 drops under the tongue. You can also take them in herbal tea or fruit juice.

In the bath: A couple of drops will be enough when the bath has finished running.

On your altar: Place the bottles on your altar to effect a certain aspect of your spiritual practice.

Combination Integrate and Transmute Treatment Kit Many of us and our clients are experiencing difficulty in regaining our balance as a direct result of the Earth wobbling on its axis. As our usual point of reference has been shifted it is important to reset our vibrational patterning to the new matrix. With this in mind the Integrate and Transmute Kit has been developed with a treatment pattern included.

K.

CRYSTAL AND GEM ESSENCES

These are another very important area of essence making, which are invaluable in their support in combination when blending with flower essences as well as a powerful tool in their own right.

Here I will let Andreas elaborate on the history and use of these elixirs.

GEMS AND THEIR ESSENCES

The history of gems

The gems are an invaluable gift of the Earth. For millions of years they were forming themselves in the Earth until Man discovered them and exposed them to daylight. Every developed civilization values their beauty and their healing power.

Old legends tell us about their harmonious healing effect on people, animals and even plants. Ninety years ago, Hildegard of Bingen compiled precise information on the medical applications of plants and gems. According to her teachings, body, spirit and soul are a complex unit of treatment. Many of these old traditions have been lost over the centuries. Man gave up integral thought and centred on division and intellectual exploration of the body. Today, at the beginning of the Age of Aquarius, integral thought is being considered again. Gems too are gaining more importance in the world of healing.

Health is a state of perfect equilibrium. Gems, with their beauty of colour, shape and shine, provide especially pleasant possibilities to approach this equilibrium and to reach harmony.

Gems' effect

Gems are not, as is often considered, dead objects. They grow and develop following natural laws though decidedly slower than plants, animals or people. Geologists have identified seven gem formation patterns, the so-called crystal system. The formation of crystals is the following one:

Cubic = in the shape of a dice.

Tetragonal = four-sided.

Hexagonal = six-sided.

Trigonal = three-sided.

Rhomboid = in the shape of a diamond.

Monoclinic = simple inclined.

Triclinic = triple inclined.

All gems with the exception of the amorphous (formless non-crystalline) stones (for example, Amber, Opal, Obsidian, Moldavian and jet) are assigned to these seven crystal systems.

When energy is brought into contact with crystals, they react in an interesting way: the transmitted energy is altered and discharged again. If electricity is applied to a crystal, this is transformed into vibrations which are completely uniform when the electricity applied is constant. This phenomenon is used in quartz clocks to measure time. If a crystal is subjected to pressure, this energy is transformed into electricity. This reaction also has a specific technical application. It is used

461

in lighters to create the spark with crystals (piezoelectricity).

Crystals modify the energies that they receive. If we carry or hold a gem, the crystal will direct or modify our energies accordingly. This can be easily verified with a rock crystal (carved in the shape of point, sphere or in any other shape). Take the crystal in your hand, be relaxed and pay attention to the way you react. Do you perceive a pulsating energy? Do you become quiet and feel balanced? Most people immediately feel the change that is taking place inside them.

This energy transformation is only one of the effects of the gems. Just as people don't have only one capacity or characteristic of personality, the gems also possess multiple aspects. They act through their colour, chemical composition, shape, through their crystalline system, their electromagnetic vibrations, transparency and their hardness.

Colour

This is the language of light. The colours arise from the light. White light consists of electromagnetic vibrations and contains all colours. If some of the white light is absorbed, its rate of vibration is reduced and colours are created. When the light falls on a gem it can either go right through it or be completely or partly absorbed.

A colourless gem allows all light through, while a black gem absorbs it. However, when a gem absorbs just one or a few colours, it will carry a mixture of the non-absorbed colours. Amethyst for example absorbs all colours except violet. Violet has a very short vibration and acts mainly on the spiritual level, while red has a vibration that it is twice as long and acts chiefly on the corporal level. Body, spirit and soul can be harmonized if they are illuminated with the colours they lack.

This is used in chromatic therapy. Gems too work through their luminous colours. They especially speak to the feelings. Different colours can be assigned to the different energy centres of the human body.

Chemical composition

Most gems are composed of silicic acid. However, there are many other elements present in gems. People can absorb missing substances dissolved and diluted in the essence through the skin. For example, Hematites contain iron, Pearls are rich in calcium, Malachite contains copper, and Rock Crystal is composed of silicic acid. The chemical composition especially affects the blood and the body of people.

Crystal system and shape

Mineral shapes contain many symbols and provide different impressions and effects to people. The shape of a gem is often changed or perfected through cutting and polishing to emphasize its chromatic effect, its sparkle and its fire. Shape and the crystal system influence the creation of cells and the person's spirituality.

Electromagnetic vibrations of crystals

This varies for different gemstones and can be made visible through Kirlian photography. We could also describe these vibrations as the gems' aura. They have an effect on the person's energy.

Transparency

The transparency of gems is varied. Transparent gems act on our ability to think, translucent ones act on the energy-providing organs (such as the heart or the lungs) and opaque gems act on processing organs, such as the stomach and the intestines.

Hardness

Hard gems (e.g. diamond, ruby, sapphire, topaz) strengthen and define character and thought. Soft gems (e.g. calcite, fluorite, turquoise and azurite) loosen too-fixed personality characteristics and impart tolerance.

Health is the state of perfect equilibrium in the person. Gems, with their beauty of colour, shape and sparkle, offer especially pleasant possibilities to be in contact with this equilibrium and to attain harmony.

ANDREAS KORTE (PHI) GEM AND CRYSTAL ESSENCES (AK GEM)

1. Amazonite A potassium aluminium silicate that belongs to the mineral group of the feldspars. It is opaque and it can be found in greenish blue and green colours. Its name means 'from the Amazonia'. Among the natives it is considered as healing and sacred. In the chakras system, it corresponds to the heart chakra (fourth chakra), to the third eye chakra (sixth chakra) and to the crown chakra (seventh chakra). It has a positive effect on the aura.
Essence effect: Amazonite essence encourages links to the environment, a deeper understanding of nature and makes it easier to connect with mineral as well as plant essences. An energy aid when there is a sensation of tension, oppression and restlessness. Dissolves disharmony, creates calm, balances mood, helps to overcome sadness. It has a balancing and soothing effect. Regains clarity, self-realization. Stimulates confidence, happiness and vitality and improves sleep.
Corresponding Orchid: Deva Orchid.
Affirmation: I am immersed in the flow of life.

2. Amethyst A transparent silicon dioxide that can be found in violet, clear violet and reddish violet tones. It forms beautiful crystals full of energy. The Greek denomination *amethystos* means 'not drunken'. In Ancient Greece, this mineral was carried to avoid spells, nostalgia and bad thoughts, especially in states of drunkenness. Hildegard of Bingen applied the Amethyst to cure freckles and recent tumescence and she used it as dermatological treatment to obtain a finer facial skin.

Buddhist monks in India have some kind of Amethyst rosary and they use it to meditate.
Essence effect: With its delicate and soothing vibrations the essence contributes to reaching a deeper state of relaxation, for when agitation and stressful influences of the body 'govern us'. Helps overcome stress and relax after a stressful day, aiding sleep and supporting work on the levels of your dream. For lack of concentration and poor memory, engendering a new clarity of thought that aids mental work and a sense of reality. Aids understanding grief and losses and changing them into happiness and harmony. It helps to redirect aggressive feelings and stimulates pure thoughts; it is an ideal preparation for meditation. It intensifies intuition and encourages and promotes spiritual development as it stimulates the brow chakra (third eye) (sixth chakra) and the crown chakra (seventh chakra).
Corresponding Orchid: Psyche Orchid.
Affirmation: I have a greater awareness of myself.

3. Aquamarine A beryllium aluminium silicate. The name comes from Latin and it means 'water of the sea'. In the 12th century, Hildegard of Bingen included it in the list of the curative minerals. Its changes of colour from clearer to darker are indicators of truth and falsehood. When it acquires a practically white tone it lets us know about false friends. It corresponds to the throat chakra (fifth chakra) and the third eye chakra (sixth chakra); in the aura level it acts especially on the ethereal and mental body.
Essence effect: It has a refreshing and purifying effect on body, aura, spirit and soul, providing clear and harmonious expression of feelings, serenity and clarity. Calms the spirit in emotional situations. Fosters expression, steady flow of thought and mental acumen. Gives energy to the eliminative organs so is a great additional aid in fasting or any changes in eating habits. Relaxes the eyes after close work in front of the computer. It reinforces intuition and the intuitive vision establishing

the development of a conscience link with our Higher Self. Complete revitalization for the body and aura by means of the progressive dissolving of the blocks to regeneration.

Corresponding Orchid: Amazon River Preparation.

Affirmation: My thought and my feelings are clear and free, and I can express them with affection.

4. Rock Crystal A silicon dioxide. It is clear, transparent and colourless. Its original denomination, *krystallos*, derives from Greek and it means 'ice' because it was believed that this mineral was petrified ice. Rock Crystal generally appears in groups inside caves or bedrock chasms. For the Romans in the legends related to Rock Crystal, it was the gem of wisdom, courage, confidence and love. The Rock Crystal is the mineral that clarifies all the chakras, the emotional and ethereal bodies of our aura.

Essence effect: Detox purifying effect on the mind, body and spirit. The luminous vibration of this essence reinforces the aura's protective effect. Stimulates detoxifying, purifying functions of the body on the energy level and balancing all the chakras. Organizes received energies and transmits positive energy. Activates spiritual detoxification process, freeing psychic blockages. The emotions undergo a filtering process, clarifying them. Tangible access to intuition, the Higher Self and more receptive to receiving higher knowledge. While recognizing our own vulnerability, we are protected and feel safe and secure.

Corresponding Orchid: Higher Superior Orchid.

Affirmation: The luminous vibrations illuminate and purify me and my Higher Self is my guide.

5. Diamond Crystallized carbon. It is the hardest gem, transparent with many tones: colourless, yellow, brown, blue, pink, black. Its Greek denomination *adamas* means 'the invincible one'. Considered the king of the gems due to its shine and refraction. It can be generated in different forms, from an octahedron to a bucket.

Essence effect: Radiates light in the dark side of the soul. Clarity and knowledge are born from its essence. It has the greatest positive healing potential and has an invigorating, clarifying effect over the organs of the whole body. Impurities of the body can be eliminated. Protects from negativity. Brings mental clarity to situations, independent thought, concentration and balances the personality. Dissolves jealousy, fear, envy and insecurity, so wholesome relationships are developed through insight, understanding and tolerance. This essence enlightens the body, aura, spirit and soul, and protects them from negative influences. The intense energy of Diamond essence liberates our spirit and we perceive our connection with the cosmos and are able to identify ourselves as a part of the whole.

Corresponding Orchid: Channel Orchid.

Affirmation: The light of the cosmos shines inside me dissolving darkness. I am at the source of my energy and I transmit it as love.

6. Elestial Crystal A silicon dioxide also known as Skeletal Quartz. Transparent or opaque with colours varying from clear to smoky quartz, or from light brown to dark brown. Points and facets are arranged over rock, either singly or in several rows. This crystal is assigned to the chakras of the feet, the root chakra (first chakra), the solar plexus chakra (third chakra) and, finally, the crown chakra (seventh chakra).

Essence effect: The essence makes it clear where our truth is at odds with universal truth. Its effect is felt in the feet and most effective when massaged on reflex zones of the feet and it acts on every organ in the body. Eliminates physical blockages produced as a result of stored anger so the body is able to reach an energetic equilibrium. By letting go of old patterns of thought and preconceived ideas the next step in personal development can be taken. When brain activity is energetically balanced, blockages in the chakras dissolved, and preparation for some new energetic equilibrium is achieved, transformation can then occur. As inner harmony is regained, it aligns our truth with universal truth and with the purpose of our life.

Corresponding Orchid: Aggression Orchid.

Affirmation: I get free of my stagnant energy and emotions and I open myself to new experiences.

7. Hematites A ferric oxide. Opaque and black with a black silver, brown reddish or metallic shine. Its former name, *Haima*, has Greek origins meaning 'Bloodstone' found in the form of a kidney or flat crystal shaped structure. Although it reflects silver black tones, it is really red (striped red). During the carving process, the water used is stained blood red, therefore it has always been related to blood. In terms of the chakras, it is related to the root chakra (first chakra).

Essence effect: Hematite essence activates our being and bonds us to the Earth. Strengthens self-confidence and energetically improves the intellect. Transforms negative pessimistic attitudes and emotions into vital positive energy. Positive effect on the blood and at the same time invigorates and refreshes the whole body. Stimulates self-healing processes and complements fasting and detoxifying. Increases personal courage and mental strength to overcome obstacles and any self-imposed limits that constrain your freedom of spirit. The intense regenerative effects are due to release of the aura from negative vibrations and we feel spontaneous and vivacious and in harmony with ourselves. The aura feels protected and expands during meditation, and sleep is more refreshing. The physical and spiritual effects of Hematite essence are perceived as the fullness of universe spirit.

Corresponding Orchid: Abundance Orchid.

Affirmation: The fullness of life and universe prompt me, and I live and I emanate my inner joy.

8. Moonstone A potassium aluminium silicate of the feldspars family. Translucent and colourless or a slight pale blue resembling the shine on pearls, found in soft pink, orange or yellow. Inspires legends, mainly because of its secret glow, which is more pronounced when carved. The chakras it corresponds to are the solar plexus chakra (third chakra), the throat chakra (fifth chakra) and the third eye chakra (sixth chakra).

Essence effect: The 'Female Stone', the essence brings our inspirational female side to light. Stimulates body detoxification and promotes strength, harmonizes feelings at all levels and treats emotional blockages, fears, for example, fear of the future, the dentist, etc. Draws out the femininity, sensitivity and tender behaviour towards others. Helps the understanding of our emotions and gathering crucial information and inspiration during dreaming process. Purifies the subconscious to be able to develop clairvoyance.

Encourages creativity awareness, self-recognition and a deep love of nature, so we can hear its message, feel its inspiration and realize our spiritual goals.

Corresponding Orchid: Inspiration Orchid.

Affirmation: My feelings and I am a unit and I can understand others.

9. Olivine (Peridot, Chrysolite) Also known as chrysolite or peridot; a magnesium iron silicate which forms small diamond prisms. St Hildegard appreciated its power and strength and its ability to activate natural development. She recommended it for cardiac pain, fever and to resist negative energies and to strengthen knowledge. The chakras it corresponds to are the heart chakra (fourth chakra) and the solar plexus chakra (third chakra).

Essence effect: This essence stimulates the heart and solar plexus, which are purified and opened to joy and self-love as well as towards others. Helpful for inner tension, emotional coldness, selfishness, sadness and jealousy. Harmonizes energy, creating positive changes in feelings and emotions. Stimulates the body's energy flow, with a favourable impact on the whole body. As inner stability increases, sensations of weakness, tensions and spasms dissipate. It promotes positive long-term life planning. Supports increased mental energy to develop the awareness needed to increase visualization, which is required to clearly set goals, and also encourages us to listen to our inner voice and know intuitively what needs to be done. As it clarifies and stabilizes states of spiritual confusion it supports wise use of clairvoyance as a guide.

Corresponding Orchid: Fun Orchid.

Affirmation: I feel lighter and my joy is expanded naturally to the outside.

10. Smoky Quartz A silicon dioxide that can be opaque to translucent, found in various colours, ranging from brown to black, smoke grey or light grey. Sometimes it has rutile inlays and it usually forms crystals. Since ancient times, Smoky Quartz has been considered a protective stone. Corresponding chakras are root chakra (first chakra), prostate or uterine chakra (second chakra) and solar plexus chakra (third chakra). In the aura, it acts on the astral body, the emotional body and mental body.

Essence effect: Provides the stability needed to embrace our dark side. Detoxifies, cleanses and boosts our energy, providing a balancing effect when there are physical imbalances. Any emotional overload is assisted by dispelling fears, neurosis, depression, sadness or long periods of grief, and it can help recognize that even painful learning processes are necessary in life. Gives courage to live and find new goals. Provides a mentally secure base and allows us to identify our life's purpose and pursue it creatively and joyfully. Brings joy of living and helps to start over and live more of a spiritual life. Purifying the aura results in a complete freedom of the body, mind and soul, and a new equilibrium is reached; we are able to reorganize our life, to meditate and be in contact with nature.

Corresponding Orchid: Past Life Orchid.

Affirmation: With each new experience I learn to know myself better and I catch a glimpse of the purpose of my life.

11. Rose Quartz A silicon dioxide, which gives it its pink colour. It can be translucent to opaque with shades ranging from pale to strong. Grows in various micro-crystalline formations, but rarely as a large crystal. Since ancient times this crystal was said to have been put on Earth by Amor and Eros and awakens love and desire through its gentle colour. The corresponding chakra is the heart chakra (fourth chakra).

Essence effect: Conveys a gentle, calm and affectionate vibration dispelling negativity. Draws out the tenderness of love and has a harmonizing effect on the emotions. Dissolves worry, fears or nervousness, and helps overcome the pain of heartbreak to find strength within ourselves. Works in healing the emotional body, creating inner balance and emotional control and an understanding of many highly charged emotional situations. We develop self-respect and an understanding of others. Substitutes negative thoughts with positive ones, refining our actions and improving the creativity in dealing with ourselves. Protects the second chakra and at the same time it provides for feeling comfortable in our sexuality. We will develop a sense of the arts and be receptive to feelings on a higher plane and to all things beautiful and will experience a new facet of love and connection with nature.

Corresponding Orchid: Heart Orchid.

Affirmation: I open my heart to beauty and the joy of living.

12. Ruby An aluminium monoxide that derives its name from its colour (in Latin *rubeus* means 'red'). Rutilated in layers sometimes causing the iridescent cat's eye or the six beams star effect. Polishing gives Ruby a sparkle similar to that of a diamond. The Greeks considered it 'the mother of the gems' because of its beauty and rarity. St Hildegard recommended Ruby to treat infections, chills, weakness, headaches and sensitivity to weather changes.

Essence effect: A lucky stone in the realms of love! The essence stimulates and stabilizes the base chakra (first chakra) and the heart chakra (fourth chakra). Physical and spiritual love are harmoniously combined, stimulating the energy to live with sensitivity within close relationships. New passion, enthusiasm and faithfulness is created. Invigorates our vital Qi, especially when feeling lazy and when heaviness creates overweight issues. Gives us the ability to stay true to our courage, self-awareness and flexibility and remain in contact with our inner fire and to be ready to act in the moment. A powerful motivator that drives the spiritual development of our consciousness. Links to Mother Earth are balanced and we are opened to inspiration and Divine Love.

Corresponding Orchid: Victoria Regia.

Affirmation: The joy of living gives me wings and I live my inner truth intensely.

13. Rutilated Quartz Made up of titanium dioxide and the result of metal deposits (titanium, copper, gold) in Rock Crystal or Smoky Quartz (silicon dioxide). Colourless and clear or of different shades of brown with black, reddish brown or with golden inlays. Rutilated Quartz is considered the mineral of truth and protection. It helps to keep promises. Corresponds to the solar plexus (third chakra). Acts on the energy body.

Essence effect: The essence helps to get to the root of our problems, brings light to the darkest corners of the soul. It soothes the mind and harmonizes opposites. Has an effect on breathing, calms the mind, overcomes nervousness. Rutile fibres are likened to sun rays and illuminate our feelings to identify and free ourselves from negative situations. The solar plexus as the centre of feelings is strengthened and emotional clarity is gained. Mentally stimulating, it improves memory. Free of aggressive tendencies, it is a great ally in understanding the messages shown through our dreams. Intensely enlightening, it aids in the development of consciousness and clairvoyant ability and connection with nature and the ability to astral travel.

Corresponding Orchid: Sun Orchid.

Affirmation: I'm full of radiant thoughts. Clarity and harmony are inside me.

14. Emerald A beryllium aluminium silicate with distinctive green hues, in many shades from transparent to opaque. The presence of chromium and vanadium gives it its colour, and it is found in the shape of elongated hexahedral prisms. The Colombian Emerald is one of the most spectacular formations found because it contains a six-ray star. During the 12th century, Hildegard of Bingen recommended the Emerald to treat heart and stomach problems as well as epilepsy. Corresponds to the heart chakra (fourth chakra) and to the third eye chakra (sixth chakra).

Essence effect: Emerald essence opens our heart to the diversity of life. Activates intuition and connection with the Higher Self. Gives us the energy to find our inner balance when applied energetically to the heart chakra. It invigorates the whole body and strengthens and stimulates our self-healing energy. Helps overcome and deal with the emotions we experience around negative karma/acts of fate. Activates the third eye as a gateway to unknown abilities and intuition. It's easier to accept energies that are not in accordance with our own perceptions, as we realize that mental variety enriches our lives, and our heart will overflow with love as we feel a connection with all. Refreshes and regenerates our body, spirit and soul as it supports meditation, strengthening our connection to the Higher Self. Enables us to tap into spiritual knowledge, accumulate renewed energy and a new sensation of spiritual freshness. Encourages a deep vision of love, hope, healing and wisdom allowing us to investigate the mysteries of life.

Corresponding Orchid: Venus Orchid.

Affirmation: I feel great love and a wonderful freshness inside me that dissipates all my fears and allows me to explore the mysteries of life.

15. Topaz An aluminium silicate that contains fluorite. Its intense tones of golden yellow to golden orange and brown remind us of the colours of the sun. It appearance is transparent to dense and it grows in the form of prismatic crystals. Grows in varieties of yellow pink and brown pink colours. It corresponds to the solar plexus chakra (third chakra) and the third eye chakra (sixth chakra).

Essence effect: Topaz essence turns negativity into happiness and love. Our feelings travel from solar plexus to the third eye, connecting inner wisdom with higher intuition. Dissipates and eliminates nervous tension that's reflected in discomfort in the solar plexus, such as suppressed anger, emotional exhaustion, jealousy and envy. Stress, mental exhaustion, restlessness, worries and many other burdens that weigh heavily on our mind will be resolved by its cleansing power. Emotions will be expressed with intelligence and thoughtfulness and the solar plexus is imbibed with great strength and warmth and will overflow with a kind of solar energy. With the 'pure sunlight' of this essence, the world will seem more colourful and lively, and a feeling of lightness will guide us. Balances where there is a lack of rapport between the body, mind and soul in the ethereal body, resulting in addictive compulsive behaviour such as gambling and sleepwalking. NB, helps overcome anxiety and fear of examinations.

Corresponding Orchid: Colour Orchid.

Affirmation: Energy similar to the sun rays overflows me and my feelings and it fills my life with joy.

16. Blue Tourmaline An aluminium borosilicate found in all shades of blue ranging from translucent to opaque. Grows forming long rods of varying strength. During the Germany Middle Ages romantic period, Tourmaline was the most loved gem. It corresponds to the solar plexus and throat chakra and third eye.

Essence effect: As an essence it dissipates stagnant blocked emotions held in the solar plexus, preventing us being or expressing ourselves. Counteracts stress and helps to 'survive' in a hostile environment by remaining positive. It strengthens the feminine part of our being and we learn to act from the heart not only to receive but also to give. By verbally expressing our feminine side it improves concentration, inner balance, tranquillity, freedom of choice and free thought,

social skills, independence and ability to be self-fulfilled and creative in our thinking.

Spiritually leads to inner peace so we can be ourselves; we recognize our spiritual goals and pursue them.

Corresponding Orchid: Angel Orchid.

Affirmation: I express my feelings and allow myself to be free. I have the ability to achieve self-fulfilment.

17. Pink Tourmaline (Rubellite) An aluminium borosilicate found in beautiful pink and red or purple tones. It can be translucent or opaque and usually grows in long rods. Of Sinhalese origin, Pink Tourmaline is a fairly new mineral which in these hectic and problem-filled days has great appeal. It corresponds to the second chakra, third chakra and fourth chakra.

Essence effect: Its essence frees the heart from blockages caused by or related to negative life experiences. It opens and enhances the energy held in the heart, creating a wholly harmonizing effect. Psychic overload can weigh heavily on the heart as it lies like a stone in the chest as we are unable to express emotions. Influences the heart chakra, frees the heart from emotional blockages, heals old wounds, clears prejudices so joy and lightness return. Ideal for those who sacrifice themselves for others, i.e. in friendship, helps to identify boundaries and define limits so sympathy does not degenerate into self-sacrifice, enhances self-confidence and clears away unhealthy relationships. It promotes detoxification and purification of the body leading to a feeling of wellbeing. Through the processes of purification and change, we free our spiritual energy to allow a fresh start.

Corresponding Orchid: Love Orchid.

Affirmation: I open my heart and I accept myself and other people with affection and find the energy to start again.

18. Black Tourmaline (Schorl) An aluminium borosilicate formed by creating long rods of varying diameters. Opaque with a shiny black colour recognized by its striated mineral structure. Traditionally mothers make their children wear it to prevent falling and stumbling. It corresponds to the feet chakra and to the root chakra (first chakra).

Essence effect: Black Tourmaline essence reinforces grounding stability and security and is especially useful for people who do not live in the present. Allows us to be aware of our dark side, to accept it and to deal with it. Aids detoxification of the body and is often compared to rejuvenation or spring clean as it strengthens and invigorates body, soul and senses. It helps to remove negative vibrations from the body and soul and is useful for reactions caused by computer radiation and sensitivity to weather changes. It offers protection against both and also electrical appliances. In naturopathy, the electroconductive glass rods of Black Tourmaline are used to increase the sensitivity to the brain's impulses. This gem essence also establishes an ethereal connection with the brain and teaches mental reactivity, skill, self-discipline and focus on objectives. When spiritual guidance is hampered by negative vibrations and radiation applied, this essence will purify the ethereal level, allowing spiritual energy to develop and increase.

Corresponding Orchid: Angel-of-Protection Orchid.

Affirmation: A protective halo surrounds me, I perceive the energy of the Earth and I am fervently devoted to my objectives.

19. Watermelon Tourmaline An aluminium borosilicate of incomparable beauty with a pink centre surrounded by a green border that gives this mineral the aspect of a cut watermelon. Formed in long rods that show great beauty when cut and polished into thin slices. It corresponds to the second chakra, third chakra and fourth chakra.

Essence effect: The healing colours green and pink act especially on the heart chakra (fourth chakra) and stimulate integral renewal. Its essence stimulates healthy cell formation and boosts cell renewal. It stimulates the structuring process and promotes self-healing energy. Disturbances on the spiritual level may

be the root cause of physical problems. By eliminating the spiritual causes, self-healing of our body can begin A sad heart, melancholy or anxiety may cause harmful emotions and burdens. Helps to identify and treat these emotional wounds which gives a new freshness, courage and hope. It stimulates spiritual growth and development, intuition, creativity and self-determination. It is also a good aid in examinations, as it helps to overcome fear of failure.

Corresponding Orchid: Coordination Orchid.

Affirmation: I gently get rid of my burdens and feel included in God's love.

20. Citrine A translucent silicon dioxide, which ranges from light yellow to golden brown colour. Genuine citrine gets its colour from trivalent iron, which gives it a light yellow tone. Because of its colour, this mineral is known as the stone of light, sun and life. Through the solar plexus (third chakra) it acts on the involuntary nervous system. It corresponds to the second and third Chakras as well as the sixth and seventh ones.

Essence effect: Citrine essence conveys individuality and personal security. Stress and sadness are energetically balanced and the emotional level of the solar plexus is strengthened so courage, self-confidence, intuition and common sense are prominent. The self-healing process with physical illness is supported and the eliminative organs enhanced in their function. Supports mental clarity and the integration between the two halves of the brain, intuition and understanding. It strengthens concentration in those who already have a goal (e.g. a professional goal) and are looking for help to achieve it. This essence provides emotional balance when in team work: this process starts among children in kindergarten and is invaluable for the classroom, the office or the family.

With stimulation of the third eye chakra and crown chakra, we experience beauty and joy of life and moments of enlightenment, where we feel included in the protection of the Earth. From this spiritual trust grows, and

a deep affection for ourselves, others and for the small things in life.
Corresponding Orchid: Chocolate Orchid.
Affirmation: Joy is inside me and it opens every door.

Sabina of Pacific Essences has also come out with her own range of gem essences to work in harmony with her flower essence range.

PACIFIC GEM ESSENCES OF CANADA (Pac G)

Amber Illumination of mind and heart.
Resonance: Light.
Attractors: Digestion, flowing, ease, magnetism.
Challenges: Darkness, stuckness.
Meridian: Stomach.
Chakra: Solar plexus.

Amethyst Transformation of energy, protection.
Resonance: Protection.
Attractors: Intuition, peacefulness.
Challenges: Depression, fear, guilt.
Meridian: Lung.
Chakra: Crown.

Apophyllite Cleanses resonances of 'old stuff', physical or mental.
Resonance: Detoxification.
Attractors: Homeostasis, purification.
Challenges: Toxicity.
Meridian: Kidney.
Chakra: Navel.

Aquamarine Peaceful, calming and soothing, balances thymus.
Resonance: Tranquillity.
Attractors: Self-love, meditation, inner peace.
Challenges: Aggravation, agitation, hysteria.
Meridian: Heart protector.
Chakra: Throat.

Aragonite Promotes self-reliance and inner security.
Resonance: Being who we can be.
Attractors: Empowerment.

Challenges: Self-doubt, indecisiveness.
Meridian: Lung.
Chakras: Third eye/ajna, throat, heart.

Aventurine Aids with meditation and visualization.
Resonance: Healing the inner child.
Attractors: Possibility, choices.
Challenges: Restrictions, self-imposed limitations.
Meridian: Heart.
Chakras: Crown, back, head.

Azurite 'Gentling' of attitudes, awareness of perfect essence of all things.
Resonance: Kindly.
Attractors: Insight, vision, patience.
Challenges: Mental chatter, idle thoughts.
Meridians: Liver, kidney.
Chakra: Third eye/ajna.

Bloodstone Alignment of energy centres.
Resonance: Wholeness.
Attractors: Vitality, circulation, strength.
Challenges: Isolation, depletion.
Meridian: Conception vessel.
Chakra: Root/basic.

Blue Lace Agate Connects sixth and seventh chakras, inspiration and grace.
Resonance: Unexpected blessings.
Attractors: Encouragement, support.
Challenges: Despair, disconnected.
Meridian: Liver.
Chakra: Throat.

Calcite Decreases fear, increases dream memory.
Resonance: Knowingness.
Attractors: Guidance, clarity.
Challenges: Resentment, envy, arrogance.
Meridian: Kidney.
Chakra: Root/basic.

Carnelian Increases vitality, stimulates the liver to throw off impurities.
Resonance: Vitality.
Attractors: Creating, purpose, adventure.
Challenges: Fear of change, addictions, frustration, depression.
Meridians: Liver, kidney.

Chakra: Solar plexus.

Celestite Transports consciousness to celestial realms, enhances perception.
Resonance: Perception.
Attractor: Sensory expansion.
Challenges: Fear of change, fear of new experiences, fear of flying.
Meridian: Spleen.
Chakra: Forehead.

Chrysocolla Harmony, balance, wholeness, integration; unifies fourth and fifth chakras.
Resonance: Loving-kindness.
Attractors: Self-expression, unconditional love.
Challenges: Stress, chaos, confusion.
Meridian: Kidney
Chakras: Heart, throat.

Citrine Clearing of thought patterns to manifest what you want by attuning to creative light.
Resonance: Will.
Attractors: Attention, focus, manifestation.
Challenges: Elimination, fogginess, sluggishness, overthinking.
Meridian: Large intestine.
Chakra: Spleen.

Coral Connects us with our depths, symbolizes life force energy.
Resonance: Embodiment.
Attractors: Sensuality, grace.
Challenges: Intimacy.
Meridian: Kidney.
Chakra: Sacral/sex.

Crocoite To let go of worry, to recognize thoughts before emotional reaction.
Resonance: Responsive.
Attractors: Presence, centred, undaunted.
Challenges: Worry, anxiousness.
Meridian: Stomach.
Chakra: Solar plexus.

Emerald Enhances wisdom and projects love.
Resonance: Wisdom.
Attractors: Inner knowing, compassion, abundance.

Challenges: Fighting, arguments, hostility, unworthiness.
Meridian: Heart.
Chakra: Heart.

Fire Agate Transformation towards harmony and love, heart tonic.
Resonance: 'Inter-being'.
Attractors: Encouragement, support, interconnectedness, passion, enthusiasm.
Challenges: Alienation, fear of connection with others, fear of success.
Meridian: Triple warmer.
Chakra: Heart.

Fluorite Transformation and devotion; links matter with spirit via the crown chakra.
Resonance: Quickening.
Attractors: Lightness, extra-sensory perception, expanded consciousness.
Challenges: Rigidity, heaviness, mass consciousness, limited thinking.
Meridian: Spleen.
Chakra: Third eye/ajna.

Galena Receptivity and microscopic intensity; helps to transmit thoughts.
Resonance: Telepathy.
Attractor: Attuned.
Challenges: Blocked, isolated.
Meridian: Stomach.
Chakra: Third eye/ajna.

Green Garnet Purifies thoughts.
Resonance: Now.
Attractors: Qi, light, *prana*.
Challenges: Anger, resentment.
Meridian: Liver.
Chakra: Third eye/ajna.

Green Tourmaline Eliminates mental and emotional toxins, a spiritual cleanser, detoxification.
Resonance: Nourishing.
Attractors: Potential, possibility.
Challenges: Anger, hostility, criticism.
Meridian: Bladder.
Chakra: Solar plexus.

Hematite Augments meridian flows.
Resonance: Connectedness.

Attractor: Balance between yin and yang.
Challenges: Shadow, inner darkness, fear.
Meridian: Kidney.
Chakra: Spleen.

Iolite Links up vision and communication.
Resonance: Discernment.
Attractors: Higher perceptions, intuition.
Challenges: Limitations, limited vision.
Meridians: Stomach.
Chakra: Sacral/sex.

Jade Emotional grounding; healing deep emotional hurts.
Resonance: Renewal.
Attractors: Rejuvenation, emotional healing, tranquillity, abundance.
Challenges: Alcoholism, abuse, bitterness, co-dependence.
Meridians: Large intestine, gallbladder.
Chakras: Solar plexus, heart.

Jasper Physical tonic; balances body energies.
Resonance: Digestion.
Attractor: Embodiment.
Challenges: Worry, obsessions, shame, guilt, ancestral emotional patterns.
Meridians: Stomach, spleen, liver, gallbladder.
Chakra: Solar plexus.

Kunzite Stabilizes pure love and joy in the heart.
Resonance: Tenderness.
Attractors: Kindness, gentleness, serenity.
Challenges: Abandonment, grief, loss, misunderstanding.
Meridian: Heart.
Chakra: Heart.

Lapis Lazuli Transcendence of the ego, assists one to become a clear channel and to see others without judgement.
Resonance: Initiation.
Attractors: Awareness, self-discovery.
Challenges: Separation, judgement, ego.
Meridian: Kidney.
Chakra: Forehead.

Larimar To become as a little child; delight and joy, wisdom and innocence.
Resonance: Childlike.
Attractors: Humour, perspective, delight, wonder.
Challenges: Overfocused, tunnel vision.
Meridian: Heart protector.
Chakra: Heart.

Lepidolite Brain hemisphere integration; alleviates depression and allows for greater perspective.
Resonance: Unboundedness.
Attractors: Wholeness, possibility, expansion.
Challenges: Depression, limited thinking.
Meridian: Kidney.
Chakra: Crown.

Malachite Reflects and mirrors that which is within.
Resonance: Creative coherent expression.
Attractors: Creativity, self-expression.
Challenges: Stiffness, tightness, limitations, anger, frustration.
Meridian: Gallbladder.
Chakra: Solar plexus.

Moonstone Promotes vision and self-awareness.
Resonance: Dreamtime.
Attractors: Feminine, receptive.
Challenges: Aggressive, pushy, external focus.
Meridian: Spleen.
Chakra: Third eye/ajna.

Muscovite Aligns the endocrine system and chakras.
Resonance: Unification.
Attractor: Spiritual certainty.
Challenge: Stuck energy.
Meridian: Kidney.
Chakra: Sacral/sex.

Obsidian Grounding and making manifest spiritual qualities.
Resonance: Transmutation
Attractors: Open heart, light.
Challenges: Darkness, fear, grief.
Meridian: Large intestine.

Chakra: Solar plexus.

Onyx Absorption and transmutation of vibrations.
Resonance: Shielding.
Attractors: Listening, inner strength, self-mastery.
Challenges: Sponge, sensitivity, sympathy.
Meridians: Lung, kidney.
Chakra: Root/basic.

Opal Enhances feelings of 'at-one-ment' between physical and spiritual; enhanced awareness.
Resonance: Mystery.
Attractors: Integration, circulation.
Challenges: Hardness, separation.
Meridians: Spleen, kidney.
Chakra: Navel.

Pearl Absorbs and holds love energy; purity, beauty, compassion.
Resonance: Beauty.
Attractors: Love, compassion, vision.
Challenges: Ugliness, horror, conflict.
Meridian: Heart.
Chakra: Heart.

Peridot Dissolves spiritual uncertainty.
Resonance: Faith.
Attractors: Christ consciousness, grace, gratitude, abundance, success, prosperity.
Challenges: Uncertainty, doubt.
Meridian: Gallbladder.
Chakra: Spleen.

Quartz Amplifies thoughts and feelings; acts on the thymus to balance the immune system; assists with the retention of information; decrystallizes congestion.
Resonance: Broadcasting.
Attractor: Expansion.
Challenges: Unconsciousness, uncertainty.
Meridian: Small intestine.
Chakra: Heart.

Red Garnet Awakens great love and compassion.
Resonance: Worldly pleasures.
Attractors: Abundance, sexuality and sensuality, self-love, self-confidence.

Challenges: Creative blocks, poverty consciousness.
Meridians: Heart, kidney.
Chakras: Root/basic, heart.

Rhodochrosite Connector of chakras via the solar plexus.
Resonance: Self-love.
Attractors: Gentleness, tolerance, acceptance.
Challenges: Emotional traumas, healing the inner child, inner darkness.
Meridians: Spleen, kidney.
Chakra: Solar plexus.

Rhodonite Impacts breathing and speaking.
Resonance: Aspiration.
Attractors: Personal power, eloquence.
Challenge: Hanging on to the past.
Meridian: Lung.
Chakra: Throat.

Rose Quartz Self-fulfilment and inner peace, teaches the power of forgiveness and re-patterns the heart to love of self, dissolves burdens which suppress the heart's ability to give and to receive.
Resonance: Forgiveness.
Attractor: Awakening.
Challenge: Self-pity.
Meridian: Heart protector.
Chakra: Heart.

Rubellite To express the exuberance and joy of love.
Resonance: Divine love.
Attractor: Compassion.
Challenges: Depression, obsessions, hysteria.
Meridian: Heart.
Chakra: Heart.

Ruby Love and courage to express one's highest potential.
Resonance: Intrepid.
Attractors: Inspiration, enthusiasm.
Challenges: Overwhelm, fear.
Meridian: Small intestine.
Chakra: Heart.

Rutile To relieve fear and anxiety, balances disturbed energy patterns.
Resonance: Directed.
Attractors: Purposeful, homeostasis.
Challenges: Stress, tension.
Meridian: Kidney.
Chakra: Sacral/sex.

Sapphire Awakens us to our spiritual nature.
Resonance: Impeccability.
Attractors: Inspiration, guidance, walking our talk.
Challenges: Fear, ego, control.
Meridian: Conception vessel.
Chakras: Throat, back neck.

Selenite To focus one's own sense of inner truth, being in touch with thoughts at their source.
Resonance: Holy instant.
Attractors: Attention, focus, integrity.
Challenges: Distractions, choices, decisions.
Meridian: Kidney.
Chakra: Root/basic.

Serpentine Stimulates psychic abilities and alleviates fear in relation to greater vision.
Resonance: Humility.
Attractors: Infinite possibility, serenity, tranquillity.
Challenges: Anger, fear, judgement.
Meridians: Liver, gallbladder.
Chakra: Third eye/ajna.

Silica Clears mental confusion.
Resonance: Acumen.
Attractors: Clarity, focus, remembering.
Challenges: Confusion, fogginess, forgetfulness, frustration.
Meridian: Stomach.
Chakra: Solar plexus.

Smoky Quartz Balances adrenal energy, purifies cloudy thought forms, uplifts level of consciousness.
Resonance: Manifestation.
Attractors: Discernment, protection, shielding.
Challenges: Stress, chaos, flight/fight triggers.

Meridian: Kidney.
Chakra: Meng Mein.

Sugellite Creating the physical problem, awakens innocence and wisdom.
Resonance: Awareness.
Attractors: Synergy, humour, acceptance.
Challenges: Hopelessness, despair.
Meridian: Kidney.
Chakra: Third eye/ajna.

Sulphur Softens rigidity and increases flexibility, both physically and mentally.
Resonance: Adaptability.
Attractors: Flexibility, digestion.
Challenges: Habits, brainwashing, mass consciousness.
Meridian: Kidney.
Chakra: Solar plexus.

Tiger's Eye Seeing and accepting diversity in oneness leading to right action.
Resonance: Diversity.
Attractors: Tact, equanimity.
Challenges: Anxiety, criticism.
Meridians: Stomach, spleen.
Chakra: Solar plexus.

Topaz Light, joy, love, brings out Christ-like qualities.
Resonance: Christ consciousness.
Attractors: Love, joy, light, vulnerability, defencelessness.
Challenges: Argumentative, opinionated, conflicts, being right.
Meridian: Kidney.
Chakra: Crown.

Tourmaline Balances chakras and meridians.
Resonance: Emergence.
Attractor: Inner radiance.
Challenges: Obsessions, compulsions, inner darkness.
Meridian: Governing vessel.
Chakras: All chakras.

Turquoise Strength, balance, vitality.
Resonance: Peace.
Attractors: Calmness, equanimity.
Challenges: Inflammatory, conflictive, argumentative.

Meridian: Kidney.
Chakra: Sacral/sex.

Unakite Right-mindedness leading to right action.
Resonance: Right-ness.
Attractors: Personal integrity, right-mindedness, right action.
Challenges: Perception, tunnel vision, limited thinking.
Meridian: Kidney.
Chakra: Crown.

Wavellite Being willing to give up resistance and to attune with the flow of life.
Resonance: Fluidity.
Attractors: Yielding, flowing, receptive.
Challenges: Resistance, stubbornness.
Meridian: Kidney.
Chakra: Third eye/ajna.

FINDHORN GEM ESSSENCES (FH Gem)
Gem essences of the Seven Rays

Diamond *Spiritual Alignment* The essence of Diamond focuses the first ray energies of will and power. Its purpose may assist to align to the vision and purpose of your Higher Self, and to attain through concentration of will. With a clear vision of the purpose you can prioritize, set objectives and focus on essentials. Expansion of the capacity to love develops the virtues of tenderness, compassion, tolerance and fearlessness.

Sapphire *Clarity and Intuition* Essence of Sapphire focuses the second ray energies of love and wisdom. These energies can help you to be calm and clear, and find peace of mind. Purity of thought and an expanded understanding and awareness will lead to illumination, insight and intuition. Compassion for and selfless service to others evokes the power to heal, teach and inspire through love.

Emerald *Balance and Communication* The essence of Emerald focuses the third ray energies of active, creative intelligence. These energies facilitate accessing the intelligent and intuitive mind that aids you in manifesting your plan. With devotion to concentration, you may attain right understanding and enhanced communication skills. Realize the will to succeed by tolerance, accuracy, creative adaptability and practical, planned activity.

Jasper *Imagination and Creativity* Essence of Jasper focuses the fourth ray energies of harmony through conflict. Realize beauty and harmony by unifying opposing forces. Cultivate stamina for ongoing projects through mental and emotional balance and serenity. By inner harmony and unity, the will to harmonize and make peace is evoked along with the confidence to express yourself creatively through the power of beauty.

Topaz *Lucidity and Inventiveness* The essence of Topaz focuses the fifth ray energies of concrete knowledge and science. Access the higher mind and think with clarity. Invoke the will to patience, persistence and wide-mindedness and keep all aspects of yourself in balance. Through concentration, observation and practical inventiveness, achieve mastery in a field of knowledge, and the power to realize great plans.

Ruby *Faith and Inspiration* The essence of Ruby focuses the sixth ray energies of devotion and idealism. Arouse inspired commitment and attain through one-pointed aspiration, fearlessness and endurance. The will to realize emotional health and intelligence stems from your awareness of, and influence over, instinctual orientations. With heartfelt devotion, and a serene, sunny outlook on life, comes the power to excite, persuade and inspire.

Amethyst *Order and Practicality* The essence of Amethyst focuses the seventh ray energies of order and organization. Manifest skill in action and bring order and organization to all areas of living. Find the will to perfect expression through humility, wide-mindedness, perseverance and high intuition. Achieve through practicality and graceful, rhythmic activity. Discover the power to translate plans into physical reality through the magical work of interpretation and the synthesizing ability.

CONCLUSION
Medicine of the Future

It is time to realize that we must take responsibility for our own wellbeing. This is perhaps the hardest lesson to learn. How much easier it is to place the blame for our unhappiness and failing health on to something extraneous to ourselves.

In reality, how we feel is a reflection of the way we live our lives, how we think and act, and how we respond to other people and events. Anyone who is constantly anxious, irritable, frustrated or depressed should heed these signs and look inwards to discover the real source of his or her discomfort.

Flower essences enhance self-knowledge and understanding, helping us to take back responsibility for our own health, happiness and fulfilment. This is tremendously empowering. Knowing you are able to take care of yourself brings great rewards. As your confidence and inner strength flourish you will feel more in control of life and of your own destiny. Deep down you will experience a sense of safety and security that does not hinge upon anyone or anything else.

In the search for inner harmony we become aware that our own welfare is inextricably linked and interconnected to the wellbeing of everything else that exists in nature. Essentially what this means is that if we fail to respect and care for our home, the planet and all living creatures, we in turn will suffer the consequences. Clearly, we can no longer afford to see ourselves as separate from everything around us.

As a race we seem to have forgotten this sense of duty and are threatening the very existence of life on Earth. The World Conservation Centre in Cambridge, England, tells us that of the 270,000 species of flora inhabiting the Earth, 41,000 are under threat. In Britain alone 27,000 flowering plants are struggling for survival, accounting for a staggering ten per cent of the entire global population, and we are now experiencing a dramatic fall in our bee population, the very creatures that pollinated our flowering plants and trees!

Survivors of certain indigenous peoples such as the Native Americans and Australian Aborigines, who have a long tradition of living in harmony with the natural environment, regard the Earth as a gift from the creator to be tended, nurtured and protected for future generations. Indeed, Native American peoples always think ahead for 'seven generations' to come before taking any action that may affect the course of nature. The wise men or spiritual leaders of such peoples are so alarmed at the way we are treating our home that they are finally breaking their silence and are now prepared to share their wisdom and knowledge with us.

The most dramatic instance of this occurred back in 1988, when Alan Ereira was in Colombia researching a documentary and chanced upon the Lost City of Taironas, as well as the descendants of those who had once inhabited this remarkable place – the Kogi. Breaking their 400 years of self-imposed isolation, the Kogi priests, or Mamas, asked him to film a message to give to the world, an urgent warning about the destruction of the planet: 'You are killing the Earth and we must teach you how to stop.'

The Kogi live in the Sierra Nevada de Santa Marta, hidden away at the remote northern tip of Colombia. They call their home 'the heart of the world'. The Sierra could easily be described as a Garden of Eden. It is like the planet in miniature, boasting the whole spectrum of landscapes and climates. Its lush Caribbean coastline gives way to tropical rain-forests, mountainous peaks and even desert in some areas. Every animal and every plant has its ecological niche in this equatorial zone.

Long ago the Sierra was inhabited by the Taironas – Indians who dressed in gold and lived in magnificent cities amid fields and or-chards. They were all but annihilated by the Spanish conquistadors in the 16th century. Some survivors managed to flee up into the mountains where they settled and remained hidden from the world. The Kogi are directly descended from these people and are living proof that a harmonious existence with nature is neither fanciful, unrealistic nor something that belongs to a bygone age. They are intel-ligent, sensitive people who dress in white; they walk barefoot to keep in touch with the Earth. They see those of us in Western society as primitive and uncouth, calling us the igno-rant 'Younger Brother'.

According to the Kogi story of creation, in the beginning was the mother. She is spirit, she is water, the life force that makes things alive – she is Aluna. The mother conceives all possibilities, everything that can be. Aluna gave birth to nine daughters or worlds, of which only one was capable of fertile growth, the Earth. She then created humans to look after this world. But then 'Younger Brother' was created in the heart of the world. He was too dangerous to live among the Kogi, so he was given knowledge of machinery and sent far away across the sea. The Kogi believe that if Younger Brother returns to the heart of the world, then the whole world will die.

During the last 30 years the Kogi have witnessed what they regard as the return of Younger Brother. They have watched settlers move into the Sierra, forcing them to move higher and higher up into the mountains. They see the havoc these intruders are wreak-ing on the land by ripping down trees and digging up the earth, and this simply recon-firms their own beliefs. As the elder broth-ers they see themselves as the caretakers or gardeners of the Earth who are responsible for looking after nature. The philosophy of harmony underpins everything that they do. The Kogi Mamas, the priests, the enlightened ones, mentally work with Aluna to keep eve-rything in balance, viewing themselves as guardians of the planet with a duty to keep humanity's spirituality alive. They believe that if we fail to be in harmony with our-selves we jeopardize not only our own health but also the harmony of the world. When this happens the life energy will become dan-gerous and uncontrolled. 'You will see new diseases appearing for which you have no medicine,' the Kogi tell us. They do not know about AIDS or BSE or the other diseases af-fecting people, animals and plants, but they know that new diseases have arisen because they are in touch with the deeper instincts of the world.

We do not have to have to look far afield to realize the truth in what the Kogi are say-ing. Throughout the world the indigenous countryside is slowly and insidiously chang-ing. Fields and hedgerows, woodlands and forests are constantly being demolished to make way for new houses, roads and other 'developments'. We have allowed such chang-es to take place because of our desire for an increasingly materialistic society. We are now paying the price for our greed, as stress and pollution take their toll on our health.

We may feel that we are powerless to avert such global tragedy. However, just as we are capable of taking charge of our own wellbe-ing, so too can we take back responsibility for looking after the planet. Time and again it has been shown that when one person changes his or her perceptions and starts to see new solutions to personal and world problems, there is a knock-on effect, instigating a shift in the collective consciousness of the rest of humanity.

The Kogi do not see the death of the planet as an inevitability. They believe there are other options open to us. This is echoed by a Mayan elder priest, Apolinario – Achi Ijatz – fifth generation of the Kaqchikel lineage. As a time keeper of the sacred ancestral wisdom carried down by the Mayan elders since the Lemurian and Atlantean times, Apolinario recounts that the ancient Mayan prophecy predicts that now the 13th B'aqtun cycle has drawn to an end, a new cycle of great economic, social, political and spiritual change is occurring, with major climatic changes already being experienced. He emphasizes that if a rapid shift in our consciousness is translated into positive global action, the inevitability of the Mayan prophecy can be averted.

When in Africa I was told a beautifully insightful story by an African shaman. He said that when he was a young boy at the missionary school he was asked by the teachers to describe God, so he replied 'The trees, flowers, rivers, mountains, animals, the skies and the sun!' He was of course laughed at and sent to stand in the corner.

They thought he was mad. On the contrary, he was so alive and awake to the living magic of nature and the world around him. It is this awareness of the living magic of the world, that we are very much a part of, that is one day going to save us all!

The rediscovery of flower remedies has come at a time when it is most needed, as the future of the planet hangs precariously in the balance. It is only by experiencing how they can help us to alter our perceptions and create that shift in our consciousness that enables us to take back our own power that will we really appreciate the value, importance and magic of the world around us.

At the same time, flower essences appear to be offering us a way of finding inner balance by enhancing our wellbeing at a time when many other systems are failing us. In this respect they may truly be the medicine of the future.

AILMENT CHART

ESSENCE KEY
Africa and the Amazon

PHI Essences by Andreas Korte Essences (AK)

Amazonian Shamanic Sacred Tree Essences (AmT)

Spirit of Makasutu Essences (SME)

Australia

Flower Essences of Australia (FE Aus)

Living Essences of Australia (Aus L)

New Zealand

First Light Flower Essences of New Zealand (NZ)

Europe
BRITAIN

Bach Flower Remedies (B)

Bailey Flower Essences (Bal)

Findhorn Flower Essences of Scotland (F)

Harebell Remedies (Hb)

Green Man Tree Essences (GM)

Sun Essences (Sun)

Wildflower Essences of England (WF)

Habundia Flower Essences (HUB)

CHANNEL ISLANDS

Channel Island Flower Essences (Chi)

FRANCE

Deva Essences (Dv)

Mediterranean Essences (Med)

NETHERLANDS

Bloesem Remedies Nederland (Blos)

Russia

Russian Essences (Aus L Rus)

Japan

Japanese Essences (Australian Living Essences, Japan) (Aus LJ)

India

Himalayan Aditi Flower Essences (Him A)

Himalayan Enhancers (Him E)

Thailand

Flowers of the Orient (FO)

Spirit of Beauty Skincare (SB)

USA

ALASKA

Alaskan Essences (Ask)

Alaskan Environmental Essences (Ask E)

Dancing Light Orchid Essences (DL)

Wild Divine (WD)

ARIZONA

Desert Alchemy Flower Essences (DAl)

CALIFORNIA

Flower Essence Society (FES)

Spirit in Nature/Master's Flower Essences (Ma)

COLORADO

Pegasus Flower and Rose Essences (Peg)

HAWAIIAN

Hawaiian Gaia Flower Essences (Haii)

TEXAS

Petite Fleur Essences (PF)

Canada

Pacific Flower and Sea Essences (Pac)

Central/South America

Bermuda Essences (GHBm)

Star Peruvian Essences (Peru)

Other essences

Butterfly Essences (Bfy)

Jaguar Calling Essences (Jag)

Environmental and sound essences

Sound Wave Essences (SW)

Alaskan Environmental Essences (Ask E)

Babies and children essences

Spirit in Nature/Master's Mother and Child Essences (*Please refer to section in Encyclopedia*)

Animal essences

Alaskan Animal Essences

Sun Animal Essences (*Please refer to section in Encyclopedia*)

Gem and crystal essences

Andreas Korte PHI Gem and Crystal Essences (AKGem)

Pacific Gem Essences of Canada (Pac G)

Findhorn Gem Essences (FH Gem)

Physical

Abuse: Emergency Rescue (FE Aus); Cotton Grass, Tundra Twayblade (Ask); Letting Go, I Like Being Me, Unveiling Self (DL); Mother's Arms, Protective Shield, Young Heart, Wise Woman (WD).

Accidents: Rose Bay Willow Herb (Ask); Emergency Rescue, Fringed Violet, Mountain Devil (FE Aus); Rock Rose, Star of Bethlehem (B); Arnica (Dv); Dogwood, Love Lies Bleeding (FES); 'Uala (Haii); Pear (Ma); Grape Hyacinth, Weigela (Pac); Magic Healer (Peru); Acceptance, Earth Mother Nurtures, Mother's Arms, On Angels' Wings, Birch Forest (WD).

Aches: Crowea, Five Corners, Tall Yellow Top (FE Aus); Earth Mother Nurtures, My own Pure Light (DL); Dandelion (FES); Mussel (Pac); Solar Power (Peru); Birch Forest, On Angels' Wings (WD).

Acidity (Excessive) *See also* **Digestive problems:** Crowea (FE Aus); Chamomile (FES); Curry Leaf (Him A); Narcissus (Pac).

Acne *See also* **Skin problems:** Detox, Billy Goat Plum, Five Corners (FE Aus); Dandelion, Cherry, Self-Heal Cream (FES); Formula 20 Acne (Him A); Mussel (Pac); Salvia (PF).

Addictions (Symptoms): Bush Iris (FE Aus); Hedgehog Cactus (DAl); Morning Glory (FES, Him A, Him E); Fairy Lantern, Five Flower Formula (B); Mallow, California Valerian, Nicotiana (FES); Pua Kenikeni (Haii); Forsythia, Nootka Rose, Urchin (Pac); Craving Combo and Spray, Stop Smoking Combo and Spray (PF); Emancipation, Inocencia Coca (Peru).

Addictions (Withdrawal) *See also* **Caffeine Problems:** Boab, Boronia, Bottlebrush, Waratah, Wedding Bush (FE Aus); Morning Glory (AK); Harmonizing Addictive Patterning (DAl); Angelica, Nicotiana (FES); Pua-kenikeni (Haii); Anti-Addiction Remedy (Him A); Forsythia (Pac); Purple Nightshade (Peg); Craving Combo and Spray (PF); Sober Up (Him E); Master Teacher (Peru).

Adrenals: Black-Eyed Susan, Macrocarpa (FE Aus); Chamomile (FES); Rainbow Kelp (Pac); Shrimp Flower, White Carnation (PF); Still Mind (WD); Strength and Qi (Peru).

Ageing: Bottlebrush, Five Corners, Mulla Mulla, She Oak (FE Aus); Almond Tree, Forever Young (AK); Almond (Dv); Mallow (Dv, Hb); California Wild Rose, Hibiscus, St John's Wort, Star Tulip, Corn Lily (FES); Country Marilou (PF); Spirit of Beauty Skincare (SB).

Allergies: Bush Iris, Dagger Hakea, Fringed Violet, Tall Mulla Mulla (FE Aus); Sneezease (Aus L); Yarrow Environmental Solution (FES); Manifesting Thought Forms (DL); Grass Widow (Pac); Balance and Stability (Peru); Allergy Combo and Spray, Lantana (PF); Skrew Pine (GH).

Altitude Sickness: Inocencia Coca, Purification (Peru); Travel-well (FE Aus).

Anaemia: Five Corners, Kapok Bush, Red Grevillea, Waratah (FE Aus); I Like Being Me, Gossamer Steel (DL); Dianthus, Sunflower (PF).

Anorexia Nervosa: Boab, Dagger Hakea, Five Corners, Paw Paw, Waratah (FE Aus); Black-Eyed Susan, Fairy Lantern, Manzanita, Pretty Face, Madrone (FES); Sea Palm, Sea Urchin (Pac).

Appetite Disorders: Peach-Flowered Tea-Tree (FE Aus); Urchin (Pac); Craving Combo (PF); Inocencia Coco (Peru); Oil Palm (SME).

Arthritis: Detox Essence, Mountain Devil (FE Aus); Azurite, Ohai-ali'i (Haii); Snowdrop (Pac); Managed Pain Combo, Zinnia (PF).

Assimilation/Absorption (of Nutrients): Paw Paw, Peach-Flowered Tea-Tree (FE Aus); Centred Love, Earth Mother Nurtures (DL); Self-Heal (Dv, Hb); Blackthorn (GM); Star Jasmine (Hb); Sublime Chocolate (Peru); Magnolia, Autumn Damask (PF).

Asthma: Bush Iris, Dagger Hakea, Fringed Violet, Sturt Desert Pea, Tall Mulla Mulla (FE Aus); Eucalyptus (FES); Sand Dollar (Pac); Babies' Breath, Allergy Combo (PF).

Bacterial and Viral Infections: Black-Eyed Susan, Dagger Hakea, Mountain Devil, Dynamic Recovery, Sturt Desert Pea (FE Aus); Manifesting Thought Forms (DL); Wild Garlic (Dv); Brown Kelp (Pac); Colds and Flu Combo, Thyme, Onion (PF); Vitex (GH).

Back Problems: Amazon River, Noble Heart Cactus (AK); Menzies Banksia (Aus L); Centaury, Vine (B); Lilac, Red Oak (GM); Brown Kelp (Pac); Indian Pipe (Peg); Cinnamon Basil (PF); Deep Breath (Peru).

Blood Disorders: Cherry (FES); Bluebell, Bottlebrush, Little Flannel Flower, Pink Mulla Mulla (FE Aus); Blackthorn (GM); Awapuhi-melemele/Yellow Ginger (Haii); Periwinkle, Plantain (Pac); Basil, Salad Burnet, Louis Philippe (PF).

Blood Pressure – High: Crowea, Five Corners, Little Flannel Flower, Mountain Devil, Mulla Mulla (FE Aus); Vine (B); Periwinkle (Pac); Rain Lily (PF).

Blood Pressure – Low: Five Corners, Kapok Bush, Tall Mulla Mulla (FE Aus); Banana (GH); Papaya (FO).

Blood Sugar (Balance): Peach-Flowered Tea-Tree (FE Aus); Iris (FES); Delphinium, Primrose, Weight Combo (PF).

Boils/Abscesses: Billy Goat Plum, Dagger Hakea, Mountain Devil (FE Aus).

Bones (Healing): Gymea Lily and Sturt Desert Rose (FE Aus); Pink Seaweed, Salmonberry (Pac); Jasmine, Inner Strength Combo (PF); Boneset (GH).

Breast Feeding: Chocolate Lily (FES); Babies' Breath (PF).

Breathing Troubles: Sneezease (Aus L); Five Corners, Tall Mulla Mulla, Tall Yellow Top (FE Aus); Eucalyptus, Rhododendron (Dv); Yerba Santa, California Valerian (FES); Fairy Bell, Polyanthus, Sand Dollar (Pac); Allergy Combo (PF); Horn of Plenty (AK).

Bronchial Conditions: Dagger Hakea, Crowea, Sturt Desert Pea (FE Aus); California Pitcher Plant (FES); Drum Stick (Him A); Deep Breath (Peru); Polyanthus, Sand Dollar (Pac); Allergy Combo, Babies' Breath, Spike Lavender (PF); Smiles and Giggles, Young Heart (WD).

Bulimia: Crowea, Five Corners, Grey Spider Flower, Paw Paw, Sturt Desert Rose (FE Aus); Black-Eyed Susan, Manzanita (FES); Sea Palm, Urchin (Pac).

Burns: Mulla Mulla (FE Aus); Aloe Vera (FES); Flora P Gel (Him A); Anemone, Regenerate Combo (PF).

Caffeine Problems *See also* **Addictions:** Coffee (Haii); Morning Glory (Him A, AK); Purple Nightshade (Peg); Sublime Chocolate (Peru); Cravings Combo (PF).

Cancer: Detox Essence before and after chemotherapy, Emergency Rescue, Electroguard before and after radiation therapy (FE Aus); My Song Calls Me Home (DL); Lilac, Harmony Blend Combo, Periwinkle, Recovery Combo (PF) (see Chapter 8 with reference to Petite Fleur); Diatoms (Pac); Super Immune (Peru).

Catarrh: Bush Iris, Dagger Hakea, Fringed Violet (FE Aus); Yerba Santa (FES); Polyanthus (Pac); Eucalyptus, Jasmine (PF).

Cellulite: Bottlebrush, Bush Iris, Dagger Hakea, Detox Essence, Tall Mulla Mulla (FE Aus); Pink Rose Soapwort (PF).

Chemical Sensitivities: Detox Combo, Wild Potato (FE Aus); Allergy Combo, Daylily (PF).

Childbirth: Balsam Poplar, Green Bells of Ireland, Shooting Star, Sticky Geranium (Ask); Billy Goat Plum, Bottlebrush, Crowea, Emergency Rescue, Kapok Bush, Macrocarpa, Wild Potato Bush (FE Aus); Star of Bethlehem (B); Angelica (Bal); Pomegranate (FES); Pear (Ma); Barnacle, Candystick, Hookers Onion, Jelly Fish (Pac); Divine Goddess, Sweet New Beginnings (Peru); Maternity Combo (PF); Sacred Void (SW); Wise Woman (WD); Birthing, Babies Blues (F); Delph + Horn of Plenty (AK).

Childbirth – Premature/Trauma: Emergency Rescue, Fringed Violet, Sturt Desert Rose, Sunshine Wattle, Waratah (FE Aus);

Poison Hemlock (Pac); Ranunculus (PF); Sacred Space (WD); Dune Primrose (FES).

Circulation Problems: Tall Mulla Mulla (FE Aus); Queen Anne's Lace (FES); Blackthorn (GM); Awapuhi-melemele/Yellow Ginger (Haii); Fireweed (Pac); Morning Glory, Soapwort, Louis Philippe (PF); Stepping Ahead Now, Unveiling Self (DL); Calliardra, Ice Plant (GH).

Cleansing: Butterwort, Inside/Outside Cactus, Sage (AK); Detox (FE Aus); Expansive Embodiment, Graceful Transformations, Letting Go (DL); Ragged Robin (F); Lungwort, Primrose, Yarrow in Seawater (Hb); Formula 19 Cleansing Aid (Him A); Apple, Blackberry (Ma); Moonsnail (Pac); Dutchman's Breeches, Sourgrass, Swamp Onion (Peg); Wise Woman (WD); Spanish Bayonet, Lemon (GH); Clear and Detox (FO).

Colic: Black-Eyed Susan, Crowea, Paw Paw (FE Aus); Chamomile (FES); Sage (PF).

Colon Spasm: Bottlebrush, Crowea, Grey Spider Flower (FE Aus); Barnacle (Pac); Bamboo (PF).

Common Cold: Black-Eyed Susan, Bush Iris (Fe Aus); Yerba Santa (FES); Radiant Strength (DL); Formula 43 Sinus/Cold (Him A); Colds and Flu Combo (PF).

Constipation: Bottlebrush (FE Aus); Letting Go (DL); Barnacle, Pink Seaweed, Poison Hemlock (Pac); Poppy (PF).

Convalescence/Recuperation: Dynamic Recovery (FE Aus); Golden Waitsia (Aus L); Hornbeam (B); Radiant Strength (DL); Elder (F); Self-Heal (FES); Lotus, Peacock Flower (Him A); Magic Healer, Integration (Peru); Recovery Combo (PF); Happy Pet (WD).

Cramps (Muscle): Black-Eyed Susan, Bottlebrush, Crowea, Grey Spider Flower, Tall Mulla Mulla (FE Aus); Impatiens (B); Anemone (Pac).

Crohn's Disease: Crowea, Paw Paw (FE Aus); Snapdragon, Yarrow (PF).

Cystitis: Surfgrass (Pac); Bottlebrush, Dagger Hakea, Mountain Devil, Mulla Mulla (FE Aus).

Cysts (on Ovaries)/Fibroids: Bush Iris, Mountain Devil, She Oak (ovarian), Sturt Desert Rose (FE Aus); Pomegranate (FES); Barnacle (Pac).

Detoxification: Arnica, Inner Cleansing Cactus, Inside/Outside Cactus (AK); Purification (Ask, Peru); Detox (FE Aus); Clearing Energy Fields, Letting Go (DL); Apple, Laburnum (GM); Awapuhi-melemele/Yellow Ginger (Haii); Primrose (Hb); Morning Glory (Him A); Apple, Blackberry (Ma); Blue Lupin, Moonsnail, Sea Lettuce (Pac); Coralroot (spotted), Pine Drops, Sourgrass (Peg); Daylily, Soapwort, Clearing Mist (PF); Ramson's Wild Garlic (Sun).

Diarrhoea: Black-Eyed Susan, Bottlebrush, Kapok Bush, Paw Paw (FE Aus); Acceptance, Heart of Nature (DL); Barnacle (Pac); Detox (FE Aus).

Digestive Problems: Crowea, Peach-Flowered Tea-Tree (FE Aus); Peppermint (BaL); Chamomile, Sage (FES, AK); California Pitcher Plant (FES); Mango, Naio (Haii); Orange Honeysuckle (Pac); Red Spider Lily (Peg); Moss Rose (PF); Loquat (GH); Yellow Oleande (SME).

Dizziness/Faintness: Bush Fuchsia, Crowea (FE Aus); Aspen, Clematis (B); Expansive Embodiment, Radiant Strength (DL); Sober Up (Him E); Mussel (Pac); Red Torch Ginger (FO).

Drug Toxins (Discharging): Detox (FE Aus); Arnica (AK); Morning Glory (FES); Apple (GM); Inocencia Coca (Peru).

Dyslexia: Bush Fuchsia (Fe Aus); Young Heart (DL); Blue Camas (Pac); White Petunia, Enhance Learning Combo and Spray (PF); Attention Formula (Peru).

Ear Problems: Bush Fuchsia, Bush Iris, Spinifex (FE Aus); Star Tulip (FES); Brown Kelp, Ox-Eye Daisy, Viburnum (Pac); French Lavender (PF).

Eczema: Billy Goat Plum, Spinifex (FE Aus); Vanilla Leaf (Pac); Salvia (PF); Cherry (FES); Self-Heal (AK, FES).

Elimination *See also* **Digestive Problems:** Detox, Crowea, Bottlebrush (FE Aus); Star Jasmine (Hb); Narcissus, Polyanthus (Pac); Chocolate Lily (FES).

Endocrine System: Dynamic Recovery (FE Aus).
Adrenals: Macrocarpa, Black-Eyed Susan (FE Aus).
Hypothalamus: Bush Fuchsia (FE Aus).
Ovaries: She Oak (FE Aus).
Pancreas: Peach-Flowered Tea-Tree (FE Aus); Papaya (FO).
Pineal: Bush Iris (FE Aus).
Pituitary: Yellow Cowslip Orchid (FE Aus).
Thymus: Illawarra Flame Tree (FE Aus).
Thyroid: Old Man Banksia (FE Aus).
Testes: Flannel Flower (FE Aus); Lotus (AK, FES); Cherokee Rose (PF).

Energy: Life Force Cactus (AK); Dynamic Recovery, Macrocarpa, Old Man Banksia (FE Aus); Essences of Energy, Leafless Orchid (Aus L); Gossamer Steel, Manifesting Thought Forms, Lotus Petals of the Heart (DL); Life Force (F); California Pitcher Plant (FES); Bay (GM); Flowering Currant, Nasturtium (Hb); Longevity, Vital Spark (Him E); Cherry, Corn (Ma); Bluebell, Goatsbeard (Pac); Cape Honeysuckle (Peg); Tonic – Energy Combo (PF).

Environmental Cleansing: Aura Cleansing Cactus, Delph, Formation Cactus, Life Force Cactus, Ti (AK); Grass of Parnassus, Sweetgrass, Yarrow (Ask); Clear and Protect Spritz (FE Aus); Reading Energy Fields, Clearing Energy Fields (DL); Ti, Kamani (Haii); Madame Louise Levique (PF); Sacred Space, Protective Shield, On Angels' Wings (WD); Red Torch Ginger (FO).

Epstein-Barr Virus (ME): K9 (AK); Banksia Robur, Macrocarpa, Peach-Flowered Tea-Tree, Sturt Desert Pea (FE Aus); Diatoms, Snowberry (Pac); Fatigue Combo, Marie Pavie (PF).

Exhaustion: K9, Aloe Vera (AK); Macrocarpa (FE Aus); Elm, Vervain (B); Staghorn Cholla Cactus, Whitehorn, Woven Spine Pineapple (DAl); Radiant Strength, Reading Energy Fields (DL); Sterlitzia/Bird of Paradise (Haii); Artichoke, Ground Ivy (HUB); Corn (Ma); Fatigue (PF).

Eye Problems: Alder (Ask); Bush Fuchsia, Red Suva Frangipani, Sunshine Wattle, Waratah (FE Aus); Queen Anne's Lace, Star Tulip (FES); Cotton (Haii); Nasturtium, Speedwell (Hb); Anemone, Ox-eye Daisy (Pac).

Fatigue: Dynamic Recovery (FE Aus); Radiant Strength, Reading Energy Fields (DL); Life Force (F); California Wild Rose, Indian Paintbrush, Lavender, Yerba Santa (FES); Corn (Ma); Diatoms, Snowberry, Bluebell (Pac); Fatigue Combo (PF).

Fertility (Problems): She Oak, Woman Balance (FE Aus); Pomegranate (FES); She Oak/Ironwood (Haii); Blackberry, Lady's Mantle, Rose-red (Hb); Barnacle (Pac); Borage (Bal); Carrot (PF).

Fevers *See also* **Common Cold:** Mulla Mulla (FE Aus); Onion (PF).

Fibromyalgia: Self-Image Combo (PF).

Fluid Retention: Wild Potato Bush, Bottlebrush, Bush Iris, She Oak (FE Aus); California Pitcher Plant (FES); Papaya (FO); Poison Hemlock (Pac); Bachelor's Button, Japanese Magnolia, Yarrow (PF); Wild Feminine (Peru).

Frigidity: Canary Island Bellflower, Courgette (AK); Sensuality (FO); Intimacy,

Wisteria (FE Aus); Lehur (Haii); Cannon Ball Tree, Ixora (Him A); Barnacle (Pac); Marigold (PF).

Gall Stones: Dagger Hakea, Mountain Devil (FE Aus); Mussel (Pac); Garden Mum (PF).

Glandular Fever *See also* **Epstein-Barr Virus:** K9 (AK); Formula 38 (Him A).

Hair Loss/Baldness: Red Carnation (PF); Detox (FE Aus); Cotton + Cedar (GH).

Hay Fever: K9 (AK); Black-Eyed Susan, Bush Iris, Dagger Hakea, Fringed Violet (FE Aus); Sneezease (Aus L); Allergy Combo (PF).

Headaches: Black-Eyed Susan, Emergency Rescue (FE Aus); Aspen, Vervain, White Chestnut (B); My Own Pure Light (DL); Awapuhi-melemele/Yellow Ginger (Haii); Meadowsweet (Hb); Clarity (Him E); Orange (Ma); Blue Lupin, Mussel, Plantain (Pac); Abate Anger Combo, Anise Hyssop, Curry, Japanese Magnolia (PF); Grapefruit (GH).

Healing (Self): Coordination Orchid, Wise Woman (AK); Self-Heal (AK, Dv, FES, Hb); Magenta Self-Healer (FES); Bog Rosemary (Ask); Spinifex (FE Aus); Star of Bethlehem (B); Aloe (DAl); Manifesting Thought Forms, New Perceptions (DL); Star Tulip (FES); Gean/Wild Cherry, Norway Maple (GM); Healing (Him E); Cellular Memory, Fairy Bell (Pac); Creeping Thistle, Milkmaid (Peg); Master Teacher, Magic Healer (Peru); African Violet, Bouquet of Harmony Combo, Madame Alfred Carriere (PF); Birch Forest, On Angels' Wings (WD).

Heart Irregularity: Emergencies (FE Aus); Foxglove (PF).

Heart Problems: Foxglove (Ask, Hb); Bluebell, Flannel Flower, Waratah (FE Aus); Borage, Rosemary (Hb); Jelly Fish (Pac); Radiant Strength (DL); Rose of Sharon (PF); Young Heart (WD).

Herpes: Spinifex (FE Aus); Marigold, Reduce Stress Combo (PF).

Hormone Imbalance – Female: She Oak, Woman Balance (FE Aus); Evening Primrose, Mala Mujer (DAl); Pomegranate (FES); Barnacle (Pac); Cherokee Rose, Female Balance Combo, Marigold (PF); Strength and Qi (Peru).

Hormone Imbalance – Male: Flannel Flower (FE Aus); Marigold (PF); Banana (FO).

Hyperactivity: Learning & Focus (FE Aus); Chamomile (Dv); Nasturtium (FES); Hibiscus (FO); Banana Poka (Passion Flower) (Haii); Lettuce (Ma); Stock (PF); Hibiscus (FO).

Hypertension (Stress related): Periwinkle, Surfgrass (Pac); Abate Anger Combo & Spray, Fortune's Double Yellow (PF).

Immune System (Boosting): K9 (AK); Wild Garlic (AK, Dv); Macrocarpa (FE Aus); My Own Pure Light (DL); Gorse, Watercress (F); Echinacea, Garlic, Lavender, Love Lies Bleeding, Morning Glory, Magenta Self-Healer (FES); Ivy, Yew (GM); Mountain Apple/Ohi a-ai (Haii); Hawthorn, Pansy (Hb); Formula 38 Immunity Booster (Him A); Fleabane (HUB); Optimal Immunity (Pac); Super Immune Combo & Spray (Peru); Gaillardia, Echinacea, Silverlace, Snapdragon (PF); Be Resistant (Sun); Smiles and Giggles (WD).

Impotence: Banana (AK, FO); Swiss Cheese Plant (AK); Boronia, Crowea, Five Corners, Flannel Flower (FE Aus); Earth Mother Nurtures (DL); Larch (B); Queen of the Night (DAl); Ixora (Him A); Grape (Ma); Marigold (PF).

Incontinence: Bottlebrush, Crowea (FE Aus); Manifesting Light Forms (DL); St John's Wort (FES); Surfgrass (Pac); Tiger's Jaw Cactus (PF).

Indigestion (Dyspepsia): Sage (AK); Crowea, Paw Paw, Peach-Flowered

Tea-Tree (FE Aus); Chamomile (FES, PF, AK); Sea Palm (Pac); Ligustrum (PF).

Inflammations: Surfgrass (Pac); Manage Pain Combo, Red Carnation, Yarrow (PF); Aloe Vera (GH).

Influenza: Bush Iris, Flannel Flower, Jacaranda, Paw Paw (FE Aus); Super Immunity (Pac); Colds and Flu Combo & Spray, Lily (PF).

Injuries: Cotton Grass (Ask); Emergency Rescue (FE Aus); Crisis Relief Essences (Aus L); Love Lies Bleeding (FES); Earth Mother Nurtures (DL); Pear (Ma).

Insomnia: Valerian (AK, Dv); Boronia, Calm & Relax Essence (FE Aus); Hibiscus (FO); Hops Bush (Aus L); White Chestnut (B); Heart of Nature, Meditative Mind (DL); Chamomile (Dv, FES); Sweet Dreams (F); Black-Eyed Susan, Dill, Lavender, Mugwort, St John's Wort, Flora-Sleep (FES); Awapuhi-melemele/Yellow Ginger (Haii); Formula 17 Sleep (Him A); Lettuce (Ma); Full Moonlight (Peru); Deep Sleep Combo (PF); Alaska Birch Forest, Still Mind (WD); Turnera (GH); Sweet Dreams (F).

Itching: Black-Eyed Susan, Dagger Hakea, Fringed Violet, Red Grevillea, Rough Bluebell (FE Aus); Floral Pain Gel (Him A); Vanilla Leaf (Pac).

Jet Lag: Travel-Well (FE Aus); Jetstream (F); Travel (Hb); Travel Solution (Peru); Fatigue Combo (PF); Sacred Space (WD); Bon Voyage (F).

Kidney Problems: Grey Spider Flower (FE Aus); My Heart Knows, Higher Levels (DL); Surfgrass, Coral, Fuchsia (Pac); Red Spider Lily (Peg); Begonia, Pansy (PF); Fungus Amazonas No. 1 (AK).

Laryngitis: Bush Fuchsia, Flannel Flower, Mountain Devil (FE Aus); Purpose Flows (DL); Snapdragon (Hb); Sand Dollar (Pac).

Liver Disorders: Detox, Dagger Hakea, Mountain Devil, Sunshine Wattle (FE Aus); Awapuhi-melemele/Yellow Ginger (Haii); Speedwell (Hb); Forsythia, Plantain (Pac); Ligustrum (PF); Red Torch Ginger (FO).

Long-Term Illness: Bottlebrush, Kapok Bush, Waratah, Wild Potato Bush (FE Aus); Acceptance, Clearing Blockages, Higher Levels, Manifesting Thought Forms, Stepping Ahead Now (DL); Peacock Flower (Him A); Coralroot (spotted) (Peg); Alaskan Birch Forest, Mother's Arms, On Angels' Wings, Smiles and Giggles, Wise Woman, Young Heart (WD); Magenta Self-Healing (FES).

Lung Imbalance: Sturt Desert Pea, Tall Mulla Mulla (FE Aus); Eucalyptus, Yerba Santa (FES); Flowering Currant (Hb); Arbutus, Fairy Bell (Pac); Spike Lavender (PF).

Menopause: She Oak, Woman Balance, Woman Balance Kit (FE Aus); Heart Wings (DL); Alpine Lily, Borage, Easter Lily, Fuchsia, Hibiscus, Mariposa Lily, Pomegranate, Rosemary, Tiger Lily (FES); Orange Honeysuckle (Pac); Female Balance Combo and Spray (PF); Smooth Hawksbeard (Bal); Divine Goddess, Strength and Qi (Peru); Formula 23 Menopause (Him A); Cardinal Flower (DAl); Calabash (SME).

Menstruation – Absence of: She Oak, Woman Balance (FE Aus); Evening Primrose, Fairy Lantern, Mugwort, Pomegranate (FES); Female Balance Combo (PF).

Menstruation – Irregular: Woman Essence (FE Aus); Evening Primrose, Fairy Lantern, Mugwort, Pomegranate (FES); Female Balance Combo (PF); Wise Woman (WD).

Menstruation – Pains: She Oak, Woman Balance (FE Aus); Black Cohosh, Love Lies Bleeding, Pomegranate (FES); Sublime Chocolate (Peru); Manage Pain Combo (PF).

Meridian Balance: Northern Lady's Slipper (Ask); Crowea (FE Aus); Clearing Blockages (DL); Silver Maple (GM).

Metabolism (Rebalancing): Black-Eyed Susan, Crowea, Mulla Mulla, Old Man Banksia (FE Aus); Nasturtium, Peppermint, Rosemary, Snapdragon (FES); Sublime Chocolate (Peru); Cherokee Rose (PF).

Miasms: Boab (FE Aus); Lotus Essence (AK, Dv, FES, Him A); Clearing Energy Fields (DL).
Heavy Metals: Purification (Ask); Detox, Wild Potato Bush (FE Aus); Letting Go (DL); Awapuhi-melemele/Yellow Ginger (Haii); Bloodroot, Daffodil (Peg); Daylily (PF).
Lymphatic System: Bush Iris, Wild Potato Bush, Detox (FE Aus); Clearing Energy Fields (DL); Awapuhi-melemele/Yellow Ginger (Haii); Red Carnation (PF).
Petrochemical: Detox (FE Aus); Garlic (FES); Almond (Peg); Daylily (PF).
Psora: Dagger Hakea, Mountain Devil (FE Aus); Eucalyptus, Garlic (FES); Camphor (Peg).
Radiation and Electromagnetic: Electro-guard (FE Aus); Radiant Strength, Reading Energy Fields, Clearing Energy Fields (DL); Garlic (FES); Bloodroot (Peg); Faith and Courage (Peru); Recovery Combo (PF); Protective Shield, Sacred Space (WD); T1 (AK).
Syphilitic: Boab, She Oak, Sturt Desert Rose (FE Aus); California Poppy, Chaparral, Iris-Blue Flag (FES); Bells of Ireland, Celandine, Four-leaf Clover (Peg).
Syscosis: Black-Eyed Susan, Dagger Hakea, Mountain Devil, Sturt Desert Pea (FE Aus); Dandelion, Lilac (FES).
Thyroid: Old Man Banksia (FE Aus); Chiton (Pac).
Tuberculosis: Sturt Desert Pea, Waratah (FE Aus); Blackberry, Eucalyptus (FES); Cotton, Hops, Live Forever, Red Clover (Peg).

Migraine: Emergency Rescue (FE Aus); Awapuhi-melemele/Yellow Ginger (Haii); Orange (Ma); Plantain (Pac); Narcissus, Curry (PF).

Miscarriage/Termination: Candystick, Sea Lettuce (Pac).

Morning Lethargy: Banksia Robur, Dynamis Essence (FE Aus); Hornbeam (B); Centred Love, Walking Out of Patterns, Manifesting Thought Forms, Meditative Mind (DL); Morning Glory (FES, Him E); Rosemary, Tansy (FES); Energy Combo and Spray (PF); Young Heart, Smiles and Giggles (WD).

Mosquito Bites: Mountain Devil, Mulla Mulla, Paw Paw, Spinifex (FE Aus); Garlic (FES).

Mucous Colitis: Bottlebrush, Peach-Flowered Tea-Tree (FE Aus); I Like Being Me (DL); Snapdragon (FES).

Multiple Sclerosis: Gymea Lily, Hibbertia, Isopogon, Rough Bluebell, Southern Cross, Spinifex (FE Aus); Dandelion, Snowdrop (Pac).

Muscular Disorders: Crowea (FE Aus); Dandelion (AK, Ask, Dv, FES, Hb); Vervain (B); Anemone, Salmonberry (Pac); Champney's Pink Cluster, Manage Pain Combo and Spray, Pink Geranium (PF).

Nasal Congestion: Bush Iris, Dagger Hakea, Fringed Violet, Tall Mulla Mulla (FE Aus); California Pitcher Plant, Eucalyptus, Jasmine, Yerba Santa (FES); Colds and Flu Combo, Purple Garden Sage (PF).

Nausea: Crowea, Dagger Hakea, Dog Rose, Paw Paw (FE Aus); Chamomile (FES); Corn (Ma); Harmony Blend Combo (PF); Windflower (Pac).

Neck and Back Stiffness/Whip Lash: Noble Heart Cactus (AK); Crowea, Black-Eyed Susan, Gymea Lily, Southern Cross, Tall Yellow Top (FE Aus); Dandelion (Dv, FES); Iris (FES); Pau Pilo (Haii); Meadowsweet (Hb); Chiton, Mussel (Pac); Manage Pain Combo (PF); Dandelion (WF).

Nervous Exhaustion: Angelsword, Black-Eyed Susan, Fringed Violet, Jacaranda, Old Man Banksia, Paw Paw (FE Aus); Buffalo

Gourd, Fairy Duster (DAl); New Perceptions, Clearing Energy Fields (DL); Lady's Slipper (FES); Alder (GM); Artichoke (HUB); Fatigue Combo (PF).

Nervousness: Hibiscus (FO); Black-Eyed Susan, Jacaranda (FE Aus); Aspen (B); Whitehorn (DAl); Idiot Glee (DL); Chamomile (Dv, FES); Wild Garlic (Dv); Comfrey (FES); Hau (Haii); Almond, Banana, Lettuce, Pear (Ma); Alaskan Birch Forest, Still Mind, Mother's Arms, On Angels' Wings (WD); Yellow Oleande (SME).

Nervous System (Tonic): Bush Fuchsia, Crowea (FE Aus); Fairy Duster (DAl); Angelica Comfrey (Dv, FES); Morning Glory (Dv, FES, Him E); Arnica (FES); Hibiscus (FO); Pear (GM); Hau (Haii); Viburnum (Pac); Madame Alfred Carriere (PF); Chinese Fan Palm (GH); Grey Coral Fungus (AK).

Neuritis: Country Marilou (PF).

Obesity: Detox, Bush Iris, Crowea, Five Corners, Fringed Violet, Old Man Banksia, Wild Potato Bush (FE Aus); I Like Being Me, Letting Go (DL); Evening Primrose, Golden Rod, Hound's Tongue, Nicotiana, Pink Monkeyflower, Tansy (FES); Poison Hemlock (Pac); Craving Combo, Pink Rose, Gruss an Aachen, Weight Combo (PF); Wise Woman, Still Mind, Sacred Space, Protective Shield (WD).

Pain (Relief): Cotton Grass (Ask); Bottlebrush + Emergency Rescue (FE Aus); Illyarrie, Menzies Banksia (Aus L); Heart of Nature, Clearing Energy Fields (DL); Love Lies Bleeding (FES); Gean/Wild Cherry (GM); Foxglove (Hb); Floral P Gel, Dayblooming Jessamine (Him A); First Aid + Gel (F); Pear (Ma); Anemone (Pac); Bougainvillea, Manage Pain (PF); Happy Pet, Still Mind, Mother's Arms (WD).

Paralysis: Bush Fuchsia, Crowea, Grey Spider Flower, Wild Potato Bush (FE Aus); Radiant Strength, Earth Mother Nurtures (DL); Scottish Primrose (F); Poison Hemlock, Snowdrop (Pac).

Parasites: Life Force Cactus (AK); Detox (FE Aus); Garlic (FES); Fleabane (HUB); Amaryllis (PF).

Pelvic Inflammatory Disease (PID): Billy Goat Plum, Fringed Violet, Woman Balance (FE Aus); Pomegranate (FES); Snowdrop (Hb).

Physical Strength/Growth: Dynamic Recovery (FE Aus); Milky Nipple Cactus (DAl); Higher Levels, My Own Pure Light, Unveiling Self (DL); Tomato (Ma); Inner Strength Combo and Spray (PF); Smiles and Giggles, Wise Woman, Young Heart (WD).

Postnatal: Woman Balance (FE Aus).

Post Trauma: Post Trauma Stabilizer (FES).

Pregnancy and Problems (e.g. Morning Sickness): Courgette (AK); Pregnancy Support (Ask); Bottlebrush, Dagger Hakea, She Oak (FE Aus); Earth Mother Nurtures, Heart of Nature (DL); Watermelon (Dv, FES); Forget-me-not, Zucchini (Dv); Chamomile, California Wild Rose, Calla Lily, Evening Primrose, Mugwort, Pomegranate (FES); Rosebud-white (Hb); Corn, Pear (Ma); Pregnancy Partner (Peg); Maternity Combo and Spray (PF); Divine Child (Peru), Delph and Horn of Plenty (AK).

Premenstrual Syndrome: Woman Balance (FE Aus); Immortal, Mala Mujer, Tar Bush (DAl); Pomegranate (FES); Pear, Grape (Ma); Easter Lily (Pac); Female Balance Combo (PF); Wise Woman (WD).

Protection From – Pollution: Guardian (Ask); Angelsword, Fringed Violet, Clear and Protect (FE Aus); Sneezease (Aus L); Radiant Strength, Earth Mother Nurtures, Letting Go (DL); White Yarrow (Dv); Clearing Spray, Reduce Stress Combo, Tansy (PF); Alaskan Birch Forest, Protective Shield, Sacred Space (WD).

Protection From – Radiation: White Yarrow (AK, Dv); T1 (AK); Guardian (Ask); Electro-Guard (FE Aus); Radiant Strength, Earth Mother Nurtures, Letting Go (DL); Environmental Solution (FES); Yarrow in seawater (Hb); Regenerate Combo (PF); Alaskan Birch Forest, Protective Shield, SacredSpace (WD); Cell Phone Combo (Blos).

Psoriasis: Aloe Vera (AK, FES); Billy Goat Plum (FE Aus); Vanilla Leaf (Pac); Salvia (PF).

Psychosomatic Illness: Peach-Flowered Tea-Tree (FE Aus); Strawberry Cactus (DAl); Reading Energy Fields, Walking Out of Patterns, Earth Mother Nurtures, Manifesting Thought Forms (DL); Canyon Dudleya, Fuchsia, Purple Monkeyflower, Yerba Santa (FES); Apple (Ma); Still Mind (WD).

Puberty: Blackboy, Bottlebrush (FE Aus); Walnut (B); Fairy Lantern, Sagebrush, Saguaro, Sticky Monkeyflower, Kinder Garden (FES); Mallow, Rosebud-Red (Hb); Almond (Ma); Orange Honeysuckle (Pac).

Radiation Problems and the Effects of Cancer Treatments: Radiation Cactus, T1 (AK); Electro-Guard, Mulla Mulla (FE Aus); Yarrow Special Formulae (FES); Recovery Combo (PF).

Regeneration: Champney's Pink Cluster, Country Marilou, Regeneration Combo (PF).

Reproductive Problems – Female: She Oak, Woman Balance (FE Aus); Alpine Lily, Pomegranate (FES); Candysticks, Silver Birch (Pac); Red Spider Lily (Peg); Female Balance Combo (PF); Wise Woman (WD).

Reproductive Problems – Male: Flannel Flower (FE Aus); Pomegranate (FES); Red Spider Lily (Peg).

Respiratory System: Five Corners, Tall Mulla Mulla, Tall Yellow Top (FE Aus); Acceptance, Lotus Petals of the Heart (DL); Eucalyptus (FES); Grape Hyacinth (Pac); Babies' Breath (PF).

SAD (Seasonal Affective Disorder): Lighten Up (Ask); Seasonal Affections (F); Diatoms, Grape Hyacinth, Periwinkle, Red Huckleberry, Snowberry (Pac).

Scar Tissue: Little Flannel Flower (FE Aus); Aloe Vera (FES); Anemone, Regenerate Combo (PF).

Sexual Diseases (Chlamydia, Herpes): K9 (AK); Billy Goat Plum (FE Aus); Pomegranate (FES).

Shingles: Manage Pain Combo (PF).

Shock: Arnica (AK, FES); Cotton Grass, Fireweed, Soul Support (Ask); Emergency Essence, Fringed Violet (FE Aus); Rescue Remedy (B); Gossamer Steel, My Song Calls Me Home (DL); First Aid (F); Self-Heal (FES); Privet (GM); 'Ulua (Haii); First Aid Remedy (Him A); Grape Hyacinth (Pac); White Hyacinth (PF); Mother's Arms (WD).

Sight (Enhancing): Eyebright (AK); Waratah (FE Aus); Dancing Light Spirit (DL); Queen Anne's Lace (FES); Cotton (Haii); Anemone, Ox-Eye Daisy (Pac).

Sinusitis: Bush Iris, Dagger Hakea, Fringed Violet (FE Aus); Sneezease (Aus L); Eucalyptus (FES); Formula 43 Sinus/Cold (Him A); Allergy Combo (PF).

Skin Lesions/Scar Tissue: Mulla Mulla (FE Aus); Lemon (GH); Defining Edges (DL); Anemone, Regenerate Combo (PF); Protective Shield (WD).

Skin Problems: Inside/Outside Cactus (AK); Detox, Billy Goat Plum (FE Aus); Office Flower (Him A); Gilia Scarlet, Red Spider Lily (Peg); Archduke Charles, Lily, Salvia (PF); Lichen (AK); Jewel Weed (GH).

Smoking (Effects of): Morning Glory (AK, FES, Him E); Detox (FE Aus); Nicotiana (FES); Drum Stick (Him A); Stop Smoking Combo (PF).

Speech Problems: Bush Fuchsia, Flannel Flower, Red Grevillea (FE Aus); Mimulus (B); I Like Being Me (DL); Petunia, Snapdragon (Hb); Parrot Tree (Him A); Anise Hyssop, White Petunia (PF).

Spinal and Structural Problems: Noble Heart Cactus, Valerian (AK); Black-Eyed Susan, Gymea Lily, Tall Yellow Top (FE Aus); Lilac (Dv); Corn (FES); Laburnum (GM); Ma'o, Ohai-ali'i (Haii); Sunflower (Hb); Indian Pipe, Salmonberry (Peg); Borage, Cinnamon Basil, Inner Strength Combo, Mushroom, Orchid (PF).

Spleen: Boronia, Dog Rose, Pink Mulla Mulla (FE Aus); Goatsbeard (Pac).

Sunburn: Mulla Mulla (FE Aus).

Swelling: Bush Iris, Old Man Banksia, She Oak (FE Aus); Bachelor's Button, Red Carnation (PF).

Teeth-Grinding: Black-Eyed Susan, Dagger Hakea, Red Grevillea (FE Aus); Morning Glory (FES); Hibiscus (FO).

Teething (Babies): Emergency Essence (FE Aus); Pink Seaweed (Pac).

Tension: Dandelion (AK, Dv, FES, Hb); Emergency Rescue (FE Aus); Purple Flag Flower, Rose Cone Flower (Aus L); Impatiens, Vervain, Water Violet (B); Cherry Plum (B, GM); Comfrey, Forget-Me-Not, Spruce (Dv); First Aid (F); Chamomile (FES, Hb); Lavender (FES); Fig, Pear (Ma); Abate Anger Combo and Spray (PF); Alaskan Birch Forest, Smiles and Giggles (WD); Fly Agaric (AK).

Throat (Sore): Bush Fuchsia, Bush Iris, Flannel Flower, Dagger Hakea, Mountain Devil, Old Man Banksia, Sturt Desert Pea (FE Aus); Blue Camas, Sand Dollar (Pac); Colds and Flu Combo (PF).

Tiredness: Dynamic Recovery (FE Aus); Leafless Orchid (Aus L); Aspen, Hornbeam, Pine (B); Tansy (FES); Almond, Corn (Ma); Fatigue Combo (PF).

Travel Sickness: Travel Ease (Ask); Travel-Well (FE Aus); Travelease (Aus L); Jetstream (F); Travel (Hb); Formula 14 Travel Aid (Him A); Corn (Ma); Travel Mate (CHI).

Tonsillitis: Bush Fuchsia, Bush Iris, Flannel Flower (FE Aus); Sand Dollar (Pac).

Toxicity/Toxaemia: Purification (Ask); Bottlebrush, Detox (FE Aus); Reading Energy Fields (DL); Ragged Robin (F); Chaparral (FES); Coffee (Haii); Apple, Blackberry (Ma); Blue Lupin (Pac); Coralroot (Spotted) (Peg); Crossandra, Pansy, Daylily (PF); Alaskan Birch Forest (WD); Fly Agaric (AK).

Ulcers: Peppermint (Pac); Crowea and Paw Paw (FE Aus).

Vitality/Revitalization/Wellbeing: Zest and Vitality (FO); Alpine Mint Bush, Crowea, Dynamic Recovery, Macrocarpa, Wild Bush Potato (FE Aus); Essences of Energy, Leafless Orchid, Pink Fountain Triggerplant (Aus L); Smooth Hawksbeard (Bal); Dancing Light Spirit (DL); Almond, Morning Glory (Dv); Nasturtium (Dv, Hb, FES); Gorse, Sycamore (F); Tansy (FES); Blackberry (Hb); Endurance (Him A); Apple (Ma); Super Vitality (Pac); Energy Combo (PF); Orange Hawkweed (Sun); Young Heart, Coconut Palm (SME); Happy Pet (WD).

Viral Infections: K9 (AK); Black-Eyed Susan (FE Aus); Wild Garlic (Dv, FES); Pansy (Hb); Colds and Flu Combo and Spray, Echinacea, Purple Garden Sage, Onion, Thyme (PF).

Warts: Billy Goat Plum, Five Corners (FE Aus); Salvia, Wild Wood Violets (PF).

Weight Control: Detox Essence and Kit, Wild Potato Bush Boronia, Bottlebrush, Peach-Flowered Tea-Tree (FE Aus); Expansive Embodiment, Manifesting Thought Forms (DL); Hound's Tongue, Yerba Santa, Madrone (FES); Mango, Naio (Haii); Tomato (Ma); Chickweed, Chiton, Poison

Hemlock, Urchin (Pac); Dayflower (Peg); Inocencia Coca, Sublime Chocolate (Peru); Craving Combo and Spray, Gruss an Aachen, Weight Combo (PF); Papaya (FO).

Psychological

Abandonment: Tall Yellow Top, Illawarra Flame Tree (FE Aus); White Hibiscus, Fremont Pincushion (GH); Mesquite, Milky Nipple Cactus (DAl); Acceptance, Gossamer Steel, Heart to Heart (DL); Tall Grape, Strawberry (Ma); Arbutus, Nootka Rose, Sea Palm (Pac); Mother's Arms, On Angels' Wings, Smiles and Giggles (WD).

Abundance: Positivity, Southern Cross (FE Aus); Ground Ivy (Bal); Prosperity, Sea Rocket (F); Double Daffodil (Sun); Cyclamen (Med); Rain of Gold (GH); Guernsey Lily (CHI).

Abuse (Emotional): White Fireweed (Ask); Confidence Boost, Emergency Rescue (FE Aus); Mountain Mahogany (DAl); Earth Mother Nurtures (DL); Martagon Lily, Scarlet Monkeyflower (Dv); Black Cohosh, Black-Eyed Susan, Bleeding Heart, Echinacea, Morning Glory, Oregon Grape, Purple Monkeyflower, Snapdragon, Tiger Lily (FES); Elder, Italian Alder (GM); Elder (Hb); Orange, Strawberry (Ma); Urchin (Pac); Happy Pet, Mother's Arms, Sacred Space, On Angels' Wings, Protective Shield (WD); Brown Eyed Evening Primrose (GH).

Abuse (Self): Billy Goat Plum, Five Corners (FE Aus); Bisbee Beehive Cactus, Kleins Pencil Cholla Cactus (DAl); Clearing Energy Fields, I Like Being Me, Lotus Petals of the Heart, Stepping Ahead Now (DL); Dogwood (FES); Fig (Ma); Forsythia, Nootka Rose (Pac).

Accident, Prone to: Jacaranda, Kangaroo Paw, Red Lily (FE Aus); Impatiens (B); Ulua (Haii); Pill Bearing Spurge (Him A); Avocado (Ma); Still Mind (WD).

Adaptability: Angel of Protection Orchid (AK); Bauhinia, Freshwater Mangrove, Slender Rice Flower, Waratah (FE Aus); Prickly Pear Cactus (DAl); Clearing Energy Fields, Graceful Transformations, Higher Levels, Reading Energy Fields, Manifesting Thought Forms (DL); Aloe Vera, Golden Yarrow, Redbud (FES); Healer (Him E); Fig (Ma); Douglas Aster, Coral, Diatom (Pac); Summer Snowflake (GH).

ADD/ADHD (Attention Deficit Disorder/Attention Deficit Hyperactivity Disorder): Learning and Focus (FE Aus); Blue Camus (Pac); Attention Formula (Peru); Dowry Avens (FES); ADD/ADHD (PF).

Addiction Withdrawal Symptoms: Morning Glory (AK); Boab, Boronia, Bottlebrush, Dog Rose of the Wild Forces, Sundew, Waratah, Wedding Bush (FE Aus); Letting Go (DL); Angelica, Sagebrush (FES); Nirjara (Him E); Tomato (Ma); Nootka Rose, Urchin (Pac); Purple Nightshade, Rosa Damascena Bifera (Peg); Positive Change (FO).

Addictive Behaviour: Boab, Boronia, Bottlebrush, Monga Waratah, Waratah (FE Aus); Blue China Orchid (Aus L); Rose Damacea, Hedgehog Cactus, Tarbrush (DAl); Gossamer Steel, Unveiling Self (DL); Morning Glory (Dv, FES); Nicotiana, Scarlet Monkeyflower (FES); Tulip Tree (GM); Morning Glory, Pua kenikeni (Haii); Drum Stick, Opium Poppy (Him A); Almond, Tomato (Ma); Forsythia, Urchin (Pac); Monkeyflower Bush, Rosa Damascena Bifera (Peg); Emancipation (Peru); Craving Combo, Stop Smoking Combo (PF); Still Mind, Wise Woman (WD); Coffee (GH); Un-Believe (DL).

Adolescence: Blackboy (FE Aus); Banana Poka/Passion Flower, Kukui (Haii); Lilac (Bal); Cherry (FES).

Ageing (in Women): Corn Lily, Red Bud (FES).

Aggression: Aggression Orchid (AK); Mountain Devil (FE Aus); Buffalo Gourd (DAl); Centred Love, Higher Levels (DL); Grape (Ma).

Alcoholism: Morning Glory (AK); Boab, Boronia, Bottlebrush, Waratah (FE Aus); Clearing Energy Fields, Radiant Strength (DL); Chrysanthemum, Mountain Pennyroyal (FES); Kou (Haii); Sober Up (Him E); Nootka Rose, Urchin (Pac); Craving Combo (PF).

Anger: Blue Elf Viola (Ask); Mountain Devil (FE Aus); Fuchsia Grevillea, Orange Spiked Peaflower (Aus L); Holly (B); Compass Barrel Cactus, Foothills Paloverde, Star Primrose (DAl); Gossamer Steel (DL); Fuchsia, Scarlet Monkeyflower (Dv, FES); Willowherb (F); Snapdragon (FES); Kukui, Impatiens (Haii); Nettle (Hb); Wellbeing (Him E); Almond, Apple, Lettuce (Ma); Mussel (Pac); Orange Flame Flower Cactus (Peg); Abate Anger Combo (PF); Smiles and Giggles (WD); Bramble (WF); Avocado (GH).

Anorexia Nervosa: Hibiscus, Female, Papaya (FO); Boab, Five Corners, Peach-Flowered Tea-Tree, Dagger Hakea, Waratah (FE Aus); Manifesting Thought Forms, Radiant Strength (DL); Black-Eyed Susan, Manzanita (FES).

Anxiety: Emergency Rescue, Calm & Relax (FE Aus); Hibiscus, Stressless (FO); Purple Flag Flower, Woolly Smoke-Bush (Aus L); Red Chestnut (B); Hoptree, Strawberry Cactus (DAl); Clearing Energy Fields (DL); Wild Garlic (Dv); Scottish Primrose (F); Filagree (FES); Alder (GM); Kukui, Plemomele Fragrans (Haii); Chamomile (Hb); Banana, Tomato (Ma); Periwinkle (Pac); Mother's Arms, On Angels' Wings, Smiles and Giggles, Still Mind (WD).

Apathy: Dynamis Recovery (FE Aus); My Own Pure Light (DL); Gorse (F); Blackberry, California Wild Rose, Tansy (FES); Tulip (Him A); Orange (Ma).

Apprehension: Water Violet (Aus L); Calm & Relax, Crowea, Tall Mulla Mulla (FE Aus); Aspen (B); Cotton/Ma'o (Haii); Tomato (Ma); Mother's Arms, Wise Woman (WD).

Argumentativeness: Dagger Hakea, Isopogon, Rough Bluebell (FE Aus); Expansive Embodiment, Acceptance (DL); Banana (Ma); Still Mind (WD).

Arrogance: Rough Bluebell (FE Aus); Larkspur (FES).

Attachment: Cotton Grass, River Beauty, Sweetgale (Ask); Bottlebrush (FE Aus); Letting Go (DL); Banana (Ma); Douglas Aster, Yellow Pond Lily (Pac); Sea Holly (Med).

Attention Seeking: Heliconia (Haii); Blackboy (FE Aus).

Autism: Boronia, Flannel Flower, Lotus/Red Lily (FE Aus); Expanding Awareness, I Like Being Me (DL); Bluebell, Blue Lupin, Wallflower (Pac); Lewisa (FES).

Balance (Emotional): Labrador Tree (Ask); Crowea, Calm & Relax (FE Aus); Hops Bush (Aus L); Scleranthus (B); Smooth Hawksbeard (Bal); Buffalo Gourd, Fairy Duster, Fire Prickly Pear Cactus (DAl); Balancing Extremes (DL); Chamomile (FES); Forget-Me-Not, Red Tulip (Hb); Almond, Apple, Pear (Ma); Fuchsia, Balancer (Pac); Balanced (Sun).

Bereavement: Emergency Rescue and later Sturt Desert Rose and Sturt Desert Pea (FE Aus); Acceptance, Earth Mother Nurtures, Graceful Transformations, Infinite Patience, Lotus Petals of the Heart, Stepping Ahead Now (DL); Grief Relief, Forget-Me-Not (FES); Radish (Him A); Grape (Ma); Purple Crocus, Starfish (Pac); Be Comforted (Sun).

Bitterness: Dagger Hakea, Southern Cross (FE Aus); Holly (B); Willow (B, FES); Clearing Blockages, My Heart Knows, Unveiling Self (DL); Mugwort (Hb); Bearing

Spurge, Drum Stick, Slow Match, Ukshi (Him A); Raspberry (Ma); Jelly Fish (Pac); Avocado (GH); Buttercup (Bal); Panama Pacific Waterlily (Haii).

Blame: Dagger Hakea, Mountain Devil, Southern Cross (FE Aus); Green Rose (Aus L); Star Primrose, Rue (DAl); Infinite Patience, Softening the Edges (DL); Grape, Raspberry (Ma).

Bonding (Developing): Soul Support (Ask); Bottlebrush, Red Helmet Orchid, Woman Balance (FE Aus); Radiant Strength and Centred Love, Lotus Petals of the Heart (DL); Linden (Dv); Mariposa Lily (FES); Plumeria (Peg).

Brain (Left and Right Imbalance): Bush Fuchsia (FE Aus); Balancing Extremes, Expanding Awareness (DL); Rainbow Kelp (Pac); Koenign Van Daenmark (Peg).

Breaking Bad Habits/Addictions: Bottlebrush, Boronia, Isopogan, Learning and Focus (FE Aus); Hairy Larkspur (DAl); Cravings Combo and Spray (PF).

Broken Hearted: Bleeding Heart (AK, FES); Boronia, Waratah, Sturt Desert Pea (FE Aus); Acceptance, Clearing Inner Pathways, Gossamer Steel, Heart Wings, Higher Levels, Light Hearted, My Heart Knows, Stepping Ahead Now (DL); Heart Support (F); Love Lies Bleeding (FES); Field Maple (GM); Heartsease (Hb); Autumn Damask (PF); Honeysuckle (WF); Red Torch Ginger (FO).

Burnout: Dynamic Recovery, Banksia Robur, Black-Eyed Susan, Macrocarpa, Old Man Banksia (FE Aus); Earth Mother Nurtures, Meditative Mind (DL); Fairy Duster, Whitehorn, Woven Spine Pineapple Cactus (DAl); Gorse, Life Force (F); Aloe Vera, Lavender (FES); Hibiscus (FO); Purple Nightshade (Peg); Mother's Arms, Protective Shield (WD); Sea Grape (GHBm).

Calming – Emotions: Lavender, Red Clover, Valerian, Wild Garlic (AK); Calm & Relax

(FE Aus); Many-Headed Dryandra, Yellow Flag Flower (Aus L); Fairy Duster, Indian Tobacco (DAl); Nettles (Dv); Chamomile (Dv, FES, Hb); Lettuce (Dv, Ma); Daisy (F); Indian Pink (FES); Gean/Wild Cherry (GM); Bluebell, Lavender, Marjoram, Red Clover (Hb); Lotus (Him A); Yellow Poppy (HUB); Purple Nightshade (Peg); Bobinsana (AmT).

Calming – The Mind: Lavender (AK); Calm & Relax (FE Aus); White Chestnut (B); Candy Barrel Cactus (DAl); Meditative Mind (DL); Ragwort (Hb); Yellow Poppy (HUB); Bobinsana (AmT); Almond, Banana, Lettuce (Ma).

Caring: Flannel Flower (FE Aus); Immortal, Mesquite (DAl); Centred Love, Earth Mother Nurtures, Lotus Petals of the Heart (DL); Poison Oak, Sunflower (FES); Lucombe Oak (GM); Peach (Ma); Mother's Arms, Wise Woman (WD).

Change: Giant Bluebell (Bal); Sacred Banyan Tree, Positive Change (FO).

Childbirth (Attitude Towards) *See also* **Pregnancy:** Delph (AK); Grove Sandwort (Ask); Bottlebrush, She Oak (FE Aus); Earth Mother Nurtures, Radiant Strength and Centred Love (DL); Evening Primrose (FES); Noni (Haii); Maternity Combo (PF); Positive Change (FE Aus).

City Stress: Corn (AK); Calm and Clear (FE Aus); Antiseptic Bush, Pink Fairy Orchid (Aus L); Radiant Strength, Sacred Sphere (DL); Pink Yarrow, Sweet Corn (Dv); Environmental Solution Special Formula, Indian Pink, Nicotiana, Sweet Pea, Yarrow (FES); Office Flower, Torroyia Rorshi Plant, Urban Stress Remedy (Him A); Beauty Secret, Buff Beauty (Peg); Reduce Stress Combo and Spray (PF); Sacred Space, Protective Shield (WD).

Clarity (of Mind): Eyebright (AK, Sun); Bladderwort, Bunch-Berry Twinflower (Ask); Alder (Ask, GM); Boronia, Bush Fuchsia, Isopogon (FE Aus); Essences of

Clarity, Pink Trumpet Flower, White Eremophila (Aus L); White Chestnut (B); Red Henbit (Bal); Candy Barrel Cactus, Star Primrose (DAl); Dill, Fig Tree, Peppermint (Dv); Expansive Awareness, Meditative Mind, New Perceptions (DL); Daisy (Dv, Hb); Deerbrush, Madia, Mountain Pennyroyal (FES); Box, Pittespora (GM); Kou, Nana-honua (Haii); Apple, Avocado, Banana, Blackberry, Lettuce, Pineapple (Ma); Brown Kelp, Blue Lupin (Pac); Learning Skills Combo (PF); Still Mind (WD); Lepista Irina (AK).

Claustrophobia: Grey Spider Flower (FE Aus); Fuchsia Gum, W.A. Christmas Tree (Aus L); Balancing Extremes, Clearing Energy Fields, Expanding Awareness, Expansive Embodiment (DL); Glastonbury Thorn (GM); Authenticity (Him E); Apple (Ma); Prickly Pear (SME).

Commitment: Relate Well (FE Aus); Compass Barrel Cactus, Prickly Pear Cactus (DAl); Basil, Evening Primrose (FES); Acceptance, Centred Love, Heart to Heart, Purpose Flows, Internal Marriage, My Heart Knows (DL); Pearly Everlasting (Pac).

Communication: Bush Fuchsia, Flannel Flower, Relate Well (FE Aus); Fishhook Cactus (DAl); Centred Love, Heart to Heart (DL); Cosmos, Linden, Zinnia (Dv); Calendula (Dv, FES); Broom (F); Scarlet Monkeyflower (FES); Jade Vine, 'Ula (Haii); Authenticity (Him E); Lettuce (Ma); Gentian (Peg).

Complaining: Dagger Hakea, Mountain Devil, Paw Paw, Southern Cross (FE Aus); One-Sided Bottlebrush, Wild Violet (Aus L); Higher Levels, Infinite Patience, Wise Action (DL); Bluebell (WF); Hawaiian Bell (SME).

Compulsiveness: Boronia (FE Aus); Filagree (FES); Clearing Energy Fields, Light Hearted, Stepping Ahead Now (DL).

Concentration: Rosemary (AK); Learning and Focus, Jacaranda (FE Aus); Essences of Clarity (Aus L); Scleranthus (B); New Perceptions (DL); Broom (F); Madia, Peppermint (FES); Teak Wood Flower (Him A); Avocado, Lettuce (Ma); Learning Skills Combo (PF); Still Mind (WD).

Confidence (Increasing): Buttercup, Self-Esteem Cactus, Sunflower (AK); Confidence Boost, Five Corners (FE Aus); Snake Vine (Aus L); Larch (B); Cerato (B, FES); Buffalo Gourd, Cardon, Ephedra, Hedgehog Cactus (DAl); My Heart Knows, My Own Pure Light, Radiant Strength, Wise Action (DL); Borage (Dv, Hb); Bell Heather, Voice Confidence (F); Mullein, Trumpet Vine (FES); Catalpa, Cherry Plum (GM); Cymbidium (Hb); Pineapple (Ma); Be Confident (Sun).

Confusion: Bauhinia (FE Aus); White Chestnut (B); Blackberry (Dv); Broom, Daisy (F); Dill (FES); Higher Levels, My Heart Knows, New Perceptions, Unveiling Self (DL); Box (GM); Stick Rorrish (Haii); Teak Wood Flower (Him A); Avocado, Corn (Ma); Still Mind, On Angels' Wings (WD); Purple Foxglove (WF).

Contempt: Mountain Devil, Rough Bluebell (FE Aus); Cowslip Orchid (Aus L); Holly (B); Softening the Edges (DL).

Contentment: Christmas Tree (Aus L); Bluebell, Rose – wild (Hb); Acceptance, Reveals Mystery Within, Purpose Flows (DL); Chickweed (HUB); Purplemat (GH).

Control (Loss of): Red Clover (AK); Southern Cross (FE Aus); Cherry Plum, Rock Rose (B); Desert Marigold, Hop Tree, Sacred Datura, Star Primrose, Strawberry Cactus (DAl); Balancing Extremes, Wise Action (DL); Daisy (F); Chinese Violet (Haii); Self-Heal (Hb); Almond, Fig (Ma); Sea Palm (Pac).

Coping (with Problems/Challenges/Change): Bauhinia, Paw Paw, Waratah (FE Aus); Rose Cone Flower, Yellow Flag

Flower (Aus L); Peppermint (Bal); Cow Parsnip, Immortal, Jojoba, Spineless Prickly Pear (DAl); Defining Edges, Expanding Awareness, Infinite Patience, New Perceptions, Meditative Mind (DL); Fig Tree (Dv); Milkweed (FES); White Poplar (GM); Dandelion (Hb); Chinese Violet, Ohai Lehua (Haii); Radish (Him A); About Space (Peru); Pomegranate (SME).

Courage: Borage (AK, Dv, Hb); Monkshood, Prickly Wild Rose (Ask); Dog Rose, Green Spider Orchid, Grey Spider Flower, Waratah (FE Aus); Menzies Banksia (Aus L); Mimulus (B); Sacred Datura, Saguaro (DAl); My Heart Knows, Purpose Flows (DL); Thistle (F); Black Cohosh, Mountain Pride, Penstemon, Fear-Less (FES); Italian Alder, White Poplar (GM); Wiliwili (Haii); Swallow Wort (Him A); Tomato (Ma); Surfgrass (Pac); Be Courageous (Sun); Iron (Med); Lupuna Blanca (AmT).

Cravings: Paw Paw, Peach-Flowered Tea-Tree (FE Aus); Craving Combo (PF).

Creativity: Iris (AK, Dv, FES); Inspiration Cactus, Inspiration Orchid (AK); Golden Corydalis, Sticky Geranium, Wild Iris (Ask); Turkey Bush (FE Aus); Essences of Creativity, Pink Impatiens (Aus L); Rainbow (Bal); Indian Root (DAl); Dance of Creation, Expansive Embodiment, New Perceptions (DL); Broom, Garden Pea, Holy Thorn (F); Indian Paintbrush, Columbine (FES); Holm Oak, Lucombe Oak (GM); Creative/Focus (Peru); Crocodiles of Katchikally (SME).

Crisis: Emergency Rescue, Waratah (FE Aus); Cowkicks, Crisis Relief (Aus L); Aloe, Ephedra (DAl); Lucid Dreaming (DL); Angelica (Dv); First Aid (F); Speedwell (Hb); Pear (Ma); Be Calm (Sun); Mother's Arms, Protective Shield (WD); Help (CHI).

Criticism: Sphagnum Moss (Ask); Yellow Cowslip Orchid (FE Aus); Brachycome, Yellow and Green Kangaroo Paw (Aus L); Beech, Chicory, Impatiens (B); Aloe,

Foothills Paloverde, Mala Mujer (DAl); I Like Being Me, Meditative Mind, Sacred Sphere (DL); Calendula, Snapdragon (FES); Ulua (Haii); White Coral Tree (Him A); Date, Figs, Grape (Ma); Garden Mum (PF).

Cynicism: Sunshine Wattle (FE Aus); Ursinia, Wallflower Donkey Orchid (Aus L); Wondrous Heart (DL); Spotted Orchid (F); Baby Blue Eyes (FES); Blackberry (Ma); Jelly Fish (Pac); Young Heart (WD).

Daydreaming: Red Lily/Lotus (FE Aus); Clematis (B, FES); Sacred Datura (DAl); Lucid Dreaming (DL); Rosemary (Dv); St John's Wort (FES); Avocado (Ma); Still Mind (WD); Angel Trumpet (SME).

Death: Cardon, Klein's Cholla Cactus (DAl); Henbane (HUB); Sierra Rein Orchid (Peg); Dill, Transitions Combo and Spray (PF); Soul Family (Peru).

Decision-Making: Lesser Toad Flax, Focus (CHI); Corn Poppy (SME); Tansy, Clematis (Blos).

Delinquency: Blackboy, Red Helmet Orchid (FE Aus); Unveiling Self (DL); Saguaro (FES); Macadamia, Stick Rorrish (Haii).

Denial: Sturt Desert Rose (FE Aus); Cardon, Klein's Cholla Cactus (DAl); Clearing Inner Pathways, New Perceptions, Reveals Mystery Within (DL); Sierra Rein Orchid (Peg); Dill (PF).

Dependency: Red Grevillea, Southern Cross (FE Aus); Canyon Grape Vine (DAl); Expansive Embodiment, Letting Go, My Heart Knows, Stepping Ahead Now (DL); Black Cohosh, Bleeding Heart, Fairy Lantern, Milkweed (FES); Chenille (Haii); Orange (Ma).

Depression: St John's Wort (AK); Borage (AK, Dv); Dynamic Recovery, Waratah (FE Aus); Essences of Positivity, Red Beak Orchid (Aus L); Mustard (B, FES); Larch, Pine (B); Bisbee Beehive Cactus, Immortal, Rainbow Cactus (DAl); Higher Levels,

Idiot Glee, Light Hearted, Manifesting Thought Forms (DL); Zinnia (Dv); Black Cohosh, Olive, Scotch Broom, Yerba Santa (FES); Copper Beech, Sycamore (GM); Blackberry, Daffodil, Primrose (Hb); Orange, Peach (Ma); Grape Hyacinth, Periwinkle, Rainbow Kelp (Pac); Red Rose (PF); Smiles and Giggles (WD); Orange (SME).

Deprogramming Dysfunctional Patterns: Northern Lights (Ask); Nijara (Him E); Fuchsia, Weigela (Pac); Velvet Shank (AK); Sacred Banyan Tree (FO).

Despair: Waratah (FE Aus); Cherry Plum, Gorse, Sweet Chestnut (B); Pine (B, FES); Indian Tobacco (DAl); Heart to Heart, Heart Wings, My Heart Knows, Wondrous Heart (DL); Scotch Broom (Dv); Elm (FES); Broom (Hb); Mother's Arms, Smiles and Giggles (WD); Sea Campion (CHI).

Determination (Lack of): Inspiration Cactus (AK); Peach-Flowered Tea-Tree (FE Aus); Pink Impatiens (Aus L); Uguisukazura – Flower (Aus LJ); Cardon, Ephedra (DAl); Purpose Flows, Stepping Ahead Now (DL); Penstemon (FES); Ohia Lehua (Haii); Coconut (Ma); Iron (Med); Activ-8 (FES); Una de Gato (AmT).

Dishonesty: Flannel Flower, Sturt Desert Rose (FE Aus); Fuchsia Grevillea, Red Feather Flower (Aus L); Devil's Claw, Syrian Rue (DAl); Higher Levels, Unveiling Self (DL); Basil, Deerbrush (FES); Manna Ash (GM); Wiliwili (Haii); Honesty (Hb); Autumn Damask (PF).

Disillusionment/Disappointments: Southern Cross (FE Aus); Snake Bush, Wallflower Donkey Orchid (Aus L); Sacred Datura (DAl); Centred Love, Expanding Awareness, Light Hearted, Lotus Petals of the Heart, Wondrous Heart (DL); Gentian, Star Tulip (FES); Pink Pond Lily (PF).

Disorientation: River Beauty (Ask); Bush Fuchsia (FE Aus); Pencil Cholla Cactus, Queen of the Night, Staghorn Cholla

Cactus (DAl); Heart Wings, Expanding Awareness (DL); Corn, Indian Pink, Madia (FES); Stick Rorrish (Haii); Avocado (Ma).

Divorce: Bleeding Heart (AK); Emergency Rescue, Relate Well (FE Aus); Pear (Ma).

Dogmatic: Hibbertia (FE Aus); Vine (B); White Coral Tree (Him A); Soaptree Yucca (DAl); Heart of Nature, Lotus Petals of the Heart (DL); Willowherb (F); Tiger Lily (FES); Hinahina-ku-kahakai (Haii); Houndstongue (HUB); Anemone, Sea Palm (Pac).

Dominating/Dominated: Relate Well (FE Aus); Vine (B); Soaptree Yucca (DAl); Heart to Heart (DL); Willowherb (F); Tiger Lily (FES); Hinahina-ku-kahakai, Jacaranda (Haii); Grape, Peach (Ma); Anemone, Sea Palm (Pac).

Doubt/Despondency: Mauve Melaleuca (Aus L); Larch (B); Hornbeam (B, FES); Tansy (Bal); White Desert Zinnia (DAl); Scotch Broom (FES); Cherry (Ma); Mother's Arms (WD).

Dreams – Disturbed: Forget-Me-Not (AK); Grey Spider Flower (FE Aus); Lucid Dreaming, Meditative Mind (DL); Sweet Dreams (F); Black-Eyed Susan, Chaparral (FES); Pa-nini-o-ka (Haii); Texas Dandelion (PF); Still Mind (WD).

Ego (Balance): Sun Orchid (AK); Isopogon, Rough Bluebell (FE Aus); Lace Flower, Round-Leaved Sundew, Sitka Spruce Pollen (Ask); Foothills Paloverde, Mountain Mahogany (DAl); Balancing Extremes, Higher Levels (DL); Sunflower (Dv); Chrysanthemum, Larkspur, Sunflower (FES); Weeping Willow, White Willow (GM); Thanksgiving Cactus, Water Poppy (Haii); White Narcissus (Hb); Flight (Him E); Dock (HUB); Douglas Aster (Pac); Charles de Mills (Peg); Still Mind, Wise Woman (WD); Goldenrod (Blos).

Emergencies: Arnica (AK); Soul Support, Fireweed, Labrador Tree, River Beauty, White Fireweed (Ask); Emergency Rescue

(FE Aus); Crisis Relief (Aus L); Rock Rose (B); Red Clover (Dv); Pear (Ma); Mother's Arms (WD).

Emotional Blockages: Shadow Cactus, Earth Star Cactus (AK); Wild Potato Bush (FE Aus); Compass Barrel Cactus (DAl); Clearing Blockages, Clearing Energy Fields (DL); Baby Blue Eyes, Dandelion, Golden Ear Drops (FES); Bay (GM); Amazon Swordplant (Haii); Apple, Grape, Lettuce, Orange (Ma); A'Ali'i (Haii); Dutchman's Pipe (SME); Giant Echium (CHI); Ground Ivy (Blos).

Emotional Cleansing/Release: Borage, Inner Cleansing Cactus, Neottia, Release Cactus, Tree Heather, Fungus Amazonas No. 1 (AK); Fireweed (Ask); Detox, Wild Potato Bush (FE Aus); Emotions in Balance (Aus L); Mycena (Bal); Clearing Inner Pathways (DL); Lavender, Onion (Dv); Chaparral, Deer Bush, Evening Primrose, Golden Ear Drops, Self-Heal, Yerba Santa (FES); Apple (GM); Chenille (Haii); Marjoram (Hb); Moonsnail (Pac); Monkeyflower Bush, Swamp Onion (Peg); Ground Ivy (Blos).

Emotional Detachment: Pink Yarrow (AK); Sweetgale (Ask); Emotions in Balance (Aus L); Mesquite (DAl); Heart Wings, Radiant Strength amd Centred Love (DL); Bleeding Heart, Love Lies Bleeding, Tansy (FES); Sweet Chestnut (GM); Cup of Gold, Kukui (Haii); Green Rein Orchid (Peg).

Endurance: Banksia Robur, Macrocarpa (FE Aus); Willow (Ask); Cardon, Soaptree Yucca (DAl); Radiant Strength, Expansive Embodiment (DL); Penstemon (FES); White Poplar (GM); Endurance (Him E); Coconut, Corn, Orange (Ma); Olive (Med).

Energy Boost: Amazon River, Victoria Regina Orchid (AK); Lady's Slipper, Lighten Up (Ask); Banksia Robur, Dynamic Recovery, Old Man Banksia (FE Aus); Fire Prickly Pear Cactus (DAl); Earth Mother Nurtures, Radiant Strength (DL); Arnica,

California Wild Rose, Cayenne (FES); Bay, Buffalo Cactus, Hornbeam (GM); Pukiawe, Pua Pilo (Haii); Healing (Him E); Red Spider Lily (Peg); Young Heart (WD); Energy Combo (PF); English Elm, Medlar (GM); Cherry, Corn (Ma); Olive (Med).

Enthusiasm: Joyful Opuntia (AK); Old Man Banksia (FE Aus); Wondrous Heart, I Like Being Me, My Own Pure Light (DL); Gorse (F); Bougainvillea (Haii); Cherry, Corn, Orange, Spinach (Ma).

Escapism: Bunchberry (Ask); Bauhinia, Red Lily/Lotus (FE Aus); Blue-Topped Cow Weed (Aus L Rus); Essence of the Edge, Lucid Dreaming (DL); Basil, Blackberry, California Poppy, Canyon Dudleya, Milkweed (FES); Oriental Poppy (Hb); Coconut (Ma).

Expressing – Feelings: Poinsettia (AK); Dagger Hakea, Flannel Flower (FE Aus); Fishhook Cactus, Ocotillo, Rainbow Cactus (DAl); Reading Energy Fields, Heart to Heart (DL); Fuchsia, Onion, Scarlet Monkeyflower (Dv); Snapdragon (Dv, Hb); Golden Ear Drops, Indian Paintbrush, Pink Monkeyflower, Trumpet Vine (FES); Birch, Holm Oak, Ivy, Larch, Mimosa (GM); Crepe Myrtle (Haii); Bluebell, Weigela (Pac); Blazing Star, Owl's Clover (Peg); Marie Pavie (PF); Harmony of the Heart (DL).

Expressing – Ideas: Bush Fuchsia, Turkey Bush (FE Aus); Defining Edges, Reveals Mystery Within (DL); Cosmos (FES); Parrot (Him A); Owl's Clover, Trillium Red (Peg); Crepe Myrtle (Haii); Field Scabious (Med).

Expansion: Essence of the Edge (DL); Sacred Banyan Tree, Positive Change (FO).

Extroversion *See* **Introversion.**

Family Pressures/Stress: Boab, Dagger Hakea, Relate Well (FE Aus); Cat's Paw (Aus L); Canyon Grapevine, Mesquite, Organ Pipe Cactus (DAl); Expanding

Awareness, Infinite Patience, My Heart Knows, Softening the Edges (DL); Nettles (Dv); Fairy Lantern, Red Clover, Sweet Pea, Tansy, Walnut (FES); Chenille, Chinese Violet, Plumbago (Haii); Plumeria (Peg); Parasol (AK); Carob (Med).

Fathering: Sunflower (AK); Flannel Flower, Red Helmet Orchid (FE Aus); Mountain Mahogany (DAl); Baby Blue Eyes, Quince, Sage, Saguaro (FES); Solar Power (Peru).

Fear – General: Queen of the Night Cactus (AK); Grey Spider Flower, Tall Mulla Mulla (FE Aus); Dampiera (Aus L); Cherry Plum, Red Chestnut, Rock Rose (B); Scorpion Weed (DAl); Clearing Blockages (DL); Scottish Primrose, Thistle (F); Blue Ginger, Cup of Gold (Haii); Chamomile, Sweet Pea (Hb); Day-blooming Jessamine (Him A); Apple, Spinach, Tomato (Ma); Fearlessness (Pac); Rosa Complicata (Peg); Mother's Arms, On Angels' Wings, Protective Shield (WD).

Fear – Specific: Bog Rosemary, Tundra Rose (Ask); Green Spider Orchid, Mulla Mulla (FE Aus); Menzies Banksia (Aus L); Mimulus (B); Indian Root, Thurber's Gilia (DAl); St John's Wort (Dv); Black-Eyed Susan, California Pitcher Plant, Fawn Lily, Pink Monkeyflower, Free-Less (FES); Red Chestnut (GM); Avocado, Bougainvillea, Cotton, Ma'o (Haii); Cymbidium, Heather (Hb); Protective Shield, Still Mind (WD); Red Archangel (WF).

Flexibility: Lamb's Quarters, Wild Rhubarb, Willow (Ask); Glacier River, Greenland Icecap (Ask E); Bauhinia, Isopogon (FE Aus); Rock Water, Vine (B); Desert Willow, Foothills Paloverde (DAl); Dance of Creation, Graceful Transformations, Reading Energy Fields, Softening the Edges (DL); Quaking Grass, Rabbit Bush (FES); Ash (GM); Ili'ahi (Haii); White Coral Tree (Him A); Fig (Ma); Feverfew (Sun); Blue (Med).

Focus (Mental): Bunchberry, Golden Corydalis (Ask); Sundew (FE Aus, Aus L); Essences of Clarity, Hops Bush, Pink Trumpet Flower, Yellow Boronia (Aus L); Fire Prickly Pear Cactus, Hedgehog Cactus (DAl); New Perceptions (DL); Madia, Peppermint, Shasta Daisy (FES); Hazel (GM); Avocado, Blackberry (Ma); Learning Skills Combo (PF); Be Focused (Sun); Still Mind (WD).

Forgiveness: Blue Elf Viola, Mountain Wormwood (Ask); Dagger Hakea, Mountain Devil, Slender Rice Flower (FE Aus); Correa, Pixie Mope (Aus L); Pine (B); Immortal (DAl); Letting Go, Lotus Petals of the Heart, Softening the Edges (DL); Rowan (F); Elder, Hawthorn (GM); Hyssop (Hb); Raspberry (Ma); Salal (Pac); Clarkia, Prickly Poppy (Peg); Lilac (PF); Forgiveness (F); For Giving (Peru); Hyssop (FES); Agave (Med); Yellow Trumpet Bush (SME).

Freedom: Mountain Wormwood (Ask); Bottlebrush, Wild Potato Bush (FE Aus); Rainbow Cactus, Tarbrush (DAl); Hearts' Wings, Unveiling Self, Wondrous Heart (DL); Sea Holly (F); Leyland Cypress (GM); Spinach (Ma); Be Free (Sun); Freedom (Peru); Gateway (Med); Harmony of the Heart (DL).

Frustration: Blue Elf Viola (Ask); Banksia Robur, Wild Potato Bush (FE Aus); Silver Princess Gum, Snake Bush, Ursinia (Aus L); Holly (B); Acceptance (DL); Blackberry, Indian Paintbrush, Iris, Wild Oat (FES); Gorse (GM); Ulua (Haii); Cymbidium (Hb); Almond, Blackberry (Ma); Mussel (Pac); Verbena (PF).

Greed: Bush Iris (FE Aus); Lotus Petals of the Heart (DL); Goldenrod, Star Thistle, Trillium (FES); Grape, Peach (Ma).

Grief: Sturt Desert Pea (FE Aus); Honeysuckle, Star of Bethlehem (B); Hackberry (DAl); Bleeding Heart (Dv, FES); Borage, Golden Ear Drops, Grief Relief (FES); Hawthorn (Hb); Ashoka Tree, Radish (Him A); Grape, Orange, Pear (Ma); Starfish (Pac); Be Comforted (Sun); On Angels' Wings (WD);

Snowdrop, Bramble (WF); Slippery Jack (AK).

Group Dynamics: Scarlet Pimpernel, Violet (AK); Martagon Lily, Mullein (Dv); Sea Quill (WF).

Guilt: Sturt Desert Rose (FE Aus); Pine (B); Jumping Cholla Cactus (DAl); Golden Ear Drops, Mullein, Pink Monkeyflower (FES); Sweet Chestnut (GM); Bougainvillea (Haii); Hyssop (Hb); Meenalih (Him A); Peach, Strawberry (Ma); Rosa Alba (Peg).

Happiness: Joyful Opuntia (AK); Mountain Devil, Sunshine Wattle (FE Aus); Cherry, Apple Star of Bethlehem (Aus L); Heart Wings, Idiot Glee, I Like Being Me (DL); Valerian (F); Manna Ash, Norway Maple (GM); Happiness (Him E); Peach (Ma); Cumaceba (AmT); Palmer's Penstemon (GH).

Hate: Mountain Devil (FE Aus); Black Kangaroo Paw, Cape Bluebell (Aus L); Holly (B); Black Cohosh, Oregon Grape, Snapdragon (FES); Indian Mulberry (Him A); Grape (Ma).

Healthy Mindset: Boronia, Crowea (FE Aus); Apple (Ma).

Honesty See also **Dishonesty:** My Heart Knows, Reveals Mystery Within, Wise Action (DL); Pineapple, Spinach (Ma).

Hope: Cinnamon Rose, Japanese Rose (AK); Waratah (FE Aus); Star of Bethlehem (Aus L); Gorse, Sweet Chestnut (B); New Perceptions, Wondrous Heart (DL); Snowdrop (F); Cherry, Orange, Tomato (Ma); Beech, Young Heart, On Angels' Wings (WD).

Humour (Lack of): Zinnia, Vipers Burgloss (AK); Little Flannel Flower (FE Aus); Compass Barrel Cactus (DAl); Idiot Glee, Wondrous Heart (DL); Valerian (F); Leyland Cypress, Pittospora (GM); Blackberry, Fig, Spinach (Ma); Zania (Peru); Smiles and Giggles (WD).

Hurt/Pain: Cotton Grass, Ladies' Tresses, River Beauty, White Fireweed (Ask); Sturt Desert Pea (FE Aus); Illyarrie, Mauve Melaleuca, Menzies Banksia, Violet Butterfly (Aus L); Aloe (DAl); Hawthorn May (Dv); Heart Support (F); California Wild Rose, Chamomile, Golden Ear Drops, Pink Monkeyflower, Yerba Santa (FES); Beech, Field Maple, Mulberry (GM); Comfrey, Heartsease, Nettle (Hb); Tassel Flower (Him A); Raspberry (Ma); Weigela (Pac); Mother's Arms, On Angels' Wings (WD); Red Torch Ginger (FO); Jaboticaba (SME); Bramble (WF).

Hyperactivity: Black-Eyed Susan, Jacaranda (FE Aus); Dance of Creation, Infinite Patience (DL); Morning Glory (FES); Hibiscus (FO); Cow Parsley (WF).

Hypochondria: Peach-Flowered Tea-Tree (FE Aus); Heather (B); Earth Mother Nurtures, My Own Pure Light (DL); Fuchsia, Purple Monkeyflower (FES); Apple, Fig (Ma); Tiger's Jaw Cactus (PF); Mother's Arms (WD).

Identity Crisis: Violet (AK); Columbine, Monkshood, Tamarack, Yellow Dryas (Ask); Five Corners, Philotheca (FE Aus); Kasumisakura Flower (Aus LJ); My Heart Knows, My Own Pure Light, Unveiling Self and Gossamer Steel (DL); Milkweed, Quaking Grass (FES); Magnolia (GM); Strength (Him E); Lesser Celendine (CHI).

Immaturity: Kangaroo Paw (FE Aus); Unveiling Self (DL); Fairy Lantern (FES); Young Heart (WD); Blackboy (FE Aus).

Impatience: Aggression Orchid (AK); Black-Eyed Susan (FE Aus); Impatiens (B, Haii); Aloe (DAl); Infinite Patience, Meditative Mind (DL); Calendula, Poison Oak (FES); Lettuce (Ma); Jewelweed (GH); Prickly Pear (SME).

Impetuousness: Kangaroo Paw (FE Aus); Impatiens (B, FES); Wise Action, Infinite Patience (DL); Verbena (PF).

Inadequacy: Confidence Boost (FE Aus); Evening Star, Hackberry, Immortal, Queen of the Night (DAl); Acceptance, I Like Being Me, Internal Marriage, Unveiling Self and Gossamer Steel (DL); Buttercup, Evening Primrose, Goldenrod, Star Thistle (FES); Peach, Strawberry (Ma).

Incest (Effects of): Bottlebrush, Dagger Hakea, Flannel Flower, Red Helmet Orchid, Wisteria (FE Aus); Macrozamia (Aus L); Balancing Extremes, Clearing Blockages, Clearing Energy Fields, I Like Being Me, Letting Go, Reading Energy Fields (DL); Black Cohosh (FES); Mother's Arms, Protective Shield, Sacred Space (WD).

Indecision: Jacaranda, Paw Paw (FE Aus); Centaury, Scleranthus (B); Ratany, Soaptree Yucca (DAl); My Heart Knows, New Perceptions, Purpose Flows, Reading Energy Fields (DL); Cayenne (Dv); Cayenne, Mullein, Tansy (FES); English Elm, Glastonbury Thorn, Pittospora (GM); Coffee, Papaya (Haii); Apple, Lettuce, Strawberry (Ma); Pipsissewa (Pac); White Petunia (PF); Still Mind (WD).

Independence: Angelsword, Southern Cross (FE Aus); Kasumisakura Flower (Aus LJ); Defining Edges, Essence of the Edge, Expansive Embodiment, Walking Out of Patterns (DL); Box (Dv); Bleeding Heart, Fairy Lantern, Milkweed (FES); Crown Flower (Haii).

Inferiority: Buttercup (AK, FES); Five Corners, Hibbertia (FE Aus); Urchin Dryandra, Yellow Cone Flower (Aus L); Cardon (DAl); Defining Edges, I Like Being Me, Unveiling Self (DL); Spindle (GM); Vilayati Amli (Him A); Pineapple (Ma).

Infertility Distress: She Oak, Woman Balance (FE Aus); She Oak/Ironwood (Haii); White Flower from Druid Rock (GH).

Inherited Behaviour Patterns: Fireweed (Ask); Boab (FE Aus); Larch (B); Tarbrush (DAl); Black Cohosh (FES); Macadamia, Ohai-ali (Haii); Nirjara (Him E); Agave

Yaquinana (Peg); Reveals Mystery Within and Walking Out of Patterns (DL); Release Cactus (AK); Inocenicia Coco (Peru).

Inner Child: Spider Lily (Haii); Cyclamen (HUB); Kids' Stuff (Pac); Primrose (Sun); Sacred Void (SW); Lilac (Bal); Cumaceba (AmT); Inner Child (F); Kinder Garden (FES).

Inner Strength: Southern Cross, Waratah (FE Aus); Essence of Inner Strength (Aus L); Pink Orchid (FO); Inner Strength Combo (PF); Iron (Med).

Insecurity: Tall Mulla Mulla (FE Aus); Happy Wanderer (Aus L); Bouvardia, Cow Parsnip, Mala Mujer (DAl); Wild Garlic (Dv); Mallow (Dv, FES); Rosemary, Star Thistle (FES); Goldenrod (Him A); Strength (Him E); Strawberry (Ma); Viburnum (Pac); Field Scabious (Med).

Insensitivity: Flannel Flower, Kangaroo Paw (FE Aus); Orange Leschenaultia, Red and Green Kangaroo Paw, Red Leschenaultia (Aus L); Heart to Heart, Reading Energy Fields, Softening the Edges (DL); Calendula (Dv); Yellow Star Tulip (FES); Awapuhi Melemele, Kamani (Haii); Lady's Smock (Hb); Indian Coral, Sithihea (Him A); Peach, Raspberry (Ma).

Inspiration: Iris, Inspiration Cactus (AK); Boronia, Turkey Bush (FE Aus); Parakeelya (Aus L); Dance of Creation, Dancing Light Spirit Wondrous Heart (DL); Iris (Dv, FES); Revelation (F); Rose White (Hb); Blackberry, Cherry, Grape (Ma); Choke Cherry (Peg).

Integrity: Sturt Desert Rose (FE Aus); Liquid Amber (GM).

Intellect (IQ Booster): Learning and Focus, Isopogon (FE Aus); Purpose Flows and New Perceptions (DL); Lemon (Dv); Cosmos, Nasturtium, Peppermint (FES); Avocado (Ma).

Intimacy: Orange Lily (AK); Flannel Flower (FE Aus); Fishhook Cactus, Klein's Pencil

Cholla Cactus, Teddy Bear Cholla Cactus (DAl); Gossamer Steel, Radiant Strength and Centred Love (DL); Sticky Monkeyflower (Dv, FES); Eros, Holy Thorn (F); Hibiscus, Pink Monkeyflower (FES); Sensuality Blend, Spirit Lift Spritz, Waterlily (FO); Pink Ginger, Pink Waterlily (Day Blooming) (Haii); Grape (Ma); Cabbage Rose (Peg); Archduke Charles, Passion, Passion Combo (PF); Cistus (Med); Amazon Lily, Red Hibiscus (SME).

Intolerance: Bauhinia (FE Aus); Green Rose, Yellow and Green Kangaroo Paw, Yellow Leschenaultia (Aus L); Beech (B); Impatiens (B, Haii); New Perceptions, Expanding Awareness, Infinite Patience (DL); Yellow Star Tulip (FES); Date (Ma).

Introversion: Five Corners, Gymea Lily, Tall Mulla Mulla (FE Aus); White Spider Orchid (Aus L); Expansive Embodiment, My Own Pure Light, Unveiling Self (DL); Mallow, Rosemary (Dv); Fawn Lily (FES); Plane Tree (GM); Rhubarb (Hb).

Intuition: White Spruce (Ask); Bush Fuchsia, Bush Iris (FE Aus); Queen of the Night (DAl); Lotus Petals of the Heart, My Heart Knows (DL); Mimosa, Stag's Horn Sumach (GM); Fig (Ma); Viburnum (Pac); Pomegranate (SME).

Irrational Behaviour: Shadow Cactus (AK); Aspen (B); Scarlet Monkeyflower (FES); Box (GM); Stick Rorrish (Haii).

Irresponsible Behaviour *See also* **Responsibility:** Wise Action (DL).

Irritability: Black-Eyed Susan (FE Aus); Leafless Orchid (Aus L); Beech, Impatiens (B); Light Hearted (DL); Poison Oak, Snapdragon (FES); Mussel (Pac); Vanilla (PF); Date (Ma); Smiles and Giggles (WD).

Isolation: Single Delight (Ask); Illawarra Flame Tree, Tall Mulla Mulla (FE Aus); Green Rose, Veronica (Aus L); Water Violet (B); Creosote Bush, Mariposa Lily (DAl); Stonecrop (F); Love Lies Bleeding, Sweet Pea (FES); Persian Iron Wood (GM); Flight (Him E); Hermit Crab (Pac); Cape Honeysuckle (Peg).

Jealousy: Mountain Devil (FE Aus); Red Feather Flower (Aus L); Holly (B, FES); Desert Holly (DAl); Centred Love, I Like Being Me, Walking Out of Patterns (DL); Pretty Face, Trillium (FES); Holm Oak (GM); Apple, Grape (Ma); Fortunes Double Yellow (PF); Still Mind (WD).

Joy: Borage, Chocolate Orchid, Joyful Opuntia (AK); Churning Bell, Tundra Rose (Ask); Little Flannel Flower, Sunshine Wattle (FE Aus); Essences of Positivity, Pink Everlasting Straw Flower, Red and Green Kangaroo Paw (Aus L); Aloe, Strawberry Cactus (DAl); Idiot Glee, Dance of Creation, Lotus Petals of the Heart (DL); Rhododendron (Dv); Gorse (F); Angel Trumpet, California Wild Rose (FES); Catalpa, Gorse (GM); Ashoka Tree, Parval (Him A); Happiness (Him E); Apple, Orange, Spinach (Ma); Vanilla Leaf (Pac); Rosa Hardii (Peg); Pure Joy (Peru); Young Heart, Smiles and Giggles (WD); Jaboticaba (SME).

Lack of Commitment: Inspiration Cactus (AK); Kapok Bush, Peach-Flowered Tea-Tree (FE Aus).

Lack of Direction: Inspiration Cactus (AK); Silver Princess (FE Aus); Wild Oat (B); Bamboo Orchid (Haii); Warrior's Path (SW).

Laughter (Tonic): Fun Orchid (AK); Little Flannel Flower (FE Aus); Zinnia (AK, Dv, FES); Strawberry Cactus (DAl); Idiot Glee (DL); Spirit Lift Spritz (FO); Cherry (Ma); Smiles and Giggles (WD).

Laziness: Kapok Bush (FE Aus); Red Feather Flower (Aus L); Purpose Flows (DL); Peppermint (Dv); Corn (Ma); Sycamore (Peg); Tiger's Jaw Cactus (PF).

Learning Ability: Daisy (AK); Bush Fuchsia, Learning and Focus, Isopogon (FE Aus); Chestnut Bud (B); New Perceptions

(DL); California Wild Rose, Cosmos, Madia, Peppermint, Rabbit Bush (FES); Hazel, Judas Tree (GM); Blue Camas, Optimal Learning (Pac); Silver Lace, Learning Skill Combo (PF).

Lethargy (Mental): Banksia Robur, Macrocarpa, Old Man Banksia, Dynamic Recovery (FE Aus); Corn (Ma); Red Beak Orchid (Aus L); Blackberry (Dv); Peppermint (Dv, FES); Broom (F); Cosmos, Tansy Mind-Field (FES); Sycamore (GM); Pua-kenikeni (Haii); Tiger's Jaw Cactus (PF).

Lighten Up: St John's Wort (WF); Lighten Up (Ask).

Listening: Listening Heart (SW).

Loneliness: Violet (AK); Tall Yellow Top (FE Aus); Parakeelya, Veronica (Aus L); Chaparral, Mesquite (DAl); My Song Calls Me Home (DL); Bleeding Heart, California Wild Rose, Nicotiana (FES); Heartsease (Hb); Grape, Date, Peach (Ma); Alaskan Birch Forest, Mother's Arms (WD); The Desert (Med); Field Violet (CHI).

Love (Ability to): Heart Orchid, Love Cactus, Love Orchid (AK); Tundra Rose (Ask); Mountain Devil, Rough Bluebell (FE Aus); Black Kangaroo Paw, Mauve Melaleuca, Pink Everlasting Straw Flower (Aus L); Organ Pipe Cactus, Teddy Bear Cholla Cactus (DAl); Centred Love (DL); Field Maple, Hawthorn (GM); Daffodil, Rosebud-Red, Self-Heal (Hb); Malabar Nut Flower, Neem (Him A); Grape, Peach, Pear, Raspberry (Ma); Reine de Violettes Rose (Peg); Cecil Brunner, Champney's Pink Cluster (PF); Mother's Arms (WD); Love (CHI).

Major Change: Positive Change, Sacred Banyan Tree (FO); Conifer Mazegill (Bal).

Male/Female Balance *See also* **Sexuality, Acceptance of:** Calla Lily, Male and Woman Energy Balancer (AK); Green Fairy Orchid, Sitka Spruce Pollen (Ask); Internal Marriage (DL); Niu (Haii); Rattlesnake Plantain Orchid, Red Ginger (Peg); Spiritual Marriage (F); God/Goddess Unity (Peru); Male Vitality and Felame (FO); Anthurium (GH); Blazing Star (FES).

Manic Depression: Black-Eyed Susan, Peach-Flowered Tea-Tree, Emergency Rescue (FE Aus); Balancing Extremes (DL); Chamomile, Mustard (FES); Copper Beech (GM); Stick Rorrish (Haii); Orange (Ma); Periwinkle (Pac).

Manipulative Behaviour: Isopogon (FE Aus); Fringed Lily Twiner, Pale Sundew (Aus L); Chicory (B, FES); Devil's Claw, Klein's Pencil Cholla Cactus (DAl); Wise Woman (DL); Chenille, Crown Flower (Haii); Grape (Ma); Viper's Bugloss (Sun).

Marital Harmony: Internal Marriage (DL); Pua Male (Haii); Indian Pipe (Pac); Spiritual Marriage (F).

Maternal Instincts, Lack of: Bottlebrush (FE Aus); Quince (Dv); Mariposa Lily (FES).

Maternal Instincts, Unfulfilled *See also* **Mothering:** Evening Primrose (FES); Earth Mother Nurtures (DL); She Oak/Ironwood (Haii); Slippery Jack (AK).

Memory (Improving): Rosemary (AK, FES); Isopogon, Learning & Focus (FE Aus); Comfrey, Fig Tree, Forget-Me-Not (Dv); Broom (F); Rabbit Bush (FES); Yew (GM); Comfrey, Eyebright (Hb); Ulei (Haii); Teakwood Flower (Him A); Avocado (Ma); Periwinkle (Pac); Still Mind (WD); Harry Sedge (Bal).

Male: Inner Strength: Banana (FO, Haii); Male Vitality (FO); Male Strength (Peru); Male Power Combo (PF).

Men – Relating to Women: Relate Well (FE Aus); Milky Nipple Cactus (DAl); Heart to Heart, Softening the Edges (DL); Mai'a/Banana, Spider Lily (Haii); Rattlesnake Plantain Orchid (Peg); California Peony (FES).

Mental Chatter: Knotgrass, Wild Carrot (AK); Boronia (FE Aus); White Chestnut (B, FES); Star Primrose (DAl); Meditative Mind (DL); Cosmos (FES); Papaya (Haii); Lettuce (Ma).

Mental Harmony: Jacob's Ladder, Willow (Ask); Boronia, Crowea, Jacaranda (FE Aus); Alaskan Birch Forest, Still Mind (DL); Nasturtium (FES); Cherry Laurel (GM); Spider Lily (Haii); Curry Leaf, Red Hibiscus (Him A); Iris (PF); Pear (Ma); Dark Mullein (Sun).

Mental Illness: Emergency Rescue (FE Aus); W.A. Smoke Bush (Aus L); Indian Root, Sacred Datura (DAl); Yerba Santa (FES); Stick Rorrish (Haii).

Mood Swings: Crowea, Peach-Flowered Tea-Tree (FE Aus); Scleranthus (B); Cherry (Ma); Buffalo Gourd (DAl); Balancing Extremes (DL); Chamomile (Dv); Bell Heather, Femininity (F); Mustard (FES); Silver Maple (GM); Cherry (Ma); Stock (PF); Papaya, Female (FO).

Mothering: Nursing Courgette, Pumpkin (AK); Grove Sandwort, Northern Lady's Slipper, Spiraea (Ask); Bottlebrush (FE Aus); Goddess Grasstree (Aus L); Desert Holly, Mala Mujer, Milky Nipple Cactus (DAl); Mariposa Lily (DAl, FES); Earth Mother Nurtures (DL); Linden (Dv); Iris, Milkweed, Pomegranate (FES); Niu, Noni, Pohuehue (Haii); Peach (Ma); Barnacle (Pac); Mother's Arms, Wise Woman (WD); Motherwort (GH).

Motivation: Inspiration Cactus (AK); Dynamic Recovery (FE Aus); Mountain Mahogany, Tarbrush (DAl); Purpose Flows (DL); Neoporteria Cactus (Peg); Freesia Rainbow (CHI); Positive Change (FO).

Negativity (Clearing, Including Negative Thoughts): Inner Cleansing Cactus, Inspirational Cactus, Life Force Cactus, Release Cactus (AK); Clear and Protect Spritz (FE Aus); Eclipse Spritz (SW); Antiseptic Bush, Essences of Positivity, Purple and Red Kangaroo Paw (Aus L); Crab Apple (B); Crown of Thorns, Ephedra (DAl); Clearing Blockages, Clearing Energy Fields, Clearing Inner Pathways, Letting Go (DL); Black Cohosh, Mountain Pennyroyal, Pink Yarrow, Yarrow (FES); Holm Oak (GM); Kamani, Spider Lily (Haii); Forget-Me-Not, Lungwort, Snapdragon (Hb); Christ's Thorn (Him A); Blackberry, Banana, Cherry, Orange (Ma); Sand Dollar (Pac); Sacred Space, Protective Shield (WD); Huaira Caspi (AmT); Ben Tree (SME).

Nervous Breakdown: Emergency Rescue, Waratah (FE Aus); Cherry Plum (B); Fairy Duster (DAl); Hau (Haii); Orange (Ma); Periwinkle (Pac); Hibiscus (FO).

Nervousness: Emergency Rescue, Waratah (FE Aus); Fairy Duster (DAl); Chamomile, Dill, Garlic, Lady's Slipper, Lavender, Nicotiana (FES); Hibiscus (FO); Horse Chestnut, Pear (GM); Hau (Haii); Almond, Banana, Lettuce, Pear (Ma); Purple Nightshade (Peg); Still Mind (WD).

Newborn Babies: Navelwort (HUB); Pear (Ma); Delph (AK); Stress-Less (FO).

Night Fears: Emergency Rescue (FE Aus); St John's Wort (Dv, Hb); On Angels' Wings (WD).

Nightmares: St John's Wort (AK, Dv, FES); Green Spider Orchid, Grey Spider Flower (FE Aus); Rock Rose (B); Crab Apple (B, FES); Jumping Cholla Cactus, Whitehorn (DAl); Lucid Dreaming (DL); Pa-nini-o-ka, Passion Flower (Haii); Swallow Wort (Him A); Tomato (Ma); Barnacle, Urchin (Pac); Rose of Sharon (PF).

Nurturing *See also* **Mothering:** Earth Mother Nurtures (DL); Mother's Arms, Self-Nurture (WD); Ginger (GH); Purple Foxglove (WF).

Obsession: Boronia (FE Aus); Rock Water (B).

Oppression: Boab, Southern Cross (FE Aus); Clearing Energy Fields, Expanding Awareness, New Perceptions, Walking Out of Patterns (DL); Tormentil (Hb).

Optimism: Inspiration Cactus, Joyful Opuntia Cactus (AK); Sunshine Wattle (FE Aus); Wild Violet (Aus L); Gorse (B, FES); Strawberry Cactus (DAl); Heart Wings, Wondrous Heart, Young Heart (DL); Scotch Broom (Dv); Spotted Orchid (F); Gentian, Penstemon, Illumine (FES); Blackberry, Cherry (Ma).

Overexcitement: Calm & Relax (FE Aus); Meditative Mind, Dancing Light Spirit (DL); Lavender (Dv); Canyon Dudleya (FES); Potato (Hb); Lettuce (Ma).

Overintellectual Behaviour: Crown of Thorns, Desert Holly (DAl); Nasturtium (FES); Spinach (Ma); Rosa Damascena Versicolor (Peg).

Overreacting: Crowea (FE Aus); Emotions in Balance (Aus L); Vervain (B); Jumping Cholla Cactus, Ocotillo, Saguaro Cactus (DAl); Balancing Extremes, Essence of the Edge, Wise Action (DL); Love Lies Bleeding (FES); Raspberry (Ma).

Oversensitivity: Aura Cleansing Cactus, Inner Cleansing Cactus, Blueberry Cactus (AK); Angelsword, Fringed Violet, Pink Mulla Mulla (FE Aus); Common White Spider, Hybrid Pink Fairy (Cowslip) Orchid, Pixie Mope (Aus L); Mimulus (B); Balancing Extremes, Defining Edges, Radiant Strength, Sacred Sphere (DL); Pink Yarrow, Zinnia (Dv); Daisy (F); Lady's Smock (Hb); Strawberry (Ma); Protective Mind, Sacred Space (WD); Field Scabious (Med).

Overwhelmed (Feeling): Dill (AK, Dv, FES, Hb); Paw Paw (FE Aus); Essence of Relaxation, One-Sided Bottlebrush, Pink Fairy Orchid (Aus L); Elm, Hornbeam (B); Buffalo Gourd, Jumping Cholla Cactus, Immortal (DAl); Clearing Energy Fields, Radiant Strength, Reading Energy Fields (DL); Daisy (F); Cosmos, Hornbeam, Larkspur, Red Clover, Scotch Broom (FES); Chinese Violet, Nani-ahiahi, Akia (Haii); Almond, Spinach (Ma); Protective Shield, Sacred Space (WD).

Panic: Red Clover (AK, FES); Calm & Relax, Emergency Rescue (FE Aus); Pink Fairy Orchid, Yellow Leschenaultia (Aus L); Pencil Cholla Cactus (DAl); Buttercup (Hb); Sithihea (Him A); Vital Spark (Him E); Pear (Ma); Bluebell, Urchin (Pac).

Paranoia: Red Clover (AK); Angelsword, Mountain Devil (FE Aus); Hybrid Pink Fairy (Cowslip) Orchid (Aus L); Oregon Grape, Purple Monkeyflower (FES); Cup of Gold (Haii); St John's Wort (Hb); Spinach (Ma).

Patience: Rock Spring (Ask); Black-Eyed Susan (FE Aus); Brown Boronia, Yellow Leschenaultia (Aus L); Impatiens (B); Indian Tobacco (DAl); Infinite Patience (DL); Pine (GM); Buttercup (Hb); Ivy (HUB); Sithihea (Him A); Pink Seaweed (Pac); Coconut, Grape, Lettuce (Ma).

Perfectionism: Boronia, Hibbertia, Yellow Cowslip Orchid (FE Aus); Golden Waitsia, Yellow and Green Kangaroo Paw (Aus L); Acceptance (DL); Star Jasmine (Haii); Fuchsia (Hb); Fig (Ma); Solandra (GH).

Perseverance: Kapok Bush (FE Aus); Kolokoltchik (Aus L Rus), Woolly Banksia (Aus L); Gentian (B, FES); Soaptree Yucca (DAl); Purpose Flows (DL); Scotch Broom (Dv, FES); Mountain Pride, Penstemon (FES); Nui/Coconut (Haii); Broom (Hb); Orange (Ma); Washington Lily (Peg); Baobab (SME).

Pessimism *See also* **Optimism:** Sunshine Wattle (FE Aus); Water Violet (B, FES); Heart Wings, Wondrous Heart (DL); Indian Mulberry, Malabar Nut Flower (Him A).

Poor Mother/Father Image: Sunflower (AK, FES, Dv); Grove Sandwort (Ask); Bottlebrush (FE Aus); Milky Nipple Cactus,

Mountain Mahogany (DAl); Mariposa Lily (DAl, FES); Baby Blue Eyes, Quince, Saguaro, Scarlet Monkeyflower (FES); Strawberry (Ma); Barnacle (Pac); Old Maid Pink/White (Peg).

Positivity: Essences of Positivity (Aus L); Cotton/Ma'o, Bougainvillea (Haii); Be Positive (Sun); Positivity (FE Aus); Positive Change (FO).

Possessiveness: Chicory (B); Harebell (F); Bleeding Heart, Trillium (FES); Grape (Ma).

Pre-Cancerous Emotional State: Release Cactus (AK); Dagger Hakea, Southern Cross, Sturt Desert Rose (FE Aus); Clearing Blockages, Clearing Energy Fields, Clearing Inner Pathways, Manifesting Thought Forms, Shadow Cactus (DL); Nani-ahiahi (Haii); Purple Crocus (Pac); Healing the Cause (F).

Prejudice: Bauhinia, Boab, Freshwater Mangrove, Slender Rice Flower (FE Aus); Acceptance, New Perceptions (DL).

Pride: Five Corners, Gymea Lily, Slender Rice Flower (FE Aus); Vine (B); Poppy (Hb); Malabar Nut Flower (Him A); Banana, Pineapple (Ma).

Procrastination: Jacaranda, Paw Paw, Red Grevillea, Sundew (FE Aus); Fuderindou Flower (Aus LJ); Larch (B); Pencil Cholla Cactus (DAl); Purpose Flows, Stepping Ahead Now (DL); Cabbage (F); Cayenne, Tansy, Active-8 (FES); Blackberry (FES, Ma); Coconut, Corn (Ma).

Protection from Negative Emotions/Thoughts: Aura Cactus, Earth Star Cactus, Golden Barrel Cactus, Life Force Cactus, Many Zoned Polypore (AK); Angelsword, Fringed Violet (FE Aus); Walnut (B); Sacred Sphere (DL); Pennyroyal, White Yarrow (Dv); Pink Yarrow (Dv, FES); Psychic Protection (F); Mountain Pennyroyal, Oregon Grape (FES); Yarrow (FES, Hb);

Kamani (Haii); White Rose (PF); Protective Shield, Sacred Space (WD).

Protection from Others' Negativity: Aura Cleansing Cactus, Inspiration Cactus, Life Force Cactus, Angel of Protection Orchid, Many Zoned Polypore (AK); Angelsword, Fringed Violet, Clear & Protection (FE Aus); Shy Blue Orchid (Aus L); Walnut (B); Sacred Sphere (DL); Psychic Protection (F); Fawn Lily (FES); Kamani (Haii); Tomato (Ma); Protection (Blos); Protective Shield, Sacred Space (WD).

Protection from Stress: Angel of Protection (AK); Yarrow (Ask); Black-Eyed Susan, Calm and Clear (FE Aus); Earth Mother Nurtures, Essence the Edge, Meditative Mind (DL); Pink Yarrow (Dv); Corn, Fawn Lily, Sweet Pea (FES); Kamani, Ti (Haii); Urban Stress Remedy (Him A).

Puberty: Blackboy (FE Aus); Expansive Embodiment, Graceful Transformations, Unveiling Self (DL); Alpine Lily, Angelica, Calla Lily, Fairy Lantern, Morning Glory, Pretty Face, Cherry (FES); Almond (Ma); Adolescence Teens (F).

Purification: Aura Cleansing Cactus, Inner Cleansing Cactus, Formation Cactus, Inside Outside Cactus (AK); Purification (Ask); Detox, Clear & Protect Spritz (FE Aus); Eclipse Clear & Protect Spritz (SW); Purifying (Peru).

Public Speaking: Hawaiian Bell (SME).

Radiation Problems: Radiation Protection Cactus, T1 (AK); Electro-Guard (FE Aus).

Rape (Effects of): Billy Goat Plum, Emergency Rescue (FE Aus); Macrozamia (Aus L); Clearing Energy Fields, Defining Edges, Letting Go, Radiant Strength (DL); Rippy Hillox (Him A); Pear (Ma); Mussel (Pac); Wise Woman (WD).

Rebelliousness: Blackboy (FE Aus); Red Beak Orchid, Silver Princess Gum (Aus L); Dogbane (DAl); Balancing Extremes, Wise

Action (DL); Saguaro (FES); Almond (Ma); Young Heart (WD).

Rejection: I Like Being Me, My Own Purple Light (DL); Black Cohosh, Bleeding Heart, Evening Primrose, Holly, Oregon Grape, Pink Monkeyflower (FES); Ukshi (Him A); Raspberry (Ma); Lemon Grass (PF); On Angels' Wings (WD).

Relationship to Oneself: Beauty Cactus, Bird of Paradise, Love Cactus (AK); Relate Well (FE Aus); Milk Thistle (Bal); Hardhack (GM); White Desert Primrose (DAl); I Like Being Me, Internal Marriage, Unveiling Self (DL).

Relationship Problems: Mountain Wormwood, Sweetgale (Ask); Relate Well (FE Aus); Emotions in Balance, Purple Eremophila, Rabbit Orchid (Aus L); Gossamer Steel, Heart to Heart, Internal Marriage (DL); Hawthorn May (Dv); Scottish Primrose (F); Bleeding Hearts (FES); Day-Blooming Water Lily, Jade Vine, Kukui, Night-Blooming Water Lily (Haii); Sweet Pea (Hb); Slow Match, Vilayati Amli (Him A); Almond, Grape, Lettuce, Pear, Strawberry (Ma); Alum Root (Pac); Sterling Silver Rose (Peg); Mari Pavie (PF); Relate (CHI); Honeysuckle (WF); Asclepia (GH).

Relationships – Breakups: Bleeding Heart (AK); Twinflower (Ask); Emergency Rescue, Relate Well (FE Aus); Snake Vine, Violet Butterfly (Aus L); Heart Klein's Pencil Cholla Cactus (DAl); Acceptance, Letting Go, Light Hearted (DL); Bleeding Heart, Hawthorn May, Nettles (Dv); Support (F); Amazon Sword Plant (Haii); Raspberry, Strawberry (Ma).

Relaxation: Zinnia (AK); Calm & Relax (FE Aus); Essences of Relaxation, Dampiera, Hop's Bush, Purple Flag Flower (Aus L); Vervain (B); Indian Root, Indian Tobacco (DAl); Dancing Light Spirit (DL); Dandelion (Dv, FES); Dill, Lavender (FES); Buttercup, Meadowsweet, Sage (Hb); Curry Leaf (Him A); Lettuce, Fig (Ma); Mussel (Pac); Zania (Peru); Relaxation Combo (PF); Be Relaxed (Sun); Alaskan Birch Forest, Mother's Arms (WD).

Repressed Emotions: Red Gravillea (FE Aus); Rainbow Cactus (DAl); Chaparral (DAl, FES); Balancing Extremes, Clearing Blockages, Unveiling Self, Walking Out of Patterns (DL); Black-Eyed Susan, Fuchsia, Golden Ear Drops (FES); Awapuhi Melemele, Nani-ahiahi (Haii); Red Hibiscus (Him A); Snowdrop (Sun).

Resentment: Mountain Wormwood (Ask); Dagger Hakea (FE Aus); Black Kangaroo Paw, Geraldton Wax (Aus L); Compass Barrel Cactus (DAl); Gossamer Steel, Letting Go (DL); Oregon Grape, Scarlet Monkeyflower (FES); Drum Stick, Slow Match, Ukshi (Him A); Raspberry (Ma).

Resignation: Kapok Bush (FE Aus); Star of Bethlehem (Aus L); Gorse (B); Tarbrush (DAl); Heart Wings, Perceptions, Wondrous Heart (DL); Wild Rose (FES); Plantain (Hb).

Resolution: Desert Broom (DAl).

Respect: Hitorisizuka Flower (Aus LJ); Bramble (HUB).

Responsibility: Colour Orchid, Golden Barrel Cactus (AK); Many-Headed Dryandra, Southern Cross, Yellow Cowslip Orchid (FE Aus); Blue-Topped Cow Weed (Aus L Rus), Red Feather Flower, Wallflower Donkey Orchid (Aus L); Kobushi (Magnolia) Flower (Aus LJ); Scleranthus (B); Ocotillo (DAl); Giant Redwood (GM); Strawberry (Ma).

Restlessness: Black-Eyed Susan, Red Grevillea, Wild Potato Bush (FE Aus); Christmas Tree, Red Beak Orchid (Aus L); Agrimony, Scleranthus (B); Meditative Mind (DL); Zinnia (Dv); California Poppy, Morning Glory (FES); Hibiscus (FO); Magnolia (GM); Swallow Wort (Him A); Be Restful (Sun); Hibiscus (FO).

Rigidity: Bog Blueberry (Ask); Bauhinia, Isopogon (FE Aus); Beech, Rock Water, Water Violet (B); Prickly Pear Cactus (DAl); Expansive Embodiment, Letting Go (DL); Spruce (Dv); Cherry Plum (GM); Ohai-ali'i (Haii); Nilgiri Longy/St John's Lily/Cape Lily (Him A); Fig (Ma); Mussel, Twinflower (Pac).

Sadness: Colour Orchid, Geranium, Queen of the Night Cactus (AK); Sturt Desert Pea (FE Aus); Cat's Paw, Mauve Melaleuca (Aus L); Gentian, Mustard (B); Rhododendron (Dv); Idiot Glee (DL); Borage (Dv); Wolfberry (DAl); Blackberry, Cherry (Ma); Smiles and Giggles (WD).

Safety and Security: Old Blush China Rose (GH).

Sarcasm: Snapdragon (FES); Blackberry (Ma).

Scattered Thinking *See also* **Focus (Mental):** Jacaranda (FE Aus); Golden Barrel Cactus (AK); New Perceptions (DL); Peppermint (Sun); Still Mind (WD).

Self-Critical Behaviour: Bird of Paradise (AK); Alpine Azalea, Columbine, Lace Flower (Ask); Yellow Cowslip Orchid, Billy Goat Plum, Confidence Boost (FE Aus); Pine (B); Foothills Paloverde, Indian Tobacco (DAl); I Like Being Me (DL); Buttercup (FES); Giant Redwood (GM); Star Jasmine (Haii); Pineapple (Ma); Twinflower (Pac); Milkmaids (Peg); Bladder Senna (Bal); Olympos Laurel (Med).

Self-Discipline: Hibbertia (FE Aus); Blue China Orchid (Aus L); Rock Water (B); New Perceptions, Purpose Flows (DL); Lawson Cypress (GM); Almond, Fig (Ma); Surfgrass (Pac); Sycamore (Peg).

Self-Esteem: Beauty Cactus, Self-Esteem Cactus (AK); Buttercup (AK, FES, Sun); Columbine, Tamarack (Ask); Confidence Boost, Five Corners, Sturt Desert Rose (FE Aus); Yellow Cone Flower (Aus L); Evening Star, Immortal (DAl); My Heart Knows, Unveiling Self (DL); Echinacea, Sagebrush, Sunflower (FES); Red Oak (GM); Milo (Haii); Daffodil, Star Jasmine, Thistle (Hb); Ukshi (Him A); Hidden Splendour, Strength (Him E); Sea Palm, Vanilla Leaf (Pac); Milkmaids (Peg); Self Image Combo (PF); Fremont Pincushion (GH); Yellow Hibiscus (SME); Lupura Blanca (AmT).

Selfishness: Rough Bluebell (FE Aus); Blue Leschenaultia, Fringed Lily Twiner (Aus L); Yamabuki Flower (Aus LJ); Heather (B); Mala Mujer (DAl); Silverweed (F); Fawn Lily, Trillium (FES); Peach (Ma).

Self-Pity: Southern Cross (FE Aus); One-Sided Bottlebrush (Aus L); Chicory (B).

Self-Shame/Disgust: Billy Goat Plum (FE Aus).

Sensitivity to Emotionalism: Angel of Protection Orchid (AK); Pink Yarrow (AK, FES); Angelsword and Fringed Violet (FE Aus); Reading Energy Fields (DL); Golden Yarrow (FES); Nui/Coconut (Haii); Protective Shield (WD).

Sensitivity to the Environment: Aura-Cleansing Cactus, Formation Cactus, Radiation Cactus (AK); Electro-Guard (FE Aus); Pink Fairy Orchid (Aus L); Sacred Sphere (DL); Yarrow Special Formula (FES); Nui/Coconut (Haii); Environmental Stress Remedy (Him A); Tomato (Ma); Protective Shield, Sacred Space (WD).

Sensitivity to Negative Thought Forms: Angel of Protection Orchid, Aura-Cleansing Cactus, Inspiration Cactus, Pennyroyal (AK); Red Grevillea, Clear & Protect Spritz (FE Aus); Clearing Energy Fields (DL); Chaparral, Golden Yarrow, Mountain Pennyroyal, Oregon Grape (FES); Sacred Space, Protective Shield (WD); Eclipse Clear & Protect Spritz (SW).

Separation/Loss: Murasakikeman Flower (Aus LJ); Grief Relief (FES).

Sexual Abuse: Balsam Poplar (Ask); Emergency Rescue, Flannel Flower, Intimacy

(FE Aus); Macrozamia (Aus L); Bisbee Beehive Cactus (DAl); Clearing Energy Fields, Graceful Transformations, I Like Being Me, Letting Go, Radiant Strength (DL); Onion (Dv); Dogwood, Evening Primrose, Mariposa Lily, Pink Monkeyflower, Purple Monkeyflower (FES); Hibiscus, Mai'a/Banana (Haii); Prickly Poppy, Rippy Hillox (Him A); Orange, Strawberry (Ma); Nootka Rose (Pac); Snowdrop (Sun); Mother's Arms, Protective Shield (WD).

Sexual Hang-Ups: Intimacy (FE Aus); Clearing Inner Pathways (DL); Basil, California Pitcher Plant, Evening Primrose, California Peony (FES); Day-Blooming Water Lily, Mai'a/Banana (Haii); Water Lily (Him A); Down to Earth (Him E); Grape (Ma); Mussel (Pac); Marigold (PF); Dwarf Purple Vetch (Bal).

Sexual Insecurity/Inhibitions: Aggression Orchid, Basil, Fire Lily (AK); Balsam Poplar (Ask); Intimacy (FE Aus); Expansive Embodiment, New Perceptions (DL); Hibiscus, Martagon Lily, Sticky Monkeyflower (Dv); Calla Lily, Easter Lily, Rosemary, Sticky Monkeyflower (FES); Bird Cherry (GM); Day-Blooming Water Lily, Pua Kenikeni (Haii); Karvi, Meenalih, Old Maid – white and pink (Him A); Madonna Lily (HUB); Purple Magnolia (Pac); Cistus (Med).

Sexuality, Acceptance of: Arum Lily, Banana, Calla Lily, Red Hibiscus (AK); Billy Goat Plum, Intimacy (FE Aus); Acceptance, I Like Being Me (DL); Basil, Pomegranate (Dv); Eros (F); Alpine Lily, Manzanita (FES); Bird Cherry (GM); Niu, Lehur (Haii); Courgette, Rose – red (Hb); Madonna Lily (HUB); Candystick (Pac); Lobivia Cactus, Mountain Pride (Peg).

Sexual/Sensuality Revitalization: Canary Island Bellflower (AK); Sensuality Mist (FE Aus); Queen of the Night (DAl); Dance of Creation (DL); Hibiscus, Lady's Slipper (FES); Sensuality, Spirit Lift, Water Lily, Red Frangipani (FO); Red Ginger,

Night-Blooming Water Lily (Haii); Ixora, Night Jasmine, Water Lily (Him A); Red Ginger, Shasta Lily (Peg); Passion Combo (PF); Mango Paradise, Red Union (Peru).

Sharing: Purple Nymph Water Lily, Christmas Tree (Aus L); Zazensou Flower (Aus LJ); Jjoba, Star Primrose (DAl); Earth Mother Nurtures, Heart to Heart (DL).

Shattered Feelings: Emergency Rescue, Sturt Desert Pea, Waratah (FE Aus); Cowkicks, Violet Butterfly (Aus L); Lotus Petals of the Heart (DL); Echinacea, Sagebrush (FES); Strength, Vital Spark (Him E); Purple Crocus (Pac); Mother's Arms, On Angels' Wings (WD).

Shock: River Beauty, White Fireweed (Ask); Emergency Rescue (FE Aus); Crisis Relief (Aus L); Five Flower Remedy, Star of Bethlehem (B); Sacred Sphere (DL); Arnica (Dv, FES); Ulua (Haii); Red Clover (Hb); First Aid Remedy, Radish (Him A); Vital Spark (Him E);]Pear (Ma); Mother's Arms, On Angels' Wings (WD); Ayahuma (AmT).

Shyness: Confidence Boost (FE Aus); Mimulus (B); My Own Pure Light, Unveiling Self (DL); Box, Buttercup (Dv); Sea Holly (F); Mallow, Violet (FES); Cherry Plum (GM); Red Tulip (Hb); Pineapple, Strawberry, Tomato (Ma); Cistus (Med).

Sleep (Disturbed): Boronia, Calm & Relax (FE Aus); Lucid Dreaming (DL); Sweet Dreams (F); Chamomile (FES); Awapuhimelemele/Yellow Ginger (Haii); Formula 17 Sleep (Him A); Lettuce (Ma); Deep Sleep Combo (PF); Mimose (SME).

Spaced-Out (Feeling): Clematis (B, FES); Pink Fairy Duster (DAl); Rosemary (FES); Avocado (Ma); Sea Turtle (Pac); Copper Beech (Sun); Alaskan Birch Forest, Still Mind (WD).

Stability/Strength: Noble Heart Cactus, Grounding Pountia (AK); Emergency Rescue (FE Aus); Essences of Inner Strength, W.A. Smoke Bush (Aus L); Red Henbit

(Bal); Radiant Strength (DL); Black Poplar, Horse Chestnut (GM); Coffee (Haii); Cedar (Him E); Cherry, Pear, Tomato (Ma); Narcissus, Pink Seaweed, Surfgrass (Pac); Inner Strength Combo (PF).

Strength: Red Grevillea, Waratah (FE Aus); Goddess Grass Tree, Happy Wanderer, Russian Forget-Me-Not (Aus L); Mimulus (B); Organ Pipe Cactus, Spineless Prickly Pear (DAl); Radiant Strength (DL); Box (Dv); Cymbidium, Elder, Red Tulip (Hb); Apple, Banana, Coconut, Date, Tomato (Ma); Inner Strength Combo (PF); Baobab (SME).

Stress: Dandelion (AK); Labrador Tea (Ask); Crowea, Emergency Rescue (FE Aus); Purple Flag Flower, Yellow Flag Flower (Aus L); Staghorn Cholla Cactus (DAl); Dill, Nettles, Valerian (Dv); Stress Release (F); Aloe Vera, Corn, Nicotiana, Self-Heal, Sweet Pea (FES); Alder (GM); Cotton, Hau (Haii); Dandelion (Hb); Almond, Spinach, Tomato (Ma); Goatsbeard, Surfgrass (Pac); Mock Orange, Sycamore (Peg); Harmony and Balance, Reduce Stress Combo (PF); Stressless (FO); First Aid (F); Edge (DL).

Stuttering: Learning & Focus, Boab (FE Aus); Silver Moon (PF).

Subconscious (Clearing): Queen of the Night Cactus, Epipactis, Sage (AK); Horsetail (Ask); Forget-Me-Not (AK, Ask); Tarbrush (DAl); Clearing Blockages, Clearing Energy Fields, Clearing Inner Pathways, Reveals Mystery Within and Walking Out of Patterns (DL); Chaparral, Mugwort (FES); Awapuhi-melemele/Yellow Ginger (Haii); Swallow Wort (Him A); Lily of the Valley (HUB); Blackberry (Ma); Moonsnail, Poison Hemlock (Pac); Agave, Yaquinana (Peg).

Success Consciousness: Positivity, Bauhinia, Southern Cross (FE Aus); Olympus Laural (Med).

Suicidal Thoughts: Waratah (FE Aus); Cherry Plum (B); Higher Levels, Lotus Petals of the Heart (DL); Orange (Ma); Urchin (Pac); Sunflower (PF); On Angels' Wings (WD).

Superiority: Hibbertia, Yellow Cowslip Orchid (FE Aus); Mitsubatsutsuji Flower (Aus LJ); Heart Wings (DL); Malabar Nut Flower (Him A); Banana, Pineapple (Ma).

Tantrums: Dog Rose of the Wild Forces, Kangaroo Paw, Mountain Devil, Rough Bluebell (FE Aus); Smiles and Giggles (DL); Grape (Ma); Scarlet Monkeyflower (FES).

Tenderness: Venus Orchid (AK); Flannel Flower (FE Aus); Softening the Edges (DL); Noni (Haii); Date (Ma).

Tension: Dandelion (AK); Emergency Essence (FE Aus).

Terror: Emergency Rescue, Green Spider Orchid, Grey Spider Flower (FE Aus); Rock Rose (B); Rainbow Cactus, Teddy Bear Cholla Cactus (DAl); Tomato (Ma); Cyprus Rock Rose (Bal).

Tolerance *See also* **Intolerance:** Black-Eyed Susan (FE Aus); Acceptance, Infinite Patience (DL); Mitsubatsutsuji Flower (Aus LJ).

Trapped (Feeling): Venus Fly Trap (AK); Red Grevillea, Geraldton Wax, Russian Centaurea (Aus L Rus); Honeysuckle, Larch (B); Arizona Sycamore (DAl); Expansive Embodiment, Heart Wings, Higher Levels (DL); Cayenne (Dv); Stonecrop (F); Corn (Ma).

Trauma: Northern Lady's Slipper, River Beauty, Soul Support (Ask); Emergency Rescue, Fringed Violet (FE Aus); Star of Bethlehem (B); Snowdrop (Bal); Zephyr Lily (DAl); Fireweed (Dv); Arnica (Dv, FES, AK); Dogwood, Echinacea, Golden Ear Drops, Post Trauma Stabilizer (FES); Beech, Larch, Monterey Pine (GM); Awapuhi Melemele, Kamani, Ulua (Haii); Ashoka Tree, Radish (Him A); Pear (Ma); Hyacinth (Pac); White Hyacinth (PF);

Mother's Arms, On Angels' Wings (WD); Ayahuma (AmT).

Travel: Travel Ease (Ask); Travel-Well (FE Aus); Travelease (Aus L); Jetstream (F); Fatigue Combo and Spray (PF); Travel (CHI).

Trust, Lack of: Flannel Flower, Southern Cross (FE Aus); Bog Rosemary, Prickly Wild Rose, White Violet (Ask); Flannel Flower (FE Aus); Golden Glory Grevillea (Aus L); Centaury, Red Chestnut (B); Ephedra, Saguaro Cactus, Syrian Rose (DAl); Reading Energy Fields, My Heart Knows (DL); Angelica, Buttercup, Mallow (Dv); Baby Blue Eyes, Oregon Grape (FES); Hawthorn, Norway Spruce (GM); Bamboo Orchid (Haii); Marjoram, Ragwort, Rosemary, Snowdrop, White Narcissus (Hb); Slow Match (Him A); Lettuce, Spinach (Ma); Camellia (Pac); Let Go and Trust (Peru).

Turmoil: Crowea, Emergency Rescue (FE Aus); Ephedra (DAl); Higher Levels, Graceful Transformations, Meditative Mind (DL); Red Clover (FES); Tormentil (Hb); Christ's Thorn (Him A).

Understanding Problems/Illness: Shadow Cactus (AK); One-Sided Wintergreen (Ask); Bush Iris, Pink Flannel Flower (FE Aus); Pine (B); Bisbee Beehive Cactus (DAl); New Perceptions, Reading Energy Fields (DL); Love Lies Bleeding (FES); Indian Coral, Malabar Nut Flower, Neem, White Coral Tree (Him A); Raspberry (Ma); Milkmaids, Pine Drops (Peg); Still Mind (WD); Common Puffball (AK).

Unloved (Feeling): Sturt Desert Pea (FE Aus); Mauve Melaleuca (Aus L); Holly (B, FES); Crown of Thorns, Mariposa Lily, Mesquite (DAl); My Own Pure Light, My Song Calls Me Home (DL); Grape (Ma); Sea Palm (Pac); Mother's Arms, On Angel's Wings (WD).

Victim Mentality: Southern Cross (FE Aus); Charlock, Urchin Dryandra (Aus L); Centuary (B); Coral Bean, Immortal, Ocotillo,

Star Primrose, Woven Spine Pineapple Cactus (DAl); New Perceptions, Radiant Strength (DL); Canyon Dudleya, Larkspur, Love Lies Bleeding (FES); Strawberry (Ma); Mussel (Pac); Viper's Bugloss (Sun); Wintergreen (GH); Mexican Creeper (Haii).

Violence: Soul Support (Ask); Emergency Rescue, Mountain Devil, Rough Bluebell (FE Aus); Orange Spiked Pea Flower (Aus L); Black Cohosh, Dogwood, Scarlet Monkeyflower (FES); Stick Rorrish (Haii); Mussel (Pac).

Vitality/Uplifting: Life Force Cactus (AK); Lighten Up (Ask); Dynamis Essence (FE Aus); Essences of Energy (Aus L); Life Force (F); Spirit Lift Spritz (FO); Puklawe (Haii); Energy Combo (PF); Be Vitalized (Sun); Flame Azalea (Bal); Chia (GH).

Vulnerability: Angel of Protection Orchid (AK); Emergency Rescue (FE Aus); Buffalo Gourd, Pencil Cholla Cactus, Spineless Prickly Pear (DAl); White Yarrow (Dv); Grass of Parnassus (F); Golden Yarrow, Pink Monkeyflower, Sticky Monkeyflower, Fiesta Flower (FES); Viburnum (GM); Mountain Apple/Ohi-a-'ai (Haii); Pansy (Hb); Cowslip (HUB); Apple, Grape (Ma); Lady's Mantle (Sun); Mother's Arms, On Angels' Wings, Protective Shield (WD); Honeysuckle (WF); Saw Palmetto (SME).

Willpower: Blackberry, Summer Cep (AK); Bunchberry (Ask); Boronia, Bottlebrush, Southern Cross (FE Aus); Blue China Orchid (Aus L); Mitsubatsutsuji Flower (Aus LJ); Aloe, Coral Bean, Desert Marigold, Pencil Cholla Cactus (DAl); Manifesting Thought Forms (DL); Box (Dv, GM); Cayenne (Dv, FES); Blackberry, Mountain Pride, Tansy (FES); Willowherb (F); Hinahina-ku-kahakai (Haii); Broom, Pansy, Sunflower (Hb); Solomon's Seal (HUB); Corn, Tomato (Ma); Snowdrop, Surfgrass (Pac); Ettringite (Peg).

Women – Accepting Femininity: Beauty Cactus (AK); Woman Balance (FE Aus); Acceptance, Dance of Creation, I Like

Being Me (DL); Quince (Dv); Femininity (F); Pomegranate (FES, Med); Frangipani, Orchid Queen, Sensuality Blend, Spirit Lift Spritz (FO); Hinahina-ku-kahakai, La'au'-aila, Lehua (Haii); Rattlesnake Plantain Orchid (Peg); Wild Feminine (Peru); Sacred Void (SW); Wise Woman (WD).

Women – Relating to Men: Relate Well (FE Aus); Internal Marriage, Gossamer Steel (DL); Baby Blue Eyes (FES); Water Lily, Sensuality Blend, Spirit Lift Spritz (FO); Hinahina-ku-kahakai (Haii); Rattlesnake Plantain Orchid (Peg).

Women – Strengthening Femininity: Bellflower, Canary Island Pumpkin, Venus Orchid (AK); Woman Balance (FE Aus); Queen of the Night, Star Primrose (DAl); I Like Being Me, Radiant Strength (DL); Zucchini (Dv); Femininity (F); Alpine Lily, Mariposa Lily, Pomegranate, Shasta Lily, Grace (FES); Red Frangipani, Orchid Queen, Sensuality Blend, Spirit Lift Spritz (FO); La'au'-aila, Lehua (Haii); Lady's Mantle (Hb); Wise Woman (WD).

Working Harmony: Calm & Relax Spritz, Clear and Protect Spritz (FE Aus); Clearing Mist, Harmonize and Balance Mist (PF).

Worry: Crowea, Emergency Rescue (FE Aus); Brown Boronia, Golden Waitsia (Aus L); Agrimony, White Chestnut (B); Jumping Cholla Cactus, Melon Loco (DAl); Filaree, Garlic (FES); St John's Wort (Hb); Apple, Spinach (Ma); Narcissus, Pipsissewa, Urchin (Pac); Dandelion (WF).

Spiritual

Abandoned (Feeling): Chalice Well (Ask E); Tall Yellow Top (FE Aus); Mesquite, Queen of the Night, Saguaro Cactus (DAl); Earth Mother Nurtures (DL); Angelica (FES); Persian Ironwood (GM); Grape, Strawberry (Ma); Mother's Arms, On Angels' Wings (WD); Locust and Wild Honey (GH).

Abundance: Positivity (FE Aus); Bluebell (HUB); Abundance Program (Pac); I Am Generous (Peru); Desert Gold (GH).

Acashic Records: Sacred Banyan Tree, Pink Lotus (FO); Machu Picchu, Double Helix (Jag).

Acceptance: Tidal Forces (Ask E); Five Corners, Bauhinia, Bottlebrush (FE Aus); Eucalyptus (AK); Green Fairy Orchid, Icelandic Poppy (Ask); Pin Cushion Hakea (Aus L); Acceptance, Dancing Light Spirit, My Heart Knows (DL); Mallow (Dv); Shooting Star, Corn Lily (FES); Norway Maple (GM); Rose Apple/Ohi'a loke (Haii); Chamomile (Hb); Day-Blooming Jasmine (Him A); Apple, Date (Ma); Anemone, Snowberry, Windflower (Pac); Sterling Silver Rose (Peg); White Violet (Sun).

Alignment: Chiming Bells, Paper Birch (Ask); Angelsword, Bush Iris, Crowea (FE Aus); Internal Marriage (DL); Lotus (Dv, FES); Apple, Harebell, Sea Pink (F); Pine (GM); Hawaiian Tree, Passion Flower (Haii); Gulaga (Him E); Almond, Strawberry (Ma); Viridiflora (PF); Still Mind (WD); White Frangipani (GHBm); Chuchuhuasi (AmT).

Astral Travel: Orchis (AK); Red Lily/Lotus (FE Aus); Lucid Dreaming (DL); Wayfaring Tree (GM); Kou (Haii); Mouse Ear Chickweed (Hb); Foxglove, Mugwort, Periwinkle (HUB); Strawberry (Ma); Rosa Ecae (Peg).

Attunement (Higher Realms): Angel Orchid, Angel of Protection Orchid, Channelling Orchid, Deva Orchid (AK); Arnica (Dv); Clear Light (F); Angelica, Forget-Me-Not (FES); Judas Tree (GM); Nana-honua, Nani-ahiahi, Pa'u-o-hi-iaka (Haii); Dittany of Crete (HUB); Staghorn Algae, Poplar (Pac); Angel Face Rose, Holy Thorn, Indian Pipe, Rosa Chinensis Minima, Spider Lily, Tagua (Peg); High Frequency, Purification (Peru); Heart of Nature, Meditative

Mind (WD); Autumn Squill (Med); White Archangel (WF); Pink Lotus, Lotus (FO).

Aura: Aura-Cleansing Cactus, White Yarrow (AK); Aloe Vera, Pennyroyal (AK, FES); Guardian (Ask); Angelsword, Crowea, Fringed Violet, Grey Spider Flower (FE Aus); Clearing Energy Fields, Radiant Strength, Reading Energy Fields, Sacred Sphere (DL); Arnica, Yarrow Special Formula (FES); Pink Orchid (FO); Panini-awa'awa (Haii); St John's Wort, Yarrow (Hb); Ben Tree, Orange Jasmine (SME); Eclipse Clear & Protect Spritz (SW); Aura Balancing and Strengthening Formula (Him A); Aura Cleansing (Him E); Pear (Ma); Aloe Eru, Dutchman's Breeches, Okenite, Snowdrop (Peg); Angel Rejuvenation Spray, Crystal Clear Spray (Peru); Ligustrum, Vanilla (PF); Protective Shield (WD).

Awareness: Rosemary (AK); Full Moon Reflection (Ask E); Expanding Awareness, Higher Levels, New Perceptions (DL); Forget-Me-Not, Mullein (Dv); Wild Service Tree, Wych Elm (GM); Anemone, Viburnum (Pac); Unbelieve (DL); Machu Picchu (Jag).

Balance – Male/Female: Calla Lily (AK); Green Fairy Orchid, Sitka Spruce Pollen (Ask); Bush Fuchsia, Crowea (FE Aus); Centred Love, Gossamer Steel, Internal Marriage (DL); Niu (Haii); Almond (Ma); Red Ginger (Peg).

Balance – Sexuality/Spirituality: Bush Iris, Flannel Flower, Red Lily, Wisteria (FE Aus); Star Primrose (DAl); Internal Marriage (DL); Water Lily (FO); Red Ginger (Peg).

Being Here, Resistance to: Here and Now Cactus (AK); I Like Being Me, My Song Calls Me Home (DL); Fawn Lily, Manzanita, Milkweed, Shooting Star (FES); Awapuhi-melemele/Yellow Ginger (Haii); Oriental Poppy (Hb).

Belonging: Chalice Well (Ask E); Cow Parsnip (Ask); Jojoba, Milky Nipple Cactus, Star Primrose (DAl); Earth Mother Nurtures, My Heart Knows (DL); Baby Blue Eyes, Sweet Pea (FES); Monterey Pine (GM); Maize (Hb); Arbutus (Pac); Chin Cactus (Peg); Alaskan Birch Forest (WD).

Blocked Spirituality: Indian Root (DAl); Clearing Blockages, Heart Wings, Lotus Petals of the Heart (DL); Cayenne, Lotus, Star Tulip (FES); White Hibiscus (Him A); Pink Lotus (FO); Amethyst Deceiver (AK).

Body/Soul Balance: Apple Rose Hybrid (AK); Pineapple Weed (Ask); Billy Goat Plum, Bush Iris (FE Aus); Expansive Embodiment (DL); Great Sallow (GM); Red Hibiscus (Him A).

Boundaries: Blueberry Cactus, Inside/Outside Cactus (AK); Guardian (Ask); Angelsword, Boab, Flannel Flower, Fringed Violet (FE Aus); Defining Edges (DL); Corn (FES); Kou (Haii); Rhubarb (Hb); Isan (Him E); Strawberry (Ma).

Catalyst: Dynamic Recovery (FE Aus); Stepping Ahead Now (DL); Cayenne, Tansy (FES); Gratefulness (Him E); Camellia (Pac); Curry Leaf Tree, Hooded Ladies' Tresses (Peg); Singapore Orchid (FO).

Centring: Red Clover (AK); Crowea (FE Aus); Alternanthera (Bal); Buffalo Gourd, Candy Barrel Cactus, Whitehorn (DAl); Centred Love, Balancing Extremes (DL); Daisy (F); Indian Pink, Lotus, Yerba Santa (FES); Sweet Chestnut (GM); Alkanet, Gypsy Rose, Potato (Hb); VitalSpark, Well-Being (Him E); Pear, Tomato (Ma); Douglas Aster, Ox-Eye Daisy, Viburnum (Pac).

Chakra Balance: Delph (AK); Crowea (FE Aus); Lady's Slipper, Lotus (FES); Lilac (GM); Lilac, Rhubarb (Hb); Chakra Tonic Formula (Him A); Balancer (Pac); Blue Witch, Hydrangea, Indian Pipe, Red Spider Lily (Peg); Higher Chakra Trilogy (Peru); All Sound Wave Essences (SW);

Early Purple Orchid (Bal); Purity (DL); Corn Poppy (SME).

Channelling: Channelling Orchid (AK); Judas Tree (GM); Astral Orchid (Him E).

Change (Major): Mistletoe (AK); Bauhinia, Bottlebrush (FE Aus); Buffalo Gourd, Tarbrush (DAl); Acceptance, Higher Levels, Transformations, Unbelieve (DL); Graceful Heart Support (F); Elder, Lawson Cypress (GM); Wiliwili (Haii); Ixora (orange, white, pink) (Him A); Corn, Tomato (Ma); Brown Kelp, Poison Hemlock (Pac); Tree Opuntia, Washington Lily (Peg); Graceful Shifts, Sweet New Beginnings (Peru); Bistort (Bal); Cielo Ayahuasca (AmT); Sacred Bayan Tree (FO).

Cleansing: Delph, Inner Cleansing Cactus, Inside/Outside Cactus (AK); Fireweed, Laird Hot Springs, Portage Glacier (Ask); Detox, Clear & Protect Spritz (FE Aus); Clearing Blockages, Clearing Energy Fields, Clearing Inner Pathways (DL); White Willow (GM); Lotus (Haii); Apple, Blackberry (Ma); Runga Amanlla (AmT).

Commitment: Here and Now Cactus (AK); Prickly Pear Cactus, Teddy Bear Cholla Cactus (DAl); Peach (Ma).

Compassion: Love Orchid (AK); Rough Bluebell (FE Aus); Pink Lotus (FO); Beech (B); Immortal, Mesquite (DAl); Lotus Petals of the Heart (DL); Cherry (F); Poison Oak, Sunflower, Yellow Star Tulip (FES); Lucombe Oak, Monkey Puzzle Tree (GM); Ohai-ali'i/Empathy (Haii); Parval (Him A); Peach, Date, Raspberry (Ma).

Confidence: Paper Birch (Ask); Confidence Boost (FE Aus); My Heart Knows, Purpose Flows (DL); Red Oak, Spindle (GM); Pineapple (Ma).

Courage: Cattail Pollen, Yellow Dryas (Ask); Black-Eyed Susan, Borage (FES); White Poplar (GM); Wiliwili (Haii) Tomato (Ma); Warriors' Path (SW).

Death and Dying: Victoria Regina Orchid (AK); Forget-Me-Not (AK, FES); Bottlebrush, Bush Iris (FE Aus); Hackberry, Sacred Datura (DAl); Graceful Transformation, Letting Go (DL); Snowdrop (F); Angels' Trumpet, Chrysanthemum (FES); Blackberry (Hb); Soul Family (Peru).

Denial: Bluebell, Bush Fuchsia, Pink Mulla Mulla (FE Aus); Wolfberry (DAl); Unveiling Self (DL); Deerbrush, Nicotiana (FES); Blackberry (Ma); Sierra Rein Orchid (Peg).

Destiny: Inspiration Cactus (AK); Pink Mulla Mulla (FE Aus); Lady's Slipper, Shooting Star, Explorer's Gentian (FES); Autumn Squill (Med); Road Less Travelled (DL).

Dignity: Confidence Boost (FE Aus); My Own Pure Light, Radiant Strength (DL); Lady's Slipper, Shooting Star (FES); Banana, Strawberry (Ma); Wise Woman (WD).

Direction: Orchid (Bal); Pencil Cholla Cactus, Spanish Bayonet Yucca, White Desert Primrose (DAl); Purpose Flows, Stepping Ahead Now (DL); California Wild Rose, Chrysanthemum (FES); Glastonbury Thorn, Lawson Cypress, Tamarisk (GM); Bamboo Orchid (Haii); Gypsy Rose, Speedwell (Hb); Avocado (Ma); Surfgrass (Pac); Yellow Archangel (Sun); Warriors Path (SW).

DNA/Blueprint: Sacred Banyan Tree (FO); Sago Palm, Date Palm (GH); Machu Picchu, Double Helix (Jag).

Dreamtime: Lucid Dreaming (DL); Madame Alfred Carriere (PF).

Empathy: Common White Spider Orchid (Aus L); Heart to Heart, Reading Energy Fields (DL); Raspberry (Ma).

Empowerment – General: Beauty Cactus (AK); Sitka Spruce Pollen (Ask); Confidence Boost (FE Aus); Desert Marigold, Klein's Pencil Cholla Cactus, Silverleaf Nightshade, Saguaro Cactus, Thurber's Gilia (DAl); My Own Pure Light (DL);

Laurel, Monkey Flower, Thistle (F); Norway Maple, Plum (GM); Pua Melia/Frangipani (Haii); Mandrake, Marjoram (HUB); Tomato (Ma); Solar Power (Peru); Warriors' Path (SW); Remo Caspi (AmT); Spirit of the Jaguar (Jag); Magical Me/I Am Infinite (DL).

Empowerment – as a Woman (Femininity): Confidence Boost, Southern Cross (FE Aus); Mala Mujer, Melon Loco, Queen of the Night (DAl); Pomegranate (Dv); Calla Lily, Mountain Pride, Grace, Pomegranate (FES); Frangipani, Orchid Queen (FO); Hinahina-ku-kahakai (Haii); Goddess (Him E); Wise Woman (WD); Pomegranate (SME).

Empowerment – as a Man (Masculinity): Confidence Boost, Southern Cross (FE Aus); Mountain Mahogany (DAl); Agrimony, Calla Lilly, Larkspur, Mountain Pride, Nicotiana, Sunflower (FES); Solar Power (Peru); Male Power Combo (PF); Banana, Male Vitality (FO).

Emptiness: Sunflower (AK, Sun); Positivity (FE Aus); Mauve Melaleuca, Wallflower Donkey Orchid (Aus L); Spineless Prickly Pear (DAl); Meditative Mind (DL); Sagebush (FES); Osier (GM); Grape (Ma); Alaskan Birch Forest, Still Mind (WD).

Energy Balance: Birds of Bakau (SME).

Enlightenment: Bush Iris (FE Aus); Lotus Petals of the Heart, Meditative Mind (DL); 'Ili'ahi, Lotus (Haii); Indian Paintbrush (PF); Alaskan Birch Forest, Still Mind (WD); Pink Lotus (FO); Cielo Ayahausca (AmT).

Etheric Body: Red-Purple Poppy, Sweetgrass (Ask); Banksia Robur, Fringed Violet (FE Aus); Expansive Embodiment, Sacred Sphere (DL); Panini-O-ka (Haii); Shasta Lily, Sourgrass (Peg); Protective Shield, Sacred Space (WD).

Evolution: Consenting (DL); Sacred Banyan Tree, Pink Lotus (FO).

Faith: Waratah (FE Aus); Higher Levels (DL); Harebell (F); Angelica, Baby Blue Eyes, Borage, Gorse (FES); Bamboo Orchid (Haii); Broom (Hb); Red-hot Cattail (Him A); Spinach (Ma).

Freedom: Stinking Hellebore (HUB); Harmony of the Heart (DL).

Focus: Learning and Focus (FE Aus); Cephalanthera (AK); Ixora (Haii); Avocado (Ma).

Getting Out of Your Own Way: Shadow Cactus (AK); Black-Eyed Susan (FE Aus); Stepping Ahead Now (DL); Canyon Dudleya, Fawn Lily, Sagebrush (FES); Hoptree, Teddy Bear Cholla Cactus (DAl); Revelation (F); Tree of Heaven (GM); Banana (Ma); Brown Kelp (Pac); Blue (Med); Goldenrod (Blos).

Grounded (Feeling): Earth Star Cactus, Grounding Opuntia, Here and Now Cactus, Porling – fungus Amazonas No. 2 (AK); Northern Twayblade (Ask); Melon Loco, Milky Nipple Cactus (DAl); Bell Heather (F); Corn, Fawn Lily, Rosemary, Shooting Star, St John's Wort, Sweet Pea, Grounding Green (FES); Black Poplar, Persian Iron Wood (GM); Buttercup, Maize, Plantain (Hb); Strawberry (Ma); Anchoring Light, Balance and Stability (Peru); Narcissus, Pink Seaweed, Windflower (Pac); Heart of the Earth (SW); Alaskan Birch Forest (WD); Wisteria (CHI); Angel's Trumpet (SME); White Foxglove (WF).

Growth: Inside/Outside Cactus, Mullein (AK); Golden Corydalis, Fireweed Combo, Spiraea (Ask); Bush Iris, Yellow Cowslip Orchid (FE Aus); Arizona White Oak, Indian Tobacco, Teddy Bear Cholla Cactus (DAl); Graceful Transformations, New Perceptions, Stepping Ahead Now, Edge (DL); Scotch Broom (FES); Gorse (GM); Mango (Haii); Bindweed (Hb); Tree Mallow (HUB); Heavenly Bamboo (GH); Double Helix (Jag); Yellow Frangipani Flower (SME).

Guidance: Rose of Sharon, Deva Orchid (AK); Mullein (AK, FES); Calling All Angels, Hairy Butterworth, Monkshood, Shooting Star (Ask); Angelica (FES); My Heart Knows, My Own Pure Light (DL); Coconut, Spinach (Ma); Inner Guru (Peru); Still Mind, Wise Woman (WD); The Road Less Travelled (DL); Allamanda (GH).

Humanitarian Feelings: Amazon River (AK); Yellow Cowslip Orchid (FE Aus); Common White Spider Orchid (Aus L); Ocotillo (DAl); Expanding Awareness (DL); Naupaka-kahakai (Haii); Parval (Him A); Yellow Silk Cotton Tree (Him E); Yellow Rose (PF); Green Rein Orchid (FES).

Humility: Japanese Rose (AK); Woolly Smokebush (Aus L); Wondrous Heart (DL); Golden Rod, Yellow Silk Cotton Tree (Him A); Banana (Ma).

Incarnation: Here and Now Cactus, Psyche Orchid (AK); Iceland Poppy (Ask); Flannel Flower, Bush Iris, She Oak (FE Aus); Defining Edges, Expansive Embodiment, I Like Being Me, Vastness (DL); Lotus, Shooting Star, Almond, Dune Primrose (FES); Mamane (Haii); Arizona Fir (Bal).

Independence: Confid Essence (FE Aus); Uguisukazura Flower (Aus LJ); Evening Star (DAl); Tree Lichen (GM); The Desert (Med).

Inner Beauty: Bird of Paradise (AK); Paw Paw, Wild Potato Bush (FE Aus); Frangipani, Orchid Queen (FO); Rock Primula (Him E); Radiant Strength (Pac); Beauty Cactus, Bella Portugaise Rose (Peg); Spirit of Beauty Skincare.

Inner Conflict: Blue Elf Viola (Ask); Ratany (DAl); Internal Marriage (DL); Fawn Lily (FES); Pear (GM); Noho Malie (Haii); Gateway (Him E); Blackberry (Ma).

Inner Harmony: Aloe Vera, Sun Orchid Love Cactus, Lavender (AK); Lotus (AK, FES); Shooting Star, Twinflower (Ask); Black-Eyed Susan (FE Aus); Immortal (DAl); Lotus Petals of the Heart (DL); Sea Pink (F); California Poppy, Star Tulip (FES); Ash, Foxglove Tree (GM); Pear (Ma); Etna (Med); Tortuga (AmT).

Inner Strength: Golden Barrel Cactus (AK); Wild Sweet Pea (Ask); Confidence Boost (FE Aus); Agave, Arizona White Oak (DAl); Radiant Strength (DL); Globe Thistle (F); Penstemon (FES); Pink Orchid (FO); Ash (GM); Hidden Splendour, Well-Being (Him E); Inner Strength Combo and Spray, Christmas Cactus (PF); Tomato (Ma); The Desert (Med).

Innocence: Forget-Me-Not (Ask); Devil's Claw (DAl); Wondrous Heart (DL); Deer Bush, Cherry (FES); Blackberry, Spinach (Ma); Lily of the Valley, Moonsnail (Pac); Young Heart (WD); Desert Forget-Me-Not (GH).

Insight/Clairvoyance: Hoop Petticoat Daffodil, Platanthera, Fly Agaric (AK); Heart Wings, Meditative Mind, New Perceptions, Reading Energy Fields (DL); Pine (GM); Black Tulip, Wild Thyme (HUB); Blackberry (Ma); Chiton, Virburnum (Pac); Madame Alfred Carriere (PF); Almond (Bal); Tansy (NZ).

Integration: Passion Flower, Sage, Tibetan White Rose, Wild Rose Hybrid (AK); Golden Corydalis, Opium Poppy, Sweetgale, Solstice Sun, White Spruce (Ask); Queen of the Night (DAl); Graceful Transformations (DL); Holy Grail (F); Basil, Lotus, Lady's Slipper, Shasta Daisy (FES); Gorse, Spindle (GM); Angel's Trumpet (Haii); Isan (Him E); Apple, Orange (Ma); Integration (Peru); Lady Eubanksia (PF); Blaze Improved Climbing Rose, Integration Combination, Integrate Spritz (SW); Claret Cup Cactus (GH).

Integrity: Love Cactus, Noble Heart Cactus (AK); Sturt Desert Rose (FE Aus); Deer Bush, Echinacea (FES); Tree of Heaven (GM); Sithihea (Him A); Thistle (HUB); Strawberry (Ma); Jaguar (Jag).

Intuition: Lamb's Quarters, White Spruce (Ask); Bush Fuchsia, Bush Iris (FE Aus); Queen of the Night (DAl); Expanding Awareness, Meditative Mind, New Perceptions, Reading Energy Fields (DL); Eyebright (Dv); Elecampane (F); Forget-Me-Not (FES); Horse Chestnut, Mimosa, Stag's Horn Sumach (GM); Sunflower (Hb); Neem (Him A); Fig (Ma); Poplar, Viburnum (Pac); Inner Guru (Peru); Bracken Aq (Bal); Grey Coral Fungus (AK); Coyote Mint (SME).

Journey (Spiritual): Lotus (AK, FES); Chocolate Orchid (AK); Teddy Bear Cholla Cactus (DAl); Lawson Cypress (GM); Cup of Gold, Lotus (Haii); Calypso Orchid, Star Thistle (Peg); Divine Purpose (SW); Road Less Travelled (DL); Explorer's Gentian, Speeding Phlox (FES).

Karmic Problems: Sundew (AK); Boab (karma between individual people); Red Lily/Lotus, Waratah (karma generally) (FE Aus); Lucid Dreaming (DL); Karma Clear (F); Forget-Me-Not, Joshua Tree (FES); Awapuhi-melemele/Yellow Ginger (Haii); Rose Campion (PF); Ground Ivy (NZ); Sacred Banyan Tree (FO).

Kundalini: Clitoria (GH).

Learning Life's Lessons: Isopogon, Bottlebrush (FE Aus); Sage (FES); Magnolia (GM); Coral Root (Spotted) (Peg).

Letting Go: Dampiera, Wallflower Donkey Orchid (Aus L); Agave, Indian Root, Lilac, Rainbow Cactus, Strawberry Cactus (DAl); Expanding Awareness, Letting Go (DL); Bleeding Heart, Sage Brush (FES); Crack Willow, Privet, Tree Lichen (GM); Marsh Woundwort, Ragwort (Hb); Let Go (Him E); Fig, Raspberry (Ma); Salal, Sea Palm (Pac); Sycamore (Peg); Madame Louise Levique (PF); Autumn Crocus, Gateway (Med).

Listening (Inner Voice): Higher Self Orchid, Mullein (AK); Twinflower (Ask); Bush Fuchsia (FE Aus); Candy Barrel Cactus (DAl); Heart of Nature, My Heart Knows (DL); Calendula, Star Tulip (FES); Banana, Date, Peach (Ma); Listening Heart (SW).

Manifestation: Early Purple Orchid, Enchanter's Nightshade (HUB); Rosa Coriifolia Froebelii (Peg); Vastness (DL); Ggantija (Med).

Materialism: Bush Iris (FE Aus); Hedgehog Cactus (DAl); Rose Water Lily, Silverweed (F); Chrysanthemum, Hound's Tongue, Trillium (FES); Foxglove (HUB).

Meditation (Aid): Horsetail, Paper Birch (Ask); Angelsword (FE Aus); White Nymph Waterlily (Aus L); Meditative Mind (DL); Blackberry (Dv); Clear Light (F); Angel's Trumpet, Fawn Lily, Star Tulip, Alpine Aster (FES); Lotus (FES, Him A); Stag's Horn Sumach, Tulip Tree (GM); 'Ili'ahi, Koa (Haii); Bougainvillea (Haii, Him A); Chamomile, Lavender, Nasturtium, Salpglossis, Scarlet Pimpernel (Hb); Blue Dragon, Isan, Lotus, Sat-Chit-Ananda (Him E); Pink Oleander (SME); Chill (CHI); Banana, Grape, Lettuce (Ma); Deer's Tongue (Peg); Higher Frequency, Light Navigator (Peru); Still Mind (WD).

Meridian Balance: Northern Lady's Slipper (Ask); Crowea, Silver Maple (GM).

Motivation: Opium Poppy, Tundra Rose (Ask); Dynamic Recovery (FE Aus); Mountain Mahogany (DAl); Purpose Flows (DL); California Wild Rose, Tansy (FES); Thornapple (HUB); Vesuvius Snow Lichen (AK).

Nature Awareness/Attunement: Alpine Azalea, Chiming Bells, Cassandra, Green Bells of Ireland, Green Bog Orchid, Moschatel, Northern Twayblade, Spiraea (Ask); Bush Fuchsia (FE Aus); Deer Bush (B); Heart of Nature (DL); Sweet Corn (Dv); Poison Oak, Yellow Star Tulip, Green Bells of Ireland (FES); Ash, Lilac, Rowan, Whitebeam, Yellow Buckeye (GM); Harebell (Hb); Four-Leafed Clover (HUB); Spinach (Ma); Poplar (Pac); Gilia Scarlet

(Peg); Nature Communication (Peru); Alaskan Birch Forest (WD); Desert Garden (GH).

Nurturing: Grass of Parnassus, Lighten Up, Spiraea (Ask); Hedgehog Cactus, Mariposa Lily (DAl, FES); Earth Mother Nurtures (DL); Quince (FES); Tulip Tree (GM); Water Lily (HUB); Grape (Ma); Be Nurtured (Peru); Mother's Arms, On Angel's Wings (WD); Autumn Crocus (Mcd).

Oneness (Universal): Green Fairy Orchid (Ask); Organ Pipe Cactus, Queen of the Night (DAl); Expanding Awareness, Lotus Petals of the Heart, Vastness, Magical Me/I Am Infinite (DL); Crack Willow (GM).

Opening Up: French Lavender, Passion Flower, Viper's Bugloss (AK); Icelandic Poppy (Ask); Pink Mulla Mulla (FE Aus); Dampiera (Aus L); Unveiling Self (DL); Dandelion Lotus, Passion Flower (Dv); Lime, Scots Pine (F); Mugwort (FES); Ilima (Haii); Jacob's Ladder (Hb); Wild Pansy (HUB); Avocado, Tomato (Ma); Poplar (Pac).

Passion: Pink Orchid (FO); Samanbaia (SME); Fairy Rose, Passion Combo (PF); Sensuality, Spirit Lift, Pink Waterlily (FO); Etna (Med).

Past (Letting Go): Release Cactus, Shadow Cactus (AK); Bottlebrush (FE Aus); Cape Bluebell (Aus L); Honeysuckle (B, FES); Indian Tobacco, Wolfberry (DAl); Letting Go, Reveals Mystery Within, Walking Out of Patterns (DL); Rowan (F); Chrysanthemum, Forget-Me-Not (FES); Juniper, Mulberry (GM); Ixora (Haii); Marsh Woundwort, Mugwort, Rosebay Willowherb (Hb); Prickly Poppy (Peg).

Past Life (Overspill): Green Spider Orchid (FE Aus); Clearing Energy Fields, Reading Energy Fields (DL); Kukui, Noho Malie (Haii); Agave Yaquinana, Caterpillar Plant (Peg); Sacred Banyan Tree (FO).

Past Life (Problems): Past Life Orchid (AK); Black and White Spruce (Ask); Pink Mulla Mulla (FE Aus); Clearing Energy Fields, Lucid Dreaming (DL); Evening Primrose (FES); Monterey Pine (GM); Naupaka-kahakai (Haii); Gul Mohar, Red-Hot Cattail (Him A); Cuckoo Pint (HUB); Agave Yaquiana, Everlasting, Prickly Poppy (Peg).

Peace (Inner): Chiming Bells, Cow Parsnip (Ask); Black-Eyed Susan, Crowea (FE Aus); White Nymph Waterlily (Aus L); Agrimony (B); I Like Being Me, Lotus Petals of the Heart (DL); Scottish Primrose (F); Sage (FES); Black Poplar, Holly, Italian Alder (GM); Naupaka-kahakai (Haii); Lavender (Hb); Butterfly Lily, Gulmohar, Indian Coral (Him A); Pear (Ma); On Angels' Wings (WD).

Perception: Bush Iris (FE Aus); Cane Cholla Cactus, Indian Root Sacred Datura (DAl); Expanding Awareness, New Perceptions (DL); Sagebush, Shasta Daisy (FES); Lani ali'i/Alamanda (Haii); Brown Kelp (Pac); Choke Cherry (Peg); Maggie (PF).

Perseverance: Kapok Bush (FE Aus); Teddy Bear Cholla Cactus (DAl); Wondrous Heart (DL); Mountain Pride (FES); Coconut, Orange (Ma); Washington Lily (Peg); Lesser Celandine (WF).

Perspective: Valerian (Ask); Bauhinia, Freshwater Mangrove, Paw Paw (FE Aus); Cane Cholla Cactus (DAl); New Perceptions (DL); Rabbitbrush (FES); Jacaranda (Haii); Sea Buckthorn (GM); Banana (Ma); Death Camas, Twin Flower, Pearly Everlasting (Pac); Green Rein Orchid (Peg); Perceiving Spirit (Peru); Grey Coral Fungus (AK); Pink Purslane (WF).

Power: Sitka Spruce Pollen, Soapberry (Ask); Southern Cross, Waratah (FE Aus); Desert Marigold, Spineless Prickly Pear (DAl); Radiant Strength (DL); Rose Alba (F); Mountain Pride, Quince, Trillium (FES); Plum (GM); Ivy-Leafed Toadflax (HUB);

Tomato (Ma); Mountain Apus (Jag); Nasturtum, Power (CHI).

Preparation: Mint Bush, Sundew, Yellow Cowslip Orchid (FE Aus); Wise Action (DL); Marsh Woundwort (Hb).

Pretending: Boronia, Little Flannel Flower (FE Aus); Cane Cholla Cactus (DAl); Canyon Dudleya (FES).

Protection – General: Angel of Protection Orchid, White Yarrow (AK); White Violet (Ask); Angelsword, Fringed Violet (FE Aus); Sacred Sphere (DL); Angelica (Dv); Psychic Protection (F); Mountain Pennyroyal (FES); Yarrow (FES, Hb); Italian Alder (GM); Kamani (Haii); Monkshood, St John's Wort (Hb); Lemon (HUB); Tomato (Ma); Urchin (Pac); Nettle (WF); Protective Shield, Sacred Space (WD).

Protection – From Psychic Attack: Aura-Cleansing Cactus (AK); Yarrow (Ask); Angelsword, Boab, Fringed Violet, Grey Spider Flower (FE Aus); Radiant Strength, Reading Energy, Sacred Sphere (DL); Red Clover (Dv); Psychic Protection (F); Garlic, Pennyroyal, Purple Monkeyflower, St John's Wort, Rue (FES); Yew (GM); Pa'u-o-hi-iaka, Ti (Haii); Elder (Hb); Deadly Nightshade, Larkspur (HUB); Tomato (Ma); Urchin (Pac); Rosa Sericea Pteracantha (Peg); Vanilla (PF); Protective Shield, Sacred Space (WD); Black Locust (Bal).

Psycho-Spiritual Balance: Victoria Regina Orchid, Paradise Lily (AK); Angelsword, Bush Fuchsia, Crowea (FE Aus); Balancing Extremes (DL); Creeping Thistle, Green Rose (Peg).

Purification/Purity: Five-Leafed Clover (HUB); Fly Agaric (AK); Purity (DL).

Purpose: Inspirational Cactus (AK); Ladies' Tresses, Paper Birch, Shooting Star (Ask); Orchid (Bal); Hoptree, Soapberry Yucca, Spineless Prickly Pear (DAl); Purpose Flows (DL); Ancient Yew, Apple, Bell Heather (F); Buttercup (FES); Great Sallow (GM); Bougainvillea, Plumeria (Haii); Geranium, Monkshood (Hb); Avocado (Ma); Cellular Memory (Pac); California Buckeye, Pegasus Orchid Cactus, Sulcorebutia Cactus (Peg); Ancient Wisdom (Peru); Viridiflora (PF); Divine Purpose (SW); Meadow Rue (Bal), Himalayan Blue Poppy (Bal); Coyote Mint (SME); Jaguar (Jag).

Quest: Wild Oat (B); Red Oak (GM).

Quietness: Twinflower (Ask); Black-Eyed Susan (FE Aus); Meditative Mind, Sacred Sphere (DL); Strawberry Tree (GM); Almond, Banana, Lettuce, Strawberry (Ma).

Reality: Willow (Ask); Angelica (FES); Oak (GM); Nijara 2 (Him E).

Rebuilding/Repatterning Life: Prickly Wild Rose (Ask); Bottlebrush (FE Aus); Cowkicks (Aus L); Echinacea (FES); Repatterning (Him E); Sacred Banyan Tree (FO); Unbelieve (DL).

Regeneration/Recharge: Alma Kee Orchid (FO); Fireweed (FES).

Relationships: Heart Orchid (AK); Relate Well (FE Aus); Gossamer Steel, Heart to Heart, Unveiling Self (DL); Plumbago, Red Ginger (Haii); Almond, Grape, Lettuce, Pear, Strawberry (Ma); Pegasus Orchid Cactus (Peg); Red Union (Peru); Amazon Lily (SME).

Releasing Old Patterns: Inner Cleansing Cactus, Inspirational Cactus, Releasing Cactus (AK); Blueberry Pollen (Ask); Boronia, Bottlebrush (FE Aus); Foothills Paloverde, Immortal, Tar Bush, Whitehorn (DAl); Walking Out of Patterns (DL); Ancient Yew, Lichen (F); Fairy Lantern (FES); Lime (GM); Rosebay Willowherb (Hb); Nijara 2 (Him E); Raspberry (Ma); Fuchsia (Pac).

Self-Acceptance: Here and Now Cactus, Self-Esteem Cactus, Spring Gold, Sun Orchid (AK); Tamarack (Ask); Five Corners (FE Aus); Aloe, Hedgehog Cactus, Ocotillo, Teddy Bear Cholla Cactus (DAl);

Acceptance, I Like Being Me (DL); Black-Eyed Susan (Dv); Holy Thorn (F); Baby Blue Eyes, Buttercup, Purple Monkeyflower (FES); Gean Wood Cherry, Norway Maple, White Willow (GM); Cornflower, Heather (Hb); Fig (Ma); Indian Pipe, Windflower (Pac); Creeping Thistle, Milkmaids (Peg); Borage (CHI).

Self-Doubt: Alpine Azalea (Ask); Confidence Boost (FE Aus); Happy Wanderer, Snake Vine (Aus L); Evening Star (DAl); My Heart Knows (DL); Buttercup, Mullein (Dv); Bell Heather (F); Elder (GM); Pineapple (Ma); Mimosa (CHI).

Self-Forgiveness: Sturt Desert Rose (FE Aus); Foothills Paloverde (DAl); Acceptance, I Like Being Me (DL); Birch (GM); Raspberry (Ma); Prickly Poppy (Peg).

Self-Healing: Coordination Orchid (AK); Self-Heal (AK, FES); Bog Rosemary, Soul Support (Ask); Five Corners (FE Aus); Manifesting Thought Forms (DL); Tracking (Him E); Fairy Bell, Rosa Hemispherica (Pac); Rosa Laevegata (Peg); Master Teacher, Strength and Qi (Peru); Lady's Mantle (FES).

Shadow (Dark Side): Cinnamon Rose, Shadow Cactus, Horn of Plenty (AK); Bush Iris (FE Aus); Sweet Chestnut (B, FES); Cardon, Crown of Thorns, Mesquite (DAl); My Own Pure Light, Unveiling Self (DL); Black Cohosh, Scarlet Monkeyflower, Glassy Hyacinth (FES); Ohelo (Haii); Heather (Hb).

Soul – Awakening: Psyche Orchid (AK); Bush Iris (FE Aus); Expanding Awareness, Unveiling Self (DL); Black-Eyed Susan, Cayenne (Dv); Wintergreen (F); Great Sallow (GM); Avocado, Coconut (Ma); Listening Heart (SW); Blazing Star (FES); 4 Elements (Bal).

Soul – Damage: Soul Support (Ask); Sacred Sphere (DL); Ancient Yew, Iona Pennywort (F); Hibiscus, Stick Rorrish (Haii);

On Angels' Wings (WD); Swamp Candles (GH); Great Willow Herb (WF).

Soul – Retrieval: Calling the Jaguar Essences (Jag); White Ginger (Haii).

Soul – Listening to: Jacob's Ladder (Ask); Angelsword (FE Aus); Mesquite, White Desert Primrose (DAl); Lotus Petals of the Heart (DL); California Poppy (Dv); Wintergreen (F); Mullein, Yellow Star Tulip, Cassiope Spreading Phlox (FES); Great Sallow (GM); Nana-honua (Haii); Still Mind (WD).

Spiritual Balance/Cleansing: Piatanthera (AK); Lotus (AK, FES); Chiming Bell (Ask); Angelsword, Crowea (FE Aus); Expansive Embodiment, Lotus Petals of the Heart (DL); Pine, Tulip Tree (GM); Rosa Gallica Officinalis (Peg); Pink Horse Chestnut and Briza Maxma (CHI); Blue Pimpernel (Bal); Festa Flower (FES).

Spiritual Glamour: Bush Iris (FE Aus); Radiant Strength (DL); California Poppy, Canyon Dudleya (FES); Robinia (GM); Ragoon Creeper, Red Silk Cotton Tree (Him A).

Stability: Formation Cactus, Grounding Opuntia (AK); Crowea (FE Aus); Ash (GM); Cherry, Pear, Tomato (Ma); Balance and Stability (Peru); Uchu Sanango (AmT).

Subconscious/Superconscious: Full Moon Reflection (Ask E); Angelsword, Paw Paw (FE Aus); Rainbow Cactus (DAl); Lime (GM); Moon Soundwave Essence (SW); Epipactis (AK).

Subtle Body Balance: Delph (AK); Grass of Parnassus, Lady's Slipper, Sweetgrass (Ask); Angelsword, Crowea (FE Aus); Expansive Embodiment, Sacred Sphere (DL); Holy Grail, Sea Pink (F); Lotus (FES); Privet (GM); Marquis Boccela, Wisteria (PF); Protective Shield (WD); Nettle, Purple and White Clover (WF); Rebalancer Sun Moon Rebalancers (SW).

Surrender: Kapok Bush (FE Aus); Arizona White Oak, Hoptree, Prickly Pear Cactus (DAl); Acceptance, Letting Go (DL); Snowdrop (F); Angel's Trumpet, Love Lies Bleeding (FES); Naupaka Kahakai (Haii); Grape, Banana (Ma); Madame Louis Levique (PF).

Therapist/Healer's Balance: Lady's Slipper, Northern Lady's Slipper (Ask); Leafless Orchid, Snake Bush (Aus L); Purple Flower (Bal); Cardon, Crown of Thorns, Desert Holly (DAl); Balancing Extremes, Sacred Sphere (DL); Eyebright (Dv); Calendula, Mallow (FES); Strawberry Tree (GM); Frangipani/Plumeria, Pua Melia (Haii); Bougainvillea (Him A); Healing, Tracking (Him E); Grape (Ma); Leopard Lily, Washington Lily (Peg); India Hawthorn, The Fairy Rose (PF); Alaskan Birch Forest, Sacred Space (WD); Agrippina Rose, Lime (GH).

Transcendence: Transmute (SW); Immortal, Rainbow Cactus, Wolfberry (DAl); Graceful Transformations, Higher Levels, Stepping Ahead Now (DL); Birch, Revelation, Stonecrop (F); Love Lies Bleeding (FES); Lotus (Him A); Grape (Ma); Angel's Trumpet, Star Traveller (SW).

Transformation: Mistletoe (AK); Fireweed Combo (Ask); Bottlebrush (FE Aus); Positive Change (FO); Chiming Bells, Fireweed, River Beauty (Ask); Bisbee Beehive Cactus, Sacred Datura (DAl); Graceful Transformations, Manifesting Thought Forms, Unveiling Self (DL); Black-Eyed Susan, Cayenne, Fireweed, Mallow (Dv); Transformation (F); Love Lies Bleeding (FES); Elder, Tamarisk (GM); Koa (Haii); Day-Blooming Jessamine (Him A); Stinking Iris (HUB); Pearly Everlasting (Pac); Butterfly Lily, Sulcorebutia Cactus, Tree Opuntia (Peg); Graceful Shifts (Peru); Transmute Combination (SW); Tall Mountain Larkspur (FES); Shiwawaka (AmT).

Transition: Cow Parsnip, Purple Poppy (Ask); Fireweed Combo, Polar Ice, Soul Support (Ask E); Bauhinia, Bottlebrush (FE Aus); Rainbow Cactus, Ratany (DAl); Graceful Transformations (DL); Stonecrop (F); Angel's Trumpet, Filaree, Mugwort, Star Tulip, Illumine (FES); Gateway (Him E); Corn (Ma); Poison Hemlock (Pac); Autumn Leaves (Sun); Amethyst Deceiver (AK); Bougainvillea (SME); Angelica (Bal).

Transparent Shield: Coconut Palm, White Yarrow (AK); Green Spider Orchid (FE Aus); Sacred Sphere, Radiant Strength (DL); Pink Orchid (FO); Protective Shield (WD).

Truth: Bladderwort, Cattail Pollen (Ask); Angelsword, Sturt Desert Rose (FE Aus); Ratany, Syrian Rue (DAl); My Heart Knows, My Own Pure Light (DL); Plane Tree (GM); Ilima (Haii); Butterfly Orchid (HUB); Blackberry (Ma); Maggie (PF); Purity (DL).

Unconditional Love: Delph, Horn of Plenty Orchid, Sarah van Fleet, Love Cactus, Love Orchid (AK); Alpine Azalea, Harebell, Sphagnum Moss (Ask); Bluebell, Dagger Hakea, Mountain Devil, Rough Bluebell (FE Aus); Uguisukazura Flower (Aus LJ); Heart to Heart (DL); Rose Chinensis Serratipetala (Peg); One Heart (Peru); On Angels' Wings (WD); Magnolia (Bal).

Understanding Why: Psyche/Soul Orchid (AK); Sweet Chestnut (B); Expanding Awareness, Lucid Dreaming, My Heart Knows (DL); Sage (Dv); Birch (F); Rowan (GM); Coconut (Ma); Coral Root (Spotted) (Peg); Madam Alfred Carriere (PF); Perceiving Spirit (SW); Wise Woman (WD).

Universal Being (Connection): Channelling Orchid (AK); Bog Rosemary (Ask); Angelsword, Green Spider Orchid, Paw Paw (FE Aus); Meditative Mind, Vastness (DL); Star Tulip (FES); Ginkgo (GM); Nana-honua/Angel's Trumpet (Haii); Calypso Orchid, Christ Thorn (Peg); Alaskan Birch Forest, Still Mind (WD).

Universal Timing: Pink Flannel Flower (FE Aus); Mountain Mahogany (DAl); Infinite Patience (DL); Star Traveller (SW).

Universal Will: Hoptree (DAl); Heart of Nature, My Own Pure Light (DL).

Uplifting: Lighten Up (Ask); Spirit Lift Spritz (FO).

Vision: Boronia, Turkey Bush (FE Aus); Dance of Creation (DL); Birch (F); Queen Anne's Lace (FES); Hawkweed, Nasturtium (Hb); Gulaga Crystal (Him E); Ox-Eye Daisy (Pac); Rosa Hugonis (Peg); Creation/Focus, Open-minded/Future Vision (Peru); Red Condor (Jag).

Vision Quest: Devil's Trumpet (SME).

Visualization: Boronia (FE Aus); Blackberry (Dv); Lotus, Fireweed (FES); Wolfsbane (HUB); Goatsbeard (Pac); Hydrangea (green) (Peg); Creation/Focus (Peru).

Warrior Spirit: Pyramidal Orchid (HUB); Warriors' Path (SW); Warrior (Him E); Iron (Med); Jaguar (Jag).

Wisdom: Lotus (AK, FES, Haii); Black Spruce, Purple Mountain Saxifrage, Red Elder, Sitka Spruce Pollen, White Spruce (Ask); Angelsword, Bush Fuchsia, Paw Paw (FE Aus); My Heart Knows, Wise Action (DL); Clear Light, Scots Pine (F); California Poppy, Sage, Saguaro (FES); Hazel, Tree of Heaven, Tree Lichen (GM); Sage (Hb); Indian Coral, Spotted Gliciridia (Him A); Date, Pineapple, Raspberry (Ma); California Baylaurel, Elephant's Head, Old Blush China Rose (Peg); Ancient Wisdom (Peru); Sage (Sun); Wise Woman (WD); Red Condor, Jaguar (Jag).

Worthlessness: Beauty Cactus, Sensitive Plant, Self-Esteem Cactus (AK); Five Corners, Sturt Desert Rose (FE Aus); Candy Barrel Cactus, Hedgehog Cactus, Immortal, White Desert Primrose (DAl); I Like Being Me, My Own Pure Light, Unveiling Self (DL); Elder (GM); Daffodil (Hb); Alfalfa (HUB); Pineapple, Strawberry (Ma); Being True Worth, Indian Pipe (Pac).

APPENDIX 2

USEFUL ADDRESSES

THE RESOURCE REPERTOIRE
Consultations with Clare G. Harvey
Flower Essence Clinic
Suite 14
103–105 Harley Street
London
WIG 6AJ
UK
Tel: +44 (0) 7778 059660

    Email: flowersenseinfo@googlemail.com
    Website: www.flowersense.co.uk

Diploma courses in flower essences with Clare
International Federation for Vibrational Medicine
Flower Essence Institute
10 Lauder Court
Milborne Port
Sherborne
Dorset
DT9 5EL
UK
Tel: +44 (0) 1963 250 750

    Email: flowersenseinfo@googlemail.com
    Website: www.flowersense.co.uk

PROFESSIONAL ORGANIZATIONS
British Flower & Vibrational Essences Association (BFVEA)
The BFVEA is supported by well-known essence enthusiasts such as lifetime presidents Martin Shaw (the actor) and Dr Andrew Tressider.

The BFVEA is a friendly association which was established in 1998 to support and serve the best interests of all practitioners of flower and vibrational essence therapy as well as providing an information resource for the general public. In 2013 it helped form the essence therapy lead body – the Confederation of Registered Essence Practitioners (www.corep.net), which now serves as the knowledge base for essence practice in the UK.

BFVEA
London
WC1N 3XX
UK
Mobile: +44 (0) 7950 142512

    Email: info@bfvea.com
    Website: www.bfvea.com

British Flower Vibrational Resources
Ainsworth Homeopathic Pharmacy
38 New Cavendish Street
London
W1M 7LH
UK
Tel: +44 (0) 20 7935 5330

The Confederation of Registered Essence Practitioners (COREP)
This collaborative venture between the two main essence professional bodies, the British Flower & Vibrational Essences Association (BFVEA) and the Bach Centre, is the UK lead body for essence therapy, giving members the right to a listing on the GRCCT (General Regulatory Council for Complementary Therapies) National Register and a National Registration Number.

SUPPLIERS UK
FlowerEssences CGH
10 Lauder Court
Milborne Port
Sherborne
Dorset
DT9 5EL
UK
Tel: +44 (0) 1963 250750

Email: flowersenseinfo@googlemail.com
Website: www.flowersense.co.uk

Lines available: Flower Essences of Australia, Flower Essence Society, Flowers of the Orient, PHI Essences by Andreas Korte, Spirit in Nature/ Master's Flower Essences, Sound Wave Essences, 'Spirit of Beauty' Skincare Range; and Laminine, Maximol, Glyconutrients.
Courses also available.

FLOWER ESSENCES OF AUSTRALIA
Wholesale distribution
Cress Ltd
Unit B1 Street Farm
North Street
Hundon
Sudbury
Suffolk
CO10 8EE
UK
Tel: +44 (0) 1440 786 644

Website: http://cressuk.com

Retail shops
The Nutri Centre
7 Park Crescent
London
W18 1PF
UK
Tel: +44 (0) 20 7436 5122

Email: info@nutricentre.com

Food for Thought
38 Market Place
Town Centre
Kingston upon Thames
KT1 1JQ
UK
Tel: +44 (0) 20 8546 7806

Website: www.foodforthoughtuk.com

Food for Thought
2–6 Haydon Place
Guildford
Surrey
GU1 4LL
UK
Tel: +44 (0) 1483 533841

Food for All
3 Cazenove Road
London
N16 6PA
UK
Tel: +44 (0) 20 8806 4138

Website: www.foodforall.co.uk

Revital Health Centre
78 High Street
Ruislip
Middlesex
HA4 7AA
UK
Tel: +44 (0) 1895 630869

Online and list of shops: www.revital.co.uk

PRACTITIONERS' SUPPLY
Flower Essences of Australia and organic essential oils
New Directions UK
Unit 19 Sandleheath Industrial Estate
Fordingbridge
Hampshire
SP6 1PA
UK
Tel: +44 (0) 1425 655555
Fax: +44 (0) 1425 658182

Email: info@newdirectionsUK.com
Website: www.newdirectionsUK.com

The Natural Dispensary Ltd
26 Church Street
Stroud
Gloucestershire
GL5 1JL
UK
Tel: +44 (0) 1453 757792

Email: enquiries@naturaldispensary.co.uk
Website: www.naturaldispensary.co.uk

Retail online
Victoria Health

Website: www.victoriahealth.com

SUPPLIERS WORLDWIDE
Flower Essences of Australia
Southern Ireland
New Vistas Health Care
Plassey Tec Park
Limerick
Ireland
Tel: +353 61334455
Fax: +353 61331515

Email: info@newvistashealthcare.com
Website: www.newvistashealthcare.com

Netherlands
PHI Essences by Andreas Korte
PHI Essences BV
Rijksweg Zuid 1
5951 AM Belfeld
Netherlands
Tel: +31 (0) 77 475 42 52
Fax: +31 (0) 77 475 41 31

Email: info@phiessences.com
Website: www.phiessences.com

United Kingdom
Eriksessences
Erik Pelham
Cooks Farm
Tothill
Alford
Lincolnshire
LN13 0NJ
UK
Tel: +44 (0) 1507 450 382

Email: erik@eriksessences.co.uk
Website: www.eriksessences.com

Gems and crystal essences
Please see producers' contact details.

Other ranges
United Kingdom
Universal Essences
Longueville House
35a Ayling Lane
Aldershot
Hampshire

GU11 3LZ
UK
Tel: 0844 854 2929/0871 872 4122

Email: essences@universalessences.com
Website: www.universalessences.com

France
Fleurs de Vie
Boite Postale 2
01170 Chevry
France
Tel: +33 4 50 426 232

Website: www.fleursdevie.com

Green Hope Farm Essences
Spain
Milagra Flower Essences
Saladavicosa
E-11391 Facinas
Spain
Tel: +34 956 687 703

Italy
Spiritual Remedies
Via Settembrini 1
20124 Milano
Italy
Tel: +39 026 693950

USA
Flower Essence Pharmacy
6265 Barlow St
West Linn
Oregon OR 97068
USA
Tel: +1 503 650 6015/Fax: 6298

Email: info@floweressences.com

Switzerland
Chruter-Drogerie Egger
Uiterstadt 28
CH -8202 Schaffhausen
Switzerland
Tel: +41 (0) 52 624 5030

Norway
Spiren a/s
Postboks 2527
N-7701 Steinkjer
Norway
Tel: +47 167 960

Japan
Masanobui Ogawa
A10S 8F, i-10-7 Higashigotanda
Shinagawa-Ru
Tokyo 141-0022
Japan
Tel: +81 (0) 3 5447 7477

PRODUCERS BY COUNTRY OF ORIGIN OF ESSENCE
Australia
Flower Essences of Australia
Flower Essence CGH
10 Lauder Court
Milborne Port
Sherborne
Dorset
DT9 5EL
UK
Tel/Fax: +44 (0) 1963 250750

Email: flowersenseinfo@googlemail.com
Website: www.flowersense.co.uk

Living Essences of Australia
Academy
Box 355
Scarborough
Perth
W. Australia 6019
Tel: +61 8 9443 5600
Fax: +61 8 9443 5610

Website: www.livingessences.com.au

Africa
Spirit of Makasutu
Sheila Hicks Balgobin
London
NW6 7NU
Tel: 077 4867 8571

Email: shbalgobin@the-healing-garden.me.uk
www.the-healing-garden.me.uk

USA
Alaskan Flower Essences
PO Box 1090
Victor
MT 59875
USA
Tel: +1 406 642 3670/Fax: 3672

Email: afep@alaskanessences.com
Website: www.alaskanessences.com

Dancing Light Orchid Essences (and Wild Divine)
823 Goldfinch Rd.
Fairbanks
AR 99709
USA
+1 907 687-3268

Email: ssk@orchidessences.com
Website: www.orchidessences.com

FES (Flower Essences Society)
PO Box 459
Nevada City
CA 95959
USA
Tel: +1 530 265 9163

Email: info@fesflowers.com
Website: www.fesflowers.com

Spirit in Nature/Master's Flower Essences
14618 Tyler Foote Rd
Nevada City
CA 95959
USA
Tel: +1 530 478 7655
Fax: +1 530 478 7652

Email: mfe@mastersfloweressences.com
Website: www.mastersessences.com

Petite Fleur Essences
8524 Whispering Creek Trail
Fort Worth
TX 76134
USA
Tel: +1 817 293 5410/Fax: 5410
Tel: +1 800 496 2125 (orders)

Email: info@petitefl@aromahealthtexas.com
Website: http://aromahealthtexas.com

Desert Alchemy
PO Box 44189
Tucson
AZ 85733
USA
Tel: +1 520 325 1545
Fax: +1 520 325 8405
Toll Free: (800) 736 3382 (USA and Canada)

Email: info@desert-alchemy.com
Website: www.desert-alchemy.com

Pegasus Products
PO Box 228
Boulder
CO 80306
USA
Tel: +1 303 667 3019
Toll Free: (800) 527 6104 (USA and Canada)

Star Peruvian Essences
130 W. Figueroa
Santa Barbara
CA 93101
USA
Tel: +1 805 962 7827
Fax: +1 805 965 1619

Website: www.starfloweressences.com

Gaia Hawaiian Essences
28 Glebelands Rd
Tiverton
Devon
EX16 4EB
UK
Tel: +44 (0) 1884 259130

Website: www.gaiaessences.com

Canada
Pacific Essences
PO Box 8317
Victoria
BC V8W3R9
Canada
Tel: +1 250 384 5560
Fax: +1 250 595 7700

Email: info@pacificessences.com
Website: www.pacificessences.com

United Kingdom
Bach/Healing Herbs
The Flower Remedy Programme
PO Box 65
Hereford
HR2 0UW
UK
Tel: +44 (0) 1873 890218

Website: www.healingherbs.co.uk

Healing Herbs remedies are also available from most healthfood stores and chemists in the UK.

Bailey Essences
7/8 Nelson Road
Ilkley
West Yorkshire
LS29 8HH
UK
Tel: +44 (0) 1943 432 012
Fax: +44 (0) 1943 432 011

Website: www.baileyessences.com

Butterfly Essences/Erik's Essences
Cooks Farm
Tothill
Alford
Lincolnshire
LN13 0NJ
UK
Tel: +44 (0) 1507 450 382

Email: Erik_pelham@yahoo.com
Website: www.eriksessences.com

Sun Essences
Well Cottage
7 Church Road
Colby
Norwich
Norfolk
NR11 7AB
UK
Tel: +44 (0) 1263 732942/Fax: 73225

Email: enquiries@sunessence.co.uk

Website: www.sunessence.co.uk

Sun Animal Essences
15 Connaught Road
Suffield Park
Cromer
Norfolk
NR27 0BZ
UK

Tel: +44 (0) 1263 732942
Helpline: 07000 785337

Email: jane@sunessence.co.uk
Website: www.cresturecomforters.org

Green Man Tree Essences
2 Kerswell Cottages
Exminster
Exeter
Devon
EX6 8AY
UK
Tel: +44 (0) 1392 832005

Website: www.greenmantrees.demon.co.uk

Habundia Flower Essences
Peter Aziz
20 Furlong Close
Buckfast
Devon
TQ11 0ER
UK
Tel: +44 (0) 1364 643127

Email: peter@azizshamanism.com

Channel Island Flower Essences
Ennio Morricone House
Abbotsfield Road
St Helens
Merseyside
WA9 4HU
UK
Tel: + 44 (0) 1942 868555

Email: susie.morvan@cife.co.uk
Website: www.cife.com

Flower essence workshops and courses
Soundwave Essences
Hertfield Cottage
Holwell
Sherborne
Dorset
DT9 5LM
UK
Tel: +44 (0) 1963 250750

Email: soundwave@p-brune.fsnet.co.uk

Harebell Remedies
Ellie Davidson
45 Main Street
Auchencairn

Castle Douglas
Galloway
DG7 1QU
UK
Tel: +44 (0) 1556 640099

Email: ellie@harebellremedies.co.uk
Website: www.harebellremedies.co.uk

The essences are available by mail order only. SAE (or international reply coupons) for catalogue appreciated.

Findhorn Flower Essences
Cullerne House
Findhorn
Forres
IV36 3YY
Morayshire
UK
Tel: +44 (0) 1309 690129

Email: sales@findhornessences.com
Website: www.findhornessences.com

Wildflower Essences
Complementary Health Partnership
5–6 Sydney Terrace
Claygate
Surrey
KT10 0JJ
UK
Clinic tel: +44 (0) 1372 464659
Direct tel: +44 (0) 7896 218359

Email: sales@wildfloweressences.co.uk
Website: www.wildfloweressences.co.uk

France
Deva Laboratoire
BP 3
38880 Autrans
France
Tel: +33 (0) 4 76 953 587
Fax: +33 (0) 4 76 953 702

Email: infofleur@lab.deva.com
Website: www.lab-deva.com

Mediterranean Essences
Healthlines
The Courtyard
Howestone
Whinfell
Kendal
Cumbria

LA8 9EQ
UK
Tel: +44 (0) 1539 824776

> Website: www.healthlines.co.uk

Netherlands
Bloesem Remedies Nederland
Postbus 6139
5960 AC Horst
Tel: +31 (0) 77 398 7826
Fax: +31 (0) 77 398 7827

> Email: info@bloesemremedies.com
> Website: www.bloesem-remedies.com

Amazon
PHI Essences by Andreas Korte
Rijksweg Zuid I
NL 5951
AM Belfeld
Tel: +31 (0) 77 475 4252

> Email: info@PHIessences.com
> Website: www.PHIessences.com

Sacred Amazonian Tree Essences

> Website: www.SacredTreeEssences.com

India
AUM Himalayan Essences
Himalayan Aditi Flower Essences
Complementary Medicine Research Centre
15(E) Jaybahrat Society
3rd Road
Khar West
Bombay 400 052
Tel: +91 22 648 6819

> Email: info@aumhimalaya.com
> Website: www.aumhimalaya.com

Himalayan Flower Enhancers
PO Box 43
Central Tilba
NSW 2546
Australia
Tel: +61 2 4473 7131

> Email: info@himalaya.com.au
> Website: http://himalaya.com.au

Flowers of the Orient
10 Lauder Court
Milborne Port
Sherborne
Dorset
DT9 5EL
UK
Tel: +44 (0) 1963 250750

> Email: flowersenseinfo@googlemail.com
> Website: www.flowersense.co.uk

PROFESSIONAL COURSES IN FLOWER REMEDIES
The International Federation for Vibrational Medicine
Tel: +44 (0) 1963 250750

> Email: flowersenseinfo@googlemail.com
> Website: www.flowersense.co.uk

Floweressence CGH
Tel: +44 (0) 1963250750

> Email: flowersenseinfo@googlemail.com
> Website: www.flowersense.co.uk

Living Essences of Australia
Box 355
Scarborough
Perth
W. Australia 6019
Tel: +61 8 9244 2073

Sound of Light Workshops
Soundwave Essences
Hertfield Cottage
Holwell
Sherborne
Dorset
DT9 5LM
UK
Tel: +44 (0) 1963 250750

> Email: Soundwave@p-brune.fsnet.co.uk

Also available at: www.flowersense.co.uk
Sound of Light Treatments available: a unique healing modality, designed for cellular repatterning.

Bach Healing Herbs – The Flower Remedy Programme
PO Box 65
Hereford

HR2 0UW
UK
Tel: +44 (0) 1873 890218

QUALIFIED IFVM FLOWER ESSENCE CONSULTANTS AND TRAINERS
United Kingdom
Margaret Gallier
Bath House
Denne Park
Horsham
West Sussex
RH13 0AY
UK

Email: flowertalk2@hotmail.com

Dennis Smith
247 Glyn Road
Clapton
London
E5 0JD
UK

Email: cuinja@yahoo.co.uk

Jane Thrift
Duntish Lodge
Duntish
Dorchester
DT2 8SQ
UK
Tel: +44 (0) 7732 942692 (mobile)

Email: jane@1770.co.uk

Shelly Shiston
The Energy Centre
Orchard Oast
School House Lane
Horsmonden
Tonbridge
Kent
TN12 8BN
UK
Tel: +44 (0) 7770 755951 (mobile)

Email: s.sishton@btopenworld.com

Beverley Downes
Pannells Ash Barn
Sudbury Road
Castle Hedingham
Essex

CO9 3AD
UK
Tel: +44 (0) 1787 463127
Tel: +44 (0) 7970 682574 (mobile)

Email: beverleydownes@yahoo.co.uk

ONLINE FLOWER ESSENCE COURSES
Sara Turner
Flowers 4 Health
95 Grange Rd
Ramsgate
Kent
CT11 9PB
UK
Tel: +44 (0) 7725 609873 (mobile)

Website: www.essentiallyflowers.com

Yvonne Foster-Palmer
56 Sutton Street
Flore
Northhampton
NN7 4LE
UK
Tel: +44 (0) 7803 562248 (mobile)

Email: yvonnefp@tiscali.co.uk

Louise Larchbourne
11 The Springs
Witney
Oxfordshire
OX28 4AS
UK
Tel: +44 (0) 1993 200602

Email: louisej@fastmail.fm

Sharon Keenan
Of the Essence
7 London Rd
Southampton
Hampshire
SO15 2AE
UK
Tel: +44 (0) 7899 095279 (mobile)

Email: Sharon.essence@gmail.com
Website: www.oftheessence.org

Sian Pope
55 Woodacre
Portishead
Somerset
BS20 7BS

UK
Tel: +44 (0) 7748 644888 (mobile)

Email: sianpope@btinternet.com

Laura MacKenzie
The Barn
Isle of Gigha
Argyll
PA41 7AA
UK

Email: lauraongigha@yahoo.co.uk

Andrya Prescott
1 Deanery Place
Church Street
Godalming
Surrey
GU7 1ER
UK
Tel: +44 (0) 1483 425477

Email: andrya@independentmidwife.com

Jacqui Meadows
Tyn-y-Celyn
Bwlchyddar
Llangedwyn
Powys
SY10 9LJ
UK
Tel: +44 (0) 1691 648784

Email: info@crystal-union.com

David Corr
150 Waterloo Road
London
SE1 8SB
UK
Tel: +44 (0) 20 7633 9957

Email: david@corehypnosis.co.uk
Website: www.corehypnosis.co.uk

Diane Green
Cedars
Old Church Rd
Lowers Ufford
Woodbridge
Suffolk
IP13 6DH
UK
Tel: +44 (0) 1394 460022

Email: diane949@btinternet.com

Victoria Brudal
20 Cogan Rd
Staple Hill
Bristol
BS16 4SX
UK
Tel: +44 (0) 1179 708670

Email: vicbru81@yahoo.co.uk

Shelagh Musoke
Orchard Cottage
2 Woodbridge Grove
Leatherhead
Surrey
KT22 7QJ
UK
Tel: +44 (0) 1372 812281

Email: shelagh.musoke@btclick.com

Rose Arnold
Longstone Cottage
Longstone Lane
Little Budworth
Cheshire
CW6 9ET
UK
Tel: +44 (0) 1829 760481

Email: rose.arnold4@gmail.com

Helen Ward
Guided Essences
46 Barnfield Rd
Harpenden
Hertfordshire
AL5 5TQ
UK
Tel: +44 (0) 1583 622636

Email: HelenFWard@aol.com
Website: www.guidedessences.com

Debbie Sellwood
Alton
Hampshire
GU34 9AN
UK
Tel: +44 (0) 1420 588479
Tel: +44 (0) 7940 821338 (mobile)

Email: debbie_sellwood@yahoo.co.uk

Isabel Appleby
19 Blendon Drive
Bexley

Kent
DA5 3AA
UK
Tel: +44 (0) 20 8304 2737

Email: rayappleby@tiscali.co.uk

Anne Mari Clarke
61 Granville Road
Limpsfield
Oxted
Surrey
RH8 0BY
UK
Tel: +44 (0) 1883 715977

Northern Ireland
Christine Allen
4 Dovecote Way
Castle Hume
Enniskillen
County Fermanath
UK
BT93 7FB
Tel: +44 (0) 7512 342714 (mobile)

Email: christineallen123@hotmail.co.uk

ORGANIC AROMATHERAPY AND ESSENTIAL OILS
New Directions UK
Unit 19 Sandleheath Industrial Estate
Fordingbridge
Hampshire
SP6 1PA
UK
Tel: +44 (0) 1425 655555/Fax: 658182

Email: info@newdirectionsUK.com
Website: www.newdirectionsUK.com

New Directions Australia
47 Carrington Road
Marrickville
Sydney
NSW 2204
Australia
Tel: +61 2 8577 5999/Fax: 5977
Toll Free: 1800 637 697

Email: nda@newdirections.com.au
Website: www.newdirections.com.au

New Directions USA
705 Jadecrest Court
San Ramon
CA 94582
USA
Tel: +1 800 246 7817/Fax: 8207 (Toll Free)

Email: sales@newdirectionsaromatics.com
Website: www.newdirectionsaromatics.com

New Directions Canada
6781 Columbus Road
Mississauga
Ontario
L5T 2G9
Canada
Tel: +1 905 362 1915/Fax: 1926
Order: +1 877 255 7692 (Toll Free)

Email: oils@newdirectionsaromatics.ca
Website: www.newdirectionsaromatics.ca

MEDITATION, QI GONG AND MESSAGES FROM WATER
Masaru Emoto
I.H.M. General Institute
East Side Blgs
IF, I-I-I-I Yanagibashi
Taito-ku
Tokyo 111-0052
Japan
Tel: +81 3 3863 0216

Website: www.masaru-emoto.net

Zhi-xing Wang
Chinese Heritage Institute
66 Basset Road
London
W10 6JP
UK
Tel: +44 845 0553666

Email: Catherine@chineseheritage.co.uk

The Art of Meditation by Guy Burgs

Email: enquiries@theartofmeditation.org
Website: www.theartofmeditation.org

INTUITIVE CLAIRVOYANTS
Peter Tadd
Foilnamuck
Ballydehob
County Cork
Ireland
Tel: +353 (0) 2837540

Email: ptadd@mac.com
Email: chakra@indigo.ie

SPIRITUAL MENTOR AND HEALER
Kelvin Heard
6 Violet Hill Studios
Maida Vale
London
NW8 9EB
UK
Tel: +44 (0) 7710 794627 (mobile)

Email: kelvinheardhealer@gmail.com
Website: www.kelvinheard.com

PSYCHIC ARTIST/INTUITIVE CLAIRVOYANT
Corrine Cyster
24 Trafalgar Rd
Bournemouth
Dorset
BH9 1BA
UK
Tel: +44 (0) 1202 526660

Email: Corrine-c@whale-mail.com
Website: www.corrinepsychicartist.co.uk

Kirlian and aura photography
Harry Oldfield
The School of Electro-Crystal Therapy
Oldfield Systems Ltd
PO Box 449
Telford
Shropshire
TF2 2EY
UK
Tel: +44 (0) 1952 270980

Website: www.electrocrystal.com

Erik Pelham
Flower photographer and Devic analyst
Cooks Farm
Tothill
Alford
Lincolnshire
LN13 0NJ
UK
Tel: +44 (0) 1507 450382

Email: Erik_pelham@yahoo.com

For supplies of blue dropper bottles, glycerine, laminine, glyconutrients and Maximol see FlowerEssence CGH (address on page 523).

REFERENCES AND FURTHER READING

Edward Bach, *Heal Thyself* (C.W. Daniel Co. Ltd, 1931, reprint 1996)

Arther Bailey, *The Bailey Flower Essence Handbook* (Arthur Bailey, 2004)

Vasudeva and Kadambii Barnao, *Australian Flower Essences for the 21st Century* (Living Essences, 1997)

Julian Barnard, *A Guide to the Bach Flower Remedies* (C.W. Daniel Co. Ltd, 1979; 1994)

Julian and Martine Barnard, *The Healing Herbs of Edward Bach* (Ashgrove Press, 1988)

John Beaulieu, *Music and Sound in the Healing Arts* (Barrytown/Station Hill Press, 1995)

David Bohm, *Wholeness and Implicate Order* (Routledge and Kegan Paul, 1980)

Barbara Ann Brennan, *Hands of Light* (Bantam New Age Books, 1988)

Ernst Chladni, *Discoveries Concerning the Theory of Music* (1787)

Jillie Collings, *The Ordinary Person's Guide to Extraordinary Health* (Aurum Press, 1993)

'*The Core Issue*' (a web-based publication exploring specific healing issues with flower essences)

Deborah Craydon and Warren Bellows, *Floral Acupuncture* (The Crossing Press, 2005)

John and Farida Davidson, *Harmony of Science and Nature* (Holistic Research Company, 1986–8)

Patricia Davis, *Subtle Aromatherapy* (C.W. Daniel Co. Ltd, 1991)

Lila Devi, *The Essential Flower Essence Handbook* (Hay House, 1998)

Lila Devi, *Flower Essences for Animals* (Hay House, 2000)

Lila Devi, *Flower Essences for Animals: Remedies for Helping the Pets You Love* (Spirit in Nature, 2010)

Dr Masaru Emoto, *Messages from Water 1 & 2* (Hado Kyoikusha Co. Ltd, 2002)

Dr Masaru Emoto, *Hidden Messages in Water* (Pocket Books, 2005)

Dr Masuru Emoto, *Messages from Water and the Universe* (Hay House UK, 2010)

Richard Gerber, *Vibrational Medicine* (Bear & Co., 1993)

Richard Gerber, *Vibrational Medicine: The Number 1 Handbook of Subtle Energy Therapies* (Bear & Co., 2001)

Kate Greenaway, *Language of Flowers* (F. Warne, 1977)

Dr Judy Griffin, *Remember Me to the Roses* (Herbal Essence Publications, 1997)

Dr Judy Griffin, *Flowers that Heal* (Paraview Press, 2002)

Green Hope Farm, *A Guide To Green Hope Farm, Flower Essences* (2003)

Gurudas, *Flower Essences and Vibrational Healing* (Cassandra Press, 1996)

Clare G. Harvey, *Flower Essences (Live Better Series)* (Duncan Baird Publishers, 2006)

Clare G. Harvey and Amanda Cochrane, *Healing Spirit of Plants* (Godsfield Press, 1999)

Eliana Harvey and Mary Jane Oatley, *Acupressure* (Hodder and Stoughton, 1994)

Stephen W. Hawking, *A Brief History of Time* (Paul Banton Press, 1988; 1993)

Liz Hodgkinson, *Reincarnation – The Evidence* (Piatkus, 1989)

Dr Leonard Horowitz, T*he Healing Codes of Biological Apocalypse* (Medical Veritas International, 1999)

Steve Johnson, *The Essence of Healing* (Alaskan Flower Essence Project, 1996)

Anodea Judith, *Wheels of Light* (Llewellyn, 1987)

Patricia Kaminski and Richard Katz, *The Flower Essence Repertory* (The Flower Essence Society, 1994)

Cynthia Athina Kemp Scherer, *The Alchemy of the Desert*, Second Edition (Desert Alchemy, 1993)

Cynthia Athina Kemp Scherer, *The Art & Technique of Using Flower Essences* (Desert Alchemy, 1993)

Andreas Korte, *Orchids, Gemstones and Their Healing Energies* (Bauer Berlag, 1993; Findhorn 1997)

Andreas Korte and Karin Huber, *Dolphins and Whales* (Gesundheit & Entwichlung, 1999)

Marion Leigh, *Findhorn Flower Essences Handbook* (Findhorn Press, 2012)

Jacob Liberman, *Light Medicine of the Future* (Bear & Co., 1991)

Denise Linn, *Sacred Space* (Rider, 2005)

Fabian Maman, *The Tao of Sound: Acoustic Sound Healing for the 21st Century* (Self published by Tama-Do Academy, 2011)

Lynne McTaggart, *The Field* (HarperCollins, 2002)

Sue Minter, *The Healing Garden* (Headline, 1993)

Dr. Hiroshi Motoyama, *Bridge to Higher Consciousness* (The Theosophical Publishing House, 1981)

Dr Hiroshi Motoyama, *Theories of the Chakras* (Nati Book Network, 1981)

Franchelle Ofsoské-Wyber, *The New Zealand Native Flower Essence Handbook* (self-published)

Franchelle Ofsoské-Wyber, *The Sacred Plant Medicine of Aotearoa* (Vanterra House Publishing, 2009)

Masanobu Ogawa, *Flower Essences of the World* (Tokyo, 1999)

Harry Oldfield and Roger Coghill, *The Dark Side of the Brain* (Element Books, 1988)

Erik Pelham, *Butterfly and Sea Essences – An Introductory Guide* (Self-published, 2009)

Sabina Pettitt, *Energy Medicine* (Pacific Essences, 1993)

Candace Pert, *Molecules of Emotion* (Pocket Books, 1999; First published 1995)

A.S. Presman, *Electromagnetic Fields of Life* (Nauka Press, 1968; Springer, 1970)

Drs Rupa and Atul Shar, *Aditi Himalaya Essences* (Aditi, 1993)

Machaelle Small Wright, *Flower Essences* (Perelandra, 1988)

Michael Smulkis and Fred Rubenfeld, *Starlight Elixirs and Cosmic Vibrational Healing* (C.W. Daniel Co. Limited, 1992)

M. Rudolf Steiner, *Cosmic Memory: Atlantis and Lemuria* (Harper & Row, 1981)

Rose Titchiner, Sue Monk, Rosemary Potter and Patricia Staines, *New Vibrational Essences of Britain and Ireland* (Waterlily Books, 1997)

Dr Andrew Tresidder, *Lazy Person's Guide to Emotional Healing* (Newleaf, 2000)

Gregory Vlamis, *Flowers to the Rescue* (Thorsons, 1986; 1994)

Ellie Web, *Harebell Remedies Handbook* (Harebell Remedies, 2001)

Nora Weeks, *The Medical Discoveries of Edward Bach Physician* (C.W. Daniel Co. Ltd, 1940; 1983)

Ian White, *Australian Bush Flower Essences* (Findhorn Press, 1991)

Ian White, *Bush Flower Healing* (Bantam Books, 1999)

Ruth White, *Working with your Chakras* (Piatkus, 1993

Vivien Williamson, *Bach Flower Remedies and Other Flower Essences* (Hermes House, 2012)

INDEX